Mental Health Care for Elderly People

For Churchill Livingstone:

Commissioning editor: Ellen Green
Project manager: Valerie Burgess
Project development editor: Mairi McCubbin
Design direction: Judith Wright
Project controller: Pat Miller
Copy editor: Stephanie Pickering
Illustrator: Marion Tasker
Indexer: Liz Granger
Sales promotion executive: Hilary Brown

Mental Health Care for Elderly People

Editors

Ian J. Norman BA MSc PhD DipAppSocStud CQSW RMN RNMH RGN

Senior Lecturer, Department of Nursing Studies,
King's College London, UK

Sally J. Redfern BSc PhD RGN

Director, Nursing Research Unit, King's College London, UK

Foreword by

Sally Greengross BA DLitt FRSA FRSH OBE

Director General, Age Concern England, London, UK

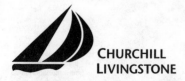

CHURCHILL
LIVINGSTONE

NEW YORK EDINBURGH LONDON MADRID MELBOURNE SAN FRANCISCO TOKYO 1997

CHURCHILL LIVINGSTONE
Medical Division of Pearson Professional Limited

Distributed in the United States of America by Churchill
Livingstone, 650 Avenue of the Americas, New York, N>Y>
10011, and by associated companies, branches and
representatives throughout the world.

First published 1997

ISBN 0 443 05173 9

British Library Cataloguing in Publication Data
A catalogue record for this book is available from the British
Library.

Library of Congress Cataloging in Publication Data
A catalog record for this book is available form the Library of
Congress.

Note
Medical knowledge is constantly changing. As new
information becomes available, changes in treatment,
procedures, equipment and the use of drugs become
necessary. The editors/authors/contributors and the
publishers have, as far as it is possible, taken care to ensure
that the information given in this text is accurate and up-to-
date. However, readers are strongly advised to confirm that
the information, especially with regard to drug usage,
complies with latest legislation and standards of practice.

The
publisher's
policy is to use
paper manufactured
from sustainable forests

Printed in Singapore.

Contents

Contributors

Trevor Adams MSc CPNCert RMN RGN RNT
Lecturer, European Institute of Health and Medical
Sciences, University of Surrey, Guildford, UK
11. Dementia

Elizabeth Armstrong RGN RHV FETC
Mental Health Training Officer, National Primary
Care Facilitation Programme, RCGP Unit for Mental
Health Education in Primary Care, UK
15. Mental health promotion in old age

Janet Askham BA PhD
Deputy Director, Age Concern Institute of
Gerontology, King's College London, UK
25. Supporting elderly people and informal carers at home

Anne Baseby BEd MRCSLT
Head of Speech and Language Therapy, Royal
Hospital for Neuro-disability, London, UK
17. Speech, language and communication

Joanna Bornat BA PhD
Senior Lecturer, School of Health and Social Welfare,
The Open University, Walton Hall, Milton Keynes, UK
22. Approaches to reminiscence

David Brandon
Professor in Community Care, Anglia Polytechnic
University, Cambridge, UK
14. Struggling with services

John Brown BSc MPhil
Senior Lecturer in Social Policy, Department of Social
Policy and Social Work, University of York, UK
5. Learning disability in later life

Eleanor J. Byrne MBChB MRCPsych
Senior Lecturer and Honorary Consultant, Old Age
Psychiatry, Withington Hospital, Manchester, UK
*10. Acute and sub-acute confusional states (delirium) in
later life*

Elizabeth Cavaglieri BSc MRCSLT
Speech and Language Therapist, Farnham Road
Hospital, Guildford, Surrey, UK
17. Speech, language and communication

Michael Farrell MRCP MRCPsych
Senior Lecturer and Consultant Psychiatrist, Maudsley
Hospital and National Addiction Centre, London, UK
12. Substance misuse in the elderly

Philip Fennell BA MPhil PhD
Senior Lecturer in Law, Cardiff Law School,
University of Wales, Cardiff, UK
*28. Legal and ethical issues in mental health care of elderly
patients*

Dinah Gould BSc PhD RGN RNT
Senior Lecturer, Department of Nursing Studies,
King's College London, UK
*23. Pharmacological treatments and electroconvulsive
therapy (ECT)*

Rosamund A. Herbert BSc MSc CertEd RGN
Head of Biological Sciences Applied to Professional
Studies, The Nightingale Institute, King's College
London, UK
3. Biological approaches to ageing and mental health

Una Holden BA PhD FBPsS
Consultant Clinical Psychologist, Lakeland Health
Authority, Garlands Hospital, Carlisle, UK
20. Reality orientation (RO) in the 1990s

Colin Hughes MA PGCE CPNCert RMN
Community Psychiatric Nurse for the Elderly, The
Dales Community Mental Health Service, Community
Health Care Service (North Derbyshire) NHS Trust, UK
8. Depression and mania in later life

Ray Jack PhD
Principal Lecturer in Social Work, Anglia Polytechnic
University, Cambridge, UK
14. *Struggling with services*

Tony Kendrick BSc PhD MBBS DRCOG DCH MRCGP
Senior Lecturer in General Practice, St. Georges
Hospital Medical School, London, UK
1. *The demography and mental health of elderly people*

James Lindesay DM MRCPsych
Professor of Psychiatry for the Elderly, University of
Leicester, Leicester, UK
9. *Suicide in later life*

Declan McLoughlin MRCPI MRCPsych
Alzheimer's Disease Society Research Fellow, Section
of Old Age Psychiatry and Department of Neurology,
Institute of Psychiatry, London, UK
12. *Substance misuse in the elderly*

Michael Morley BSc MSc PhD
Consultant Clinical Psychologist, Department of
Clinical Psychology, Central Manchester Health Care
Trust, Gaskell House Annexe, Manchester Royal
Infirmary, Manchester, UK
13. *Schizophrenia in later life*

Ian R. Morton BA RMN
Day Centre Manager, Health Care of the Elderly
Directorate, Nottingham Healthcare Trust,
Nottingham, UK
21. *Beyond validation*

Niki Muir MRCLST
Freelance Speech and Language Therapist,
specialising in Mental Health and Training. Part-time
tutor at the Department of Human Communication
Science at University College London, UK
17. *Speech, language and communication*

Ian J. Norman BA MSc PhD DipAppSocStud CQSW RMN
RNMH RGN
Senior Lecturer, Department of Nursing Studies,
King's College London, UK
26. *Supporting paid carers*
29. *Reflections*

Sally J. Redfern BSc PhD RGN
Professor of Nursing and Director, Nursing Research
Unit, King's College London, UK
27. *Supporting residents in long-stay settings*
29. *Reflections*

Lynette Rentoul BSc MSc ChartClinPsych ABPS
Psychotherapist BAP
Lecturer, Department of Nursing Studies, King's
College London, UK
2. *Psychosocial approaches to ageing and mental health*
4. *Developmental problems in later life*

Marcus Richards MA PhD
Lecturer, Section of Old Age Psychiatry, Institute of
Psychiatry, London, UK
7. *Anxiety in later life*

Susan Ritter BA MSc RMN
Lecturer in Psychiatric Nursing, Institute of
Psychiatry, London, UK
6. *Assessment of older people*

Steven Scrutton BSc MA DipEd CQSW
Social Work Manager, Northamptonshire Social
Services Department, Northampton, UK
16. *Counselling: maintaining mental health in older age*

William Sellwood BSc MSc CPsychol AFBPS
Consultant Clinical Psychologist, Department of
Clinical Psychology, Withington Hospital, Nell Lane,
Withington, Manchester, UK
13. *Schizophrenia in later life*

Tracey Sparkes MSc BA RGN HV(Dip)
Primary Care Survey Manager, Kings Fund
Organisational Audit, UK
15. *Mental health promotion in old age*

Hamish Thomson MSc DipNEd RGN RNT
Lecturer, The Nightingale Institute, King's College
London, UK
3. *Biological approaches to ageing and mental health*

Anthea Tinker BCom PhD
Professor of Social Gerontology and Director, Age
Concern Institute of Gerontology, King's College
London, UK
24. *The development of service provision*

Anthony M. Warnes BA PhD
Professor of Social Gerontology, Department of Health
Care of Elderly People, University of Sheffield,
Northern General Hospital NHS Trust, Community
Sciences Centre, Sheffield, UK
1. *The demography and mental health of elderly people*

Mary J. Watkins MN PhD DipNEd DipN RGN RMN
Head of Institute, Institute of Health Studies, Faculty
of Human Sciences, University of Plymouth,
Plymouth, UK
6. *Assessment of older people*

Catherine Wells RGN RMN PGDip
Senior Clinical Nurse Specialist in Cognitive
Behaviour Therapy, City and Hackney Community
Services Trust, London, UK
18. *Reducing challenging behaviour of elderly confused
people: a behavioural perspective*
19. *Cognitive therapy with older people*

John S. G. Wells BA MSc PGDip RMN
Lecturer, Department of Nursing Studies, King's
College London, UK
18. *Reducing challenging behaviour of elderly confused
people: a behavioural perspective*
19. *Cognitive therapy with older people*

Foreword

The increase in the number of older people in the population is, historically, an unprecedented phenomenon affecting all parts of the world. It is a triumph, mainly due to greatly improved health and social care, heralding the fact that at the end of the 20th century most of us can expect to survive to a great age and be fitter, more active and more able to participate in the life of our communities as we age than ever before.

Yet there is a darker side to the picture. Some of the intractable diseases associated with old age are still beyond our current level of knowledge and skill to prevent and, if they do attack us, to cure. Dementia is the most prevalent, particularly amongst the very elderly, but at Age Concern we receive growing numbers of enquiries from people with elderly friends and relatives experiencing a range of mental health problems, including Alzheimer's Disease, but also suffering from anxiety, confusion, depression and many other serious conditions. As the number of older people in our society increases, this trend seems set to continue, and an increasing burden of responsibility is falling upon the shoulders of doctors, nurses, social workers and other professional carers. It is, therefore, essential that adequate resources and training are provided so that the highest standards of care are available to both patients and their carers throughout the country.

I am, therefore, delighted to be associated with this exciting new textbook which should certainly play its part in improving standards of care. Drawing on the knowledge and experience of some 36 contributors – all experts within their respective fields – this book is not only extremely comprehensive in its coverage, but offers a refreshing multi-disciplinary and client-based approach reflecting the nature of elderly health care services today. As a result, it endorses the 'team' approach to care, and attempts to view the client's needs from a range of perspectives, including the client's own veiwpoint. This is so important; no care can be truly effective unless the needs of the person being cared for are fully understood.

I have already briefly touched on the size and scope of the book and would like to say a little more about this. One of the real strengths of this text is that it not only deals with the theoretical background and medical conditions which may arise (for example, schizophrenia, addictions and depression), but it also includes a range of important material on subjects such as counselling, reminiscence therapy, and health promotion. Many mental health problems need never arise in the first place, while others can be kept in check through the application of appropriate therapy. It naturally follows that a great deal of unnecessary suffering on the part of older people and their families can be avoided, while precious health and social care resources can be saved, simply by recognizing that prevention is better than cure.

In a book of this nature, there are inevitably many features which stand out as being worthy of comment. However, a few either strike a personal chord or tie in particularly with our work and experiences at Age Concern. In this context I would single out David Brandon and Ray Jack's chapter entitled Struggling with Services. Based on first hand experience, this case study describes very graphically the struggles and problems experienced by a married couple looking after an elderly relative, and the hurdles which they had to overcome before their needs were fully appreciated and eventually met. This example is very typical of huge numbers of enquiries that we receive and provides a good insight into the stresses and strains of being an informal carer.

In a similar vein is Janet Askham's chapter, entitled Supporting Elderly People and Informal Carers at

Home. The current policy of deinstitutionalisation in this country means that more will be expected of carers while greater efforts will be made to keep older people with mental health problems in their own homes. As a result, the role of professional carers has become even more challenging, for communication, perception and understanding are more important than ever. I am, therefore, delighted to see this chapter included and hope it will be an inspiration to all those reading it.

As we all become more elderly, so our vulnerability increases, particularly if this is accompanied by mental health problems. As John Brown points out in his chapter entitled Learning Disability in Later Life, we all seek to have six basic values in our autumn years, namely: dignity, privacy, independence, choice, rights and fulfilment. Providing these is a huge challenge,

but it is a challenge to which we must all rise. After all, it is only right that we should strive to offer the care that we ourselves would hope to receive in similar circumstances. This book answers an important need and I warmly commend it to you. It should encourage its readers to work together as a team, to communicate and share experiences. Above all, I hope it will play a role in improving the professional care of older people with mental health problems in this country, surely one of the most vulnerable groups among us, composed of people who depend on the readers of this book and others like them to make their lives worth living. Time for such elderly people is short – they cannot wait.

1997   S. G.

Preface

Our intention has been to produce a relatively comprehensive text which demonstrates the many facets of mental health care for elderly people and their underpinnings in theory and research. The book is written primarily for health and social care students and students of gerontology. It should also be useful reference material for professionals. The book avoids allegiance to any one discipline, so reflecting the multi-professional nature of elderly mental health care services today and the breadth and complexity of the subject. Multidisciplinary is reflected in the contributors who are drawn from a variety of professional and academic backgrounds (social gerontologists, social policy analysts, psychiatrists, nurses, social workers, health educators, clinical psychologists, speech and language therapists, lawyers and service users). All are experts in their subject, and many work every day with elderly mentally ill people and their families. The material on the organisation of mental health care and provision of services necessarily emphasises a UK perspective, but we have tried to produce a text which is not too parochial and can cross geographical boundaries.

The book is person focused and warm blooded. It regards elderly people as valued members of society and mental health care as a positive process that helps them take control of their lives and find meaning and purpose in living. These are fine statements of principle and we recognise that they are not prominent in many care environments; the reality of care for many elderly mentally disordered people is unsatisfactory.

We have coexisting in mental care for elderly people new treatments and creative, innovative, person-centred practices in some care settings and some of the worst examples of care, characterised by ritual, routine, batch treatment and psychological neglect, in others. A practical challenge for us all is to disseminate the person-centred care practices and ideas, many of which are discussed in this text, beyond conference-attending, journal-reading professionals, to those who deliver hands-on care every day to elderly mentally ill people and their families. This book will have been successful if it goes a small way towards improving the lives for elderly people who have yet to feel the benefit of person-centred care.

We are grateful to Sally Greengross for writing the Foreword. As Director of Age Concern England, she is a respected public figure whose work to improve the living conditions of elderly people in our society is well known to all in the health and social care professions and beyond.

Without the commitment and patience of each author, this book would not have been written. We are grateful to them all for taking time out of their busy lives to produce their chapters and for being prepared to write with a multi-professional audience in mind. Our thanks, too, to Gian Brown for her high quality typing and correction of the manuscript.

London
1996

I. J. N., S. J. R.

Introduction

Elderly mental health care as a field of study and a practical activity is a paradox. On the one hand it has benefited over the past 20 years from major innovations and developments in treatments and approaches to care, many of which are discussed in this volume. On the other, it is a neglected area of health and social care in which there is considerable scope for quality improvement.

The positive progress made in the field is illustrated, for example, by the considerable knowledge we now have about what forms of support are needed by elderly mentally ill people if they are to live at home (discussed by Askham in Chapter 25). Another example is the growing interest in psychological interventions in dementia that draw upon theories of disorientation which recognise the actions of dementing people as the outcome not simply of a relentless disease process but also the ways in which we, the carers, react and respond to that behaviour (discussed by Morton in Chapter 21). In contrast, the negative reality for many elderly people is perhaps best illustrated by research into continuing and long-stay hospital care for elderly people over the past 40 years (discussed by Norman in Chapter 26 and Redfern in Chapter 27) which, by and large, describes undesirable environments, activities and patterns of care, especially for patients who are perceived by staff as mentally impaired, confused or demented. The dominant picture from these studies, and also the literature on residential homes is of discouraged and disheartened direct care staff whose emotionally demanding work is undervalued by the public and other health and social care professionals.

The book is in four sections. In Section 1, the focus is on what it means to be old and the changes consequent on normal ageing. We begin with Kendrick and Warnes' (Chapter 1) account of the demography of old age and the epidemiology of mental health problems amongst elderly people. This chapter throws light on the conditions of old age in a way that illuminates the experience of old people themselves. It reveals the tendency for psychiatric epidemiological studies to underestimate the number of elderly people with mental health problems because, for every person meeting the criteria of 'caseness', there are many others with fewer or milder symptoms, who nevertheless would benefit from assessment and assistance.

In Chapter 2, Rentoul gives an overview of psychological changes in old age, drawing upon theory and research in the traditions of developmental and cognitive psychology, and the newer tradition of health psychology. The value of reminiscence in the life of older people is introduced (to be expanded by Bornat in Chapter 22). The complex association between stress, social support, personality, health and financial status are related to life events such as bereavement and widowhood, retirement and residential relocation. Rentoul highlights the importance of individual variability, the need to consider current circumstances of elderly people and the powerful influence of personal history.

The theme of individual variability is one which is underlined by Herbert and Thomson's (Chapter 3) discussion of biological changes associated with ageing and the biological basis of mental health problems. The authors point to the complexities of differentiating true ageing changes from changes that result from deconditioning (unfitness) or lack of use and those that arise from disease processes. The importance of professional carers having a good understanding of normal ageing processes is emphasised as a prerequisite of assessment and planning interventions to maintain or maximise the independence of elderly people.

Chapters 4–14 comprise Section 2. The emphasis now moves from what might be considered as normal changes and challenges of late life in Section 1, to mental health problems. In Chapter 4, Rentoul picks up some of the themes raised in her earlier chapter (Chapter 2) to provide an overview of developmental problems which may arise if the challenges and changes of late life are not successfully negotiated. This theme is pursued by Brown in Chapter 5 which focuses upon elderly people who have a learning disability, a traditionally neglected segment of the population who are now entering old age.

Ritter and Watkins' overview of assessment in old age (Chapter 6) is relevant to elderly people suffering from a variety of mental health problems. These problems are expanded in subsequent chapters in Section 2. Richards' discussion of anxiety in late life (Chapter 7) reveals that we tend to be concerned with practical issues and with the consequences of adversive events rather than the events themselves. However, against this background, anxiety in late life is often overlooked; somatic symptoms attributed to physical illness, or fears, of crime for example, are seen as normal for an elderly person. In this respect, anxiety is similar to depression which is discussed, together with mania in late life, by Hughes in Chapter 8. Depression is the most common mental illness in old age but is frequently overlooked or dismissed as a natural consequence of ageing. Mania is much less common. Hughes emphasises that both disorders demand a positive approach to detection and assessment, and to care, treatment and follow-up by multi-professional clinical teams knowledgeable about the main presenting features and effective treatments. The problem of suicide, an all too frequent outcome of depression in old age, is discussed by Lindesay in Chapter 9. He highlights the ample scope that exists for suicide prevention and the potential of this role for health care professionals.

Chapters 10 and 11 consider the care and treatment of elderly people suffering from the most common organic mental disorders of old age. Byrne (Chapter 10) discusses delirium which is especially common amongst old people living in hospital or residential care, and may often have fatal consequences. In Chapter 11, Adams introduces dementia. He presents an overview of models of dementia, touches on their implications for clinical practice and discusses some practical issues in family care and assessment. This chapter sets the scene for more detailed discussions of dementia care in some of the chapters in Section 3.

Farrell and McLoughlin's discussion of drug and alcohol misuse in old age (Chapter 12) draws attention to a problem which is barely recognised and has attracted virtually no interest from researchers; the assumption being that such problems only arise in young people. The authors point to this neglect as a glaring example of ageism. They discuss presentation of the problem, guidelines to management, and point to the potential of brief therapeutic interventions directed at modifying substance consumption to deliver a substantial degree of health and social gain to the elderly population.

Morley and Sellwood's (Chapter 13) consideration of schizophrenia distinguishes between people first diagnosed in early adulthood who have grown old and those first diagnosed later in life. The former group are more numerous; late paraphrenia or late onset schizophrenia being fairly rare. This chapter covers the important issues of institutionalisation and strategies for resettlement, community care and management. The authors highlight the danger of recreating smaller institutions 'in the community' which, like the large mental hospitals they are designed to replace, lead to institutionalisation.

Section 2 concludes with a chapter by Brandon and Jack (Chapter 14) in which Brandon describes his experience of caring for his father-in-law and Jack draws upon this account to derive lessons for professional carers. The picture drawn here is of professionals who fail to recognise the meaning of caring relationships within a family, conceiving them simply in terms of burden. This can lead to a rush into service provision in which the professionals 'colonise' the caring relationships and the family is left feeling abandoned and guilty because of what they see as enforced severance. This chapter condemns paternalistic models of formal helping relationships which rob both dependent elderly people and their families of control over their lives.

In Section 3 we turn from mental health problems in late life to consider therapeutic interventions. We begin with Armstrong and Sparks' (Chapter 15) discussion of mental health promotion in old age which challenges two myths: the inevitable link between old age and mental illness; and that older people are unable to alter their lifestyles to improve their health. The chapter discusses models of health promotion and illness prevention and, developing themes raised by Rentoul (Chapters 2 and 4), considers the links between mental and physical ability, autonomy and control, social support and stress reduction.

Chapter 16, by Scrutton, highlights the potential of counselling for: maintaining mental health by helping people manage the stresses associated with late life and living within an ageist society; and combating mental health problems by voicing unpleasant memories, raising expectations and morale and reducing fears. Counselling, as with other therapies discussed in Section 3, relies on the ability to speak, use language and communicate. But for some elderly people these skills are impaired. In Chapter 17, Muir, Baseby and Cavaglieri discuss how normal ageing changes and how acquired disorders can affect these skills in elderly people. They advocate a multidisciplinary approach to assessment and management, drawing upon the specialist knowledge of the speech and language therapist.

Chapters 18, by the husband and wife team of Wells and Wells, is written from a behavioral perspective and discusses the application of behaviourial techniques to the management of 'problem' behaviours in old age. The authors question the oft-held belief that problems such as urinary incontinence and aggression are inevitable and irreversible consequences of biophysical and cognitive degeneration. They argue for behavioural approaches founded upon thorough assessment and respect for the client's priorities and best interests. The theme of collaboration and partnership between therapist and client is again prominent in Chapter 19, also written by the Wells, which considers cognitive therapy with older people. Cognitive therapy emerges from this chapter as an intervention focused on immediate problems which can provide depressed and demoralised older people with skills that they can use in their everyday life to reinforce their self-esteem, empower them and challenge their sense of disability.

In Chapters 20 and 21 we turn to consider some of the major psychological therapies for helping dementing elderly people. The oldest of the therapies, reality orientation, is brought up to date by Holden (Chapter 20) who considers its diverse clinical manifestations and applications in the 1990s. This is followed by Morton's (Chapter 21) discussion of: validation therapy, which evolved as a reaction to reality orientation; newer arrivals on the scene, resolution therapy and pre-therapy; and also the contribution of Kitwood and his team to the theory and practice of dementia care. This chapter develops some of the issues raised by Adams in Chapter 11, and sets the theories of dementia and therapies discussed within the context of a developing new culture of dementia care.

Bornat (Chapter 22) draws together the distinct set of practices described as reminiscence and traces its development and application in diverse contexts of elderly care work, including dementing people and those with learning disability; old people who traditionally have been excluded from opportunities to reminisce. Reminiscence therapy emerges from Bornat's chapter as a powerful means of challenging the stereotypes of old age which deny individuality, and the established power relationships between younger and older people, carers and cared for.

Gould's Chapter 23 concludes Section 3 with an account of the main drugs used in the treatment of mental disorders in old age and the value of electro-convulsive therapy for elderly people.

In Section 4, we consider the issues involved in developing and delivering services for elderly mentally disordered people and their families and carers. Tinker (Chapter 24) identifies four key themes of policy change: preventing people going into institutions; resettlement into the community; improving conditions in hospital; and building up community care. These themes are picked up again in Chapter 29. The focus of Tinker's chapter is the UK, which emerges as having many lessons for health and welfare systems for other countries. Chapter 24 illuminates the complexity of present arrangements for health and social care, highlights the fundamental conditions that must be met for policies to be successful and speculates on future directions.

The next 3 chapters discuss support for elderly mentally ill people and informal carers at home (Askham, Chapter 25), for paid workers (Norman, Chapter 26) and for elderly residents in long-stay care settings (Redfern, Chapter 27). Askham considers what people who are affected personally, or as a carer, want and what kind of services can best meet their needs. She reveals that the needs of the person cared for, and the carer, may conflict, and that setting priorities for service provision means we need to know more about the varying benefits of different types of support to different kinds of people in different circumstances. Norman's starting point is the nature and causes of worker stress in mental health care settings for elderly people – particularly long-stay settings. Pathways to 'burnout' and 'rustout' are described and both are seen to have pernicious consequences for the ways in which elderly people are treated by their paid carers. The clear message is that care settings that support their care workers as much as they do their residents reap the rewards of high quality care and positive working environments. This message is reinforced by Redfern's consideration of the values that underpin a supportive approach to quality of life and quality of care in long-stay settings, and the sort of support that an old person should expect from the physical and social environment and the caring regime.

The penultimate chapter is by a lawyer (Fennell, Chapter 28) who discusses the legal and ethical issues which arise during the course of everyday care of mentally disordered elderly people. It raises the problem of how we, the carers, can reconcile respect for the free choices of others with a concern for their welfare in cases in which free choices are self-destructive or harmful. The chapter also shows how our legal framework in the UK aims to achieve a system which respects the dignity of patients, ensures that their autonomously expressed wishes are given adequate weight and that treatment is not denied to those who need it but are unable to consent.

In the final chapter (Norman and Redfern, Chapter 29) we draw upon the previous chapters to highlight some of the main issues and challenges facing workers concerned with mental health care for elderly people today.

I. J. N., S. J. R.

Mental health, old age and society

1

The demography and mental health of elderly people

Tony Kendrick
Tony Warnes

This chapter is an introduction to the demography of old age and to the epidemiology of mental health among elderly people. The opening sections concentrate on demographic change but from an unusual point of view, not that of Treasury ministers or health service planners, but that of elderly people themselves. The changing statistics of survival and life expectancy are examined less to illuminate the changing age-structure of the population and the increasing number of elderly people, but more to throw light on the changing conditions of old age. A brief and conventional presentation of past and projected changes in the population age-structure is also given. The epidemiological section provides a summary and guide to recent population-based research on the prevalence of some major psychiatric and psychological disorders among elderly people. It includes discussions of the instruments which have been most widely adopted for assessing the presence and severity of mental conditions, and reflections on current approaches in primary care to diagnosis and treatment.

BEING OLD IN AGED SOCIETIES

A widespread impression is that societal ageing is something rather new, of the last 2 decades, or a post-modern characteristic. In fact, the mean life expectancy of human beings has been increasing in irregular leaps for 100 000 years. For example, life expectancy at birth among privileged and aristocratic women increased from around the low thirties in 1600 to the low fifties by 1900. In Europe, the modern increase in the share of the population aged 60 years and more, from around 5% to around 20%, began in the early decades of this century and peaked during the period 1921–1971. We have now entered a different phase, for in the future the size of the elderly population will fluctuate rather than continuously increase. This is a direct consequence of the irregular birth rates of the 20th century, with a 'boom' during 1945–1965 and very low birth rates during the inter-war period and from the early 1970s. There are other factors, as we shall see, but it is quite wrong to regard the growth of the elderly population, especially in Europe or in other affluent world regions, as an unprecedented, hugely disruptive and limitless process (Hendricks & Hendricks 1986, Suzman et al 1992).

This section unconventionally approaches the demographic record from the perspective of the individual's actual and perceived life chances and survival. Not least among a person's concerns is how vigorous, healthy, mentally competent and socially integrated they will be in the near and distant future. If young adults normally take several decades of life for granted, by the time people reach their fifties, they are more aware of the finite nature of human life and of how fragile good health can be. Adjustment to old age involves accepting many losses in old age, as with eyesight, powers of memory, career prospects, hopes for children, and the bereavement of parents and spouses. The entire book will be a small contribu-

tion to widening awareness and debate on adjustment to such losses. Here we begin with the starkly fundamental matter of how long individuals survive.

Mortality and life expectancy of the individual

Crude death rate

Over the last 150 years the crude death rate (CDR) in England and Wales has halved, from around 22 per 1000 per year in the middle decades of the 19th century to 11.2 per 1000 in 1991 (Table 1.1). The fall has been far from continuous, most having occurred from the early 1870s to the early 1920s. The CDR of around 12 per 1000 in 1921–1925 has since changed little, apart from a slight rise during the late 1930s and early 1940s and, according to the provisional evidence, a marked decrease during the 1980s. As the vital statistics of a nation's fertility and mortality change, they impact directly on family composition and individual experience and survival. The main changes to date have been that families have become smaller (so we have fewer brothers, sisters and cousins) and that very

Table 1.1 Selected age-specific death rates (both sexes) in England and Wales 1840s–1991

Year(s)	SMR[1]	All ages	Age group (years)				
			0–1	55–64	65–74	75–84	85+
1841–1845	344	21.4	148	28.7	62.0	137.2	295.3
1851–1855	356	22.7	156	29.6	62.9	143.2	299.6
1861–1865	353	22.6	151	30.3	62.5	139.1	299.0
1871–1875	342	22.0	153	31.6	65.3	141.7	305.2
1881–1885	308	19.4	139	31.0	63.5	136.2	277.9
1891–1895	296	18.7	151	32.5	67.3	140.7	273.9
1901–1905	249	16.0	138	28.7	59.4	127.3	258.6
1911–1915	205	14.3	110	26.2	57.3	126.2	257.9
1921–1925	157	12.1	76	21.6	51.1	121.8	251.4
1931–1935	134	12.0	62	20.1	49.0	119.3	255.7
1941–1945	112	12.8	50	18.1	43.0	104.5	213.0
1951–1955	97	11.7	27	16.6	42.0	105.7	235.7
1961–1965	90	11.8	21	15.8	39.6	96.7	220.2
1971–1975	84	11.8	17	14.9	36.9	87.8	201.0
1981–1985	75	11.7	10	13.4	33.4	78.2	186.3
1991	70[2]	11.2	7	10.9	29.1	71.5	166.4
Annual rate of improvement (%)							
1843–1893	0.30	0.27	−0.04	−0.25	−0.16	−0.05	0.15
1893–1953	1.84	0.78	2.83	1.11	0.78	0.48	0.25
1953–1991	0.93[2]	0.11	3.49	1.10	0.96	1.02	0.91

Note: 1: Standardised Mortality Ratio (SMR) on death rates in 1950–1952.
2: Refers to the SMR during 1986–1990 and the rate of improvement during 1953–1988.
Sources: Office of Population Censuses and Surveys (OPCS) (1989): *Mortality Statistics 1841–1985, Serial Tables.* HMSO, London, Table 1; OPCS (1992): *Mortality Statistics 1990: England and Wales, General.* HMSO, London, Table 2; OPCS (1993): *Mortality Statistics 1991: England and Wales, General.* HMSO, London, Table 3.

few babies or very young children now die. Few of us now have to cope with a premature death in our immediate family. Brothers and sisters mostly survive to old age and marriages are rarely broken by a bereavement during working age.

Standard mortality ratio

Crude death rates understate the improvement in overall mortality, for which a better indicator is the standard mortality ratio (SMR). This applies the age-specific death rates for a reported year to a standard age–sex structure, in this case that of 1950–1952. The SMR indexes the estimated total deaths in the reported year to the total in the standard year (SMR = 100). The average annual rates of improvement of the SMR and of various death rates have been calculated for the three intervals from 1841–1845, 1891–1895, 1951–1955 and for 1991. As the lower panel of Table 1.1 shows, the SMR and the all-age death rate improved most rapidly during the first half of this century, since when both have slowed, but the former less abruptly. During this century all age-specific death rates have progressively decreased, one effect being to redistribute deaths from infancy and late-middle age to old age. Infant mortality by 1991 was only 5% of the rate for 1891–1895, and that for persons aged 65–74 years was 43% of the earlier rate. Since the early 1950s, most age-specific death rates, including all in old age, have improved faster than before. Although it remains true that the fastest recent declines have been for infant mortality (3.5% per year), the acceleration of improvement in later-life mortality is impressive (Table 1.1).

The pace and chronology of improvement in three late-age-specific death rates are compared with the CDR and infant mortality in Figure 1.1. This presents the mean rates for the first 5 years of each decade from the 1840s to the 1980s and the provisional rates for 1991 as ratios of the average rate in the early 1910s and 1920s, i.e. each rate is expressed as a ratio of the trend figure in 1918. The rapid improvement of infant mortality after the 1890s and recent moderation is evident, as also that death rates at ages 55–64 years improved fastest from the 1890s to the 1920s. On the other hand, the trends in death rates at ages 75–84 and at 85+ years both display gently accelerating improvement since the third quarter of the last century.

The period life table

Age-specific death rates are the basis of calculations about average life expectancy from birth (E_0) or from

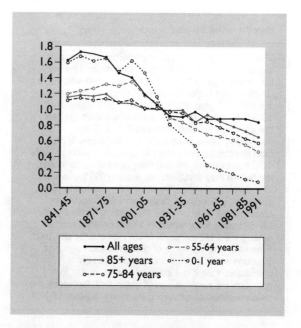

Figure 1.1 The progress of the crude death rate and selected age-specific death rates, 1841–1991.

later ages (E_x). While a statement that 'life expectancy for males is 78 years' is superficially easy to understand, it is rarely emphasised that the statistic is a complex and abstract compilation: it is based on a *period life table*, a particular form of the age-specific death rates that have just been examined, and the data are drawn from but a single year or a few years – the 'period' in question (see Box 1.1). Careful study of Box 1.1 and Table 1.2 will give a good understanding of the construction of a life table.

When the construction of the period life table has been understood, it is clear that it falsifies time. It assumes that the 10 000 males or females complete their whole lives under the mortality conditions of the period (in this case 1989–1991). Neither the unhealthier childhood conditions that today's elderly people experienced, nor any future improvements in mortality are represented. No one is actually exposed to the mortality risks expressed in a period life table, and the mean life expectancies calculated from it are abstract – nobody has the life expectancy that is usually described. This is true even when setting aside another difficulty: that is, even if someone is entirely average, it is impossible to identify them.

Mean life expectancies are frequently quoted because they summarise the mortality risks in a population and are useful comparative indicators over

---

Box 1.1 The life table

The construction of these important demographic models and their unreal representation of time may be understood by examining the abridged 1989–1991 England and Wales life table. It starts by assuming the birth in 1 year of a cohort of 10 000 males and 10 000 females. To these cohorts are then applied the age-specific death rates at 0, 1, 2, 3 and successive years of age until the last survivor has died (for this size of cohort at about 110 years) (Table 1.2). For example, among the male births, 89 would die before their first birthday, leaving 9911 survivors. The death rate at age 1 year is then applied to these survivors, producing 6 deaths and 9905 survivors. Lower in the table, we see that among those aged 55–59 years, there would in 1 year be 459 deaths among the 9112 males, a death rate of 5.04 per 100. When the entire column of deaths at each age and the numbers of survivors beyond has been calculated, then it is a straightforward matter to calculate the average age of death and, therefore, the mean duration of remaining life at age x years (E_x).

---

more for women. Since then there have been substantial increases, of 38% for males and 58% for females. By 1989–1991, the female E_{65} was 17.9 years.

While throughout most of this century survival prospects have improved, mainly because of declines in infant mortality, increasingly it is reductions in mortality in late-middle and early-old age which are increasing longevity. Certainly they are altering the survival and familial experience of people in their fifties and sixties. The improvements may be shown from the England and Wales life tables for the period since 1972 (Table 1.4). Not only can new-born individuals be increasingly confident of their own survival to 75 years (and, by inference, of a lower likelihood of ill health), they are also less likely to lose their spouse or brothers and sisters before this age. Remembering the assumption that 1989–1991 mortality conditions continue, women who reach the age of 50 years can now expect to live at least another 30 years, and men another 26 years. Over the last 17 years, the probability of a 50-year-old female surviving to 75 years has improved by 8%, to 0.72. For men, the improvement has been an impressive one-quarter, to 0.56. Indeed, it is only in the last few years that a majority of 50-year-old men in the UK could expect to live to 75 years of age (Warnes 1993).

If we assume husbands and wives (or brothers and sisters) of the same age, then the chances of a pair at age 50 years both surviving until 75 years reached 0.40 by 1989–1991, a 36% improvement over the previous 17 years. Turning to the cases in which women are 5 years younger than males aged 50 years, the chance

time or among countries or regions. The historical decline in death rates translates into substantial increases in life expectancies. The English life tables show an increase in E_0 from around 41 years in the early 1840s to 76 years by 1989–1991 (Table 1.3). Life expectancy at age 65 years (E_{65}) decreased during the second half of the 19th century, particularly for men, and in the 1890s was 10.3 years for men and 1 year

Table 1.2 Extract of the England and Wales life table 1989–1991

Age (years) expectancy	Males		Females	
	Survivors	Life expectancy	Survivors	Life expectancy
0	10 000	73.2	10 000	78.7
1	9911	72.9	9932	78.2
2	9905	71.9	9927	77.2
3	9901	71.0	9924	76.3
4	9897	70.0	9921	75.3
55	9112	21.7	9446	26.1
60	8653	17.7	9158	21.8
65	7893	14.2	8682	17.9
70	6757	11.1	7960	14.3
75	5259	8.5	6917	11.0
80	3530	6.4	5494	8.2
85	1898	4.9	3700	5.9

Source: OPCS (1993). *Mortality Statistics 1991: England and Wales, General.* HMSO, London, Table 15.

Table 1.3 Mean life expectancy at different ages by sex, England and Wales c.1840–1990 (years)

Reference years	E^0 At birth		E^1 At 1 year		E^{45} At 45 years		E^{65} At 65 years	
	M	F	M	F	M	F	M	F
1838–1844	40.4	42.0	47.0	47.4	23.1	24.2	10.9	11.6
1871–1880	41.4	44.6	48.1	50.1	22.1	24.1	10.6	11.4
1891–1900	44.1	47.8	52.2	54.5	22.2	24.2	10.3	11.3
1910–1912	51.5	55.4	57.5	60.3	23.9	26.3	11.0	12.4
1920–1922	55.6	59.6	60.1	63.0	25.2	27.7	11.4	12.9
1930–1932	58.7	62.9	62.3	65.5	25.5	28.3	11.3	13.1
1950–1952	66.4	71.5	67.7	72.4	26.5	30.8	11.7	14.3
1960–1962	68.1	74.0	68.8	74.4	27.1	32.1	12.0	15.3
1970–1972	69.0	75.2	69.4	75.4	27.4	32.9	12.2	16.1
1980–1982	71.1	77.1	71.0	76.9	28.7	34.1	13.1	17.1
1989–1991	73.2	78.7	72.9	78.2	30.5	35.2	14.2	17.9
Annual rate of improvement (%)								
1841–1895	0.17	0.24	0.20	0.26	−0.08	0.00	−0.11	−0.05
1895–1951	0.78	0.76	0.49	0.54	0.33	0.46	0.24	0.45
1951–1990	0.25	0.25	0.19	0.20	0.36	0.34	0.50	0.58

Source: OPCS (1993). *Mortality Statistics 1991: England and Wales, General.* HMSO, London, Table 15.
Note: The figures for 1980–1982 are from the full life table, for 1970–1972 from the abridged life tables, and for 1960–1962 and earlier from the successive English Life Tables.

of both surviving another 25 years has reached 0.46, a 31% improvement over the period. A third situation is that of a woman aged 50 years paired with a male 5 years older. The chance of both surviving until the woman is 75 years remains low at 0.28, although this probability has improved by as much as 49% since 1972–1974. These estimates could be refined by taking into account marital-status-specific mortality rates,

since married persons have lower age-specific mortality rates than others. It is clear, however, that by the early 1990s in England and Wales a threshold in survival had been crossed. Not only can a majority of men and women now expect to attain 75 years of age, but some time in this decade it is likely that a majority of married men who reach a half-century will survive with their wives for a further 25 years.

Table 1.4 Improving survival through later life: England and Wales 1972–1974 to 1989–1991

	Males				Females			
	1972–1974	1979–1981	1989–1991	89–91: 72–74	1972–1974	1979–1981	1987–1989	89–91: 72–74
Remaining life expectancy (years)								
.... at 50 years	23.2	24.1	26.0	1.12	28.6	29.4	30.6	1.07
.... at 75 years	7.4	7.7	8.5	1.15	9.7	10.3	11.0	1.13
Probability of surviving from birth								
.... to 50 years	0.911	0.925	0.938	1.03	0.940	0.951	0.962	1.02
.... to 75 years	0.408	0.451	0.526	1.29	0.626	0.653	0.692	1.11
Probability of surviving from 50 years of age								
.... to 75 years	0.448	0.487	0.560	1.25	0.665	0.687	0.720	1.08
Probability of joint survival for 25 years								
.... Males 50 years and females 50 years					0.297	0.335	0.403	1.36
.... Males 50 years and females 45 years					0.349	0.386	0.458	1.31
.... Males 55 years and females 50 years					0.187	0.215	0.279	1.49

Source: Office of Population Censuses and Surveys (1976): *Mortality Statistics 1974: General.* HMSO, London, Table 22; OPCS (1983a): *Mortality Statistics 1981: General.* HMSO, London, Table 23; OPCS (1993) *Mortality Statistics 1991: General.* HMSO, London, Table 15.

There is no reason to believe that we are near the end of the possible improvements in old age survival, even without major breakthroughs in our under-standing and prevention of the most common lethal disorders or of human ageing itself. There are strong differentials in mortality among income groups and social classes in the UK, and between southern England and Scotland or Northern Ireland. If the entire population enjoyed the mortality conditions of the most privileged, mean life expectancy would increase by several years. And mortality conditions are far more favourable in several other European nations, in North America and in Japan. Significant further improve-ments can and should be achieved.

THE CHANGING SIZE AND AGE-STRUCTURE OF THE UK POPULATION

The age-structure of a population is a complex record of the histories of fertility, mortality and migration. One reason Switzerland had an aged population in 1900 was because of a high rate of out-migration during the immediately preceding decades. One reason that the population of the USA is relatively young for an affluent nation is its recent history of a high rate of immigration by young adults. The principal influences on the age-structure of the UK during the past century have been the decrease in fertility during the second half of the 19th century, its low level since (moderated during the 1940s and during 1955–1970), the decreases in mortality that we have examined, and a change from net emigration in the early decades of this century to net immigration during the third quarter.

Since the second decade of this century, the 5-year totals of births have fallen irregularly, from 4.3 million during 1911–1915 to 3.0 million during the 1930s. The subsequent recovery peaked at 4.2 million in the early 1960s, after which there was a fall to 3.2 million during 1981–1985. It is this long-term fall in the rejuvenation of the population that has been the main cause of the increasing average age of the UK population and the growing share of elderly people. The share of the population who are aged 60+ years has progressed from 7.5% of the total in 1901 to 20.7% by 1991 (see Fig. 1.2). The maximum rate of growth was during 1911–1921. As has been the case in all of the most developed nations, the population of advanced old age has grown faster than the aggregate elderly population. Those aged 70+ years have increased from just over 1 million in 1901 to 6.3 million in 1991, their share rising over the same period from 2.8% to 11.4%. The decades of the fastest rates of growth in their absolute numbers were 1931–1951. Octogenarians and

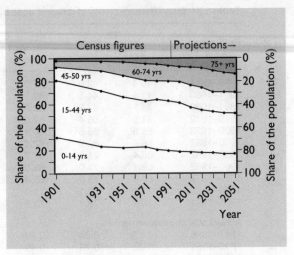

Figure 1.2   The age-structure of the United Kingdom population, 1901–1991.

older have had even faster rates of increase, peaking between 1931 and 1961, and again during the 1980s. From a population of less than a quarter of a million in 1901, they reached 2.2 million by 1991.

LATE-AGE MORTALITY TRENDS AND POPULATION PROJECTIONS

The absolute and relative size of the future elderly population cannot be known precisely. Although many projection figures are published and they are widely reproduced, actual population figures always diverge from them. Projections are as good as the assumptions (about fertility, mortality and sometimes migration) that are built into them, and therefore as good as our understanding and models of recent trends. That understanding has been improving fast but remains rudimentary. For around 20 years, population projections in both the USA and the UK have underestimated the number of survivors to advanced old age. This is because, through weak evidence and caution, the assumptions have insufficiently modelled the acceleration of late-age mortality decline that we have described (Olshansky 1988).

The perennial difficulty of population forecasters has been to anticipate fertility – birth rates in this century have been notably fickle. In comparison, demographers have generally seen mortality trends as relatively stable and one-directional, i.e. moving down. The current difficulty facing forecasters is therefore novel; to anticipate the duration, pace and age distribution of the accelerated mortality declines among the older age groups, and at what age there is a 'flip' to the less favourable trends found among middle and young adults (associated with rising accidental and violent deaths and those associated with the HIV virus). If we could achieve a more substantial understanding of the factors controlling the recent improvements in mortality, then the assumptions for the future would have more substance. Our models of mortality change are, however, becoming more powerful, and the sophistication of the guesswork behind population projection assumptions is developing rapidly.

Box 1.2 Population projection models

Population projections are built up from a life table for a base year, one for which detailed fertility and mortality rates by single years of age have been carefully checked and for which high quality estimates of the number of people alive at each age have been made. Three sets of assumptions referring to fertility, mortality and net external (international) migration are applied to the starting (base) population. For Year 1 of the projection, the number of male and female babies born is estimated from the 'fertility schedule'; secondly, the number and ages of deaths are estimated from the life table; and thirdly, the net gains or losses by age and sex from external migration are estimated from the 'migration schedule'. When all the adjustments have been made, the size and age-structure of the population after 1 year has been projected.

For Year 2 and later years of the projection, the original age-specific fertility, mortality and net migration rates are adjusted in line with the assumptions about their temporal trends. Sometimes, for example, it is expected that birth rates will rise. Usually it is expected that mortality rates will continue to fall. Normally, the best assumption that can be made about net international migration is that it will not change. Once the adjusted schedules have been calculated, they are applied to the population at the beginning of Year 2 (or a subsequent year). This process is continued for as far forward as is desired. There are technical modelling problems about the numbers who survive to extreme old age. Often refinements have to be made either to project sufficient centenarians or to prevent a few people surviving unrealistically long. Uncertainty and unreality increases with the duration of the projection. The ethos of projection methodology is however to be cautious, conservative and moderate. A spreading practice among official forecasters is to produce 'variant models', with more pessimistic and more optimistic assumptions.

Although projection methodology is a specialist technical subject, it would be valuable if a good critical understanding was more widespread. Box 1.2 outlines the construction of a simple population projection model. Careful study of this and of the fuller explanations of the most recent England and Wales projections reveals a paradox: while we have an increasingly detailed knowledge of recent fertility and mortality trends, and projection models are impressively systematic and logical, a large element of guesswork is unavoidable in the assumptions about future changes in the rate of mortality and fertility change. The actuaries and demographers who develop projection models are subtle and cautious; not all secondary users are as sophisticated.

UK population projections

Projections of the size and the age- and sex-structure of the population of the UK are produced every 2 years by the Government Actuary in collaboration with the Office of Population Censuses and Surveys (OPCS). Increasingly detailed and valuable explanations of the assumptions about future fertility, mortality and external migration are given (OPCS 1993, pp. 4–10). The latest 1991-based projections to 2031 (with extrapolations to 2061) use substantially-revised assumptions, the first since the previous interesting revision in 1985. Of most influence upon the projected size and age-structure of the UK population, 'the assumed long-term family size for the UK as a whole has been reduced from 2.00 to 1.90 children per woman'. And even more intriguingly, following the intricate analyses of cause-specific deaths by Alderson & Ashwood (1985) and others in the early 1980s, the government actuaries have now revised the mortality assumptions on the basis of a careful examination of cohort-differentials in all-cause death rates:

For men between the ages of 24 and 46 mortality rates are tending to rise at present, largely due to deaths arising from HIV infection, but also from an increasing number of suicides and accidental deaths. ... Past and current trends suggest that those now over about age 47 will continue to show, in each cohort, lower mortality rates than in the preceding cohort ... this has been their experience to date and at present their mortality rates are diminishing by between one and four per cent a year. This trend has been strong for nearly 2 decades. ... It has therefore been decided to assume, in general, rather greater improvement than in the previous projections for all those born in 1945 or earlier.
(OPCS 1993, p. 8)

The adopted mortality assumption is a middle course between high and low 'scenarios'. The high scenario, the standard assumption up to 1991, is that the current rates of age-specific mortality improvement would halve each decade for 40 years and then be constant. The low scenario is that the improved mortality experienced to date by the post-1945 cohorts would continue for the remainder of their lives. The middle course averages the high and low trends: 'Under these optimistic low mortality rate assumptions, E_0 continues to increase by nearly 2 years a decade for the best part of 4 decades – reaching $79\frac{1}{2}$ years for males and $84\frac{3}{4}$ years for females in 2041' (OPCS 1993, p. 9). The life tables for the year 2041 which would arise if mortality trends took the middle course between these scenarios would generate mean life expectancies of 77.4 years for males and 82.7 years for females.

A selection of the new official projections is given in Table 1.5. These indicate that the UK population aged 60+ years will exceed 12 million during the 1990s and in the early decades of the next century enter a period of faster growth, to 15.8 million by 2021. During the 2030s the growth phase will end, and no change is projected in the 60+ population of 18.1 million during the decade. By 2061, it is expected that the 60+ years population will have fallen by 6% from 2041 to 17.1

million. As a result of the low fertility assumption, during this period the total population is likely to be falling and the elderly population will continue to grow as a share of the total. In 2031 they are likely to form 29.1% of the total, and by 2061 to be 29.8%. An increasing average age is projected among the elderly population, and the numbers aged over 75 years and over 85 years will grow more quickly than the entire elderly population. In comparison to the 1989-based projections, the 1991-based estimates increase the number of 75+ year-olds by 1.3% in 2001, 4.9% in 2011 and 12.9%, or 633 000, in 2021.

HETEROGENEITY AND SOCIAL CHANGE

One reason for this extended treatment of the projected size and age-structure of the elderly population is that such data are commonly given undue emphasis and treated as certain predictions in the health sciences and health services. On the other hand, awareness of the variability or heterogeneity of the elderly population, and of the degree to which each successive birth-group or cohort of elderly people differs from their predecessors, is much less well developed.

Table 1.5 Population projections, United Kingdom 1991–2041

Age (years)	1991 M	1991 F	2001 M	2001 F	2011 M	2011 F	2021 M	2021 F	2041 M	2041 F
Thousands
0–15	5675	5377	6033	5726	5419	5403	5508	5250	5194	4953
16–44	12 677	12 430	12 483	12 129	12 381	11 660	11 698	11 203	11 052	10 601
45–59	4736	4776	5528	5614	6105	6203	6284	6273	5725	5584
60–64	1393	1501	1403	1457	1843	1928	1861	1956	1628	1649
65–69	1291	1503	1231	1331	1466	1566	1546	1674	1584	1653
70–74	983	1299	1048	1262	1124	1262	1494	1690	1637	1815
75–79	727	1136	811	1141	847	1048	1062	1280	1404	1692
80–84	419	829	475	843	554	855	666	907	921	1263
85–89	180	466	230	548	291	600	359	595	522	839
90+	50	201	92	332	128	426	179	494	409	863
60+	5044	6934	5291	6914	6252	7685	7167	8598	8105	9775
75+	1377	2632	1609	2864	1819	2930	2266	3277	3256	4658
Total	28 132	29 517	29 335	30 383	30 158	30 952	30 657	31 324	30 075	30 912
Percentage of total population
0–15	20.2	18.2	20.6	18.8	18.0	17.5	18.0	16.8	17.3	16.0
16–44	45.1	42.1	42.6	39.9	41.1	37.7	38.2	35.8	36.7	34.3
45–59	16.8	16.2	18.8	18.5	20.2	20.0	20.5	20.0	19.0	18.1
60–69	9.5	10.2	9.0	9.2	11.0	11.3	11.1	11.6	10.7	10.7
70–79	6.1	8.2	6.3	7.9	6.5	7.5	8.3	9.5	10.1	11.3
80–89	2.1	4.4	2.4	4.6	2.8	4.7	3.3	4.8	4.8	6.8
90+	0.2	0.7	0.3	1.1	0.4	1.4	0.6	1.6	1.4	2.8
60+	17.9	23.5	18.0	22.8	20.7	24.8	23.4	27.4	26.9	31.6
75+	4.9	8.9	5.5	9.4	6.0	9.5	7.4	10.5	10.8	15.1

Source: OPCS (1993), Appendix I.

The future personal and social situation and well-being of elderly people will, on the one hand, have much to do with people's own experience and capacities and, on the other, with societal attitudes and policies. Health and vigour, savings and income, the quality of housing, the range and responsiveness of social networks, the resources available for services for elderly people and many other factors condition old age lives. Successive cohorts of elderly people exhibit markedly different histories at all stages of their lives, from childhood nutrition and education, through marital, reproductive and occupational experiences, to the physiological, mental, familial and material resources with which they enter old age.

A 'cohort profile' of those born in 1900

In the UK, the generation born in the 1900s received no more than rudimentary education in the 'three rs' – most only ever attended one school. Their childhood nutrition was deficient by today's standards, and work commonly started at 14 years of age. As young people, retirement would have been expected only for a small middle class and not for the mass of manual and junior clerical workers. The cohort raised larger families than today in homes without modern amenities and, whether in household work or in paid occupations, except on Sundays, they worked long hours that left little time for recreation. Manual occupations were dominant, exposure to accidents and toxins was high, and housing conditions were spartan and, in some cases, sufficiently damp and unhygienic to compromise health. Many women worked as domestic servants when young, but then married and ceased paid work. The entire cohort experienced adverse economic and employment conditions during the 1920s and 1930s, and were nearing the end of their working lives when the more prosperous post-Second World War years began (Jefferys 1991).

This 'cohort profile' does not consciously over-draw the harshness and privations of that generation's lives. Sturdy survivors of the cohort are the oldest members of our society today. Are our impressions of the patients and clients of residential and welfare services informed by an appreciation of how different these people's lives have been to our own? In every dimension, from physiology to pension entitlements, future cohorts of elderly people will be different from those before. Only superficial descriptions and assessments of the importance of these changes can be made. It is possible, however, to distinguish those aspects of variability in the elderly population that are likely to endure from those that are more uncertain.

DURABLE SOCIODEMOGRAPHIC VARIATIONS

Gender

The clearest sociodemographic differential within the elderly population is the situation of men and women. A long-standing feature of contemporary affluent societies is that, on average, women live longer than men. At least until in the most recent cohorts, most women in their early adult lives married and remained so, on average to men 2 to 3 years older than themselves. Also true of all the cohorts that are presently old, most married women withdrew from employment during the years in which they were raising children and, when and if they returned to paid work, they entered lower status occupations, were paid at lower rates and accumulated fewer pension entitlements than men.

Among the many consequences in today's elderly population, we find that husbands tend to die before wives, most elderly men are relatively young and live with their wives in two-plus person households, and widowed men have a higher re-marriage rate than widowed women. It follows that the elderly population has a substantial over-representation of women, and that the oldest age groups are substantially made up of widows who predominantly live alone and have very low incomes. Old age poverty is largely a problem of low incomes among very old women in one-person households. There is no sign that the many modifications in recent decades in late-age mortality rates, in the employment histories of men and women, in people's housing preferences, or in the government's intentions concerning pensions and social security policies will quickly change these patterns (Hills 1994).

Frailty, disablement and chronic sickness

Another enduring characteristic of the elderly population is the concentration of frailty, disablement and chronic sickness at the older ages. But while these age-relationships will endure, substantial modifications in the ages of incidence of disorders and of reduced functioning have been occurring. As mean life expectancy increases, so also do the ages at which a given share of the population has a given severity of functional impairment, although the non-existence of large data sets of health and functioning variables means that few examples can be given. The general tendency is not, however, disputed; rather, current debate focuses on the relative rates at which the mean ages of death and of grades of ill-health disability are increasing. If mean life expectancy is increasing at a greater rate than the mean age of onset of given functional impairments, then disabled years will be increasing faster than healthy years. On the other hand, if the mean age of onset of a defined level of functional impairment is increasing faster than the mean age of death, i.e. the gap between the two is reducing, then the prevalence of morbidity and disablement in the population will be decreasing. Because of the obvious impacts of these trends on the need for treatment and care and upon the total cost of health and personal social services, governments are intensively interested in improved estimates and a concerted research effort is underway to monitor and project these trends (Bebbington 1991). Longer series of data will, however, be required in the UK before convincing trends can be described and before more than suppositional forward projections can be made.

Socioeconomic differentials

A third source of variability in old age is associated with socioeconomic differentials which, like 'the poor', will always be with us. Their detailed form is, however, constantly changing. Every modern society has a stratified social structure and differentials of income and wealth. An individual's relative economic position is partly endowed by their parents and childhood experience but mainly established by their income during working age. Three generalisations about elderly people's material circumstances are empirically supportable: first, real average living standards have improved substantially in recent decades; second, income declines for the great majority of people at the transition from working age to retirement; and thirdly, income and wealth differentials established during working lives tend to be magnified in the retirement years.

A large percentage of the retired population in the UK is dependent upon state benefits for their income, and a large proportion lives at no more than officially recognised poverty levels. From 1950 to 1970, income differentials tended to narrow, and this was probably true for the retired as well as for the general population because of the rising real value of state and occupational pensions and of savings. Since the mid-1970s, income differentials have tended to widen in the UK, and this again is probably true within the elderly age groups, because of the decreasing real value of the state pension, earlier and longer retirement, and the increasing number of ethnic minority elderly people (Wilkinson 1994). The income position of women is particularly disadvantageous, and recent amendments to social security legislation have weakened their entitlements to state pensions. This is another field which has recently attracted very careful and detailed high-quality research (Johnson 1991).

FIELDS OF RAPID GENERATIONAL CHANGE

Marital status

Other sociodemographic characteristics of elderly people are even more subject to change. In the case of the marital status of the elderly population and various derivative characteristics such as household composition, the patterns that will be found as little as 10 years ahead are very difficult to predict. Rapid changes will result from the entry into old age of the first cohorts to experience the higher rates of divorce and re-marriage in early adulthood which began in the 1960s. Among the prospective changes will be increasing differences in the ages of spouses and the complex derivative effects on the ages and prevalence of widowhood, widowerhood and low incomes, and more diverse kin networks with a higher percentage of children and grandchildren not in contact but more functioning step-relationships.

Ethnic groups

Equally rapid changes will occur in the next decade in the ethnic group membership of the UK's elderly population (Blakemore & Boneham 1994). The substantial flows of young adult migrants into the UK from the 'New Commonwealth' began during the 1950s. Those people and their successors will soon begin to enter the elderly age groups in large numbers. There are likely to be highly contrasted family structures and household forms among the various ethnic groups. Elderly UK citizens with origins in the Indian subcontinent will have a relatively high propensity to be living with their children in multi-generational households, while those originating from the Caribbean will sustain living arrangements much closer to national norms. In some ethnic groups, there are large numbers of multiply deprived elderly people, and their situation will be worsened by a history of low pay and incomplete employment and insurance contributions records in the UK. Some groups will also be disadvantaged, particularly with respect to their health and health care, by poor childhood nutritional and educational standards, by ignorance of UK institutions and entitlements, and by poor reading or conversational ability in the English language.

Health status and health care expectations

The third and final area of rapid change is likely to be in health status and health care expectations. The elderly cohorts born in the 1940s will be the first to have enjoyed mass school secondary education, full employment and rising prosperity during most of their working lives, mass home ownership and car ownership, several weeks of paid holidays, ample leisure hours besides, and lifetime access to the National Health Service and to contemporary social security benefits and personal social services.

How these and a host of other changes throughout the life course will translate into people's vigour, resources and demands in old age is impossible to predict. The hypothesis that there will be substantial cohort differences is, however, compelling. Improved nutrition and housing standards, and the reduction of arduous physical work will manifest in changed vulnerabilities to the disorders and diseases of later life. For the most part, people at any given age are likely to be physically healthier than their parents and grandparents. It can be expected that more discomforts, diseases and disabilities will be treated or successfully managed. Even more likely is that the new generation of elderly people will have higher expectations as to their own health and functioning. There will undoubtedly be more demands upon the health services and the caring professions.

COHORT SIZE, WELLBEING AND MENTAL HEALTH

Cohort size

Several academic disciplines have put forward propositions about connections between the size of successive cohorts and their relative material progress. A US economic historian, Richard Easterlin, studied the declining fertility of farm families in the USA during the later 19th and early 20th centuries, and constructed a thesis of the relations between the material progress made by parents, their children's expectations when they enter working life, the size of the child's cohort, the degree of competition among the children for jobs, and their occupational success (particularly how swiftly they occupy better paid positions) (Easterlin 1980). Some cohorts see their parents achieving little material progress and so enter employment with low expectations which are then surpassed. Others, noting that their parents have a sense of economic wellbeing, adopt optimistic expect-

ations for themselves and are then disappointed. Easterlin argued that there is a connection between a sense of over- or under-achievement and a cohort's marriage age and family size. Historical demographers have for long used similar ideas in linking sequences of bad harvests and famine to delayed marriages, and of good harvest years to early marriages and higher fertility.

Relative wellbeing/deprivation

Comparable reasoning in more general form is found in conceptions of relative material wellbeing. These are well set out in W. G. Runciman's (1966) much debated thesis of *relative deprivation* which, at its core, suggests that an individual's sense of wellbeing has less to do with an absolute level of wages or material possessions than with a comparative evaluation against a standard. (This may be one's own position when young, that of one's parents at the same age, or a perception of the wellbeing of one's peers.)

In the many discussions of these ideas, interesting counter-intuitive ideas can be found. One, for example, is that the greatest discontent (leading to revolts and revolutions) is found not in societies with large social and material differentials, nor necessarily when there is little economic progress. Often it occurs in societies in which there has been an actual or promised high rate of economic growth and material progress followed by stagnation or reversal. These situations raise expectations which are frustrated (Runciman 1989).

Societal wellbeing and mental states

Attempts to link the analyses of social historians and sociologists of comparative societal wellbeing with the prevalence of mental states (and particularly of depression) in the population are rare. Some connections are widely understood, e.g. that rates of suicide decline during years of full employment or during periods of exceptional common national purpose, as at the beginning of a war. Elderly people's reactions to their own old age will show some parallels. Old age involves physical, cognitive, familial and social losses, and frequent adjustments to changed capacities and horizons are made (Erikson et al 1989). An individual's reaction to a sensory decline or to bereavement will to some extent be conditioned by their expectations for later life, and in the field of health and welfare these will to some extent be a product of societal norms. They will also be influenced by comparative judgements that are made with the situation of their parents and their age peers. Mental states in old age therefore have complex and multifarious bases, from biochemical changes leading to cognitive decline to the duplicities of confidantes, and some with a foundation in sociodemographic change.

EPIDEMIOLOGY OF PSYCHIATRIC PROBLEMS IN ELDERLY PEOPLE

Information about the prevalence, distribution and associations of mental health problems may help to determine causal factors and is needed to plan the allocation of resources for treatment and support. Epidemiological studies of mental health problems in the elderly have usually been carried out by psychiatrists on community samples, selected using census lists, or by house-to-house surveys (Gurland et al 1983, Myers et al 1984, Livingston et al 1990, Hofman et al 1991). In the UK, researchers have taken advantage of the fact that 95% of people are registered with general practitioners (GPs) and have recruited subjects through general practices in some studies (Morgan et al 1987, Copeland et al 1987). Most recently, GPs themselves have begun to carry out epidemiological surveys in the UK (Iliffe et al 1991a).

Caseness

The aims of such surveys have been to identify the prevalence and incidence of mental health problems in the community, defined in terms of syndrome 'caseness'. 'Caseness' means a subject displays 'a collection of symptoms which a psychiatrist would recognise as a characteristic and abnormal mental state for which intervention would be appropriate if it were available' (Copeland 1990). The advantage of such a categorical classification is that it predicts the prognosis and the likely response to treatment in any one 'case'. However, many problems do not fit neatly into the categories devised. Alongside the 'cases' identified, many subjects are found to have similar symptoms which are not numerous or severe enough to reach 'case' level and yet may cause them significant problems. In addition, subjects with symptoms of more than one type of syndrome will be labelled as suffering from whichever is the more severe, and information about the overlap of syndromes may be lost.

Screening instruments

In order to be able to compare the results of studies in different geographical areas, researchers have tried to develop standardised reliable psychiatric interview instruments (Copeland 1990).
Examples include:

- CARE – the Comprehensive Assessment and Referral Evaluation (Gurland et al 1983)
- GMS – the Geriatric Mental State (Copeland et al 1986)
- CAMDEX – the Cambridge Examination for Mental Disorders of the Elderly (Brayne & Calloway 1989)
- DIS – the Diagnostic Interview Schedule, designed to elicit the diagnostic criteria of the American Psychiatric Association's *Diagnostic and Statistical Manual of Mental Disorders*, 3rd edition, the DSM-III (Myers et al 1984).

A further refinement has been to standardise the interpretation of the symptoms found, by using a computer program – for example the AGECAT program which is used to interpret the findings of the GMS interview (Copeland et al 1986).

Two-stage designs

However, screening all the subjects of a survey with instruments such as the GMS or CAMDEX is time-consuming, and researchers have attempted to make the process more efficient by adopting 'two-stage' designs. A brief instrument is used on the whole population initially, followed by longer interviews with those subjects found to be positive. Usually, a sample of subjects who are negative on screening is also interviewed, to check that the brief instrument is sensitive enough not to miss too many cases.
Brief screening instruments include:

- CAPE – the Clifton Assessment Procedures for the Elderly (Pattie & Gilleard 1976)
- MMSE – the Mini Mental State Examination (Folstein et al 1975, Myers et al 1984)
- the short-CARE (Livingston et al 1990).

Prevalence of mental health problems

Table 1.6 summarises data from a number of surveys using approximately equivalent diagnostic criteria for identifying dementia, depression and specific anxiety disorders in populations aged 65 years and over.

Dementia

Diagnostic criteria for case level dementia include diminished intellectual functioning to a degree that

Table 1.6 Prevalence of psychiatric disorders in the over-65s

Study	Location	Prevalence of disorder (%)		
		Dementia	Depression	Anxiety disorders*
Gurland et al 1983	London	2.3	12.4	2.0
Gurland et al 1983	New York	4.9	13.0	1.4
Myers et al 1984	3 towns in USA	4.8	2.7#	4.6
Morgan et al 1987	Nottingham	4.3	9.8	
Copeland et al 1987	Liverpool	5.2	11.3	2.4
Livingston et al 1990	London	4.7	15.9	
Iliffe et al 1991a	London	4.6	22.0	
Lobo et al 1992	Zaragoza	7.4		
Dewey et al 1993	Zaragoza		10.4	

* including generalised anxiety disorder, panic disorder, phobias and obsessive–compulsive disorder but excluding anxiety associated with depressive disorder.
# DSM-III major depression and 'dysthymia' combined.

impairs social or occupational functions, impairment of memory, impaired ability to think in abstract terms, impaired judgement, and alteration of personality.

Table 1.6 shows that the overall prevalence of cases of dementia is remarkably similar in studies carried out in the UK, USA and Europe, at around 5% of the over-65s. However, these studies have usually failed to include elderly people living in institutions in their samples. When those people are included, the prevalence increases to around 7–8% of the population over 65 (Livingston et al 1990, Hofman et al 1991).

Studies have also consistently found that the prevalence of dementia is a function of age. Hofman et al (1991), reviewing 12 European surveys, found that the prevalence at age 65 was around 1%, but that it increased exponentially through approximately 5% at age 75 and 20% at age 85, to around 33% of people in their 90s. The incidence of new cases has been estimated at around 10 to 20 per 1000 per year in the over-65s (Copeland et al 1992, Boothby et al 1994).

As well as these 'cases', studies have usually found a number of people with symptoms of dementia which do not reach case level, but nevertheless cause problems for them and their families. Myers et al (1984) found mild cognitive impairment in 11–18% of subjects in addition to the 4.8% with severe impairment, Copeland et al (1987) found that 4.9% of their Liverpool sample were 'subcases' of dementia in addition to the 5.2% who reached case level, and Iliffe et al (1990) estimated that 'possible' dementia was present in 10.5% of their north London sample in addition to the 4.6% who were 'probable' cases.

There are a number of possible causes of dementia. Copeland et al (1992) judged that in Liverpool, of the total of 4.3% of their population with case-severity dementia, 3.3% was due to Alzheimer's disease, 0.7% was due to cerebrovascular causes, and 0.3% was due to alcohol excess.

Anxiety disorders

Specific disorders include generalised anxiety disorder, phobic disorders including agoraphobia, and obsessive–compulsive disorder. The diagnostic criteria for caseness are very strict and include only those people likely to need specialist psychiatric treatment. This may explain why the reported prevalence of cases of such disorders is low, at around 2–4% of the over-65s (Table 1.6).

Symptoms of anxiety are very common indeed, however. For example, Copeland et al (1987) found that over 25% of their Liverpool sample were 'subcases' of anxiety neurosis, of whom over a third had a mixture of anxiety and depressive symptoms. Again, these symptoms are likely to cause problems for sufferers and their families, and often require help from GPs and the primary care team, despite the fact that they do not fit neatly into the categorical definitions of specialist psychiatric syndrome cases.

Alcohol misuse

Rates of alcohol use and misuse in the elderly have proved rather difficult to estimate, for a number of reasons. There may be reluctance to admit to overconsumption, which is perceived as socially undesirable, or elderly people may not be able to recall how much they have consumed (especially those who are chronic misusers who may develop memory problems). In general though, it is thought that alcohol misuse is less prevalent in elderly people than among younger subjects. Saunders et al (1989) found 'problem' drinking in only 0.9% of their Liverpool sample, although 6.1% of men and 2.4% of women exceeded the recommended daily maximum of 21 and 14 units respectively. Iliffe et al (1991c) found that 3.6% of men and 3.2% of women in their London sample exceeded recommended levels, and overall 10.5% were daily drinkers. It has been estimated that around 5–12% of men and 1–2% of women are 'problem' drinkers (Dunne 1994).

Chronic alcohol misuse is associated with liver disease, peripheral neuropathy and dementia, and the mortality is high. Long-standing misuse is associated with psychiatric illness and a family history of alcohol problems. Misuse which begins in old age is associated with bereavement, reduced social support and physical illness, and tends to respond much better to intervention (Dunne 1994).

Depression – a major public health problem

Depression of 'case' severity means low mood or loss of interest in almost all usual activities, plus 4 out of 7 symptoms, namely: change in appetite and weight, change in sleep pattern, agitation or retardation in thinking and movements, loss of energy or tiredness, feelings of guilt or worthlessness, poor concentration, and suicidal ideas (DSM-III major depression). Around two-thirds of cases of major depression will respond to treatment with antidepressants or with cognitive therapy.

As with dementia and anxiety disorders, in addition to the cases of depression identified, a proportion of subjects surveyed are found with symptoms of depression not reaching case level. Myers et al (1984) found that around 20% of their over-65-year-olds had symptoms of depression in addition to the 2.7% with DSM-III major depression or dysthymia. Copeland et al (1987) found that 10.7% of their sample were subcases of depression in addition to the 11.3% who were cases. Kay et al (1964) found that 10% of their Newcastle sample had moderate to severe depression and a further 16.2% had mild depression.

Table 1.6 shows that the prevalence of depression varies between studies more widely than for dementia. This is probably partly due to differences in the screening instruments used, giving different thresholds for caseness. It may also be due to true variation in the proportion of subjects with depression. For example, depression is usually found to be more prevalent in deprived inner city areas. The high prevalence of depression makes it a major public health problem with high economic costs alongside the suffering it causes. The incidence of depression in the elderly has been estimated to be between 15 and 30 cases per 1000 per year (Copeland et al 1992, Blanchard et al 1994). The prognosis seems to be poor; in Liverpool around two-thirds of over-65-year-old subjects with GMS–AGECAT case-level depression were either still psychiatrically ill or had died after 3 years of follow-up (Copeland et al 1992).

Unlike dementia, levels of depression have been found not to vary with age, but studies have demonstrated a consistent sex difference, with approximately double the prevalence in women compared to men. Iliffe et al (1991a) found prevalences of 25.3% in women and 13.4% in men. Dewey et al (1993) found prevalences in Liverpool and Zaragoza of 14.2% and 14.8% respectively for women, and 7.2% and 6.2% respectively for men. Whilst the prevalence of depression was very similar in Liverpool and Zaragoza, the symptom pattern varied (Dewey et al 1993). Symptoms more common in Liverpool included depressed mood, subjective slowing, lack of energy, irritability and indecisiveness. Symptoms more common in Zaragoza included difficulty concentrating, pessimism, tremulous feelings and worry about almost everything.

Social factors associated with depression. Studies of social factors and life events which might be associated with depression in the elderly have yielded conflicting results. Murphy (1982) found that the onset of depression in elderly Londoners was associated with major life events including bereavement, physical illness and financial problems. Vulnerability was increased by major social difficulties and the incidence of depression was higher in working class subjects. In addition, those without a confiding relationship seemed to be more vulnerable, echoing the findings among younger subjects (Brown & Harris 1978). Livingston et al (1990) found that being single and living alone increased the likelihood of depression, but by contrast, Iliffe et al (1991b) found no association with a lack of confiding relationships. Green et al (1992) found that depression was associated with bereavement within the previous 6 months, and with feelings of loneliness, but not with marital status, living alone, poor housing, size of social network, or physical illness.

Depression, elderly people and primary health care

Studies have suggested that, on average, GPs identify only around half of the psychological problems among the patients presenting to them (Marks et al 1979,

Freeling et al 1985). Many patients present with physical rather than psychological complaints and psychiatric problems associated with physical disease are less likely to be acknowledged as needing treatment in their own right. This is likely to be more of a problem with elderly than with younger patients, since the prevalence of physical disorders rises with age.

The available evidence suggests that many elderly people suffering from depression receive no treatment or support. Blanchard and colleagues (1994) found in the Gospel Oak ward of north London, that depression was associated with increased contact with GPs but that depressed subjects gave psychological reasons for consulting in only 3% of attendances. Just over one-third of cases had discussed their emotional problems with their family doctors but of these only half were receiving treatment with antidepressants, psychotherapy or counselling. It has been suggested that educational initiatives are needed to reduce the stigma of depression, make it more acceptable to present psychological symptoms to doctors, and to reframe depression as an illness like any other, for which treatment is available.

General practitioners may also be unaware of the development of dementia in some of their patients. Iliffe et al (1991a) found a diagnosis of dementia recorded in the GP notes in only 1 of the 11 cases which they found on screening elderly people in north London with the Mini Mental State Examination (MMSE).

The primary health care team

The primary care of mental illness should be more efficient and effective where other members of the primary health care team besides the GP are involved, including district nurses, health visitors and practice nurses. These professionals are in frequent contact with many patients and could assist the GP in preventing, identifying and managing mental illness in primary care. The World Health Organization *Working Party on Psychiatry and Primary Care* (1973) concluded that the primary medical care team is the cornerstone of community psychiatry.

Community nurses. Community nurses regularly visit old people who are physically ill or disabled, often isolated, and therefore at increased risk of depression. Such visiting may continue for months and the nurse may become very familiar with the home situation. It has been suggested that community nurses could identify depression in their patients and bring it to the attention of the GP. A study has recently been carried out in south London of the ability of 60 district nurses

to detect depression among their elderly housebound patients. Accuracy measured against a 1–2 hour diagnostic interview by a psychologist was generally poor. The nurses tended to over-diagnose depression and were therefore not able to identify very accurately which patients might benefit from extra treatment or support (Gilleard 1993).

Research has shown that training GPs in interviewing skills can improve their accuracy in the diagnosis of psychiatric disorder (Gask et al 1987). Community nurses, like GPs, probably need training in interviewing skills if they are to identify depression in their patients with accuracy. Given the high prevalence of depression reported among elderly patients, such training might be cost-effective although community nurses may not have time to do more than carry out the physical nursing tasks required of them.

Practice nurses. The rapid increase in the number of employed practice nurses has increased the potential for teamwork in the care of mental disorders in general practice in the UK. However, so far there is little evidence that practice nurses are involved at all in the management of psychiatric problems, except in a few cases where they administer depot injections to patients with chronic schizophrenia. Tudor-Hart (1985) has pointed out that they are an under-used resource and could be a valuable help if trained properly, given enough time, and allowed to maintain skills by continued experience.

Practice nurses are likely to be involved in the routine annual screening of patients over 75 years old, which has been a requirement in the UK since the 1990 GP contract was introduced. It has been suggested that such screening should include questions to detect probable depression and dementia and to assess social networks (Iliffe et al 1991a).

Wilkinson et al (1993) found that practice nurses could assist GPs in the management of depression, by advising patients about antidepressants and their side-effects, in an effort to increase compliance with treatment. The efficacy of such collaborative work remains to be established, however.

CONCLUSION

Psychiatric epidemiological studies have shown that mental health problems are common in the elderly, especially depression and dementia, together with anxiety disorders and alcohol misuse. These studies have adopted categorical definitions of mental illness corresponding to the severity seen in psychiatric specialist practice, which means that the whole range of symptoms in the population may not be described. For every subject meeting the criteria for 'caseness', there are many others with fewer or milder symptoms which nevertheless may need assessment and treatment.

At present, it seems that many elderly people are not offered any treatment or support for their mental health problems. Primary health care workers need to be aware of the prevalence of mental health problems in the community, the risk factors associated with their development, and methods of detecting them, including questionnaire and interview instruments. Members of primary care teams should organise their services between them in ways which will maximise the detection and treatment of psychological problems among their elderly patients.

REFERENCES

Alderson M, Ashwood F 1985 Projections of mortality rates for the elderly. Population Trends 42: 22–29

Bebbington A C 1991 The expectation of life without disability in England and Wales 1976–88. Population Trends 66: 26–29

Blakemore K, Boneham M 1994 Age, race and ethnicity: a comparative approach. Open University Press, Buckingham

Blanchard M R, Waterreus A, Mann A H 1994 The nature of depression among older people in Inner London, and the contact with primary care. British Journal of Psychiatry 164: 396–402

Boothby H, Blizard R, Livingstone G, Mann A H 1994 The Gospel Oak study stage III: the incidence of dementia. Psychological Medicine 24: 89–95

Brayne C, Calloway P 1989 An epidemiological study of dementia in a rural population of elderly women. British Journal of Psychiatry 155: 214–219

Brown G W, Harris T 1978 The social origins of depression: a study of psychiatric disorder in women. Tavistock, London

Copeland J R M, Dewey M E, Griffiths-Jones H M 1986 A computerised psychiatric diagnostic system and case nomenclature for elderly subjects: GMS and AGECAT. Psychological Medicine 16: 89–99

Copeland J R M, Dewey M E, Wood N, Searle R, Davidson I A, McWilliam C 1987 Range of mental illness among the elderly in the community: prevalence in Liverpool using the GMS–AGECAT package. British Journal of Psychiatry 150: 815–823

Copeland J R M 1990 Suitable instruments for detecting dementia in community samples. Age and Ageing 19: 81–83

Copeland J R M, Davidson I A, Dewey M E et al 1992 Alzheimer's disease, other dementias, depression and pseudo-dementia: prevalence, incidence and three-year outcome in Liverpool. British Journal of Psychiatry 161: 230–239

Dewey M E, Camara de la C, Copeland F R M, Lobo A, Saz P 1993 Cross-cultural comparison of depression and depressive symptoms in older people. Acta Psychiatrica Scandinavia 87: 369–373

Dunne F J 1994 Misuse of alcohol or drugs by elderly people. British Medical Journal 308: 608–609

Easterlin R A 1980 Birth and fortune: the impact of numbers on personal welfare. Grant McIntyre, London

Erikson E H, Erikson J M, Kivnick H Q 1989 Vital involvement in old age. Norton, New York

Folstein M F, Folstein S E, McHugh P R 1975 Mini mental state examination: a practical method for grading the cognitive state of patients for the clinician. Journal of Psychiatric Research 12: 189–198

Freeling P, Rao B M, Paykel E S, Sireling L I, Burton R H 1985 Unrecognised depression in general practice. British Medical Journal 290: 1880–1883

Gask L, McGrath G, Goldberg D, Millar T 1987 Improving the psychiatric skills of established general practitioners: evaluation of group teaching. Medical Education 21: 362–368

Gilleard C 1993 The elderly housebound project: final report to South West Thames Regional Health Authority. St George's Hospital Medical School, London

Green B H, Copeland J R M, Dewey M E et al 1992 Risk factors for depression in elderly people: a prospective study. Acta Psychiatrica Scandinavia 86: 213–217

Gurland B, Copeland J, Kuriansky J, Kelleher M, Sharpe, L, Dean L 1983 The mind and mood of ageing. Croom Helm, London

Hendricks J, Hendricks C D 1986 Ageing in mass society: myths and realities, 3rd edn. Little, Brown, Boston

Hills J 1994 The future of the welfare state. Joseph Rowntree Foundation, York

Hofman A, Rocca W A, Brayne C et al 1991 The prevalence of dementia in Europe: a collaborative study of 1980–1990 findings. International Journal of Epidemiology 20(3): 736–748

Iliffe S, Booroff A, Gallivan S, Goldenberg E, Morgan P, Haines A 1990 Screening for cognitive impairment in the elderly using the mini-mental state examination. British Journal of General Practice 40: 277–279

Iliffe S, Haines A, Gallivan S, Booroff A, Goldenberg E, Morgan P 1991a Assessment of elderly people in general practice, part 1: social circumstances and mental state. British Journal of General Practice 41: 9–12

Iliffe S, Haines A, Stein A, Gallivan S 1991b Assessment of elderly people in general practice, part 3: confiding relationships. British Journal of General Practice 41: 459–461

Iliffe S, Haynes A, Booroff A, Goldenberg E, Morgan P, Gallivan S 1991c Alcohol consumption by elderly people: a general practice survey. Age and Ageing 20: 120–123

Jefferys M (ed) 1991 Growing old in the twentieth century. Routledge, London

Johnson P 1991 Ageing and economic performance, discussion paper 34. Centre for Economic Performance, London

Kay D W K, Beamish P, Roth M 1964 Old age mental disorders in Newcastle-upon-Tyne, part 1: a study of prevalence. British Journal of Psychiatry 110: 146–158

Livingston G, Hawkins A, Graham N, Blizard B, Mann A 1990 The Gospel Oak study: prevalence rates of dementia, depression and activity limitation among elderly residents in Inner London. Psychological Medicine 20: 137–146

Lobo A, Dewey M, Copeland J, Dia J-L, Saz P 1992 The prevalence of dementia among elderly people living in Zaragoza and Liverpool. Psychological Medicine 22: 239–243

Marks J N, Goldberg D P, Hillier V F 1979 Determinants of the ability of general practitioners to detect psychiatric illness. Psychological Medicine 9: 337–353

Morgan K, Dalloosso H M, Arie T, Byrne E J, Jaones R, Waite J 1987 Mental health and psychological wellbeing among the old and the very old living at home. British Journal of Psychiatry 150: 801–807

Murphy E 1982 Social origins of depression in old age. British Journal of Psychiatry 141: 135–142

Myers J K, Weissman M N, Tischler G L et al 1984 Six-month prevalence of psychiatric disorders in three communities. Archives of General Psychiatry 41: 959–967

Olshansky S J 1988 On forecasting mortality. Milbank Quarterly 66: 482–530

OPCS (Office of Population Censuses and Surveys) 1992 Mortality statistics England and Wales 1990: general. HMSO, London

OPCS (Office of Population Censuses and Surveys) 1993 National population projections: 1991-based, Series PP2, No. 18. HMSO, London

Pattie A H, Gilleard C J 1976 The Clifton Assessment Schedule – a further validation of a psychogeriatric assessment schedule. British Journal of Psychiatry 129: 68–72

Runciman W G 1966 Relative deprivation and social justice: a study of attitudes to social inequality in twentieth-century England. University of California Press, Berkeley

Runciman W G 1989 A treatise on social theory, volume 2: substantive social theory. Cambridge University Press, Cambridge

Saunders P A, Copeland J R M, Dewey M E et al 1989 Alcohol use and abuse in the elderly: findings from the Liverpool longitudinal study of continuing health in the community. International Journal of Geriatric Psychiatry 4: 103–108

Suzman R, Kinsella K G, Myers G C 1992 Demography of older populations in developed countries. In: Evans J G, Williams T F (eds) Oxford textbook of geriatric medicine. Oxford University Press, Oxford

Tudor-Hart J 1985 Practice nurses: an underused resource. British Medical Journal 290: 1162–1163

Warnes A M 1993 The demography of ageing in the United Kingdom of Great Britain and Northern Ireland. Committee for International Cooperation in National Research in Demography and the United Nations Institute on Ageing, Valletta, Malta

Wilkinson G, Allen P, Marshall E, Walker J, Browne W, Mann A H 1993 The role of the practice nurse in the management of depression in general practice: treatment adherence to antidepressant medication. Psychological Medicine 23: 229–237

Wilkinson R G 1994 Divided we fall: the poor pay the price of increased social inequality with their health. British Medical Journal 308 (6937): 1113–1114

World Health Organization Working Group 1973 Psychiatry and primary medical care. WHO, Copenhagen

RECOMMENDED READING

Bebbington A C 1991 The expectation of life without disability in England and Wales 1976–88. Population Trends 66: 26–29. *Articles in this journal provide carefully written and authoritative digests of issues of concern to policy makers. This reflects the international interest in trends in the prevalence of morbidity and impairments in the elderly population.*

Blakemore K, Boneham M 1994 Age, race and ethnicity: a comparative approach. Open University Press, Buckingham. *A pioneer and very readable account of emergent issues concerning the imminence of substantial UK populations of elderly people in ethnic minorities.*

Easterlin R A 1980 Birth and fortune: the impact of numbers on personal welfare. Grant McIntyre, London. *A short popular account that introduces some fascinating reasoning about subjective wellbeing and fertility behaviours.*

Erikson E H, Erikson J M, Kivnick H Q 1989 Vital involvement in old age. Norton, New York. *Another very readable account from a major contributor to social psychology and specifically to life course studies.*

Hendricks J, Hendricks C D 1986 Ageing in mass society: myths and realities, 3rd edn. Little, Brown, Boston. *A leading US undergraduate textbook in social gerontology. Some excellent chapters on general processes of ageing.*

Hills J 1994 The future of the welfare state. Joseph Rowntree Foundation, York. *A very well produced and tightly argued dissenting argument against the dominant ideology of the last decade that western societies cannot support the present scale of state welfare and specifically retirement pensions.*

Jefferys M (ed) 1991 Growing old in the twentieth century. Routledge, London. *An excellent collection of essays by leading social gerontologists in the UK on (mainly) social policy issues and the implications for the older population.*

OPCS (Office of Population Censuses and Surveys) 1993 National population projections: 1991-based, Series PP2, No. 18. HMSO, London. *Not entirely dry statistics, for the methodological introduction is a splendid discussion of recent fertility and mortality trends.*

Olshansky S J 1988 On forecasting mortality. Milbank Quarterly 66: 482–530. *A lively and well written article by a retired population projection professional, 'outing' the intriguing mixture of sophisticated technical caution and informed guesswork which is essential for projections.*

Runciman W G 1966 Relative deprivation and social justice: a study of attitudes to social inequality in twentieth-century England. University of California Press, Berkeley. *A modern sociological classic, closely argued but readable. Best taken in short bites, but a book which delivers real dividends in understanding of social stratification in the UK.*

Runciman W G 1989 A treatise on social theory, volume 2: substantive social theory. Cambridge University Press, Cambridge. *Not for beginning students of the social sciences nor a fashionable book, but every page impresses with its erudition and rigour. Start with volume 1, and Runciman's exploration of what we understand by 'understanding'.*

Wilkinson R G 1994 Divided we fall: the poor pay the price of increased social inequality with their health. British Medical Journal 308 (6937): 1113–1114. *A 'red hot' issue in understanding variations in health and mortality in contemporary affluent countries. Bold interpretations of cross-national variations. To be read carefully, and then for us all to ask, why should large income differentials be associated with relatively high mortality?*

2

Psychosocial approaches to ageing and mental health

Lynette Rentoul

INTRODUCTION

The word ageing implies a wide variety of processes; these include the biological inevitability of growing old, the psychological reality of growing old, and the social context, which provides a wealth of meanings in which growing old is understood and made sense of. Some aspects of this process are inevitable, they are part of what the French refer to as 'la condition humaine'. We may try to ward off some of the less agreeable aspects of growing old, by means of operations to make our skin appear more youthful, or fitness regimes to maximise health and make us feel younger and fitter, but growing old, and eventually dying, is the fate of all human beings. However, some aspects of old age in our society are not intrinsic to growing old, they are simply associated with it in our current social context. The prejudice experienced by older people (ageism) is not inevitable, but nonetheless is a reality which affects the lives of many older people.

A wide range of stressful events have been researched in the context of the psychology of old age, such as the impact of bereavement, relocation, social isolation, poverty, serious illness and retirement. Individual meanings of these events differ significantly and, although they represent challenges to older people, such events cannot be regarded as inevitable and intrinsically linked to old age. Indeed, these events can occur at any point in the human life cycle and one of the difficulties for researchers in the field of stress and health psychology is to find ways of understanding and measuring the differential impact of such events as a function of age.

Defining 'oldness'

It is important, before discussing the wide range of psychosocial issues associated with old age, to attempt to define the terms of reference. Growing old may not be difficult to define but defining 'oldness' poses more problems. The process of growing old begins in adulthood and its repercussions can be seen in terms of biological, psychological and sociological markers. The point at which one can be said to be old, however, is less clear. For most researchers in developmental and health psychology, the cut-off point is normally the age of retirement; thus, the age of 65 years is arbitrarily designated as the beginning of old age, or what has more recently been referred to as the 'Third Age' (Laslett 1989). In terms of numbers, this will be 15–20% of the population by the end of the century (Office of Population Censuses and Surveys 1984, 1993), and is seen to be a significant increase on the proportion at the beginning of the century, when elderly people only represented 5% of the population. This means that developmental and health psychology, which focus upon old people, can cover an age range of up to 4 decades. It is therefore important to recognise that there are likely to be vast differences within this population, due not only to individual differences of, for example, personality and intelligence, but also related to age differences between the younger and older groups within this population and differences as a function of gender and ethnicity (see for example Bond at al 1993).

Some authors have argued that individual differences of personality and cognitive functioning among older people is greater than the differences observed among younger people (see for example, Knight 1986). However, Knight himself, persuaded by the excellent review of Bornstein and Smircana (1982), has changed his mind and now agrees that there is no empirical evidence to support the claim that there is greater individuality among elderly people. However, it is equally important to note that elderly people are no more alike than younger people, and that any approach to the psychology of old age must accommodate the significance of important individual differences.

THE SCOPE OF PSYCHOSOCIAL APPROACHES TO OLD AGE

Interest in the psychology of old age has taken place largely in the context of developmental psychology, although increasingly relevant research is being conducted within the area of health psychology. Influential in this recent development is the excellent review of the meeting point in old age research of developmental and health psychology provided by Markides and Cooper (1989).

Psychological approaches to the study of old age can be divided into those which emphasise developmental tasks which are seen to be intrinsic to old age, and thus unavoidable, and those which focus upon external stressors and factors which, although in our culture tend to be associated with old age, are not inevitably linked to it. Individual differences and contrasting contexts are emphasised from this point of view, with little attention paid to predictable tasks and transitions that are relevant to all people.

Developmental approaches to old age

Old age, seen as a stage of development with its own tasks and challenges, grew from a tradition in psychology that emphasised this approach across the whole of the human life cycle. The notion of stage is characteristic of both psychoanalytic psychology and of the cognitive–developmental approach of Piaget. These perspectives focus upon different facets of human development. The psychoanalytic view, developed originally by Freud, considers largely what has been referred to as the affective component, or emotional aspects of personality development. Piaget's work, on the other hand, largely concerned itself with the development of our capacity to understand the social and physical world, that is cognitive growth. These perspectives were not seen to be in conflict; indeed Piaget himself argued that a comprehensive understanding of human development should involve an incorporation of both points of view. However, Piaget's work focused upon cognitive development that took place during childhood and adolescence, the point at which intellectual maturity was assumed to be achieved. He did not, therefore, consider cognitive development or change in old age. It was left to subsequent researchers such as, for example, Rabbitt (1980) and Schaie (1977–1978) to consider this.

Similarly, with regard to affective development, although Freud may have set the academic scene, his stages of psychosexual development, which emphasised unconscious determinants of character and behaviour, ended in adolescence. He believed that it was during this period that mature adult character was achieved and that subsequent changes were variations on a theme laid down in early life.

Revisions and modifications to Freud's work, especially with regard to understanding developments in old age, began in the 1930s with the work of Charlotte Buhler (1933) and continued throughout subsequent years. One author who has been particularly influential in this tradition has been Erikson, who rather sketchily set out his ideas on old age with the publication of his book, *Childhood and Society* (1950), and then elaborated and developed them much more fully as an older man himself (see for example, Erikson 1978, Erikson et al 1986).

Within the psychoanalytic tradition, Erikson has been exceptional in his interest in old age. The idea, characteristic of psychoanalytic thinking, that all important developments took place early in life militated against an interest in old age. In addition to this, older people were seen, by psychotherapists, to find it very difficult to change and thus psychoanalysis as a therapy was not considered appropriate for older people. As a consequence, there was only limited case material, which was the main source of data and inspiration for theory development within this tradition. Recently this view has changed and, increasingly, psychotherapy is seen to be useful as a way of working with some older people. This provides an increasingly rich source of data for enhanced understanding of the feelings and fantasies of older people. Particularly influential in this area have been Knight (1992), Levin and Kahana (1967) and Tobin (1972, 1989).

External influences on the experience of old age

Against this backdrop of interest in predictable transitions of old age has been interest in the context of growing old, and in particular on the negative impact of environmental stressors. Although the early work in this context was not linked to health and stress psychology, the parallels of this work and the more general health psychology research on, for example, life events (Holmes & Rahe 1967) are quite clear. Researchers have looked at the impact of relocation (for example, Aldrich & Mendkoff 1968), of social isolation (Lowenthal 1968), of different housing circumstances (Rosow 1968) and of retirement (Carp 1977, Maddox 1968).

One of the flaws of this research, which was also a criticism of much of the life events work, was its failure fully to take account of individual differences and personal meaning. More recently, with the introduction of more sensitive research tools especially designed for elderly people, the criticisms of the early work are being overcome (for a review of these tools see Chiriboga 1989). For example, see the work of Baglioni (1989) on relocation and the elderly, the work of Ferraro (1989) on widowhood in old age and the work of McGoldrick (1989) on early retirement.

Dividing interest in old age into two camps, firstly work which focuses upon internal, predictable, developmental tasks or transitions, and secondly, research which considers external, often unpredictable events, and their impact in old age may be presenting a false dichotomy. It may be far more useful to develop a flexible way of thinking about the psychology of old age which incorporates developmental themes, whilst at the same time accommodating the social reality in which older people live. This must recognise that certain life events are more common during this period and that their impact may be a function of age as well as context.

LIFE SPAN DEVELOPMENTAL PSYCHOLOGY

The influence of Freud

The work of Freud at the beginning of this century revolutionised the way in which personality development is seen to take place. His ideas have not only been influential in the field of psychology but also in related disciplines, such as psychiatry, anthropology and sociology, and also in our culture more generally, for example, in art and literature. In A. N. Wilson's (1991, p. x) excellent biography of C. S. Lewis, he writes: 'Though all Freud's theories about the origins of consciousness may be disavowed, this remains the century of Freud. We have learnt that our lives are profoundly affected by what happens to us when we were very young children, and that wherever we travel in mind or body we are compelled to repeat or work out the drama of early years'. In understanding the life of C. S. Lewis this notion was seen to be particularly relevant.

Freud stressed not only the importance of early life experiences in shaping later ones, but also the importance of fantasy life and unconscious forces in mediating the impact of relationships. Freud's notion that people did not always fully comprehend their own motives, and that rational behaviour could only be understood with reference to conscious and unconscious forces, has continued to have an impact on our understanding of personality developments across the life cycle.

Psychological development and the ageing process

Freud himself was not interested in psychological developments and changes consequent upon the ageing process although some of those influenced by his ideas were. For example, Jung (1972) did place much greater emphasis upon what he referred to as the second half of life, and significant changes that took place during this period. For him, mid-life was a critical turning point, which afforded the individual opportunities for new developments. Greater emphasis was laid upon introspection during the second half of life, and the possibility of a new kind of wisdom that grew from acceptance of life, including its shortcomings as well as its opportunities. He laid much emphasis upon the value of symbolic and religious experiences in creating a state of harmony within personality, and between the individual and the outside world.

More recently, a number of researchers have attempted to look at the diversity of changes that are associated with old age. For example, Peck (1968) maintained that psychological growth during old age is characterised by three main psychological tasks of adjustment:

- ego differentiation versus work-role preoccupation
- body transcendence versus body preoccupation
- ego transcendence versus ego preoccupation.

These areas include social, psychological and biological aspects of growing old.

Ego differentiation versus work-role. This focuses upon the impact of vocational retirement and the difficulties for many older people in securing a strong and stable sense of identity and purpose in the absence of work. For many elderly people this demands a shift in individual value systems. Personal worth must be reappraised and redefined so that the retired person can take satisfaction in activities and relationships beyond those of work. A sense of self-worth derived from activities beyond work is crucial to establishing a continued, vital interest in living instead of a despairing sense of loss of meaning in life.

Body transcendence versus body preoccupation. This second psychological task refers to the increasing incidence of ill-health in later years and the impact this has on psychological wellbeing. For those who equate comfort and pleasure with bodily wellbeing, this decline in health may represent the gravest of insults. Peck suggested that the worst outcome can be seen in those whose lives seem to move in a decreasing spiral because of their continuous and ever increasing interest in, or preoccupation with, the state of their bodies. Many experience a state referred to as 'inner preoccupation' (Neugarten & Gutmann 1958). There are other people who experience declining health yet continue to enjoy life greatly.

Ego transcendence versus ego preoccupation. This final task seems to most closely relate to the develop-

mental hurdle so eloquently described by Erikson (1950) in his work on 'integrity versus despair'. For Peck, one of the greatest challenges of old age is to be able to live life fully in the realisation that not only is death an inevitable end, but also that it is not far away. Despite the proximity of death, Peck argued, it is nonetheless possible to enjoy life and continue to participate fully. He suggested that a constructive lifestyle in the face of death might be defined in the following way: 'To live so generously and unselfishly that the prospect of personal death – the night of the ego, it might be called – looks and feels less important than the secure knowledge that one has built for a broader, longer future than any one ego could encompass' (Peck 1968, cited in Neugarten 1968, p. 91).

The work of Erik Erikson

The work of Erik Erikson, who began outlining his ideas on developments in old age with the publication of the influential book *Childhood and Society* (Erikson 1950), was a further example of the application of psychoanalytic ideas to an understanding of personality development in old age. In this book he described the last developmental crisis of the life cycle, which he named 'ego integrity versus despair', and which defined the crucial elements of adjustment in old age. For Erikson, adjustment in old age was seen in terms of the integration of all aspects of personality, and a capacity to adapt to the triumphs and disappointments of both current circumstances and past life experiences. In further elaborating upon this, Erikson suggested that the capacity to find meaning in life, to make sense of one's life and relationships, is an important part of adjustment. In addition to this, it relates to the capacity to accept that the life that one had, had to be, and to realise that there could be no substitutions. In facing up to these realities, he argued, death loses its sting. As a consequence, a kind of wisdom is thus possible; a wisdom that was unlikely to prevail in earlier years, when a more defensive view of life, denying the reality of death, was likely to be adopted.

An inability to achieve a sense of self integrity, with regard to these crucial issues, is characterised by a pronounced fear of death, and a sense of increasing desperation. The despair expresses the feeling that time is too short, too short to attempt to lead a different kind of life and too short to try alternate routes to achieving a sense of personal integrity. There is a sense of being at the end of life without having lived life fully. The individual is then overwhelmed with a sense of waste, which feels as though it cannot be overcome. Such individuals are likely to have an overwhelming sense of regret, disappointment, shame, guilt or resentment when looking back over their lives. This is the state of affairs referred to in the negative end of the continuum described by Erikson and referred to simply as despair.

Erikson's ideas were only sketchily outlined in *Childhood and Society* (1950, pp. 259–291), yet they continue to be a source of inspiration to many. Coleman (1986) argued that the continuing attraction for the few pages that Erikson wrote on the characteristics of an ideal old age, indicates something of the hunger for a meaningful view of the last part of life, and the lack of more substantial and comprehensible alternatives. Yet, in the 40 years since his account was first written, we have come to realise that the characteristics of integrity that he describes are rarely achieved (Clayton 1975). This comment is not meant to be a criticism of an ideal model, rather a recognition that there was a failure in this early work to fully acknowledge the forces that militate against positive human development. For Coleman (1986), adjustment in old age is not simply coming to terms with eventual physical decline, past life and relationships, and loss of friends and loved ones. It also means coming to terms with discontinuities between the past, the present and the likely future. These challenges are all the greater during times of great social change and upheaval, as many would argue has been and still is characteristic of the 20th century.

Perhaps the emphasis simply upon the last stage of the life cycle, integrity versus despair, fails to do justice to Erikson's contribution to life-span developmental psychology or to a comprehensive understanding of the developmental tasks of old age. His theory is more sophisticated than this implies. He attempted to develop a theory of personality development across the life cycle, in which understanding of developments at one point in the life cycle could only be understood with reference to earlier developments. The negotiation of each task facing the individual at different points in life is affected by the ways in which earlier developmental crises were dealt with. It is not simply a question of resolving or failing to resolve a task, but rather of understanding the ways in which the earlier tasks were experienced and handled, and the impact this has on later development. Indeed, Erikson also argued that the way in which previous generations dealt with crises also affects subsequent generations' capacity to face the challenges of developmental tasks. In this sense, understanding the developmental task of old age, in the context of any individual, can only be

understood with reference to the whole life cycle. To quote Erikson: 'Each individual, to become a mature adult, must to a sufficient degree develop all the ego qualities mentioned, so that a wise Indian, a true gentleman, and a mature peasant share and recognize in one another the final stage of integrity'. And to complete the cycle he continued: 'And it seems possible to further paraphrase the relation of adult integrity and infantile trust by saying that healthy children will not fear life if their elders have integrity enough not to fear death' (Erikson 1950, pp. 260–261).

Towards the end of his own life, Erikson became more and more interested in developments in old age. The elaboration and discussion of these ideas with colleagues, were published in the influential volume, *Vital Involvement in Old Age: the Experience of Old Age in Our Time* (Erikson et al 1986).

Erikson can rightly be considered one of the most important precursors of what has come to be known as life span developmental psychology, a useful context to study the psychology of ageing. Within this framework there is a growing literature (see, for example, Allman & Jaffe 1978, Baltes et al 1980, Datan et al 1987). The influence of these ideas can be seen in popular literature in the USA (Sheehy 1978) and in the UK (Nicholson 1980). The main thrust of all this work is that to understand older people it is important to see them in the context of their whole life history; in particular, to look at ways in which important issues from earlier life were either resolved or inadequately dealt with. This route offers the possibility of considering both contemporary issues in old age and the legacies of earlier developmental phases, including childhood and adolescence.

This approach also takes account of intergenerational effects of life span development. Each generation can set the tone of the prevailing psychological atmosphere, which may affect the experiences of the next generation. This must have been of particular relevance for Erikson's generation because of the profound effects across Europe of the Second World War and the Holocaust.

THE IMPORTANCE OF REMINISCENCE

Published material on the developmental psychology of old age throughout this century has been sparse until the upsurge in interest during the 1970s and 1980s. However, the few seminal papers that served to inspire interest before this time focused on the related issues of reminiscence (looking back on one's life) and self-preoccupation. For example, the work of Charlotte Buhler in the 1930s, focused upon the role of reminiscence as an inevitable part of the ageing process, resulting from the individual's need to substantiate his life in the face of loss of ability. Buhler looked, too, at the increasing interest in writing autobiographical accounts of life among elderly people, in an attempt to locate themselves in their past as well as in current circumstances (Buhler 1933).

More recent interest was inspired by Robert Butler's paper, *The Life Review: an Interpretation of Reminiscence in the Aged* (Butler 1963). In this article, Butler, a psychiatrist, referred to his own clinical work and other literary authorities (although, interestingly, he did not link his ideas to those of Erikson despite some important parallels) in developing his ideas on the value of looking back over one's life in an attempt to achieve positive adjustment in later life. He made a strong case for viewing reminiscence as a normal activity in old 'age. Indeed, he went further and suggested that, for older people, it was an important component of coming to terms with, and accepting their lives. In Erikson's terms, it might be seen as one of the means to achieving a sense of ego integrity.

Coleman (1986) cites Rose Dobrof, in emphasising the extent to which this paper was seen to revolutionise the way in which many professional groups revised the way that they had traditionally thought about reminiscence among elderly people:

In a profound sense, Butler's writings liberated both the old and the nurses, doctors and social workers; the old were free to remember, regret, to look reflectively at the past and try to understand it. And we were free to listen, and to treat rememberers and remembrances with the respect they deserved, instead of trivializing them by diversion to a Bingo game.   (Dobrof 1984 cited by Coleman 1986, p. 10)

At the end of his article, Butler challenged other researchers to subject his ideas to further scrutiny and empirical review. Many rose to this challenge and, as a consequence, there is now a great deal of research evidence which throws light upon the meaning and significance of reminiscence among elderly people. For example, McMahon and Rhudick (1964), in their study of veterans of the Spanish–American war, were impressed not only with how well adjusted they appeared to be, but also by the extent of reminiscing they displayed. This was a study of men only, but it seemed clear to the researchers that the pleasure in story-telling about the past mirrored some of the anthropological material, which stressed the importance of story-telling in giving older people in primitive societies an important role in maintaining tradition and keeping alive the history of the culture. In this sample, the authors found that increased reminiscence was related to better adjustment and

freedom from depression. In addition, they found that the attempts the men made to exaggerate the importance of the past, in the face of current circumstances, placed a constructive role in old age, in the face of losses, in preserving self-respect by investing in the image of oneself as one had been.

Variables influencing the value of reminiscence

In reviewing a number of studies on the value of reminiscence, Coleman (1986) concludes that the findings are equivocal. For example, Lieberman and Falk (1971) explored the value of reminiscence in three samples of older people: those who were living in their own homes, those who were waiting to enter old people's homes, and those who had been living in such institutions for some time. They found that those in the waiting situation were involved in far more reminiscence, but that this was not related to psychological adjustment and wellbeing. Havighurst and Glaser (1972), on the other hand, did identify an associated pattern between high levels of personal adjustment, positive effect of reminiscence and high frequency of reminiscence. In looking at a range of studies, the positive effects of reminiscence have not been clearly and consistently demonstrated (see, for example, Merriam 1980, Merriam & Cross 1982). It is likely that there are many confounding variables that need to be subjected to greater scrutiny, including differences as a function of sex, individual circumstances, and individual differences of resources, personality, and personal history.

Reminiscence therapy

One of the main clinical developments following from this work is that of reminiscence therapy. However, given the equivocal nature of the findings on reminiscence, Coleman (1986, p. 11) concluded, 'Reminiscence therapy therefore cannot be said to stand on a very solid base'. It is important, as Merriam (1980) pointed out, not to talk in a simplistic way about the overall value of reminiscence, but to develop interventions which address the specific needs of individuals or particular groups. In more psychologically vulnerable older individuals, great skill is needed if the past is to be reviewed in a constructive way; indeed the warnings signalled in the early writings of people such as Erikson (1950) and Butler (1963), that reviewing life can be associated with despair and depression, as well as satisfaction, self esteem and wisdom, should be heeded. Approaches to reminiscence as therapy are discussed in detail in Chapter 22.

Functions served by reminiscence

In seeking to understand the functions that reminiscence can serve, the literature provides a wide diversity of views. For Butler, life review is a normative crisis prompted by the realisation of death (a view which owes much to the writings of Erikson). Butler stressed that reminiscence could take many forms such as day-dreaming and dreaming, as well as more clearly conscious and purposive thinking. The striving to find meaning at the end of life, indeed throughout life, has been stressed by writers, in allied disciplines, such as Frankl (1963) and Antonovsky (1979).

It is this striving which seems to underpin much of the writing about the developmental tasks of old age or, more specifically, the work on the life review. For many people this task can bring with it many satisfactions. For others it may bring, as has already been described, regret, self-hatred, guilt, shame and an overwhelming sense of waste, depression and fear. The problems that unhappy memories of the past can bring in old age was highlighted by Somerset Maugham who stated: 'What makes old age hard to bear is not a failing of one's faculties, mental and physical, but the burden of one's memory' (Maugham 1959, p. 70).

Both Erikson and Butler acknowledged the possibility of constructive and pathological outcomes of this process. For these authors the outcome is determined by the individual's capacity to accept one's one and only life and to find some meaning in it. Given the profound nature of the task, the scope for psychotherapy with this age group has traditionally been underestimated, though increasingly its value has been recognised (see, for example, the work of Levin & Kahana 1967, Knight 1992, Castelnuovo-Tedesco 1978, Zinberg & Kaufman 1963).

McMahon & Rhudick's (1964) work stressed the function of reminiscence in terms of the maintenance of self-esteem and self-worth in the face of personal losses. They, too, linked their work to the ideas of Erikson by emphasising that the adaptive functions of reminiscence can best be understood with reference to Erikson's work on the lifelong task of identity formation. For these authors, however, in looking at the value of reminiscence among elderly men, they stressed not simply individual meaning, but also the value felt by the men in terms of their contribution to society, by carrying on tradition through their knowledge of a bygone era.

In their criticism of the work of Butler, especially his emphasis upon the high order functions of accepting one's life and facing death, Lieberman & Tobin (1983) argued, from their research on elderly people moving into homes for the aged, that reminiscence often serves to create a myth or a story that places them as central to the drama. In this way, justification for present circumstances is found and their role given prominence and meaning. It is meant to be believed and represents an attempt to preserve a coherent and consistent sense of self in the face of loss and the threat of loss. Thus, the defensive functions of reminiscence are highlighted. It is important, of course, to bear in mind that the population studied by Lieberman and Tobin was not typical, since the majority of elderly people do not move into homes for the elderly. In addition, they were studied at a time of heightened stress, contingent upon relocation and loss of home, when the need for defensive strategies is likely to be greatly enhanced (see, for example, earlier work on relocation, Tobin & Lieberman 1976, as well as more recent work, Baglioni 1989).

Coleman's (1986) contribution to the study of reminiscence is immense, both in the development of ideas, and in the moving biographical accounts he provides. He ends his book with some advice for those people working with elderly clients:

It is with a sense of individual difference and variation in old age that I would like to close this book. I hope that I have demonstrated that the attitudes to reminiscence displayed by older people are worth close consideration by those in the helping professions. Disturbed memories need to be faced. Care has to be exercised though in judging whether self-accusatory memories are the symptoms of a depression that require challenging, or whether they call out instead for healing and a genuine reconciliation with people from the past. A flight from happy memories also seems to be a sign of the need for therapy, an indication of an incomplete grieving process. Memories for many people will be a treasure, a solace and a source of wonder. What we can do to strengthen bonds between the past and the present, and preserve a sense of continuity for people who are threatened by loss, will be appreciated.   (Coleman 1986, pp. 159–160)

AGEING AND PERSONALITY

Many reviews of the research findings on the relationship between personality and ageing indicate considerable stability in personality with ageing (for example, Woods & Britton 1985, Stuart-Hamilton 1991). However, the use of personality inventories does indicate a shift on the introversion–extroversion dimension towards introversion. This seems to suggest that as people grow older they become more preoccupied with their inner selves, their own thoughts and feelings, and less with the outer world and have less engagement with an active social life. Recent work carried out in the context of health psychology, rather than developmental psychology, suggests that elderly people use proportionately more passive, intrapersonal, emotion-focused forms of coping (such as distancing, acceptance of responsibility and positive reappraisal), as opposed to active, interpersonal, problem-focused forms of coping (such as confronting coping, seeking of social support, planful problem solving) (Folkman et al 1987).

The disengagement hypothesis

In the light of these studies, it is interesting to look back at earlier controversies such as the discussion and debate following the publication of Cumming & Henry's work on the disengagement hypothesis in 1961 (see, for example, Cumming & Henry 1961, Chown 1972, Cumming 1975, Cath 1975). The findings were the result of a major study of elderly people during the 1950s in Kansas, carried out by researchers from the University of Chicago. Their findings suggested that, 'Disengagement is an inevitable process in which many of the relationships between a person and other members of society are severed and those remaining are altered in quality' (Cumming & Henry 1961, p. 211).

Their work led them to conclude that the process of growing old is characterised by an increasing distance between older people and the rest of society. The process is described as one of mutuality, in which older people move away from society, and society moves away from its older members. It was also linked, by implication, to the psychological wellbeing of older people; in other words, it was seen as both a normative and optimal, healthy process.

The disengagement hypothesis – a critical review

Bond et al (1993), in their review of the disengagement hypothesis, cited three main criticisms:

1. The implication that the process of disengagement is desirable for elderly people could be seen as encouraging laissez-faire approaches to the care and support of elderly people in the community. From the point of view of many researchers in the field (for example, Shanas et al 1965) the disengagement hypothesis seemed to condone a policy of indifference towards the problems of older people.

2. Disengagement is simply not an inevitable outcome of growing old. For many people, maintaining social contacts is seen to be a priority; non-engagement in old age is likely to reflect a life-long pattern of social interaction for some people. Furthermore, there was evidence to suggest that those individuals who remained active and socially integrated enjoyed a greater degree of life satisfaction than those who disengaged from social contacts.

3. The data presented in Cumming & Henry's book (1961), *Growing Old*, has been incorrectly interpreted, since disengagement is more likely to be a consequence of cultural values and economic structure than of developmental, psychological processes. These social and economic factors combine to create a climate in which a large proportion of older people are forced to disengage. Thus, to describe the process as one of mutual withdrawal does not do justice to the evidence.

The current status of the original thesis has been considerably undermined by the impact of critical review. In an attempt to overcome some of the difficulties of the Cumming and Henry study, the same data, from Kansas City, were subjected to further analysis, in an attempt to define in more detail patterns of good and poor adjustment in old age. For example, Riechard et al (1962) attempted to do this in terms of attitudes expressed, by focusing upon the men in the study (even though they were in a minority).

From this work five typologies were described: three were seen to reflect positive adjustment in old age and poor adjustment. The three well-adjusted groups were:

- The 'mature', who adopted a flexible and positive approach to life and the changes they were facing in old age.
- The 'rocking-chair' group, who took a less active role in life and who seemed happy to allow themselves to become more dependent on others.
- The 'armoured' group, who strove to maintain high levels of activity and involvement, both at work and in their social lives, and who resisted any degree of dependence on others. This group attempted to continue with all their previous life commitments and resisted any changes contingent upon the restrictions of old age.

The two poorly adjusted groups, were referred to as:

- The 'angry', who tended to respond to changes associated with old age with increasing anger and to blame those around them for their problems. They resented others, especially their wives, they were increasingly unable to gain solace from social networks and experienced a great fear of death.

- The 'self-haters', who, on the other hand, blamed themselves for their misfortunes, and increasingly became locked in a circle of self-hatred, regret and depression. Many welcomed the prospect of death as a way out of an intolerable situation.

A few years later, the data from the Kansas study were subjected to still more analysis, and a more complex typology was developed (Neugarten 1968).

Recent studies of personality development in old age

In recent years, the large-scale, longitudinal studies which have focused upon personality development in old age (see, for example, Thomae 1976, Lehr & Thomae 1987, Schaie 1983) have confirmed the view of a high degree of stability in people's behaviour over time spans of up to 10 years and more. Individuals tend to enjoy the same interests and activities as before, and continue to hold earlier beliefs and values. Differences which are observed are more likely to reflect differences in class, education, social context and health. It may be, too, that large-scale survey methods do not tap the subtleties of changes contingent upon growing old. What may be called for are ethnographic and case study approaches which may highlight some changes obscured by survey methodologies.

COGNITIVE CHANGES IN OLD AGE

Within the study of the psychology of ageing, a great deal of attention has been paid to changes in cognitive functioning. Historically, there was a commonly held view that intellectual functioning and cognitive performance showed a general decline with age. This decline was considered to become increasingly apparent during old age. This view, however, has become increasingly subjected to critical scrutiny, in part because of the methodological shortcomings of much of the early research. The rather crude conception of intellectual decline in old age was associated with negative attitudes towards elderly people, and affected the views that younger people had of the potential contribution of elderly people to society.

Much of the research relied heavily upon the use of standard IQ tests, such as the WAIS (Wechsler Adult Intelligence Scale, 1955); the problem with this approach was that it was unlikely to assess the particular strengths of older people, such as accrued wisdom and knowledge, born of extensive life experience. In many situations, elderly people may make better judgements,

as a consequence of their experience, or may be able to bring wisdom to bear upon difficult issues such as moral and ethical dilemmas, theoretical issues and social and political controversies.

Wisdom and experience may also feed the minds of great writers or artists, facilitating creativity and productiveness. There are many famous examples of the contribution of elderly people in these spheres: the later work of Albert Einstein in science; the later work of Freud, Jung and Erikson in psychology; the novels of Mary Wesley (for example, 1988, 1992), all written after the age of 70; and many others. In reviewing the research findings on the effects of ageing on cognitive functioning, it is important to consider the different approaches to gathering data and the methodological shortcomings associated with them.

Methodological issues and cognitive change

Much of the work on cognitive functioning in old age was conducted in experimental conditions, in the laboratory rather than in real life situations, although increasingly there have been calls for observational studies of performance in naturally occurring life situations (see, for example, Neisser 1982). The main approaches to studying changes in intellectual functioning with age have been cross-sectional studies, longitudinal studies and sequential designs.

Cross-sectional studies

In cross-sectional studies, individuals of different ages are compared at one point in time. For example, data on cognitive functioning may be gained from individuals aged say, 20, 40, 60 and 80 years, and the results compared. As far as possible, the groups involved are matched on the obvious socioeconomic, demographic or other important non-experimental variables. Conclusions are then drawn from comparisons of each age group's results. The obvious advantage of this approach is that it is less time-consuming and thus cheaper to carry out than longitudinal studies; however, there are also problems. Cultural effects can be very strong and evident between different cohorts and they can confound the results. However well matched groups are, it is not possible to have a group of 20-year-olds who will have had comparable early life experiences to the 60-year-old cohort. This point is eloquently put by Rabbitt, speaking from the context of his research on cognitive functioning among the elderly:

People now aged eighty are time travellers, exiled to a foreign country which they now share with current twenty year olds. These groups have been fed, housed, and educated very differently, have received, or failed to receive, different medical treatment for different conditions, have been taught to prize different skills and attitudes, and have been shaped by dramatically different experiences.

(Rabbitt 1984a, p. 14)

Longitudinal studies

In cross-sectional studies, it is not possible to separate the effects of culture, age and cohort differences. One attempt to overcome these problems is by carrying out a longitudinal study of cognitive changes and ageing in one group over time. This involves following a group of individuals over a series of assessments over a long period of time, in an attempt to assess changes. In this way, age-related changes in an individual or an age group can be measured. To follow groups of individuals over many years clearly takes many resources, and in the current climate of research funding such studies may be seen to be too expensive. There are a number of additional problems, such as the inevitability that some subjects are not available or are unwilling to be reassessed; the problems of practice effects, that is, that some changes with age may be obscured by increasing familiarity with the tasks; and, finally, that other, extraneous factors, may influence results on any one occasion. These include factors such as the context of testing and changes in motivation, health and interest of the subject.

Sequential designs

The problems of the research strategies outlined led to serious consideration of alternative approaches and new methodologies, notably by Schaie (1967) and Baltes (1968), who produced designs aimed at distinguishing between age effects, cohort effects and time of measurement effects. These researchers carried out cross-sectional studies at different points in time (see, for example, Schaie & Labouvie-Vief 1974). Although there are methodological problems associated with this approach too, this research pointed out the dangers of simply assuming cognitive decline with old age. Indeed, they found that for most of the life cycle, cohort effects can be as large as effects that are a function of age differences.

Cognitive changes – reviewing the evidence

In reviewing the evidence on cognitive changes across the life cycle, the research evidence is equivocal,

reporting inconsistent findings. Eisdorfer & Wilkie (1973) assessed subjects initially aged 60–69 on four occasions over 10 years. They found no substantial overall decline, but a decrement in performance ability (measured on the WAIS). Blum et al (1972) carried out a 20-year follow-up on these same subjects, and reported that an overall decline was evident. Savage et al (1973), on the other hand, actually found an increase in performance ability in their sample (mean age 71 years), who were assessed four times in 7 years. The sequential studies of Schaie and his colleagues (1990) suggest that age-related decline is minimal, until the age of 75. Verbal abilities show decline later that speeded decline in performance tasks.

The extent of age-related decline in cognitive functioning in old age does not appear to be dramatic enough to affect the adaptive capacities of most elderly people, and is more likely to affect the very old (over the age of 75 years), rather than the younger old (60–75 years). In the most recent account of his research, Schaie (1990) emphasised that there is no uniform pattern of age-related changes across all intellectual abilities. After the age of 75, a number of measures do appear to indicate specific age-related changes. However, many individuals in his study did not show any evidence of decline, even after the age of 80. In the UK, Rabbitt (1984b) found from his own cross-sectional study, that 10–15% of people in their 8th decade performed on fluid intelligence tests at the same level as the best of those 20 years younger. Further research is needed to identify what underlies maintained good functioning of this order in old age.

Factors influencing intellectual functioning in old age

Psychologists have demonstrated that intellectual functioning in old age can be improved with specific interventions (see, for example, Baltes & Barton 1977, Patterson & Jackson 1980). A number of factors, too, have been associated with poor performance on tests of intellectual functioning including; tiredness (Furry & Baltes 1973), cautiousness (Birkhill & Schaie 1975), and the effects of elderly people worrying about their performance or viewing their own abilities in a negative way. Intellectual ability is not a fixed attribute, as was once thought, but a more dynamic concept. The term 'plasticity' was introduced by Baltes & Willis (1979), who emphasised that mental ability is best viewed as a growing and developing function. Indeed, Labouvie-Vief et al (1974) went as far as stating that the intellectual deficits sometimes observed among elderly subjects reflect only the lack of practice on the kind of tasks under scrutiny. Used to support this view are the intervention studies which showed that elderly people improve their performance on intelligence tests with practice.

Cognitive function and physical and mental health

A number of studies have attempted to consider the relationship between age, health, adjustment, and cognitive functioning. For example, Savage et al (1973) found that a group of elderly people who were free from physical and mental health problems and free from adjustment and social difficulties, had higher scores on tests of cognitive functioning than others who were not free. In addition, they were found to have high levels of involvement in activities within and outside their homes and they also survived longer than would have been expected.

In the over 75s, it is likely that increasing evidence of cognitive decline can be accounted for by disease processes. However, the more general relationship between health and mental functioning in later life is less widely understood (Coleman 1983). For example, many studies of cognitive functioning in older people still neglect adequately to control for the health status of their subjects, and are therefore less likely to make accurate estimates of the influence of factors, other than disease, on cognitive functioning. Bond et al (1993) suggested that the neglect of this topic is particularly surprising given that it is already 30 years since a major study, carried out by the National Institute of Mental Health in the USA (Birren et al 1963), showed that the presence of even a mild degree of chronic disease has a noticeable effect on a wide variety of mental functions in old age.

More recently, Holland & Rabbitt (1991) reviewed relevant literature, including an analysis of their own research on the effects of diabetes on cognitive performance. This is research with clear practical implications, since it is apparent from their findings that not only are there cognitive decrements associated with poorly controlled non-insulin-dependent diabetes, but also that these cognitive impairments may themselves make adherence to medical regimens less likely. To quote Coleman (1993): 'Studies that neglect the health status of their subjects thus tend to overestimate the influence of chronological age on cognitive functioning. Effects which appear age-related may in reality be health-related' (cited in Bond at al 1993, p. 71).

Intellectual performance and survival

Another area of interest has been the relationship between intellectual change and survival. In a review of research findings, Siegler (1980) noted that most longitudinal studies indicate that higher levels of intellectual performance, at the beginning of the study, are related to survival. A further tentative finding (see, for example, Savage et al 1973) is that there is a clear decline in cognitive functioning in the 2 or 3 years before death. However, the extent to which this is simply related to underlying disease processes, rather than cognitive changes associated with decline at the very end of life, is unclear. As Siegler concluded in her review, 'any large change in the cognitive capacity of an older person should be treated with suspicion – it may be a terminal sign, or it may indicate a potentially treatable illness' (Siegler 1980, cited in Bond et al 1993, p. 7).

Conclusion

In conclusion, it is important to recognise that the previously held tenet that there is inevitable cognitive decline with old age is no longer an accurate way to consider changes in intellectual functioning among older people. There are enormous methodological problems in gathering data in this area, and thus the results of early studies must be considered in the light of their research design shortcomings. Most studies emphasise the significant individual differences in the patterns of change with age. A number of factors influence cognitive performance and they may be more pertinent to older people than younger ones; for example, lack of familiarity with the kind of tests often used, lack of belief in one's intellectual abilities, the capacity to feel overwhelmed by the tester or the test situation. Schaie & Willis (1986) argued that unless tasks are framed in a way that places them in an appropriate context, elderly people will perform badly, feeling unable or unwilling to use their resources effectively and constructively. In addition to motivational and situational variables, the impact of health-related factors (both mental and physical health) must be taken into account when considering the results of testing.

The most pervasive cognitive change with ageing is the slowing of response that occurs in all tasks when speed of response is a factor (Botwinick 1984, Salthouse 1985). While reaction times can be speeded up in older adults with practice, with exercise and other interventions, the age difference is seldom completely eliminated. Furthermore, there is evidence to suggest that in tasks where attention is divided between two elements, elderly people fare less well than younger people. What appears to particularly disturb older people is information competing for their attention when they are concentrating on a specific task (Stuart-Hamilton 1991). Experiments carried out by Rabbitt (1985) led him to conclude that older people find it difficult to ignore irrelevant information.

In a thorough review of the literature, Salthouse (1985) argued that the probable locus of slowing down on speed-related tasks, is in the central nervous system. The types of task, however, most associated with adult intelligence, such as the general fund of information, vocabulary and arithmetic skills, show little change as a result of the ageing process, until the age of about 75 (Schaie 1983). Changes after the age of 75 are largely unstudied, but it is hard to disentangle the effects of changes due to underlying disease processes, such as Alzheimer's disease or other dementing illnesses in the early stages.

On a positive note, Rybash et al (1986) suggested that in some areas of cognitive functioning, elderly people are likely to outperform young people. With the accumulation of experience, older adults have a considerable store of knowledge about how things are and how things work, especially in their individual areas of expertise, either in the family context or the work environment. It is in these areas, where older people can draw on their wealth of knowledge and experience, that they are likely to excel. The kinds of things to which older people have been exposed in the course of their life may have been many and varied, and their lives have often been far less constrained than those of many young people.

In considering his psychotherapeutic work with elderly clients, Knight (1992) argued that this background of a lifetime of experiences in relationships and other areas means that often the older client has more to draw upon than the therapist. Knight suggests that, 'These experiences have led to the distillation of concepts about how life and relationships work, a kind of psychological "expert system"'(Knight 1992, p. xv).

Many studies have stressed the strengths that remain in elderly people's memory and mental functioning. Simple measures of learning show little or no decline in old age (Savage et al 1973). Many psychologists now argue that some of the differences observed between older and younger people's performance on tests of cognitive functioning reflect differences in approaching the tasks rather than differences in abilities. Those studies that report positively on the performance of older people, in comparison with younger people, emphasise the superiority of older people in dealing with personal and meaningful information. Older people can remember the gist of a story that they have been reading better than younger people, perhaps because of the meaningfulness of the story, or because they were better able to focus on the essentials of the story in their process of recall (Labouvie-Vief & Blanchard-Fields 1982).

In viewing the cognitive abilities of older people in a positive light, it is important not to gloss over individual differences. The message from the literature is that there are enormous individual differences in all age groups and that, overall, cohort differences are greater than differences that are a function of age. Among older people, there are those whose mental abilities show no evidence of decline until at least the age of 75, and there are those whose experience and wisdom mean that they have much to offer our society. However, there are also those whose cognitive abilities have been negatively affected by decline in physical and mental health status.

Memory changes and ageing

In reviewing the literature on memory changes and ageing, there is now general agreement that the differences between young and old people are not great, when the material is meaningful and relevant to the older adult, and the older adult is motivated to learn (Botwinick 1984, Craik & Trehub 1982, Light 1990, Poon 1985). Although it is a commonly held assumption that elderly people's memory for distant events is better than for more recent ones, there is no experimental evidence to support this generalisation. The literature on the subject of long-term and short-term memory indicates that older people's memories of past events, as well as of more recent ones, are remarkably accurate (Botwinick & Storandt 1980, Field & Honzik 1981).

STRESS, SOCIAL SUPPORT AND AGEING

Most of the work discussed so far has been carried out within the traditions of developmental and cognitive psychology. There is, however, increasing interest in the lives of older people within the newer discipline of health psychology. Markides and Cooper (1989, p. 2) noted that, 'it is only recently that the concept of stress has become part of the gerontological vocabulary'. This is due, in part at least, to the growing interest among researchers in the systematic study of the health of elderly people (see, for example, Ward & Tobin 1987).

Many of the epidemiological studies have focused

on predictors of mortality in older people (see, for example, Blazer 1982, Seeman et al 1987). In addition to the epidemiological studies, research in this area has focused not simply upon the social context of ageing, with its emphasis upon stressful life events commonly associated with ageing in our society, such as bereavement, retirement, loss of social status and economic and political power, but upon the inter-relationship between these variables and the health status of elderly people.

Together with the pivotal role that the concept of stress plays in health psychology, the related concept of social support is increasingly receiving much attention. Indeed, Markides and Cooper (1989, p. 5) stated that, 'the concept of "social support" is rapidly approaching the status of the concept of stress in social and behavioural research of health and illness'. As with the concept of stress, definitions of social support abound, and often leave the researcher with a sense of vagueness and confusion about precise meaning. Most definitions focus on the benefits of supportive social relationships and interactions in moderating the negative impact of stressful events and conditions. For example, Antonucci (1985) emphasised the way in which social interactions enable individuals to meet their goals and deal with the demands and challenges of their environment.

During the 1970s, a number of studies documented the positive effects on people's mental and physical health of supportive social relationships. These studies used a variety of measures of health and wellbeing and were undertaken in a number of different settings. More recently, studies have sought to demonstrate that not only do social relationships have a beneficial impact on health, but that their effect is also linked to mortality rates among older people (Blazer 1982, Seeman et al 1987). However, it has been suggested that social factors are likely to be less predictive of the health and mortality of older people than of middle-aged people, because of other, selective survival factors, which are also likely to be operating (Markides & Machalek 1984).

The relationship between stress and the moderating influences of social support in understanding the mental and physical health of older people is likely to be highly complex rather than direct. The majority of research studies in this area have focused on the indirect influences of social support in interactions with stress in understanding the ways that it influences the health status of older people. These studies will be considered in the context of the work on the transition to widowhood, the impact of retirement and relocation on health, and in understanding the social and psychological determinants of depression among elderly people.

Widowhood and health

In the early work on bereavement as a stressful life event (see, for example, Holmes & Rahe 1967), it was considered to be the most significant event in a person's life, and rated as such. Its negative impact was emphasised in most of the literature. There is little doubt that it is indeed a major life event for most elderly people, especially women, but gerontologists are increasingly beginning to conceptualise widowhood as a life transition that has implications far beyond the event of the death of one's spouse. In seeking to understand the relationship between widowhood and mortality rates, Ferraro (1989, p. 74) asked: 'Can the stress of losing a spouse be so severe that it can kill the survivor?'

Mortality

In seeking to answer this question, some interesting patterns have emerged. Widowhood does not appear to be associated with increased mortality among older women, because it is likely that they are psychologically prepared for the event. In seeking to understand male–female differences in mortality rates, it is likely that widowhood is a normative transition for women, but not for men, and in this sense the impact is likely to be much greater on men (Pearlin et al 1981). Ferraro (1989) argued that what appear to be gender differences may in fact be differences in social support. Older women, as younger women, tend to have far more extensive and elaborate networks of social support, which operate as a buffer against the negative impact on health of widowhood. Men appear to enjoy the advantages of close friendships and social support to a lesser extent, and thus the negative consequences of the stress associated with widowhood have a greater impact since there are fewer moderating factors. In addition to this, men are socialised to express their feelings to a lesser extent than women, and this may also place men at a disadvantage when considering the negative repercussions of widowhood. In the words of Ferraro (1989, p. 79): 'Expressivity as a cultural norm may predispose women to do more active grief-work and thereby avoid some of widowhood's deleterious effects'. If men are not socialised to express their sadness and loneliness, and find it difficult to use social support, then it is likely that these factors combine to explain the higher mortality risk for men, especially for suicide (Bock & Webber 1972).

Morbidity

The relationship between widowhood and morbidity rates is also interesting. Declines in health status have been observed in many studies but often only in the short term. Long-term effects are either non-existent or modest. Again, gender differences have been observed, with men at greater risk of ill-health. Age of widowhood and socioeconomic status also influence the negative impact of widowhood on health among elderly people.

Socioeconomic status and age as factors

With regard to socioeconomic status the findings are unequivocal; the higher up the socioeconomic ladder you go, the clearer are the advantages in coping with widowhood and other life stresses. They enjoy better health, larger social networks of support, and more coping resources. Ferraro therefore argued for interventions to focus largely on those lower down the socioeconomic scale.

With regard to age, the findings are less clear. Some argue that for older adults the stress of widowhood is likely to be greater, because of reduced physiologic ability (Eisdorfer & Wilkie 1977). However, Ferraro (1989) argued that there are likely to be countervailing forces which make widowhood harder to bear among younger adults. The intensity of physiological reactions observed among younger adults following bereavement has to be considered, and may serve to make the event harder to accommodate. In addition, the desperation among many younger adults for a relationship and for remarriage is much greater than among older adults. This may be because older adults have anticipated some degree of social disorganisation and isolation and, as a consequence, are less likely to desire remarriage.

Perhaps an important message from much of this work is that older adults may be more resilient than is popularly portrayed. Widowhood is an intense struggle for most people, but older adults seem no less able to deal with this challenge than younger adults, especially if they are able to draw upon resources known to facilitate the grieving process, such as the capacity to express sadness and to find help and solace in human contact and friendship.

Retirement, social support and health

Much of the early work on retirement emphasised the negative aspects (see, for example, Maddox 1968, Crawford 1972). However, increasingly researchers are struck by the positive effects experienced by many older people (Markides & Cooper 1989). Indeed, there is little strong evidence that retirement has negative health outcomes, and it is likely that this is related to the fact that it is now an expected and normal transition.

Research has also looked at the impact on health status of early retirement (McGoldrick 1989), and has concluded that, as long as retirement was not on health grounds and as long as there is adequate financial support, retirement is likely to have a beneficial impact on health. There are a number of variables which need to be taken into account when considering the relationship between retirement and health status; the most significant ones seem to be:

- whether retirement is financially viable (many older people live in dread of sudden economic inflation)
- the extent to which the older person can adjust to the changes in life style, in particular increased leisure time
- whether retirement was felt to be voluntary or involuntary
- the extent to which the older person is able to enjoy a network of social support.

Individual personality differences are likely to play a major role, though there is little emphasis in the research on this aspect. Coping with stress is determined by the way in which the stressful events, and personal resources to deal with them, are viewed. Older people's beliefs about how well equipped they feel they are to deal with the demands of change in old age, as well as their views on how much support they can call upon, are also likely to exert an important influence on their capacity to deal with change and adjusting positively to it. The sort of personality factors that have been considered include high levels of self-efficacy (Bandura 1977), internal locus of control (Rotter 1966), a belief in personal ability to face change and master new situations, and positive expectations about life's possibilities after retirement. To conclude with the words of McGoldrick:

Assessment of existing evidence would suggest that we cannot directly associate retirement with either physical or mental health decline. ... Early retirement can represent a strategic response to stresses experienced in later working years and increasing difficulties in coping with modern industrial environment. Nonetheless, not all individuals view retirement positively and for the minority adaptation problems may be severe, especially in respect of financial problems and health decline.   (McGoldrick 1989, p. 112)

Residential relocation and health

An important stressful event that has received much attention is that of relocation, especially when the relocation is from home to a long-term care setting (Lieberman & Tobin 1983). The extent to which relocation among elderly people is associated with increased morbidity and mortality rates has been the subject of much critical review (Baglioni 1989). The methodological shortcomings of much of the research is considered at length by Baglioni, as are the inherent problems in designing research which is able to disentangle the effects of of relocation from other factors.

The literature on the special case of relocation to an institutional setting, however, has portrayed a more unrelentingly negative picture. The transition from living in a community setting to a long-term care setting has been conceptualised as a life transition, which takes place over a period of time (Tobin 1989). Before the move takes place there is the anticipatory stage, when the individual has to deal with feelings of abandonment and a redefinition of one's self. Following admission, the first month is seen to be particularly stressful. During this period many residents deteriorate rapidly, others become severely depressed, others become disorientated, and others exhibit bizarre behaviours.

The culmination of many years' research (Lieberman & Tobin 1983, Tobin 1989) led Tobin to conclude that relocation to an institutional setting is a highly stressful event, and is linked to both increased mortality and increased morbidity. However, this finding must be tempered by the recognition that there are large individual differences in response to relocation. Much attention has therefore focused upon attempts to ascertain what responses are linked with positive adjustment to living in an institution when old. Tobin describes two categories of predictors: characteristics of the individual and characteristics of the institution.

The characteristics of individuals that were associated with positive adjustment to relocation to an institutional setting, after the initial settling-in period of about 1 month, were:

- maintaining a sense of self
- maintaining hope
- developing coping strategies, including 'magical mastery' of the situation (such as transforming the situation into one which is more palatable by perceiving the relocation as voluntary and ideal)
- being active in response to the move rather than passive
- showing some degree of healthy aggressiveness.

Of these, magical coping and aggressiveness appeared to be the most critical characteristics. These factors have clear implications for care in institutional settings and for the fostering of positive styles of adjustment, which include tolerating some degree of aggressiveness (for example, complaining and griping), instilling hope and encouraging active participation.

The environmental predictors listed by Tobin were:

- fostering achievement among the residents
- encouraging individuation among the residents
- fostering some degree of dependency
- the showing of warmth and humanity to residents by the staff
- the extent to which the institution fosters social interaction among the residents
- the extent to which the environment recognises and rewards achievements
- providing a stimulating environment in terms of sights, sounds and activity
- providing an environment which is physically attractive
- providing an environment which is rich in cues for perceptual orientation (such as signs)
- providing an environment which tolerates some deviance, such as wandering, complaining and drinking alcohol
- the extent to which the environment provides good health care, in the form of physical examinations, nursing care, drugs and the handling of medical emergencies.

In considering the predictive values of personal, compared to environmental, factors, the consensus of opinion is that environmental factors are more significant. Linn et al (1977) found that the most important predictor was the quality of nursing care. In the words of Tobin (1989, pp. 149–150), 'simply stated, negative environmental conditions could not be compensated for by aggressiveness and magical coping'.

Mental and physical health problems as stressors in old age

Problems of mental and physical health have been considered by researchers as significant sources of stress for elderly people. For example, being diagnosed as suffering with a major disease can be immensely stressful and lead to further deterioration in health. However, some researchers (Vernon & Jackson 1989) have demonstrated that older people often fare better in the face of life-threatening illnesses, such as breast cancer, than do younger people. The most likely explanation for this is that the diagnosis of a life-threatening illness in old age is more expected than in younger years.

A vast amount of research has focused upon the negative consequences for mental health and psychological functioning of stressful life events (see, for example, Cohen 1987). Much of the work has looked specifically at the relationship between depression among elderly people and stressful life events. The studies reveal a fairly high degree of consistency in their findings, that stress is associated with the onset of depression, and the effect is more significant in the case of chronic stress (such as chronic illness or long term financial deprivation) than in the case of sudden, stressful life events. As with younger people, the presence of support social networks acts as a buffer moderating the impact of stress among elderly people. Although there is a high degree of depressive symptoms reported, there is no evidence to suggest that elderly people are more prone than younger people to a full depressive illness.

In reviewing the literature on stress, support and depression and the extent to which these variables differ as a function of age, George (1989) concluded that the findings are somewhat fragmentary. Overall, major patterns seem to apply to both younger and older adults. The main differences are likely to be due to the interaction between age and stress and support, and few studies appear to have focused upon these interactional effects. The main differences that are likely to be a function of age relate to the normativeness of certain experiences and their perceived age-specific prevalence. For example, certain experiences are simply expected to occur among older people, such as increases in ill-health and widowhood, and this may temper their impact. This area of research, like attempting to understand differences in cognitive functioning across the life cycle, is fraught with methodological difficulties, and demands sophisticated approaches to research design.

CONCLUSION

In considering the psychosocial aspects of ageing, a number of themes emerge. Although it is important to look for trends for developing theory, it is important to recognise the significance of individual differences. Any approach to understanding old age which glosses over individual differences, in either cognitive functioning or dealing with the emotional and social challenges of old age, cannot do justice to the phenomena. Bond et al (1993, p. 338) concluded that: 'One of the major achievements of modern studies of

ageing has been to demonstrate that most of the decline in psychological functioning with age is not an inevitable product of age'.

These authors, like many others in the field, noted that one of the major failures of much of the early research was to underestimate the significance of the enormous differences in the way people age. These differences were often lost in studies that used measures of average tendencies. For example, with regard to changes in cognitive functioning, much of the research now points to the stability of cognitive performance rather than decline (see, for example, Rowe & Kahn 1987).

Furthermore, studies which focus upon means of promoting positive adjustment in later life have demonstrated ways in which increased autonomy (control) and social support, which enhances a sense of social connectedness, demonstrate a positive effect on both subjective measures of wellbeing, and physiological indicators. Indeed, Bond et al (1993) went one step further in postulating that much of the emotional disturbance and health deterioration observed in elderly people is due to the failure of modern society to satisfy their needs for autonomy and social relationships.

Although the social context in which elderly people grow old plays an important role in determining adjustment, it cannot provide the key to understanding the whole picture. Many older people become locked in unsatisfactory relationships, or become unable to free themselves from a pervasive sense of regret, fear or disappointment with their past life or current conditions. Loss of any sense of control or the ability to protest, or overwhelming despair and helplessness, can lead to decline in old age, which can be assessed in terms of both psychological and physiological markers. Increasingly, elderly people are seen to have a right to have access to psychotherapy (Levin & Kahana 1967, Knight 1992), counselling services and a range of occupational and art therapies, when they become depressed or demoralised.

Furthermore, the correlates of positive adjustment to living healthy lives in institutions are being recognised. For example, the pivotal role of high quality nursing care in institutions is seen to be important. Lieberman & Tobin (1983) also emphasised the importance of recognising the wide range of coping strategies adopted by older people, including 'magical coping', and aggressive and irritable responses to loss of freedom and autonomy associated with moving to an institution. When difficult realities have to be coped with, the research reveals that no strategy is seen to be effective for all older people. Some may need to adopt a highly 'mythical' view of their own life history, others prefer not to think about their past and engage instead in current interests, others still want to look honestly at their past in an active attempt to make sense of their lives and integrate past and present themes. This final approach was the one stressed in the early literature on effective coping when faced with the crisis of old age (see, for example, Erikson 1950, Butler 1963). However, many researchers now agree that this is simply one style that has to compete with many other, equally effective, styles of living in old age (see, for example, Coleman 1986).

The literature derived from health psychology and stress, too, reveals that older people are far more resourceful than they have been traditionally given credit for. Studies on the responses of older people to bereavement revealed, in many instances, that they are more able to deal with loss than many young people. An important caveat to this is the significant gender difference revealed in many of the studies (Stroebe & Stroebe 1983, Bock & Webber 1972). Men tend to cope less well in old age with loss because they have traditionally developed fewer social contacts and have less social support at the time of loss. In addition to this, their lifelong difficulty in expressing their emotions, in particular their grief and sadness, may make the work of mourning all the more difficult for them.

With regard to the development of major theoretical models of psychological ageing there is also a hope expressed in the literature (Bond et al 1993), that the rather narrow research, looking largely at the parameters of successful ageing (such as that outlined in Erikson 1950, Cumming & Henry 1961) will be replaced by more creative ways of thinking about the elderly. Issues like finding meaning and making sense of life, current circumstances and relationships, as well as the appreciation of the characteristic achievements of a long life (such as increased wisdom), will play a more important role in future research (Reker & Wong 1988).

There are many forces which constrain older people from living healthy and fulfilled lives. For example, public attitudes to the capacities of older people are often inaccurate and circumscribe, in an unnecessarily narrow way, what is possible. Waldman and Avolio (1983) reviewed more than a dozen studies of adult performance in the workplace and found very little evidence for any deterioration in abilities. On the contrary, many measures revealed improvements with age, especially for those working in professional jobs. However, contrary to this finding, many people believe that professional abilities deteriorate markedly with

age. This prejudice is likely to reduce the possibilities for effective working for many older people.

Most researchers in the field emphasise the need to consider emotional, cognitive, behavioural and social components of growing old, in order to do justice to the psychosocial components of adjustment and development in later years. In addition to this, there is increasing stress upon the heterogeneity of the experiences of elderly people. In the words of Coleman: 'Human beings are not born all the same, and the varying circumstances of life make them increasingly diverse as they age. By the time they are old differences are therefore maximized' (Coleman 1986, p. 152).

The challenge for researchers and practitioners is to understand common themes in the literature, whilst at the same time embracing individual differences. For example, with regard to the value of reminiscence among elderly people, the questions that used to be asked, such as, 'does reminiscence promote adjustment in later life?' are now seen as naïve. What needs to be done is to consider more specific questions, such as, 'under what conditions is reminiscence conducive to adjustment in later life?' Or, focusing upon individual differences of personality, 'what kind of people appear to find reminiscence particularly beneficial, and what kind of people appear to find it unhelpful?' Indeed, Coleman (1986) went one step further, and suggested that if we study the use of memory among older people, this may throw light upon understanding the structure of personality, and personality changes in old age, since the use of memory may reveal fundamental aspects of a person's way of thinking about themselves and their lives.

Current research also emphasises stability in personality over the life cycle, rather than thinking of old age as a time when character and cognitive functioning change rapidly. In the words of Wood and Britton (1985, p. 47): 'Current models of personality assessment suggest that there are no dramatic changes in personality in the elderly. At most there is an increase in introversion and a degree of social withdrawal. Variability between individuals is likely to increase, however.' They go on to suggest that, although for some elderly people there are problems of adjustment to the changes and challenges contingent upon growing old, the majority of elderly people are well adjusted in old age; furthermore, there is a minority of 'supernormal' elderly people, who appear to fare very well in later years, appear happier than at other periods of their lives and cope with life challenges in a more resourceful way than many younger people. For example, although elderly people suffer multiple losses there is no evidence to suggest that, as a group, they cope less well with them than other age groups. However, when elderly people are faced with increasing disability, access to social support and family support are clearly very important. Although loneliness is not a problem for most elderly people, isolation is a real problem for a minority of people in old age.

What emerges from the growing literature on psychosocial aspects of old age is a sense of increasing diversity in approaches, stressing the need to look at current circumstances and to recognise the powerful influence of personal history. There is a need to consider material gained from a variety of sources, for example from psychotherapists working with elderly people (Knight 1992), from ethnographic studies that emphasise subjective accounts of older people, from the use of psychological tests and personality inven-

tories, and from large-scale cross-sectional surveys and longitudinal studies that follow cohorts of subjects over many years.

The coming together of researchers in the field of health psychology and developmental psychology is likely to result in a fruitful collaboration, reviewing and revising theoretical perspectives on old age, coping, adjustment and health. Overall, the picture portrayed in the proliferation of material now available on this subject reveals an increasingly diverse view of older people, with much greater emphasis on positive aspects of growing old. This does not represent an increasingly sentimental view of old age and the processes inherent in growing old; rather, an honest portrayal of the diversity of experience, acknowledging the pains and challenges, which can be present at all points in the life cycle, as well as the adaptive capacities of older people to deal with them.

REFERENCES

Aldrich C K, Mendkoff E 1968 Relocation of the aged and disabled: a mortality study. In: Neugarten B L (ed) Middle age and aging. University of Chicago Press, Chicago

Allman L R, Jaffe D T (eds) 1978 Readings in adult psychology: contemporary perspectives. Harper & Row, New York

Antonovsky A 1979 Health, stress and coping. Josse Bass, San Francisco

Antonucci T 1985 Personal characteristics, social support, and social behavior. In: Binstock R H, Shanas E (eds) Handbook of aging and social sciences. Van Nostrand Reinhold, New York

Baglioni A S 1989 Residential relocation and health of the elderly. In: Markides K S, Cooper C L (eds) Aging, stress and health. John Wiley & Sons, Chichester

Baltes P B 1968 Longitudinal and cross-sectional sequences in the study of age and generational effects. Human Development 11: 145–171

Baltes M M, Barton C M 1977 New approaches to ageing: a case for the operant model. Educational Gerontology 2: 383–405

Baltes P B, Willis S L 1979 The critical importance of appropriate methodology in the study of ageing: the sample case of psychometric intelligence. In: Hoffmeister F, Muller C (eds) Brain function in old age. Springer-Verlag, Berlin

Baltes P B, Reese H W, Lipsitt L P 1980 Life-span developmental psychology. Annual Review of Psychology 31: 65–110

Bandura A 1977 Self-efficacy: towards a unifying theory of behavioral change. Psychological Review 84: 191–215

Birkhill W R, Schaie K W 1975 The effects of differential reinforcement of cautiousness in intellectual performance among the elderly. Journal of Gerontology 30: 578–583

Birren J E, Butler R N, Greenhouse S W, Sokoloff L, Yarrow M R (eds) 1963 Human aging: a biological and behavioral study. Publication No. (HSM) 71-9051. US Government Printing Office, Washington, DC

Blazer D G 1982 Social support and mortality in an elderly population. American Journal of Epidemiology 115: 684–694

Blum J E , Fosshage J L, Jarvik L F 1972 Intellectual changes and sex differences in octogenarians: a twenty-year longitudinal study of ageing. Developmental Psychology 7: 178–187

Bock E W, Webber I L 1972 Suicide among the elderly: isolating widowhood and mitigating alternatives. Journal of Marriage and the Family 34: 24–31

Bond J, Coleman P, Peace S (eds) 1993 Ageing in society, 2nd edn. Sage, London

Bornstein R, Smircana M T 1982 The status of empirical support for the hypothesis of increased variability in aging populations. The Gerontologist 22: 258–260

Botwinick J 1984 Aging and behavior: a comprehensive integration of research findings, 2nd edn. Springer, New York

Botwinick J, Storandt M 1980 Recall and recognition of old information in relation to age and sex. Journal of Gerontology 35: 70–76

Buhler C 1933 Der menschliche lebenslauf als psychologisches problem, 2nd edn. 1959 Verlag fur psychologie, Gottingen

Butler R N 1963 The life review: an interpretation of reminiscence in the aged. Psychiatry 26: 65–76

Carp F M 1977 Retirement and physical health. In: Kasl S F, Reichman F (eds) Advances in psychosomatic medicine, vol. 9: epidemiologic studies in psychosomatic medicine. S Karger, Basle

Castelnuovo-Tedesco P 1978 The mind as a stage: some comments on reminiscence and internal objects. International Journal of Psychoanalysis 59: 19–25

Cath S H 1975 The orchestration of disengagement. International Journal of Aging and Human Development 6(3): 199–213

Chiriboga D A 1989 The management of stress exposure in later life. In: Markides K S, Cooper C L (eds) Aging, stress and health. John Wiley, Chichester

Chown S (ed) 1972 Ageing. Penguin, London

Clayton V 1975 Erikson's theory of human development as it applies to the aged: wisdom as contradictive cognition. Human Development 18: 119–128

Cohen G 1987 Social change and the life course. Tavistock, London

Coleman P G 1983 Cognitive functioning and health. In: Birren J E, Munnichs J M A, Thomae H, Marois M (eds) Ageing: a challenge to science and society, vol. 3: behavioural sciences and conclusions. Oxford University Press, Oxford

Coleman P G 1986 Ageing and reminiscence processes. John Wiley, Chichester

Coleman P G 1993 Psychological ageing. In: Bond J, Coleman P, Peace S (eds) Ageing in society. Sage, London

Craik F I M, Trehub S (eds) 1982 Ageing and cognitive processes. Plenum Press, New York

Crawford M 1972 Retirement as a psychological crisis. Journal of Psychomatic Research 16: 375–380

Cumming E, Henry W E 1961 Growing old. Basic Books, New York

Cumming E 1975 Engagement with an old theory. International Journal of Aging and Human Development 6(3): 187–191

Datan N, Rodeheaver D, Hughes F 1987 Adult development and ageing. Annual Review of Psychology 38: 153–180

Dobrof R 1984 Introduction: a time for reclaiming the past. In: Kaminsky M (ed) The uses of reminiscence: new ways of working with older adults. The Hayworth Press, New York

Eisdorfer C, Wilkie F 1973 Intellectual changes with advancing age. In: Jarvik L F, Eisdorfer C, Blum J E (eds) Intellectual functioning in adults. Springer, New York

Eisdorfer C, Wilkie F 1977 Stress, disease, aging and behavior. In: Birren J E, Schaie K W (eds) Handbook of the psychology of aging. Van Nostrand Reinhold, New York

Erikson E H 1950 Childhood and society. Norton, New York. Republished (1965) Penguin Harmonsworth, London

Erikson E H (ed) 1978 Adulthood. W W Norton, New York

Erikson E H, Erikson J M, Kivnick H Q 1986 Vital involvement in old age: the experience of old age in our time. W W Norton, New York

Ferraro K F 1989 Widowhood and health. In: Markides K S, Cooper C L (eds) Aging, stress and health. John Wiley, Chichester

Field D, Honzik M P 1981 Personality and accuracy of retrospective reports of aging women. Paper presented at the International Congress of Gerontology, Hamburg, July

Folkman S, Lazarus R S, Pimley S, Novacek J 1987 Age differences in stress and coping processes. Psychology and Ageing 2: 171–184

Frankl V E 1963 Man's search for meaning: an introduction to logotherapy. Pocket Books, New York

Furry C A and Baltes P B 1973 The effect of age differences inability extraneous performance variables on the assessment of intelligence in children, adults and the elderly. Journal of Gerontology 28: 73–80

George L K 1989 Stress, social support, and depression over the life-course. In: Markides K S, Cooper C (eds) Aging, stress and health. John Wiley, Chichester

Havighurst R J, Glaser R 1972 An exploratory study of reminiscence. Journal of Gerontology 27: 235–253

Holland C A, Rabbitt P 1991 The course and causes of cognitive change with advancing age. Reviews in Clinical Gerontology 1: 79–94

Holmes T, Rahe R 1967 The social readjustment rating scales. Journal of Psychosomatic Research 11: 213–218

Jung C G 1972 The transcendent function. In: Read H, Fordham M, Adler G, McGuire W (eds) The structure and dynamics of the psyche, 2nd edn: volume 8 of the Collected Works of C G Jung. Routledge & Kegan Paul, London

Knight B G 1986 Psychotherapy with older adults. Sage, Beverley Hills

Knight B G 1992 Older adults in psychotherapy. Sage, London

Labouvie-Vief G, Hoyer W J, Baltes M M, Baltes P B 1974 Operant analysis of intellectual behaviour in old age. Human Development 17: 259–272

Labouvie-Vief G, Blanchard-Fields F 1982 Cognitive ageing and psychological growth. Ageing and Society 2: 183–209

Laslett P 1989 A fresh map of life: the emergence of the third age. Weidenfeld & Nicholson, London

Lehr U, Thomae H (eds) 1987 Formen seelischen alterns. Ferdinand Enke Verlag, Stuttgart

Levin S, Kahana R J 1967 Psychodynamic studies on aging. International Universities Press, New York

Lieberman M A, Falk J M 1971 The remembered past as a source of data for research on the life cycle. Human Development 14: 132–141

Lieberman M A, Tobin S S 1983 The experience of old age: stress, coping and survival. Basic Books, New York

Light L L 1990 Interactions between memory and language in old age. In: Birren J E, Schaie K W (eds) Handbook of the psychology of aging, 3rd edn. Academic Press, New York

Linn M W, Gurel L, Linn B S 1977 Patient outcome as a measure of quality of nursing home care. American Journal of Public Health 67: 337–344

Lowenthal M F 1968 Social isolation and mental illness in old age. In: Neugarten B L (ed) Middle age and aging. University of Chicago Press, Chicago

McGoldrick A E 1989 Stress, early retirement and health. In: Markides K S, Cooper C C (eds) Aging, stress and health. John Wiley, Chichester

McMahon A W, Rhudick P J 1964 Reminiscing: adaptational significance in the aged. Archives of General Psychiatry 10: 292–298 Republished in: Levin S, Kahana R J (eds) 1967 Pysychodynamic studies on aging: creativity, reminiscing and dying. International Universities Press, New York

Maddox K 1968 Retirement as a social event in the USA. In: Neugarten B L (ed) Middle age and aging. University of Chicago Press, Chicago

Markides K S, Machalek R 1984 Selective survival, aging and society. Archives of Gerontology and Geriatrics 3: 207–222

Markides K S, Cooper C L (eds) 1989 Aging, stress and health. Wiley, Chichester

Maugham W S 1959 Points of view. Doubleday, Garden City, New York

Merriam S 1980 The concept and function of reminiscence: a review of the research. Gerontologist 20: 604–608

Merriam S, Cross L 1982 Adulthood and reminiscence: a descriptive study. Educational Gerontology 8: 275–290

Neisser U 1982 Memory observed: remembering in natural contexts. W H Freeman, San Francisco

Neugarten B L 1968 Middle age and aging. University of Chicago Press, Chicago

Neugarten B L, Gutman D L 1958 Age-sex roles and personality in middle age: a thematic apperception study. In: Neugarten B L (ed) Middle age and aging. University of Chicago Press, Chicago

Nicholson J 1980 Seven ages. Fontana, London

Office of Population Censuses and Surveys (OPCS) 1984 Census Guide No 1 HMSO, London

Office of Population Censuses and Survey (OPCS) 1993 Population Trends, No 71 Spring

Patterson R L, Jackson G M 1980 Behaviour modification with the elderly. Progress in Behaviour Modification 9: 205–239

Pearlin L I, Lieberman M A, Menaghan E G, Mullan J T 1981 The stress process. Journal of Health and Social Behaviour 22: 337–356

Peck R C 1968 Psychological development in the second half of life. In: Neugarten B L (ed) Middle age and ageing. University of Chicago Press, Chicago

Poon L W 1985 Differences in human memory with ageing: nature, causes and clinical implications. In: Birren J E, Schaie K W (eds) Handbook of the psychology of ageing, 2nd edn. Van Nostrand Reinhold, New York

Rabbitt P M A 1980 A fresh look at changes in reaction times in old age. In: Stein D (ed) The psychobiology of ageing: problems and perspectives. Elsevier/North Holland, New York

Rabbitt P M A 1984a Investigating the grey areas. Times Higher Educational Supplement, 1 June, 14

Rabbitt P M A 1984b Memory impairment in the elderly. In: Bebbington P E and Jacoby R (eds) Psychiatric disorders in the elderly. Mental Health Foundation, London

Rabbitt P M A 1985 An age decrement in the ability to ignore irrelevant information. Journal of Gerontology 20: 233–238

Reker G T, Wong P T P 1988 Aging as an individual process: toward a theory of personal meaning. In: Birren J E, Bengston V L (eds) Emergent theories of aging. Springer, New York

Riechard S, Livson F, Peterson P G 1962 Aging and personality: a study of seventy eight older men. Wiley, New York

Rosow I 1968 Housing and local ties of the aged. In: Neugarten B L (ed) Middle age and aging. University of Chicago Press, Chicago

Rotter J B 1966 Generalized expectancies for internal versus external control of reinforcement. Psychological Monographs 80(1)(Whole No. 609): 1–28

Rowe J W, Kahn R L 1987 Human aging: usual and successful. Science 237: 143–149

Rybash J M, Hoyer W J, Roodin P A 1986 Adult cognition and ageing. Pergamon, Elmsford, New York

Salthouse T A 1985 Speed of behavior and its implications for cognition. In: Birren J E, Schaie K E (eds) Handbook of the psychology of aging, 2nd edn. Van Nostrand Reinhold, New York

Savage R D, Britton P G, Bolton N, Hall E H 1973 Intellectual functioning in the aged. Methuen, London

Schaie K W 1967 Age changes and age differences. Gerontologist 7: 128–132

Schaie K W 1977–1978 Towards a stage theory of adult cognitive development. Journal of Ageing and Human Development 8: 129–138

Schaie K W 1983 Longitudinal studies of adult psychological development. New York, Guidford

Schaie K W 1990 The optimization of cognitive functioning in old age: predictions based on cohort-sequential and longitudinal data. In: Baltes P B, Baltes M M (eds) Successful aging: perspectives from the behavioral sciences. Cambridge University Press, New York

Schaie K W, Labouvie-Vief G 1974 Generational versus ontogenetic components of change in adult cognitive behaviour: a fourteen year cross-sequential study. Developmental Psychology 10: 305–320

Schaie K W, Willis S L 1986 Can decline in intellectual functioning in the elderly be reversed? Developmental Psychology 22: 223–232

Seeman T E, Kaplan G A, Knudson L, Cohen R, Guralnick 1987 Social network ties and mortality among the elderly in the Almeda County Study. American Journal of Epidemiology 126: 714–723

Shanas E, Townsend P, Wedderburn D, Friis H, Milhoj P, Stehouwer J 1965 Old people in three industrialised societies. Routledge and Kegan Paul, London

Sheehy G 1978 Passages. Bantam Books, Toronto

Siegler I C 1980 The psychology of adult development and aging. In: Busse E W, Blazer D G (eds) Handbook of geriatric psychiatry. Van Nostrand Reinhold, New York

Stroebe M S, Stroebe W 1983 Who suffers more? Sex differences in health risks of the widowed. Psychological Bulletin 93: 279–301

Stuart-Hamilton I 1991 The psychology of ageing: an introduction. Jessica Kingsley, London

Thomae H (ed) 1976 Patterns of aging. Karger, Basle

Tobin S 1972 The earliest memory as data for research. In: Kent D, Kastenbaum R, Sherwood S (eds) Research, planning and action for the elderly: power and potential of social science. Behavioural Publications, New York

Tobin S S 1989 The effects of institutionalization. In: Markides K S, Cooper C L (eds) Ageing, stress and health. John Wiley, Chichester

Tobin S S, Lieberman M A 1976 Last home for the aged. Josse-Bass, San Francisco

Vernon S W, Jackson G L 1989 Social support, prognosis and adjustment to breast cancer. In: Markides K S, Cooper C L (eds) Ageing, stress and health. John Wiley, Chichester

Waldman D S, Avolio B S 1983 Enjoy old age. Norton, New York

Ward R A, Tobin S S (eds) 1987 Health in aging: sociological issues and policy directives. Springer, New York

Wechsler D 1955 Manual for the Wechsler Adult Intelligence Scale. Psychological Corporation, New York

Wesley M 1988 Second fiddle. McMillan, London

Wesley M 1992 A dubious legacy. Bantam Press, London

Wilson A N 1991 C S Lewis: a biography. Fontana, London

Woods R T, Britton P G 1985 Clinical psychology with the elderly. Chapman & Hall, London

Zinberg N, Kaufman I 1963 Cultural and personality factors associated with aging: an introduction. In: Zinberg N, Kaufman I (eds) Normal psychology of the aging process. International Universities Press, New York

RECOMMENDED READING

Bond J, Coleman P, Peace S 1993 Ageing in society, 2nd edn. Sage, London. *This is a highly accessible, up-to-date book covering a wide range of issues. It considers both sociological and psychological perspectives, and brings a critical eye to bear upon a range of topics, such as bereavement, retirement, poverty, inequality and later life adjustment.*

Baltes P B, Baltes M M (eds) 1990 Successful aging: perspectives from the behavioral sciences. Cambridge University Press, New York. *Extremely thorough and well documented US text, bringing together, in one source, excellent papers from well established contributors in the field of gerontology.*

Salthouse T A 1991 Theoretical perspectives on cognitive aging. Lawrence Erlbaum, Hillsdale. *Excellent, up-to date review of the main theoretical and empirical material on the cognitive aspects of ageing and old age.*

Coleman P G 1986 Ageing and reminiscence processes: social and clinical implications. Wiley, Chichester. *This book is a highly readable account of the general issues pertaining to reminiscence processes and the details of the in-depth study conducted by Coleman. It is full of interesting case material. It considers both healthy and pathological aspects of reminiscence and adjustment in old age.*

Markides K S, Cooper C L (eds) 1989 Aging, stress and health. Wiley, Chichester. *One of the few books in the field to look at ageing from the perspective of health psychology rather than developmental psychology. It includes papers from well established experts in the field of gerontology, and covers such diverse topics as; bereavement, relocation, retirement, ill-health, methodological problems in the measurement of stress exposure in later life, stress and social support among elderly people, and the impact of formal and informal support.*

Erikson E H, Erikson J M, Kivnick H Q 1986 Vital involvement in old age: the experience of old age in our time. Norton, New York. *Important contribution from one of the most influential psychoanalytic writers in the field of the psychology of old age. This represents an elaboration and update of his earlier ideas, as well as the introduction of new themes.*

Tobin S S 1991 Personhood in advanced old age: implications for practice. Springer, New York. *Important contribution from one of the influential American researchers in the field. Well written, up-to-date and importantly, much attention paid to the implication of the research for practice.*

Woods R T, Britton P G 1985 Clinical psychology with the elderly. Chapman & Hall, London. *An extremely influential UK textbook written by clinical psychologists, but aimed at a wide audience of practitioners, working with elderly people. It is particularly good on cognitive aspects of growing old and on the psychopathology of old age.*

Knight B G 1992 Older adults in psychotherapy. Sage, London. *This is an excellent book on working psychotherapeutically with older people, and the particular issues raised for practitioners in this field. It is a US book but highly relevant to the UK situation. It is well-written, full of interesting case material and provides clear guidelines for clinical work with elderly people.*

Birren J E, Bengston V L (eds) 1988 Emergent theories of ageing. Springer, New York. *This book is full of highly readable articles that cover theoretical issues and provide a wealth of empirical research findings. It covers a wide range of topics.*

3

Biological approaches to ageing and mental health

Rosamund A Herbert
Hamish Thomson

INTRODUCTION

An understanding of biological sciences has much to contribute to the care of elderly people with mental health problems. Regardless of the particular mental health problem that an individual may experience, 'underneath' is a person subject to the usual ageing processes. Knowledge of the 'normal' changes that occur with increasing age is therefore essential in understanding the physiological function of each individual and also enables assessment of changes over time and effective clinical decision-making. Without this understanding, decisions will be made from a basis of incomplete information.

In addition to the so-called 'normal' ageing changes, older people often are affected by acute or chronic medical problems and knowledge of the common pathologies and their effects in older people is helpful in planning care. In some instances, the signs and symptoms of physical and mental health problems may be similar (for instance, an anxiety attack and a myocardial infarction can be confused). It is obviously important to make the correct assessment and knowing what is 'medical' and what is 'psychiatric' in origin is often difficult (Trygstad 1994). Some medical problems precipitate psychiatric symptoms (e.g. organ failure or dehydration leading to acute confusion) and some medical illnesses have a psychiatric component (e.g. hypothyroidism and depression, or AIDS dementia). This is a complex and fascinating area.

Fields of study that are helpful are biological gerontology and biological psychiatry and some knowledge of these will have a positive impact on the quality of care that a particular elderly person receives. As both of these fields are rapidly developing areas, a chapter like this can only give a flavour of a few key issues. Biological gerontology refers to the biological basis of ageing changes, whereas the term biological psychiatry is used to convey biological causation and psychological change. Knowledge of the biological basis of mental health problems and treatment options have expanded greatly in the past few years (Trygstad 1994).

The term 'mental' means 'of the mind/pertaining to the mind/done by the mind', so, when considering mental health, anything that affects or alters the function of the mind is of relevance. Usually 'the mind' is taken to be equivalent to the higher centres of the brain. However, since the body works as an integrated whole, a change in one physiological system frequently has knock-on effects in other regions of the body. Thus just as changes in blood flow and circulation may have consequences on the brain, so alterations in brain function (whether physiological, psychological or pathological in origin) have effects on systems outside the nervous system. Traditionally, however, when referring to mental health, we tend to think more of cognitive functions of the brain. Regardless of the aspect of function being considered, the brain depends on the optimal structure and function of the cells and the chemical neurotransmitters. Changes and the consequence of these will be considered in depth later in the chapter.

Thus there are three aspects superimposed when thinking about elderly people with mental health problems. We must consider:

1. the recognised changes that seem to occur with increasing chronological age in some individuals (i.e. ageing changes)
2. the possible presence of pathology affecting the overall functioning of the individual (e.g. stroke, arthritis, anaemia)
3. changes in the normal functioning of 'the mind' (e.g. depression, dementia).

The whole issue is further complicated by the fact that sometimes 'normal' ageing changes can be difficult to distinguish from early onset, say, of dementia. For example, one aspect of the diagnosis of dementia involves showing objective evidence of impairment in long-term memory (Horvath & Davis 1990) but certain types of memory loss are common in older people (Christensen et al 1994) and are considered 'normal'. Episodes of confusion common in dementia could also arise from dehydration during an acute infection, or even from a change in environment combined with deterioration in hearing, vision and memory loss.

As discussed in Chapter 11, dementia itself can have many different aetiologies; these range from degenerative processes affecting the brain such as Alzheimer's[1], to changes in the vascular supply (multi-infarcts or inflammatory diseases of the blood vessels as in polyarteritis), chronic toxic effects from alcohol, metabolic changes such as hypothyroidism, vitamin B_{12} deficiency, or even from chronic meningitis or some tumours. One challenge for people caring for elderly people with mental health problems is differential diagnosis and the ability to distinguish specific reversible causes from those that are irreversible. Thus it is helpful to have an understanding of what the normal function is of elderly people, and how it may differ from younger adults.

The example of dementia illustrates some of the complexities, but the same principles apply to other conditions as well. If someone is showing signs of difficulty in breathing, is this due to an anxiety disorder or does it result from chronic obstructive pulmonary disease secondary to heavy smoking? Understanding when incontinence is a consequence of the ageing changes rather than a means of communication to others or manipulative behaviour would enhance care of elderly people with mental health problems. Thus the aim of this chapter is to discuss some of the general biological changes and issues associated with ageing, to consider some of the biological bases of mental health problems and to draw the two perspectives together. The impact of these changes on older people with mental health problems will then be evident.

'NORMAL AGEING' OR PATHOLOGY?

It is generally acknowledged that all physiological systems in humans show some decline in function with increasing age. However, in the majority of people the decline in physiological function seen with 'normal' ageing does not interfere with an independent lifestyle except under conditions of severe stress such as simultaneous physiological and pathological challenges. One problem with the use of the term 'normal ageing' is that it implies that because something is normal it is therefore acceptable, and nothing needs to be done about it. A simple example might be that there is often a decline in overall hearing acuity with ageing. Although this is a common occurrence it would not be acceptable to ignore it; use of a hearing aid, if appropriate, might alleviate this 'normal' problem.

Much of the difficulty in describing physiological changes with ageing comes from the problem of not having hard facts about the baseline or normal values

---

[1] For the purpose of this chapter, the term Alzheimer's disease is used to mean organic dementia illness across the age range, excluding multi-infarct dementia.

of physiological functioning for older people. In many instances it is difficult to distinguish between true ageing changes, the changes that result from deconditioning or disuse (lack of use) and those that arise from pathology or disease processes. Often several aspects interact. For example, if comparing the cardiovascular function of unfit, predominately sedentary individuals with fitter, more active people there will be marked differences, whatever the age of the people concerned. Similarly if there is an apparent decline in cardiovascular function, is this due to deconditioning or is it evidence of atherosclerosis or some other pathological process? Loss of cognitive function has also been related to lack of use of the mental faculties.

Previously held pessimistic views that declining mental and physical function were unavoidable consequences of ageing were based largely on the results of cross-sectional studies but more recent longitudinal work suggests that some of these earlier results were artefacts of the cohort effect, different lifestyle and illness experiences and the samples used (Grimley Evans et al 1992). With a cross-sectional study, individuals of different generations are being directly compared at any one point in time and so effects of different diets, educational backgrounds, work patterns, trends in smoking, etc. are not accounted for. Both cross-sectional and longitudinal studies can provide useful information and have advantages and disadvantages; the important point is that each approach needs to be subject to careful criticism and the findings evaluated in accordance with the methodology used.

Results from longitudinal studies are gradually replacing previously held stereotyped and simplified concepts about human ageing (Kalache et al 1988). Several large scale longitudinal studies have been under way for some years in the USA and in Scandinavia they are giving useful data. There are also many mini-longitudinal studies that follow a group of people for, say, 5 or 10 years over the crucial periods, such as the study in Leicestershire by Jagger et al (1989) which followed the change in mental and physical functioning in a group of 594 elderly people over 5 years.

Individual variability

The biological gerontology literature concerned with human ageing is frustrating as it is sometimes difficult to find consensus about particular changes with ageing. Some of this is due to the methodology chosen, as discussed above, but often it is due to aspects such as small sample sizes and individual variability. It is often difficult to recruit subjects for study (for example, Greig et al (1994) discuss the problem of recruiting 'fit' elderly people to study the effects of exercise) and difficult to get a disease-free sample. Hence, for understandable pragmatic reasons, some studies have small sample sizes. If this is combined with the individual variability, discussed below, it is possible to see why studies sometimes seem to contradict each other.

Individual variability is an important aspect; whether considering physical health problems or mental health problems, no two individuals will show the same degree of physiological or pathological change. Chronological age is not necessarily a good predictor of loss of physiological function or performance. The range of 'normal', i.e. the heterogeneity between individuals, is much greater in older adults than younger ones. There are people of 80+ who are physically and mentally fit and well, 80-year-olds who are physically strong but who have, say, dementia, and those who have crippling arthritis but are mentally very sharp and able. Similarly when comparing two people aged 70 and 85, it may be the 85-year-old who is able to lead the more independent life. This may be labouring the point, but it is vital to challenge the stereotyping of an older person as inactive, suffering from several medical conditions, weak, depressed and lonely, and deteriorating year by year. It is, however, true to say that as the majority of people get older there is some deterioration in physical and mental functioning. Jagger et al's short longitudinal study (1989), following elderly people in Melton Mowbray over a 5-year period, found individuals who followed the 'expected or anticipated pattern' of declining function but there were also individuals who had improved in both physical and mental functioning or had not changed over the period.

The terms 'elderly' or 'old' are used to cover a large age span from 60 or 65 up to the 'super elderly' in their 90s+. The diversity in physiological function in this age range is enormous and one useful way of considering ageing is to use the terms young old age/elderly (say 65–75), middle old age (75–85) and old old age/very old (85+). Another way of contemplating it is that people in the age range 60–90 are as heterogeneous (if not more so!) than people between 20 and 50 years of age.

Interaction between genetic and environmental factors

Much research has been done, and much is ongoing, to ascertain the aetiologies of both ageing and mental health problems and although our understanding of the processes involved has increased, there are not many definitive findings as yet. The lack of answers may be due to not researching the right areas but is much more likely due to the complex aetiologies. A strong familial tendency is found in a few instances (for example, with schizophrenia and affective disorders) and this implies a genetic component. However, in many instances there will be a combination of genetic and environmental factors leading to a change of function. A good example of this is the debate around aluminium and Alzheimer's disease (see later).

Grimley Evans (1992) discusses the possible epidemiology of Alzheimer's disease and his proposed model has similarities with our understanding of how ageing changes occur. The model (see Fig. 3.1) postulates that the brain damage that is characteristic of Alzheimer's is due to interaction between environmental agents and genetic susceptibility. It seems that most people who develop Alzheimer's have a genetic endowment which gives them 70 years or more before they accumulate a toxic dose of the environmental factors (whatever these prove to be); other people (a minority of those who develop Alzheimer's) seem to have a genetic predisposition that allows their brains to be affected earlier in life.

The second phase of this epidemiological model linking the initial brain cell damage to resulting functional impairment of the brain can also be thought of as being influenced by both genes and environment. Some work has shown that 'better brains' (whether born better or improved by education or use) may be able to compensate for damage from the disease process associated with Alzheimer's. Impaired mental function inevitably leads to alterations in social functioning. The degree of effect on social function is also influenced by environmental factors, such as the quality of input from social and health services. Thus the outcome of the same disease process can and does vary from one individual to another.

The above example is also a useful analogy for considering the ageing processes since the manifestations of ageing are a combination of intrinsic (genetic) and extrinsic (environmental) factors. In order to maximise chances of a long life expectancy, we should choose individuals whose parents live a long time! This is obviously not a feasible choice, but it again demonstrates the combination of both genes and environment. An individual can optimise the chances of reaching old age by taking note of the factors known to promote health and prevent death or disease, such as healthy eating (whatever that may be), taking regular exercise, not smoking, not drinking to excess, nor living dangerously (hang-gliding, fast driving, etc.) and so on. What we probably cannot do much about is the pre-programmed or genetic factors that will eventually undermine homeostasis. An appealing theory is that of 'metabolic switches' in ageing where, in simple terms, energy is switched from one area of metabolic activity to another (Grimley Evans 1993). For instance, energy used in repairing and maintaining cell function could be traded off against energy for reproduction. This is based on a theory of ageing proposed by Kirkwood and Holliday (1986).

Homeostasis and functional reserve

When considering ageing changes in the body, there is a tendency to look at the function of physiological systems one by one, and indeed this chapter takes this approach in some parts. However, what is most important to consider is whether an individual is capable of independent life, namely that the body function as a whole is adequate for 'normal' existence.

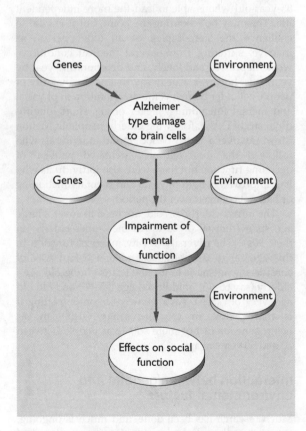

Figure 3.1   A general epidemiological model of Alzheimer's disease (after Grimley Evans 1992).

The maintenance of homeostasis (that is, the maintenance of the stability of the internal environment of the body) is vital to ensure adequate functioning of the cells and tissues in the body. Physical (and even mental) health depends on maintenance of this internal environment. Considering the body as discrete physiological systems is not always helpful, but is necessary when gaining underlying information.

There is in many systems of the body a considerable reserve in function. This functional reserve is important because there can often be situations where a significant loss of tissue or cells occurs and yet this does not adversely affect the capacity of the system. One of the most obvious examples of this spare capacity is in the renal system. It is possible to donate one kidney to a recipient without the donor having any adverse effects on her own health, i.e. losing 50% of renal capacity does not affect the donor's health. This principle of functional reserve or spare capacity holds for many other systems in the body and probably for regions of the brain too. Thus in many ways homeostatic function is more important than changes in individual systems.

Homeostasis involves a complex series of physiological and biochemical changes and responses, and many organs and systems in the body participate in this process. There is generally accepted to be a decline in homeostatic capabilities with increasing age, but in most elderly people homeostasis is maintained unless the body is particularly stressed, for example by concurrent factors such as infection, exposure to extremes of temperature, severe exercise. In many instances it takes an older person longer to re-establish resting or equilibrium levels than it would for a younger person. For example, changes in the neuroendocrine controls of salt and water homeostasis with age make elderly people more susceptible to fluid and electrolyte disturbances such as dehydration and overhydration (Phillips et al 1993). Postural hypotension is more common in elderly people because the reflexes that maintain blood pressure on changes of posture from lying to standing are less efficient. As discussed earlier, individual variability is significant too. For a fuller discussion of homeostasis and functional reserve, see Johnson (1985) and Herbert (1991).

CHANGES WITHIN THE CENTRAL NERVOUS SYSTEM

Almost all the systems in the body show structural and functional changes with age. Obviously it is those changes which affect especially the structure and function of the central nervous system (CNS) which most influence the development of mental health problems. The changes may result from innate ageing changes, for example atrophy of brain cells and changes within cells (e.g. presence of neurofibrillary tangles), vascular changes or changes in neurotransmitter activity. In many instances it is difficult to say whether changes observed are 'normal' ageing changes or due to pathology superimposed, and it is even more difficult to make causal associations between particular changes and the effects of these on brain function.

Although the majority of causes of mental health problems probably do have a central nervous system aetiology, not all do. Systemic conditions can also have an adverse effect on brain function. For example, hypothyroidism (low output of thyroid hormones) has a direct effect on many aspects of physiology and can also lead to depression, psychosis and dementia (Osterweil et al 1992). Cerebral hypoxia will also affect cognitive functions. Later sections of the chapter will consider some of these.

Neurobiology and neuropathology are rapidly developing areas of study and it is only possible in this chapter to pick out certain key issues and changes.

Normal age-related physiological changes

Mature neurones in both the central and peripheral nervous systems are generally considered postmitotic (no longer capable of cell division) and therefore cannot be replaced if they die during adult life. In contrast, the glial cells (see Fig. 3.2), which are the non-conducting cells of the brain that protect, nurture and support the neurones, not only go through cell division and replication, but they can also proliferate in response to injury or loss.

The irreplaceable nature of neurones may have been overemphasised in the past since, although they cannot divide, they remain highly active, both in metabolic terms and in response to injury. The mere presence or absence of cells may prove to be only a crude determinant of neurological integrity.

Changes in the nervous system certainly do occur over time, but the fact that neurones are unable to divide after their formation suggests that they possess a very efficient homeostatic mechanism to maintain both their integrity and function for many years. Homeostasis in the individual as a whole may depend largely on the central nervous system: the larger it is in relation to total body size, the more effective it appears

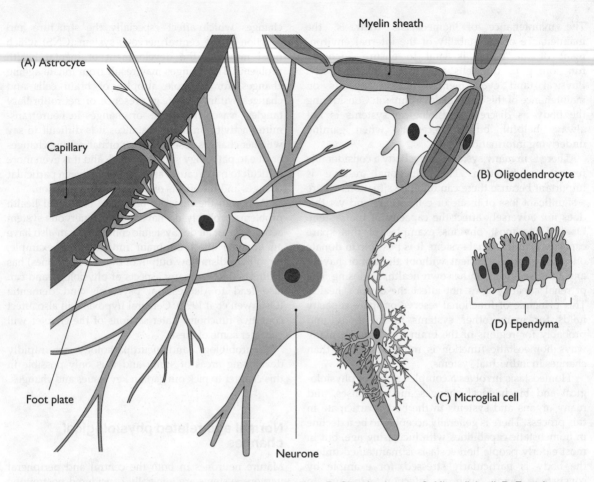

(A) Astrocyte

Capillary

Foot plate

Neurone

Myelin sheath

(B) Oligodendrocyte

(D) Ependyma

(C) Microglial cell

Figure 3.2 Glial cells: **A**: Astrocyte with foot plates on a capillary. **B**: Oligodendrocyte. **C**: Microglial cell. **D**: Ependyma.

to be in slowing the rate of homeostatic decline. The index of cephalisation (i.e. the bigger the brain is in relation to body size) is therefore a good predictor of species' life span.

During human embryonic development the brain surface is smooth in the first 4 months and then becomes irregular, producing the characteristic gyri (ridges) and sulci (troughs) on the surface. These undulations increase the surface area of the brain to about 30 times that of the internal surface of the skull, which allows for organisation and specialisation of particular areas.

Since the anatomy of the brain is complex, the reader should refer to Figure 3.3 and Table 3.1 during the following discussion, to locate the various regions of the CNS and their functions.

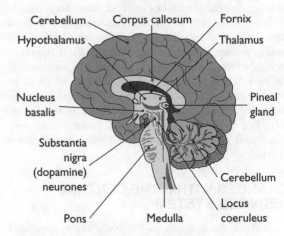

Cerebellum

Hypothalamus

Nucleus basalis

Substantia nigra (dopamine) neurones

Pons

Corpus callosum

Fornix

Thalamus

Pineal gland

Cerebellum

Locus coeruleus

Medulla

Figure 3.3 The brain: mid saggital section.

Table 3.1   Major structures of the brain and their functions (Carola et al 1992)

Structure	Description	Major functions
Basal ganglia	Large masses of gray matter contained deep within each cerebral hemisphere.	Help to coordinate skeletal muscle movements by relaying information via thalamus to motor area of cerebral cortex to influence descending motor tracts.
Brainstem*	Stemlike portion of brain continuous with diencephalon above and spinal cord below. Composed of midbrain, pons, medulla oblongata.	Relays messages between spinal cord and brain, and from brainstem cranial nerves to cerebrum. Helps control heart rate, respiratory rate, blood pressure. Involved with hearing, taste, other senses.
Cerebellum	Second largest part of brain. Located behind pons, in posterior section of cranial cavity. Composed of cerebellar cortex, two lateral lobes, central flocculonodular lobes, medial vermis, some deep nuclei.	Processing centre involved with coordination of muscular movements, balance, precision and timing of movements, body positions. Processes sensory information used by motor systems.
Cerebral cortex	Outer layer of cerebrum. Composed of gray matter and arranged in ridges (gyri), grooves (sulci), depressions (fissures).	Involved with most conscious activities of living. (See major functions of cerebral lobes.)
Cerebral lobes	Major divisions of cerebrum, consisting of frontal, parietal, temporal, occipital lobes (names for bones under which they lie), insula, and limbic lobe.	Frontal lobe involved with motor control of voluntary movements, control of emotional expression and moral behaviour. Parietal lobe involved with general senses, taste. Temporal lobe involved with hearing, equilibrium, emotion, memory. Occipital lobe organised for vision and associated forms of expression. Insula may be involved with gastrointestinal and other visceral activities. Limbic lobe (along with the limbic system) is involved with emotions, behavioural expressions, recent memory, smell.
Cerebrospinal fluid	Fluid that circulates in ventricles and subarachnoid space.	Supports and cushions brain. Helps control chemical environment of central nervous system.
Cerebrum	Largest part of brain. Divided into left and right hemispheres by longitudinal fissure and divided into lobes. Also contains cerebral cortex (gray matter), white matter, basal ganglia.	Controls voluntary movements, coordinates mental activity. Centre for all conscious living.
Corpus callosum	Bridge of nerve fibres that connects one cerebral hemisphere with the other.	Connects cerebral hemispheres, relaying sensory information between them. Allows left and right hemispheres to share information, helps to unify attention.
Cranial nerves	Twelve pairs of cranial nerves. Olfactory (I) and optic (II) arise from cerebrum; others (III through XII) arise from brainstem. Sensory, motor, or mixed.	Concerned with senses of smell, taste, vision, hearing, balance. Also involved with specialised motor activities, including eye movement, chewing, swallowing, breathing, speaking, facial expression.
Diencephalon	Deep portion of brain. Composed of thalamus, hypothalamus, epithalamus, ventral thalamus.	Connects midbrain with cerebral hemispheres. (See major functions of thalamus and hypothalamus.)
Hypothalamus	Small mass below the thalamus; forms floor and part of lateral walls of third ventricle.	Highest integrating centre for autonomic nervous system. Controls most of endocrine system through its relationship with the pituitary gland. Regulates body temperature, water balance, sleep-wake patterns, food intake, behavioural responses associated with emotion.

Table 3.1 *Cont'd*

Structure	Description	Major functions
Medulla oblongata	Lowermost portion of brainstem. Connects pons and spinal cord. Site of decussation of descending corticospinal (motor) tract and an ascending sensory pathway from spinal cord to thalamus; emergence of cranial nerves VI through XII; movement of cerebrospinal fluid from ventricle to subarachnoid space.	Contains vital centres that regulate heart rate, respiratory rate, constriction and dilation of blood vessels, blood pressure, swallowing, vomiting, sneezing, coughing.
Meningeal spaces	Spaces associated with meninges. Potential epidural space between skull and dura mater; potential subdural space between dura mater and arachnoid; subarachnoid space between arachnoid and pia mater (contains cerebrospinal fluid).	Provide subarachnoid circulatory paths for cerebrospinal fluid, protective cushion.
Meninges	Three layers of membranes covering brain. Outer tough dura mater; arachnoid; inner delicate pia mater, which adheres closely to brain.	Dura mater adds support and protection. Arachnoid provides space between the arachnoid and pia mater for circulation of cerebrospinal fluid. Choroid plexuses, at places where pia mater and ependymal cells meet, are site of formation of much cerebrospinal fluid. Pia mater contains blood vessels that supply blood to brain.
Midbrain	Located at upper end of brainstem. Connects pons and cerebellum with cerebrum. Site of emergence of cranial nerves III, IV.	Involved in visual reflexes, movement of eyes, focusing of lens, dilation of pupils.
Pons	Short, bridgelike structure composed mainly of fibres that connect midbrain and medulla oblongata, cerebellar hemispheres, and cerebellum and cerebrum. Lies anterior to cerebellum and between midbrain and medulla oblongata. Site of emergence of cranial nerve V.	Controls certain respiratory functions. Serves as relay station from medulla oblongata to higher structures in brain.
Reticular formation	Complex network of nerve cells organised into ascending (sensory) and descending (motor) pathways. Located throughout core of entire brainstem.	Specific functions for different neurones, including involvement with respiratory and cardiovascular centres, regulation of individual's level of awareness.
Thalamus	Composed of two separate bilateral masses of gray matter. Located in centre of cerebrum.	Intermediate relay structure and processing centre for all sensory information (except smell) going to cerebrum.
Ventricles	Cavities within brain that are filled with cerebrospinal fluid. Left and right lateral ventricles in cerebral hemispheres, third ventricle in diencephalon, fourth ventricle in pons and medulla oblongata.	Provide circulatory paths for cerebrospinal fluid. Choroid plexuses associated with ventricles are site of formation of most cerebrospinal fluid.

Atrophy of the brain

A review of studies by Perry and Perry (1982) confirms that brain atrophy occurs with increasing age in normal individuals. There is a decrease in the total number of nerve cells with increasing age, due initially to patchy loss of dendrite spines (the short thread-like extensions of the nerve cell body that conduct nerve impulses towards the cell body), followed by swelling of dendrite shafts and cell bodies, progressing to fragmentation and cell death (Coleman & Flood 1987). The total number of dendrites decreases with age, which may be due to a reduction in the rate at which they are renewed, or may be a genuine loss. This loss of dendrites on its own should lead to a reduction in synaptic activity, but it may be possible to generate new synaptic connections over time, compensating for at least some of this loss.

There is an overall reduction in brain weight of about 10–15% between the ages of 25 and 75 years, from about 1400 g in males in their thirties to about 1250 g in males in their eighties, and 1250 g to 1125 g in females over the same period. There is a poor correlation between such weight loss and neuro-psychological changes, i.e. no direct link between the changes observed and loss of cells. Brain weight at post-mortem is, however, subject to variability due to irregular trapping of cerebrospinal fluid (Brookbank 1990). Also we are, in general, taller and heavier than our grandparents were, and this is reflected in an increase in average brain weight of approximately 50 g during the past century (Katzman 1988). However, the observed loss of brain weight with ageing is much greater than accounted for by this physical change.

Computerised tomography examination supports the findings of a decrease in brain volume during normal ageing (Yamaura et al 1980). As the brain's weight and volume decrease there is more space for cerebrospinal fluid between the now more prominent gyri and deeper sulci and this is associated with enlargement and deformation of the cerebral ventricles, and meningeal thickening (this is particularly pronounced in Pick's disease).

It is probably not the case that many millions of neurones are lost from all parts of the brain throughout life, as once was believed (Brody 1955). It is more likely that, while some significant losses do occur in the 3rd or 4th decade onwards, they are confined to specific brain regions (Haug 1984, Terry et al 1987). For example, subcortical structures like the brainstem nuclei of the pons and medulla seem to be resistant to cell loss (Curcio et al 1982). Others seem to be more vulnerable, such as the neurones of the cerebral cortex in the parasagittal frontal and parietal areas, as well as the visual cortex, basal ganglia, cerebellar cortex, hippocampus (a structure in the limbic system, associated with memory functions) and in particular the locus cœruleus (a nucleus in the brain stem made up of millions of neurones using the neurotransmitter noradrenaline); this area is involved in the control of rapid eye movement (REM) sleep, and may be the most vulnerable. Losses are estimated to be as high as 1% per year in these regions, with a total loss as high as 60%. Pronounced cell loss in the locus cœruleus appears to be a significant feature of Alzheimer's disease (Marcyniuk et al 1986). The locus cœruleus is well suited to quantitative study because of its discrete, well defined character and large neurones which provide the noradrenergic input into the cerebral cortex and the hypothalamus (Roth et al 1985). A count of the cell population of this nucleus has indicated a 70–80% decrease in younger Alzheimer's patients (Bondareff et al 1982).

The exact extent to which the neurones of the cortex are affected by ageing is unclear, but many studies have shown a loss of large neurones which are probably pyramidal cells (i.e. those associated with motor control, for example gait) from the frontal and temporal cortex, with a significant increased loss in individuals with early onset Alzheimer's disease (Gearing et al 1988). There appears to be a correlation between a low neuronal count and a higher incidence of plaques and tangles (Mountjoy et al 1983). These changes could explain the linguistic disturbances, emotional dulling, changes in personality and loss of insight commonly observed in individuals with Alzheimer's disease.

However, in animal studies, experimentally induced 'loss' of large neurones in other areas of the brain appears to be due to shrinkage so that the neurones remain, but are smaller (Pearson et al 1983). When the morphology as well as size is taken into consideration, there appears to be a proportionally greater loss of non-pyramidal cells (Braak & Braak 1986) and this will affect cognitive function. Studies of this type depend on the examination of a relatively small area of the cortex and fail to take account of shrinkage of the total area of the cortex. The neurones of the cortex are interconnected functionally in columns arranged perpendicularly to the pial surface. In pathological conditions where cortical atrophy is prominent, and possibly also as a consequence of ageing processes, a loss of entire columns may occur and mask the true extent of cell loss unless the whole cortex is considered (Hauw et al 1986). It is important to consider age-related changes in the central nervous system as a whole, in terms of their effects on the individual, but for research purposes it is often easier to look at specific regions or functions in isolation. For obvious reasons, research is not done on humans!

Studies on age-related changes in the cerebellum in rats and mice indicate that significant decreases in synaptic density in the cerebellum occur with age (Brookbank 1990). Purkinje cells are lost, along with other cerebellar elements and neurones of the locus cœruleus (Hall et al 1975). Purkinje cells are multipolar neurones mainly in the middle layer of the cerebellum. The axons of the Purkinje cells provide the only efferent path from the cerebellar cortex. This decline in synaptic density might be the morphological basis for the decline in integrative functions of the cerebellum that have been noted to occur with age in humans and laboratory mammals. This decline has been presumed to be due to synaptic delay in neurotransmitter synthesis, but may also reflect the loss of cellular elements in the cerebellum.

Anatomically, in ageing mammals the small projections (dendrites) from the neurones of the spinal cord and brain stem nuclei seem to be lost. The dendritic surfaces appear featureless save that some dendrites appear to be shorter and thinner. The membranes of neurones may become more vulnerable to neurotoxic agents with age, and this may be significant for some elderly people who have high consumption of drugs (Bondy et al 1989).

Conversely, glial cell proliferation appears to be a consistent feature of ageing, more noticeably in the hippocampus than the neocortex, and this may be due to increased demands for metabolic support for ageing neurones. Glial cell volume is increased, but there appears to be no change in the number of astrocytes (the largest and most numerous type of glial cell) and a slight decline in the number of oligodendrocytes (smaller glial cells associated with myelin production (see Fig. 3.2)). However, glial cells fulfil a supporting role, and proliferation cannot replace lost neuronal function.

Redundancy. There are initially many more nerve cells present than are ever going to be needed, so it may be possible to make many of them redundant before any functional change is observed – another example of the functional reserve discussed earlier. The exact number of cells required for specific functions is not known so the extent of over-provision is difficult to estimate. One example that has been studied is the secretion of antidiuretic hormone (ADH) from the supraoptic and paraventricular nuclei. Lack of ADH

produces a condition called diabetes insipidus, where large volumes of dilute urine are continually produced. It is known that this form of diabetes only occurs when the number of cells in the nuclei concerned are reduced to 10–15% of normal, i.e. cell loss less than 85–90% does not have a marked effect on physiological function.

Reactive synaptogenesis. There appear to be two different processes occurring at the same time: a gradual death of nerve cells, accounting for the decreased number, associated with a lengthening and an increasing number of dendrites in the remaining nerve cells, particularly in the cerebral cortex and hippocampus. With the increase in the dendritic tree, new connections are possible, called reactive synaptogenesis, to make up for the loss in total number of cells (see reviews by Coleman & Flood 1986, Cotman et al 1981, Cotman & Anderson 1988). This is another reason why considering simple loss of cell numbers alone is unhelpful.

Intracellular changes

Much research has been carried out examining the intracellular changes in the brain with age, in an attempt to link these changes with other observed changes in function. The main intracellular changes are described below:

Lipofuscin. Various organic pigments and minerals accumulate in the brain throughout life. The most characteristic of these is the yellow pigment lipofuscin, sometimes called the 'age pigment', which is found in neurones and glial cells, and formed in degenerating cytoplasm probably from lysosomes or mitochondria (lipofuscin does also accumulate in tissues outside the CNS). The main accumulation occurs in storage vacuoles and correlates with age. The amount per cell varies, but can be enough to fill 75% of the cytoplasm.

There appears to be a variety of lipofuscins since cells in different areas of the brain contain pigments of different structure. Animal studies have shown that the amount of pigment accumulation may be modified by dietary vitamin E, with a deficient diet leading to increased accumulation (Kenney 1989). The significance of lipofuscin accumulation for human ageing is not yet fully understood, as it is not known whether it does actually interfere with cell function in any way.

Lewy bodies. These are intraneuronal spheroid substances with an affinity for monoaminergic neurones, and are commonly found in the pigmented melanin-containing cells of the locus cœruleus and substantia nigra (which are characteristically associated with idiopathic Parkinson's disease). They are also found in a small proportion of brains of healthy elderly people (Kemper 1984).

One component of the Lewy body appears to be related to filamentous proteins of the sort found in tangles, and when Lewy bodies are present, neurofibrillary tangles (associated with Alzheimer's disease) are generally not found in the same cell.

Net losses of proteins and gangliosides (a major component of the nerve sheath) only occur to a significant extent in the caudate nucleus part of the brain.

Senile amyloid plaques. Senile amyloid plaques, another common occurrence, are round or ovoid granular or filamentous structures, much larger than individual neurones and are known as argentophilic (i.e. they reduce silver salts to metallic silver) and, in silver stained sections, therefore, they appear as black foci of irregular shape and size.

These plaques contain abnormal neural processes, glial processes, macrophages (Terry 1980), and some contain a central core of amyloid material (Merz et al 1983). This amyloid material is probably an extracellular protein related to portions of the immunoglobulin molecule and is also found in cardiovascular tissue. Plaques are most frequent in the medial temporal lobe, particularly the amygdala (limbic system structure, associated with emotional state) and hippocampus but may be present in all cortical areas, particularly the limbic cortex.

The pathophysiological significance of plaques in a cognitively normal individual remains unclear, but the number of plaques correlates well with the severity of Alzheimer's dementia and with the extent of the cholinergic abnormalities. However, the work of Whitson et al (1989) suggests that amyloid protein fragments may have a non-toxic effect on hippocampal neurones in vitro.

The appearance of amyloid in the brain does, however, seem to be an age-related phenomenon. There are also indications that the brains of individuals with Pick's disease, Creutzfeldt–Jakob disease, kuru and Down's syndrome accumulate larger amounts of amyloid than the brains of elderly non-demented individuals (Kemper 1984).

Neurofibrillary protein tangles. First described by Alzheimer in 1906, neurofibrillary protein tangles are accumulations of filaments found in the cytoplasm of neurones. They are composed of twisted helical fibrils or tubules, each consisting of a pair of filaments wound round each other (Wisniewski et al 1984), which again take up silver stains heavily. These tangles are common in the limbic cortices, hippocampus, amygdala and brain stem nuclei in diseases such as: Alzheimer's disease, Down's syndrome, dementia

pugilistica, postencephalitic Parkinsonism and other degenerative disorders (Katzman & Terry 1983).

Neocortical tangles are not common in non-demented elderly brains, but tangles in areas such as the locus cœruleus and substantia nigra may be found in intellectually unimpaired individuals, particularly over the age of 80 years, and this may explain the phenomenon of short-term rather than long-term memory loss.

In experimental animals, degenerative changes in intracellular fibrils can be induced by intracranial injection of aluminium ions. Since in some studies aluminium is found in greater than normal concentrations in the plaques and tangles found in the brains of Alzheimer's sufferers, it has been suggested that aluminium, particularly when associated with cooking utensils, may be the cause of this disease. Other studies have failed to find high levels of aluminium. This kind of analysis is quite difficult to carry out, and carries a risk of accidental contamination by aluminium from other sources. Also, the investigation can only be carried out at post-mortem examination; there is no way of monitoring levels during life at the present time. Some consider that the presence of aluminium is more likely to be a result of the disease process rather than the cause (Brookbank 1990).

Goudsmit et al (1990) suggest that, while aluminium has been considered as one of the causes of Alzheimer's disease, there are many other possible factors, for example viral infections, sensory deprivation, head injury, autoimmune destruction of neurones, excitatory compounds such as glutamate and aspartate, and DNA damage caused by reducing sugars.

Doll (1993), in a comprehensive review of Alzheimer's disease and environmental aluminium, writes that the evidence to date suggests that aluminium is neurotoxic in humans, but not that it is a cause of Alzheimer's disease. The possibility that it could be a cause must be kept open until the neuropathological evidence is resolved.

Genetic predisposition to Alzheimer's disease is also a possibility. Down's syndrome has been associated with an extra copy of part of chromosome 21, a region probably containing several hundred genes. No single gene has as yet been identified with causing the disorder. Genes associated with familial Alzheimer's disease and encoding the precursor for amyloid protein have also been located in the same portion of chromosome 21. This may be why some elderly people with Down's syndrome also develop Alzheimer's disease-like neuropathology (Cheng et al 1988).

Granulovacuolar degeneration. Affected neurones show clusters of membrane-bound vacuoles in their cytoplasm, each of which has a dense, round, dark central granule and looks similar to lysosome vacuoles (Price et al 1986). It is possible that the concentration of lipofuscin decreases as the vacuoles progress, and therefore these vacuoles might constitute a mechanism by which the neurone is able to rid itself of excess lipofuscin.

These particular cellular changes occur mainly in the pyramidal nerve cells of the hippocampus where they are associated with Alzheimer's disease, Down's syndrome, progressive supranuclear palsy and the Guam ALS–Parkinsonism–dementia complex (Tomlinson 1977). However, these changes may also appear in the brains of older people with no evidence of dementia.

Neurotransmitter changes

Neurones communicate with each other using chemicals which cross the synapse; these chemicals synthesised by the neurones themselves are referred to as neurotransmitters. Neurotransmitters in the CNS act in two main ways by producing either an excitatory or an inhibitory response in the postsynaptic membrane. It is believed that an imbalance between the excitatory and inhibitory neurotransmitters can lead to conditions such as depression, anxiety and some forms of insomnia. Parkinson's disease is caused by a deficiency of one of the excitatory neurotransmitters, dopamine. Some neurotransmitters also produce broader and longer-lasting effects, similar to that of hormones, and the effects are said to be metabotrophic (for example noradrenaline, dopamine and serotonin).

The neurotransmitters considered in this section are dopamine, noradrenaline, acetylcholine, serotonin and gamma-aminobutyric acid (GABA). Table 3.2 summarises the probable function of the key neurotransmitters. Age-related changes in neurotransmitter function may have profound effects on the overall functioning of the CNS.

Noradrenaline and dopamine. Dopamine and noradrenaline are catecholamines and have excitatory

Table 3.2 Neurotransmitters with roles in the central nervous system (CNS)

Neurotransmitter	Function	Sites where secreted in CNS	Comments
Acetylcholine (ACh)	Excitatory to skeletal muscles; excitatory or inhibitory to visceral effectors, depending on receptors bound.	Basal nuclei and some neurones of motor cortex of brain.	Release increased by insecticides; decreased ACh levels in certain brain areas in Alzheimer's disease.
Noradrenaline	Excitatory or inhibitory, depending on receptor type.	Brainstem, particularly reticular activating system; limbic system; some areas of cerebral cortex.	Release enhanced by amphetamines; removal from synapse blocked by cocaine.
Dopamine	Generally excitatory; may be inhibitory in sympathetic ganglia.	Substantia nigra of midbrain; hypothalamus; is the principal neurotransmitter of extrapyramidal system.	Release enhanced by L-dopa and amphetamines; re-uptake blocked by cocaine; deficient in Parkinson's disease; may be involved in pathogenesis of schizophrenia.
Serotonin	Generally inhibitory.	Brainstem; hypothalamus; limbic system; cerebellum; pineal gland; spinal cord.	Activity blocked by LSD; may play a role in sleep.
GABA (gamma-aminobutyric acid)	Generally inhibitory.	Purkinje cells of cerebellum; spinal cord.	Important in presynaptic inhibition.
Endorphins, enkephalins	Generally inhibitory.	Widely distributed in brain; hypothalamus; limbic system; pituitary; spinal cord.	Effects mimicked by morphine, heroin and methadone.
Substance P	Excitatory.	Basal nuclei; midbrain; hypothalamus; cerebral cortex.	Mediates pain transmission.
Somatostatin	Generally inhibitory.	Hypothalamus; retina and other parts of brain. Pancreas.	Inhibits release of growth hormone; A gut-brain peptide.

functions. The locus cœruleus, a region in the floor of the fourth ventricle, contains a large number of cells that secrete catecholamines and is thought to lose cells at a rate of up to 40% per year after the age of 60, leading to lower levels of these neurotransmitters. Morgan & May (1990) suggest that noradrenaline levels decline by 20% in the hypothalamus, while remaining stable in the rest of the brain, and this might be linked to a general impairment of cortical function.

Noradrenaline is synthesised from dopamine via the enzyme dopamine beta-hydroxylase. Inactivation is also primarily by presynaptic re-uptake and by monoamine oxidase. Decreases in re-uptake have been found in the locus cœruleus. Noradrenaline receptors decrease with age in the cerebellum in association with the loss of Purkinje cells. These changes are also associated with severe Alzheimer's disease and premature death.

Changes in catecholamine activity are implicated in depression and psychosis. Some cases of depression may be the result of reduced catecholamine levels in the brain and thus antidepressants have their effect by increasing the level of the excitatory neurotransmitters. Tricyclic antidepressants block the re-uptake of neurotransmitters and so prolong the stimulatory effect.

Age-related decline in dopamine seems particularly severe in the hippocampus and hypothalamic regions. Normally, dopamine is inactivated at the synapse by re-uptake into presynaptic vesicles or by the action of the enzyme monoamine oxidase. Dopamine receptors also appear to decline with age, especially in the striatum.

Levels of monoamine oxidase (MAO), the enzyme responsible for the breakdown of catecholamines, appear to increase with age. This is the reason for the use of monoamine oxidase inhibitors (MAOIs) in the treatment of certain types of depression in some elderly people. Thus MAOIs allow the neurotransmitters to build up to a high level and produce a greater stimulation of the brain. Increased communication between brain cells via dopamine is thought to be involved in some forms of psychosis including abnormal thought processes and behaviour. Antipsychotic drugs (also known as major tranquillisers or neuroleptics) produce their effects by blocking dopamine receptors. This brings about the desired changes of stabilising mood and reducing anxiety, tension and hyperactivity but also results in a range of undesirable side-effects.

It is not surprising that an overdose of tricyclics and MAOIs produces dangerous side-effects because these drugs interfere with fundamental neurotransmitter activity in the body as a whole. MAOIs have numerous side-effects because they deactivate enzymes that normally break down chemicals such as tyramine found in some foods. MAOIs taken with certain drugs or food rich in tyramine (such as cheese, meat or yeast extracts and red wine) can produce a dramatic rise in blood pressure. Antipsychotic drugs may also block the action of noradrenaline. One side-effect is lowering of blood pressure, and dizziness is a symptom of this.

Degeneration of the dopaminergic neurones in the substantia nigra is closely associated with the development of Parkinson's disease. Teravainen & Calne (1983) have suggested that alterations in gait and posture sometimes seen in otherwise normal elderly people may also be due to the loss of dopaminergic neurones; these individuals show a loss of tyrosine hydroxylase and dopaminergic receptors. Increased levels of dopamine are associated with schizophrenia.

Acetylcholine. Although acetylcholine (ACh) is the main neurotransmitter released by neurones of the peripheral nervous system, only a restricted number of neurones in the CNS release ACh. There is a loss of function in the cholinergic system as levels of ACh decline in some regions of the brain, for example the cerebral cortex. Levels may remain unchanged in the striatum of the basal ganglia.

There is a slight decline in presynaptic choline acetyl transferase (CAT) activity in the cortex and the caudate nucleus with ageing. This enzyme is involved in the synthesis of ACh. CAT levels suffer a greater reduction in Alzheimer's disease than in normal ageing (Francis et al 1985). Deficiency of ACh innervation of the cerebral cortex may contribute to some of the behavioural, memory and cognitive abnormalities associated with Alzheimer's dementia.

The number of ACh receptor sites does decline with age. Receptor losses in healthy individuals occur throughout the brain. The alteration is in the number of binding sites and not the affinity of the site for ACh.

As we have said, in Alzheimer's disease the CAT level is lower than in normal age-matched controls, but the deficit in ACh receptors does not appear to be greater than in age-matched controls. This would indicate that the deficit in Alzheimer's disease is on the presynaptic side of the nerve junction, not on the other side of the synapse, where the receptors are located. In addition, acetylcholinesterase (a postsynaptic enzyme which breaks down ACh) activity is not altered with age, and levels in cerebrospinal fluid of Alzheimer's patients were no different from that of age-matched controls (Elbe et al 1987).

The loss of cholinergic neurones in the hippo-campus and amygdala characteristic of Alzheimer's disease correlates well with the degree of dementia characteristic of this condition (Price et al 1982). While cell loss in the hippocampus and amygdala has been well documented, the magnitude of cell loss in the cerebral cortex has been more difficult to measure in Alzheimer's disease.

In experimental animals significant improvement in recall has been observed on a choline-rich diet, a finding that is consistent with the vital role of ACh in memory functions. Similar results have not been found in humans.

The overall cholinergic deficit is probably the most consistent change in Alzheimer's disease and cellular degeneration is correlated with a decrease in presynap-tic cholinergic activity in the cortex (Mountjoy et al 1984). There is a high concentration of acetylcho-linesterase in predominantly neuritic plaques, but in those plaques where the amyloid core predominates the concentration is lower; this suggests that changes in cholinergic axons may play a part in the formation of neuritic plaques (Struble et al 1982).

Serotonin. Serotonin (5-hydroxytryptamine or 5-HT) has a generally inhibitory effect and is associated with various mood swings, including depression, elation, insomnia and hallucinations. There are not many serotonin-releasing neurones in the brain; the cell bodies are located in the brain stem but their fibres are widely distributed throughout in, for example, the brain stem, hypothalamus, limbic system and pineal gland. Serotonin levels do not decline with age, but the number of serotonin receptors does decline by up to 30% (Procter et al 1987). This is likely to affect a number of central regulatory activities such as eating and drinking, respiration and heart rate, thermoregula-tion, sleep and memory, and pain perception. The changes may also be associated with eating disorders, aggressive behaviour, sexual behaviour, changing mood states and affective disorders such as depression. Outside the CNS, 95% of the body's serotonin is found in the blood, mainly in platelets. When released from the platelets it causes vasoconstriction; it is therefore associated with the symptoms of migraine and the development of hypertension.

Gamma-aminobutyric acid. Gamma-aminobutyric acid (GABA) is one of the principal inhibitory neurotransmitters in the CNS. GABA has its inhibitory effect in a small circuit of neurones in such structures as the cerebral cortex, cerebellum and upper brainstem. Because GABA has an inhibitory effect, it reduces communication between the brain cells. Anxiety states are thought to result from excessive brain activity. The benzodiazepines, a group of drugs used in the treatment of anxiety, work by increasing the inhibitory effect of GABA on brain cells and glutamic acid as a stimulatory neurotransmitter. Older people have an increased sensitivity to benzodiazepines (Walker & Wynne 1994) although the exact cause is not known. Glutamic acid decarboxylase, the enzyme responsible for converting glutamic acid into GABA, may decrease with advancing age by 20–30% in the cortex, basal ganglia and thalamus. GABA levels have been shown to be lower in the frontal, temporal and occipital cortex (Perry et al 1987).

GABA-producing cells have a role in the processing of sensory information. A deficiency of GABA neurones in the basal caudate nucleus leads to the uncontrolled movements found in Huntington's chorea.

Vascular changes

Atherosclerosis increases with age in many individuals and affects all the blood vessels in the body including those in the brain. This process can interfere with the normal properties of the vessels. In some instances, the vertebral arteries which provide part of the arterial blood supply to the brain follow a more tortuous route due to changes in the structure of the vertebrae and intervertebral discs. This can lead to the vessels becoming kinked with movements of the neck, leading to temporary poor blood flow to the brain. These are called transient ischaemic attacks.

Several studies have been carried out to assess the extent of changes, if any, in cerebral blood flow with advancing age. Some studies show a deficiency in overall blood flow, but this may not have a direct effect on oxygen available to the brain. Cerebral blood flow may decrease with age (by 10–15%), but adequate oxygenation can be maintained as more oxygen is liberated from the haemoglobin. There is a considera-ble functional reserve or spare capacity of oxygen carriage. The capillary network of the cerebral cortex appears to increase in diameter, volume and length which may also help to compensate (Kenney 1989).

Dekoninck (1985) reports studies looking at elderly subjects rigorously selected for as great a freedom from disease as possible. In this very select group, cerebral blood flow and oxygen consumption remained unchanged from the levels in control subjects 50 years younger. However, cerebral glucose utilisation was significantly reduced, possibly due to the use of ketones as a substrate. Despite their seemingly normal cerebral blood flow and oxygen uptake, these otherwise healthy aged people still exhibited impairments of cognitive and psychomotor functions, and electroencephalogram changes. Thus it is unlikely that blood flow changes are responsible for the changes seen.

Whatever the overall changes in the vascular system with age, it is clear that normal neuronal function depends on an adequate blood supply.

Peripheral nerves

The CNS undergoes some functional and structural changes with ageing but there is also a reduction in the number of peripheral nerves and the velocity of conduction. The reduction in nerves in the autonomic, motor and sensory systems leads to reduced effectiveness; for example, reduced stimulation of muscles at motor end plates and a reduced effectiveness in reflexes or feedback mechanisms.

Conduction is most rapid in myelinated fibres and is roughly proportional to the diameter of the neurone. For example, in the ulnar nerve, the velocity is quite slow in the newborn, averaging 30 metres per second. This increases rapidly and maximal levels are reached by age 5 years of about 60 m/s. This reduces again during adult life, down to about 50 m/s by the age of 80 years, a decline in velocity in the region of 15%. Conduction velocity is slightly greater in women than men. There is likely to be about a 10% overall average reduction in conduction velocity in myelinated neurones throughout the body as a whole, but some reflex times show a marked slowing; for example, up to a 30% increase in Achilles tendon reflex time. This may, of course, be compounded by other age-related changes in muscles and joints (Collins et al 1980).

CHANGES IN SYSTEMS OUTSIDE THE NERVOUS SYSTEM

The previous sections have been considering in detail the changes in the CNS. However, maintaining an independent lifestyle also depends on systemic functioning and the physical health of the individual as a whole. This part of the chapter will consider some of the biological changes in systems other than the nervous system. Although it is important to consider the function of the body as a whole, it is sometimes necessary to consider systems separately in the first instance. The factors discussed earlier such as individual variability and lifestyle differences make any discussion of ageing changes more complex.

This section looks at the additive effects of the consequences of ageing on physical function together with mental health problems.

Changes in nutrition, metabolism and the gastrointestinal tract

With increasing age there are changes in body composition; for example, there is an increase in the percentage of body fat, reduced muscle mass and reduced mineral content of bone. As discussed in Chapter 23, percentage body fat is relevant when considering drug metabolism. Drugs that are not fat soluble will be distributed in a smaller volume of tissue whilst fat soluble drugs (e.g. some anaesthetics) will be more widely distributed in fat tissue and possibly take longer to be metabolised and excreted from the body. The reduction in lean muscle mass indicates a reduction in muscle strength affecting most parts of the body; this reduction may also be due to lowered activity and fitness levels in some older people. Mineral content of bone reduces and is one of the main reasons for the increase in osteoporosis and fractures.

Many older people have a reduced food intake; this may be a natural consequence of being less active and a reduced lean body mass, but it can lead to a lower intake of essential nutrients such as vitamins and minerals. Although frank malnutrition is rare in elderly people it is sometimes detected. What is more significant is the mild degrees of malnutrition or deficiencies in particular substances. For example, protein energy malnutrition can impair several aspects of the immune system and there are known to be relationships between immunology, nutrition and disease in elderly people (Chandra 1990). The ability to eat food properly is also essential in maintaining adequate nutrition. Dental decay, gum recession and ill-fitting dentures are not uncommon and will interfere with dietary intake. The number of taste buds dramatically decreases as a function of age and there can be loss of up to 65% between the ages of 74 and 85 years (Holmes 1994). The sensitivity to sweet and salty tastes declines particularly; we have all come across old people who add more salt and sugar to their food than they used to. Some medications, such as antihypertensives, diuretics and antidepressants, also affect taste acuity and xerostomia (dryness of the mouth from lack of normal secretions). Put all this together with a reduction in saliva production (essential for taste and starting the digestive processes) and the possible factors such as social isolation and retirement (reduced income), and it is not difficult to see why some older people both lose their appetite and do not have an adequate diet. Eating patterns also become erratic if individuals are depressed. An excessive alcohol intake may restrict nutrient consumption too. For a fuller discussion of the nutritional requirements of elderly people see Department of Health (1992).

The sense of smell also decreases with age. This may be due to a loss of cells in the olfactory bulb and, for some, the additional long-term inhalation of toxic substances, e.g. tobacco smoke. Sensory cells in the nasal passages are reduced in number. Most aromatic compounds tested, including camphor, show an increase in threshold concentration with age (Brookbank 1990); i.e. you need a stronger concentration of the substance to smell it. Reduced sense of smell may also contribute to reduced taste sensation and appetite. For a full review of the age-related changes to taste and smell perception, refer to Bartoshuk and Weiffenback (1990).

There are many changes in the gut, both structural and functional, but it is thought that overall gut function usually remains adequate. There are changes in the ability of the liver to carry out its many complex functions and an area of concern is in the metabolism of drugs. Adverse drug reactions (ADRs) are more common in elderly people; this results from aspects such as polypharmacy, individual differences and multiple pathologies, and not simply changes in metabolism and renal clearance (for a fuller discussion see Walker & Wynne 1994). There is often some atrophy (wasting) of the muscle layers in the wall of the intestine and this can lead to weaker peristalsis and be one contributing factor in the aetiology of constipation. The efficacy of the anal sphincter reflexes can be lessened and make it difficult for an individual to distinguish between pressure from flatus or faeces. This again can be one factor involved in faecal incontinence and genuine anxieties amongst some older people about control of bowel function.

Respiratory and cardiovascular systems

The widespread changes in composition of collagen and connective tissue that has an effect all over the body, have a particular effect on these systems. Lung tissue loses its elasticity as the collagen is stiffer and there are changes in lung volumes, capacity and aspects such as peak expiratory flow rate. Overall there is a reduced surface area for gas exchange. The protective mechanisms in the lungs such as the mucociliary escalator and macrophages are less efficient, which means that chest infections are likely to be more common. This age-related loss in lung function is greater in people who smoke.

It is particularly difficult to describe 'normal ageing' changes in the cardiovascular system because such a high percentage of people have some degree of pathology, such as atherosclerosis, and also because cardiovascular function depends on the fitness or training status of people; the fitter the individual, whatever her age, the better the cardiovascular function. Changes in collagen affect the structure and function of the heart and blood vessels making them less distensible. There is some loss of pacemaker cells in the heart which means that the maximum heart rate achievable decreases. An approximation to calculate the maximum heart rate for an older person is (Astrand & Rodahl 1977):

Maximum heart rate = 210 − (0.65 × age)

Thus for a person aged 70, it would be about 165. This has importance when considering, for example, the significance of a tachycardia; a young person with a heart rate of 150 would not necessarily be a cause for concern but for a person of 70 the same heart rate would mean that her heart was working near its maximum capacity.

Considering blood flow as a whole there is a tendency for reduced perfusion of many tissues, e.g. 50% reduction in blood flow to the kidneys and, as discussed earlier, a 10–15% reduction in cerebral blood flow with increasing age. A decline in blood flow does not inevitably mean that the tissue is hypoxic as there is capacity for greater extraction of oxygen from blood, but it may mean slower removal of waste products. In developed societies there seems to be an almost universal increase in blood pressure values with age, with a greater increase in systolic than diastolic pressures. It is hard to give normal ranges of blood pressure for older people due to marked individual variability but a value such as 135/90 mmHg may be normal for an individual of 60 or 70.

Endocrine system

Changes in the endocrine system with ageing are complex. The endocrine system plays a key role in regulating most aspects of body function and therefore has an important role in maintaining homeostasis. Many factors influence hormone levels (for example, disease, drugs, smoking, diet and exercise) and so it is difficult to attribute particular changes to ageing per se. Hormone levels in the blood are determined by the combined effects of secretion rates, transport around the body, binding with receptor sites on target cells, clearance (removal) or metabolism rates, the carriage of hormones in the blood and also the effectiveness of feedback or controlling mechanisms. Thus, although there are changes with ageing, there are no dramatic consequences as physiological compensation can occur. An example of this is that there may be a decline

myoedema - hypothyroidism   ataxia - lack muscle coordination

myopathy - disease of the muscle

in secretion rate of a particular hormone, but if at the same time there is reduced clearance from the blood, the end result may be a stable plasma level. Growth hormone secretion is reduced in certain circumstances, for instance there is a decline in its secretion during sleep. The capacity to secrete glucocorticoids from the adrenal cortex is not impaired; this response is an important component of the stress response.

The output of thyroid hormones has been carefully studied with ageing. At one time it was thought that there was a correlation between low output of thyroid hormones and ageing, as some of the symptoms of hypothyroidism are similar to ageing changes (e.g. drying of skin, loss of hair). This was found not to be the case, but the prevalence of hypothyroidism does increase with age. Diagnosis of hypothyroidism is important, however, as low levels of thyroid hormones can lead to, in the most extreme cases, dementia; an association between thyroid gland function and mental activity in adults has been acknowledged for over 100 years. Myxoedema may cause neurological and psychiatric abnormalities including myopathy, ataxia, psychosis and dementia (Osterweil et al 1992). Cognition is impaired in patients with hypothyroidism but it can be reversed with thyroid replacement therapy. Osterweil et al (1992) in the USA looked at cognitive function in 54 non-demented hypothyroid patients and 30 control subjects. Subjects with hypothyroidism showed impairments in learning, word fluency, visual–spatial abilities and some aspects of attention, visual scanning and motor speed when compared to the control group. As hypothyroidism is reversible with thyroid hormone supplements, it is obviously important to exclude this as a cause of mental health problems.

Another change in the endocrine system that has clinical significance is a change in glucose tolerance. There is a progressive increase in plasma glucose levels with increasing age and this can be as much as 1.5 mg/dl per decade (Holmes 1994). This impaired glucose tolerance may result from a reduced secretion of insulin in response to glucose or the tissues themselves being less sensitive or responsive to the actions of insulin. One change that could be linked is the increase in the percentage of fat tissue, since adipose tissue is very resistant to the actions of insulin. There has been debate as to whether this change is a 'normal' ageing change or whether the individual has developed mild clinical diabetes mellitus.

Hormones are widely used for the treatment of physical health problems and many hormones have a widespread effect on the physiology of the body. For example, steroids such as cortisone are used for their anti-inflammatory effects but cortisone can also induce depression, psychosis or euphoria; again the closeness of physical and mental health problems is demonstrated. Similarly, excessive insulin given to a diabetic precipitates hypoglycaemia and along with this, irritability, anxiety and/or confusion.

Genitourinary system

There are many age-related changes in the reproductive systems in both sexes. The obvious change for women is the menopause, which occurs in the early fifties for the majority of women. The changes that ensue are mainly due to reduced level of the sex hormones and lead to the uterus shrinking, the vagina becoming smaller with reduced and altered secretions (this can lead to dryness and vaginitis). Breast tissue atrophies, ligaments relax and there is a loss of muscle tone. Oestrogen depletion is also implicated in mineral loss from bone and this can lead to osteoporosis.

Men do not show the same sharp cut-off in reproductive function. The rate of spermatogenesis slows down and there is an increase in the percentage of abnormal sperm. Secretion of androgens (the male hormones) is reduced and the prostate gland enlarges. The changes that occur do not prevent sexual intercourse and people can remain sexually active during their old age.

A progressive deterioration of renal structure and function has been shown to accompany ageing (Anderson & Brenner 1987). The ageing kidney is less able to concentrate urine and there is reduced excretory capacity, characterised by reduced glomerular filtration rates (Phillips et al 1993). Disorders of micturition also become increasingly common with advancing age. Nocturia (i.e. getting up during the night to pass urine) affects most old people. Common problems include urgency, frequency and actual leakage of urine. Urinary incontinence can be defined as the passing of urine in the wrong place, unintentionally and involuntarily (Research into Ageing 1994). Because of the nature of incontinence, it causes serious social and psychological problems to sufferers. Approximately 10–20% of elderly people living in the community suffer from incontinence with higher percentages of those in hospitals or nursing homes affected (Research Into Ageing 1994). The aetiology of incontinence is often complex and multifactorial.

There are known to be changes in the bladder itself, in the urodynamics and also in the control of bladder function which occurs within the central nervous system. Unfortunately, little is known about bladder function in 'normal' elderly people as many of the studies to date have centred around people with established incontinence (Cheater 1992). The frequency of detrusor instability (sometimes referred to as the unstable bladder) rises with age. This means that the person loses the ability to reliably inhibit the detrusor (bladder muscle) contractions and so experiences urgency and frequency (Norton 1991). There is also an age-related decline in the capacity of the bladder. Another cause of urinary problems in some elderly women is associated with atrophic changes in the vagina or urethra, possibly due to oestrogen depletion, and it can lead to an incompetent urethral sphincter. Uterine prolapse can also influence this. Incompetent sphincters can lead to stress incontinence. Prostatic hypertrophy in men can cause an obstruction to urinary outflow and the individual experiences frequency and difficulty voiding. Surgery may be required to overcome these problems.

If the detrusor muscle fails to contract to produce micturition or if the contraction is not sustained until the bladder is empty, a chronic residual collection of urine may develop (Norton 1991). This is an ideal situation for an infection to develop and urinary tract infections are common in individuals where this happens. Overflow incontinence occurs too. People with dementia often suffer from these types of problems, as do others with neurological disease, for instance after strokes. Psychological motivation is a factor, too. Restricted mobility from whatever cause will also make getting to the lavatory more difficult and sometimes an individual just cannot get there in time.

It is important to remember that incontinence is not an inevitable consequence of ageing; most elderly people remain continent all their lives (Cheater 1992). Elderly people do, however, become more likely to develop incontinence because of the changes described above. Drugs can be prescribed to treat some of the contributory factors, for example infections and some other disorders. Physiotherapy can also help with improving muscle strength in the pelvic floor, but also with general mobility.[2]

Skin and appearance

The most obvious external manifestations of ageing are in the hair and skin. The classic signs of greying hair and wrinkled skin are not simply related to chronological age though. Some individuals go grey in their thirties and this may be a family trait with a genetic basis (baldness also has a genetic component).

[2] For information, contact The Continence Foundation, 2 Doughty Street, London WC1N 2PH.

Likewise, the skin of people who have spent much time in the sun during adulthood can appear to prematurely age due, in this instance, to exposure to ultraviolet radiation, which damages the soft tissues and leads to wrinkling.

Paradoxically, the hair on the head thins but there is an increase in hairs in the nose, ears and eyebrows. Scalp hair growth rate decreases, with noticeable thinning in people in their sixties. Pigmentation is determined by the activity of melanocytes in the hair and as mentioned before, is not necessarily reliably age-related; strangely, greying of pubic and axillary hair seems to be more age-related than scalp hair (Kenney 1989). The onset of hair loss occurs in their thirties for most men and after the menopause for women.

The changes in skin structure mean that the skin becomes more delicate and more prone to damage especially, for example, by shearing forces which occur when nurses drag, rather than lift, a patient up the bed. This is due to a reduced strength of attachment between the various layers of the epidermis and dermis and the supporting tissues. There are changes in the blood flow to the skin, and thus the supply of nutrients and removal of waste products is less efficient. Topically-administered drugs are not absorbed as well either for the same reason. Changes in the connective tissue in the dermis result in poor support for the capillaries and this makes the small vessels very fragile. Spontaneous or easy bruising is common in older people. The changes in sensory functions of the skin are considered in the next section.

Special senses

Vision

The diameter of the pupil is at its maximum in the early teens, reaching its minimum by age 60, reducing the amount of light entering the eye by up to two-thirds. This leads to a rise in threshold for light perception and an increase in the level of illumination necessary for function. The reduction in pupil size may prove to be a complicating factor when performing neurological observations on an elderly client. There is a link between the retina and the pineal gland in the brain; the pineal gland secretes higher levels of melatonin at low light intensity and, as the pupil is smaller and the retina less efficient, the older person may experience persistently high levels of melatonin. It is thought that this may account for the polycyclic sleeping patterns and the increased incidence of nocturia in some elderly people.

Presbyopia, the loss of ability to accommodate for

near vision, is common due to decreased flexibility of the lens in the eye and its inability to focus the image on the retina. The lens becomes thicker and more opaque with age and results in deterioration of vision and some individuals develop cataracts. Peripheral light-sensitive rods are lost from the retina, reducing peripheral vision. The older retina is less able to respond to changes from light to dark, and colour perception is also reduced. For a full review of age-related changes in the eye, refer to Weale (1989).

Hearing

Age-related physiological degeneration of the auditory system is often referred to as presbycusis and usually results in bilateral hearing loss. Hearing is at its most efficient, in both acuity and range of perceivable frequencies, at age 10 years. At that age the upper limit of perceived frequencies is as high as 20 kHz; by age 50 years this has gone down to 14 kHz, and by age 60 years there is little useful hearing above 5 kHz (Kenney 1989). This is accompanied by loss of acuity of 40–50 dB for all frequencies above 1000 Hz.

The threshold intensity for pure tones is raised and the greatest hearing loss occurs in the higher frequencies, and these together mean that the perception of speech is particularly affected. There is also impairment of discrimination, particularly between speech and background noise; this increases with age and may be due in part to slowing of information processing and impaired memory functions.

The auditory orienting reflex is used to locate a particular source of sound or a particular voice. This becomes slower and less accurate with age, and may account for some older people's difficulty in participating in multiperson conversations. For a full review of age-related changes in the ear, refer to Gilhome Herbst (1991).

Pain and touch

Pain and touch are important protective mechanisms. The threshold for cutaneous pain caused by heat increases with age, up 12% by age 70 (Brookbank 1990), even though there appears to be no loss of the free nerve endings of the C fibres (Kenney 1989). This is probably due to changes in pain receptors in the skin and to greater heat dispersion in older skin. Changes like these may lead to impairment of the behavioural response to change in environmental temperature.

The touch threshold varies all over the body surface, but when comparing equivalent skin areas, touch threshold increases with age. There is a loss of encapsulated receptors and of Merkel's disks (which respond to light touch), but there is no apparent loss of free nerve endings.

Balance

The degeneration of the vestibular system with age is considered moderate when compared with the extent of hearing loss. There is cell loss both in the organs detecting the position of the head and in the organs detecting motion change. There is little change in the number of neurones in the vestibular nerve. Elderly people are more likely to report episodes of vertigo, which could be related to processing defects in the CNS or to impaired detection of motion changes. Vestibular function is also closely associated with visual function, so defects of balance and dizziness may result from a failure of coordination with visual input or poor visual input in general. Balance also depends on proprioceptor input from joints and coordination of all sensory inputs in the cerebellum.

Speech

Unclear speech is often related to severe hearing loss, ill fitting or absent dentures, confusion, disorientation and, for some, aspects such as English as a second language. Social isolation may also lead to a lack of practice, so that conversational skills are lost. Many illnesses influence speech; strokes and Parkinson's disease are just two examples. The effect of these and other disease processes on speech and language are discussed in Chapter 17.

Sensory deprivation

As discussed earlier, sensory deprivation may in itself be a causal factor in the development of Alzheimer's disease. It can also exaggerate existing personality traits, and distort perceptions of shape, size, colour and time (Vernon 1961). Emotional changes can also occur, such as increased boredom, restlessness, irritability, anxiety and panic (Soloman 1961). In extreme hallucinations, delusions and confusion of sleeping and waking states may also occur. Hebb (1949), in a classic series of studies, was able to demonstrate that monotony produced disruption in the capacity to learn.

MOBILITY AND PHYSICAL FITNESS

Mobility is essential for a person to remain independent. Mobility can range from 70-year-olds fit enough to run a marathon to people who can just about manage activities of daily living, such as dressing themselves, and can just about walk far enough to go to the toilet. There are very many factors involved in mobility which relate to intrinsic ageing changes whilst others are more to do with lack of use or deconditioning (becoming unfit) as a consequence of a sedentary lifestyle (Bassey 1978). Of course, pathology or disease processes such as arthritis, or heart failure, are of significance too, as is poor vision.

Mobility depends on stamina, strength, suppleness and skill, and there can be changes in several of these. There is a well-documented age-related loss of muscle strength and power, due to a loss of muscle fibres. This accounts for the lower lean body muscle mass discussed in the nutrition section. Lower limb muscles, especially the large thigh (quadriceps) muscles, are important for walking, climbing stairs, getting up out of a chair and in maintaining balance. It seems that the quadriceps is particularly vulnerable to age-associated loss of strength from the 5th decade onwards (Grimley Evans et al 1992). Upper limb strength is essential for manual dexterity, dressing, feeding and everyday activities of living. This loss of strength and power is minimised by regular physical activity (Edwards & Larson 1992). The age-related changes in muscle strength and reduced exercise tolerence means that elderly people will be living at or near thresholds of physical ability, needing only a minor further reduction (due say to an episode of illness) to render them dependent (Young 1986).

The ability to sustain activity is known as stamina and depends on oxygen and nutrient delivery to the active muscles. There is a loss of stamina with increasing age and this may be due to either intrinsic metabolic changes within muscle or to possible changes in the delivery of oxygen to muscle, i.e. changes in the respiratory or cardiovascular systems. The completion of a task requires a skill, which is mainly of central nervous system origin. Walking, for example, requires coordination of muscles and nerves, feedback information from peripheral proprioceptors in the connective tissue and joints and input from the cerebellum to maintain balance and avoid falls. Reaction times are also slowed down in older people, due to a combination of slower nerve conduction and slower central processing, and so coping with an unexpected stumble takes longer and may lead to a fall in an older person. Deterioration in vision and hearing also contribute to age-associated decline in skill.

Suppleness is influenced by joint mobility, tendons, ligaments and muscles themselves. Muscle stiffness is common in older people. Many of these changes result from the change in structure of the connective tissue. Osteoarthritis is common in older people and can lead to a painful restriction of movement. This can alter the gait, especially if linked with the knee or hip, and frequently leads to problems with activities of daily living.

There is research evidence (Edwards & Larson 1992) that appropriate exercise benefits even sedentary elderly people who begin at an advanced age. Benefits appear to include increased muscle strength and power, increased stamina and suppleness. Edwards and Larson also suggest that it may slow or prevent some of the intellectual and psychomotor decline which is associated with ageing. Despite the fact that the benefits of exercise have been known about for some time (Bassey 1978) exercise does not seem to be incorporated into the care programmes by health professionals (Young 1986). If interested in exercise classes designed for elderly people contact EXTEND.[3]

RELATIONSHIP BETWEEN PHYSICAL HEALTH AND COGNITIVE FUNCTIONING

Is there any relationship between health and cognitive function? Certainly conditions such as hypoxia, anaemia, transient infection, hypothyroidism or nutritional deficiency can lead to changes, sometimes dramatic, in cognitive function (Christensen et al 1994). However, are the more subtle changes in cognitive function a result of neuropathology, ageing changes or poor physical health status? There is no clear answer to these questions and different views are held. It is obvious that mental function is crucial to a successful old age; maintaining an independent lifestyle depends on adequate cognitive function as much as maintenance of physical health. Physical and social wellbeing are inextricably interlinked. In fact Schaie (1990) goes as far as to say that an individual is able to maintain cognitive abilities provided that physical health is also maintained. Some have claimed that declines in intellectual functioning are due to the effects of ill-health rather than consequent on the biological ageing processes and others take a middle line. It is thus artificial to consider biological factors on their own; an integrated approach is needed to study this effectively. Socioeconomic and environmental factors also play a vital part in determining the physical health of any individual; these factors may

---

[3] EXTEND, 22 Maltings Drive, Wheathampstead, Hertfordshire AL4 8QJ. (Movement to music for men and women over age 60 and disabled people of all ages.)

include housing, diet, previous experiences in earlier life (including as far back as intrauterine factors (Barker 1992)) and lifestyle. This is a very complex area.

A study in Australia by Christensen et al (1994) examined the health status and cognitive performance in a sample of 708 elderly people (aged over 70) living in the community. The study aimed to investigate whether at least some of the age differences in cognitive function could be attributable to health factors. Their findings were complex, but on the whole did not support the hypothesis that health mediates declines in cognitive processing with age. These results are consistent with the view that cognitive decline may be attributed to neuropathology rather than to the secondary effects of other medical conditions.

There may also be a difference between what individuals themselves perceive as factors affecting health and what the health professionals think is important. A large Swedish study (Lindgren et al 1994) looked at the prevalence of a range of problems and their effects on wellbeing. Eyesight and hearing problems were common in the study, but they did not appear to affect perceived health to any extent. Mobility problems and sleeping problems had a greater impact. The most important factors related to perceived health were activity score, contentment and mobility problems. Contentment was affected by activity score and loneliness and the latter was in turn affected by age and type of dwelling. The implications of these findings are that possibly more attention should be focused on improving factors that improve old people's satisfaction rather than on marginal improvements in their medical situation. What matters is very individual again and so should be assessed for each person.

Another approach is to see whether any form of intervention could postpone functional decline in ageing. The large-scale longitudinal study in Gothenburg, Sweden, has shown that lifestyle factors such as smoking, alcohol abuse, social isolation and bereavement influenced both the prevalence of definable diseases, and the rate and functional consequences of ageing (Svanborg 1993). As part of the ongoing research, a multidisciplinary designed intervention study was set up to see whether the physical or mental functioning of the individuals could be maintained or improved, or at least retard the development of disablement, and increase the sense of wellbeing and quality of life. The preliminary results are encouraging (Svanborg 1993) and show that positive effects can be produced. The resources that went into the Swedish study will not be widely available, but there are valuable insights about what can be achieved.

CONCLUSION

This chapter has discussed the biological basis for ageing changes together with the biological aspects of mental health function. There is a close relationship between physical changes and mental health changes and in many instances both need to be considered simultaneously.

Knowledge of the normal ageing processes is an essential baseline for assessment and understanding effects on physical and mental capabilities. Appropriate interventions, based on aspects such as diet and exercise as discussed in the chapter, can have positive outcomes in maintaining or maximising the independence of elderly people.

REFERENCES

Anderson B, Brenner B 1987 The ageing kidney structure, functions, mechanisms and therapeutic implications. Journal of American Geriatrics Society 35: 590–593

Astrand P, Rodahl K 1977 Textbook of work physiology. McGraw-Hill, New York

Barker D (ed) 1992 Fetal and infant origins of adult disease. British Medical Journal, London

Bartoshuk L M, Weiffenbach J M 1990 Chemical senses and ageing. In: Schneider E L, Rowe J W (eds) Handbook of the biology of aging, 3rd edn. Academic Press, San Diego

Bassey E J 1978 Age, inactivity and some physiological responses to exercise. Gerontology 24: 66–77

Bondareff W, Mountjoy C Q, , Roth M 1982 Loss of neurons of origin of the adrenergic projection to cerebral cortex (nucleus locus cœruleus) in senile dementia. Neurology 32: 164–168

Bondy S C, Martin J, Halsall L C, McKee M 1989 Increased fragility of neuronal membranes with ageing. Experimental Neurology 103: 61–63

Braak H, Braak E 1986 Ratio of pyramidal cells versus non-pyramidal cells in the human frontal isocortex and changes in ratio with aging and Alzheimer's disease. In: Swaab D F, Fliers E, Mirmiran M, Van Gool W A, Van Haaren F (eds) Progress in brain research. Elsevier Science Publications, BV

Brody H 1955 Organisation of the cerebral cortex, III: a study of aging in the human cerebral cortex. Journal of Comparative Neurology 102: 511–556

Brookbank J W 1990 The biology of aging. Harper & Row, New York

Carola R, Harley J P, Noback C R 1992 Human anatomy and physiology, 2nd edn. McGraw Hill, New York

Chandra R K 1990 The relation between immunology, nutrition and disease in elderly people. Age and Ageing 19: S25–31

Cheater F 1992 The aetiology of urinary incontinence. In: Roe B (ed) Clinical nursing management – the promotion and management of continence. Prentice Hall, London

Cheng S V, Nadeau J H, Tanzi R E et al 1988 Comparative mapping of DNA markers from the familial Alzheimer's disease and Down's syndrome regions of human chromosome 21 to mouse chromosomes 16 and 17. Proceedings of the National Academy of Science 85: 6032–6036

Christensen H, Jorm A F, Henderson A S, Mackinnon A J, Korten A E, Scott L R 1994 The relationship between health and cognitive functioning in a sample of elderly people in the community. Age and Ageing 23: 204–212

Coleman P D, Flood D G 1986 Dendritic proliferation in the aging brain as a compensatory repair mechanism. In: Swaab D F, Fliers E, Mirmiran W, Van Gool W A, Van Haaren F (eds) Progress in brain research. Elsevier Science Publications, BV

Coleman P D, Flood D G 1987 Neuron numbers and dendritic extent in normal ageing and Alzheimer's disease. Neurobiology of Aging 8: 521–545

Collins K J, Exton-Smith A N, James M H, Oliver D 1980 Functional changes in autonomic nervous responses with ageing. Age and Ageing 9: 17–24

Cotman C W, Nieto-Sampedro M, Harris E 1981 Synapse replacement in the nervous system of adult vertebrates. Physiological Reviews 61: 684–784

Cotman C W, Anderson K J 1988 Synaptic plasticity and functional stabilization in the hippocampal formation: possible role in Alzheimer's disease. In: Waxman S (ed) Physiological basis for functional recovery in neurological disease. Raven, New York

Curcio C A, Buell S J, Coleman P D 1982 Morphology of the central nervous system: not all downhill. In: Mortimer J A, Pirozzolo F J, Maletta G J (eds) The ageing motor system. Praeger Press, New York

Dekoninck W J 1985 Brain metabolism and ageing. In: Bergener M, Ermini M, Stahelin H B (eds) Thresholds in ageing. Academic Press, London

Department of Health 1992 The nutrition of elderly people. HMSO, London

Doll R 1993 Review: Alzheimer's disease and environmental aluminium. Age and Ageing 22: 138–153

Edwards K E, Larson E B 1992 Benefits of exercise for older adults. Clinics in Geriatric Medicine 8: 35–50

Elbe R, Giacobini E, Scarsella G F 1987 Cholinesterases in cerebrospinal fluid: a longitudinal study in Alzheimer's disease. Archives of Neurology 44: 403–407

Francis P T, Palmer A M, Sims N R 1985 Neurochemical studies of early onset Alzheimer's disease. New England Journal of Medicine 313: 7–11

Gearing B, Johnson M, Heller T (eds) 1988 Mental health problems in old age. John Wiley, Chichester

Gilhome Herbst K 1991 Hearing. In: Redfern S J (ed) Nursing elderly people, 2nd edn. Churchill Livingstone, Edinburgh

Goudsmit E, Fliers E, Swaab D F 1990 Ageing of the brain and Alzheimer's disease. In: Horan M A, Brouwer A (eds) Gerontology: approaches to biomedical and clinical research. Edward Arnold, London

Greig C A, Young A, Skelton D A, Pippet E, Butler F M M, Mahmud S M 1994 Exercise studies with elderly volunteers. Age and Ageing 23: 185–189

Grimley Evans J 1992 From plaque to placement: a model for Alzheimer's disease. Age and Ageing 21: 77–80

Grimley Evans J 1993 Metabolic switches in ageing. Age and Ageing 22: 79–81

Grimley Evans J, Goldacre M J, Hodkinson M, Lamb S, Savory M 1992 Health: abilities and wellbeing in the third age. The Carnegie inquiry into the third age: research paper no 9. The Carnegie United Kingdom Trust, Dumfermline

Hall T C, Miller A K H, Corselis J A N 1975 Variations in the human Purkinje cell population according to age and sex. Neuropathology and Applied Neurobiology 1: 267–292

Hauw J J, Duychaerts C, Partridge M 1986 Neuropathological aspects of brain aging and SDAT. In: Courtols Y, Faucheux B, Forette B, Knook D L, Treton J A (eds) Modern trends in ageing, vol. 147. John Libby Eurotext, London

Haug H 1984 Macroscopic and microscopic morphometry of the human brain and cortex: a survey in the light of new results. Brain Pathology 1: 123–149

Hebb P O 1949 The organisation of behaviour. Wiley, New York

Herbert R A 1991 The biology of human ageing. In: Redfern S (ed) Nursing elderly people, 2nd edn. Churchill Livingstone, Edinburgh

Holmes S 1994 Nutrition and older people: a matter of concern. Nursing Times 90, 42: 31–33

Horvath T B, Davis K L 1990 Central nervous system disorders in ageing. In: Schneider E L, Rowe J W (eds) Handbook of the biology of ageing, 3rd edn. Academic Press, San Diego

Jagger C, Clarke M, Book A J 1989 Mental and physical health of elderly people: five year follow-up of a total population. Age and Ageing 18: 77–82

Johnson H A 1985 Relations between normal ageing and disease. Raven Press, New York

Kalache A, Warnes T, Hunter D 1988 Promoting health among elderly people. King Edward's Hospital Fund for London, London

Katzman R, Terry R D (eds) 1983 The neurology of ageing. Davis, Philadelphia

Katzman R 1988 Normal aging and the brain. News in Physiological Sciences 3: 197–200

Kemper T 1984 Neuroanatomical and neuropathological changes in normal aging and in dementia. In: Albert M L (ed) Clinical neurology of ageing. Oxford University Press

Kenney R A 1989 Physiology of ageing: a synopsis, 3rd edn. Year Book Medical Publishers, Chicago

Kirkwood T B L, Holliday R 1986 Ageing as a consequence of natural collection. In: Bittles A H, Collins K J (eds) The biology of human ageing. Cambridge University Press, Cambridge

Lindgren A, Svardudd K, Tibblin G 1994 Factors related to perceived health among elderly people: the Albertina project. Age and Ageing 23: 328–333

Marcyniuk B, Mann D M A, Yates P O 1986 The topography of cell loss from locus cœruleus in Alzheimer's disease. Journal of Neurological Science 76: 335–345

Merz P A, Wisniewski H M, Somerville R A 1983 Ultrastructural morphology of amyloid fibrils from neuritic and amyloid plaques. Acta Neuropathologica 60: 113–124

Morgan D G, May P C 1990 Age-related changes in synaptic neurochemistry. In: Schneider E L, Rowe J W (eds) Handbook of the biology of aging, 3rd edn. Academic Press, San Diego

Mountjoy C Q, Roth M, Evans N J R, Evans H M 1983 Cortical neuronal counts in normal elderly controls and demented patients. Neurobiology of Aging 4: 1–11

Mountjoy C Q, Rossor M N, Iversen L L, Roth M 1984 Correlation of cortical cholinergic and GABA deficits with quantitative neuropathological findings in senile dementia. Brain 107: 507–518

Norton C 1991 Eliminating. In: Redfern S (ed) Nursing elderly people, 2nd edn. Churchill Livingstone, Edinburgh

Osterweil D, Syndulko K, Cohen S et al 1992 Cognitive function in non-demented older adults with hypothyroidism. Journal of the American Geriatrics Society 40: 325–335

Pearson R C A, Gatter K C, Powell T P S 1983 Retrograde degeneration in the basal nucleus in monkey and man. Brain Research 261: 321–326

Perry R, Perry E 1982 The aging brain and its pathology. In: Levy R, Post F (eds) The psychiatry of late life. Blackwell, Oxford

Perry T L, Yong V W, Bergeron C, Hansen S, Jones K 1987 Amino acids, glutathione, and gluthatione transferase activity in the brains of patients with Alzheimer's disease. Annals of Neurology 21: 331–336

Phillips P A, Johnson C I, Gray L 1993 Disturbed fluid and electrolyte homeostasis following dehydration in elderly people. Age and Ageing 22: 26–33

Price D L, Whitehouse P J, Struble R G et al 1982 Alzheimer's disease and Down's syndrome. In: Sinex F M, Merril C R (eds) Alzheimer's disease, Down's syndrome, and aging. Annals of the New York Academy of Science 396: 145

Price D L, Altschuler R J, Struble R G 1986 Sequestration of tubulin in neurons in Alzheimer's disease. Brain Research 385: 305–310

Procter A W, Middlemiss D N, Bowen D M 1987 Selective loss of serotonin recognition sites in the parietal cortex in Alzheimer's disease. In: Gearing B, Johnson M, Heller T (eds) 1988 Mental health problems in old age. John Wiley, Chichester

Research into Ageing 1994 Urinary incontinence. Focus on Healthy Ageing Leaflet. Research into Ageing, London

Roth M, Wischik C M, Evans N, Mountjoy C Q 1985 Convergence and cohesion of recent neurobiological findings in relation to Alzheimer's disease and their bearing on its aetiological basis. In: Bergener M, Ermini M, Stahelin H B (eds) Thresholds in ageing. Academic Press, London

Schaie K 1990 Intellectual development in adulthood. In: Birren J, Schaie K (eds) Handbook of the phycology of ageing, 3rd edn. Academic Press, San Diego

Soloman P (ed) 1961 Sensory deprivation. Harvard University Press, Cambridge, Mass

Struble R G, Cash L C, Whitehouse P J, Price D L 1982 Cholinergic innervation of neuritic plaques. Science 216: 413

Svanborg A 1993 A medical-social intervention in a 70-year-old Swedish population: is it possible to postpone functional decline in ageing? The Journals of Gerontology 48 (special issue): 84–88

Teravainen H, Calne D B 1983 Motor system in normal aging and Parkinson's disease. In: Katzman R, Terry R D (eds) Neurology of aging. Davis, Philadelphia

Terry R D 1980 Structural changes in senile dementia of the Alzheimer's type. In: Amaducci L, Davison A N, Antuono P (eds) Aging of the brain and dementia. Ageing Series 13. Raven, New York

Terry R D, DeTeresa R, Hansen L A 1987 Neocortical cell counts in normal human adult aging. Annals of Neurology 21: 530–539

Tomlinson B E 1977 The pathology of dementia. In: Wells C E (ed) Dementia. Davis, Philadelphia

Trygstad L 1994 The need to know: biological learning needs identified by practicing psychiatric nurses. Journal of Psychosocial Nursing 32(2): 13–18

Vernon J 1961 The effect of human isolation on some perceptual and motor skills. In: Soloman P (ed) Sensory deprivation. Harvard University Press, Cambridge, Mass

Walker J, Wynne H 1994 Review: the frequency and severity of adverse drug reaction in elderly people. Age and Ageing 23: 255–259

Weale R 1989 Eyes and age: views on visual health promotion. In: Warnes A M (ed) 1989 Human ageing and later life: multidisciplinary perspectives. Edward Arnold, London

Whitson J S, Selkoe D J, Cotman C W 1989 Amyloid protein enhances the survival of hippocampal neurons in vitro. Science 243: 1488–1490

Wisniewski H M, Merz P A, Iqbal K 1984 Ultrastructure of paired helical filaments of Alzheimer's neurofibrillary tangle. J Neuropathol Exp Neurol 43: 643–656

Yamaura H, Ito M, Kubota K, Matsuzawa T 1980 Brain atrophy during aging: a quantitative study with computed tomography. Journal of Gerontology 35: 492–498

Young A 1986 Exercise physiology in geriatric practice. Acta Medica Scandinavica Supplement 711: 227–232

RECOMMENDED READING

Brookbank J W 1990 The biology of aging. Harper & Row, New York. *This book covers general issues related to the biology of ageing, considering effects on all the body systems. It is easy to use and well referenced.*

Department of Health 1992 The Nutrition of Elderly People. HMSO, London. *This contains a comprehensive review of all aspects of the nutritional needs of elderly people.*

Grimley Evans J, Goldacre M J, Hodkinson M, Lamb S, Savory M 1992 Health: abilities and wellbeing in the third age. The Carnegie inquiry into the third age, research paper no 9. The Carnegie United Kingdom Trust, Dumfermline. *An excellent very readable report considering all aspects of health in the third age (the age range of 50–74 years). Aspects covered include disease, active life expectancy and disability, psychological changes, fitness and exercise, special senses, physical disability, mental wellbeing and major risk factors.*

Kenney R A 1989 Physiology of ageing: a synopsis. Year Book Medical Publishers. Chicago. *Although getting rather old, this is a valuable sensible-sized book covering all aspects of the physiology of ageing. It concentrates very much on the normal ageing processes rather than diseases.*

Schneider E L, Rowe J W (eds) 1990 Handbook of the biology of ageing, 3rd edn. Academic Press, San Diego. *A detailed research-based edited book. It is not an easy book to read but it does contain up-to-date relevant (mainly animal based) research. Invaluable as a reference book but not one to browse through.*

Trygstad L 1994 The need to know: biological learning needs identified by practicing psychiatric nurses. Journal of Psychosocial Nursing 32(2): 13–18. *An enlightened article reviewing a research study undertaken on psychiatric nurses in the USA, ascertaining the biological sciences knowledge base important for working with clients with mental health problems.*

Understanding mental health problems in later life

SECTION CONTENTS

4

Developmental problems in later life

Lynette Rentoul

INTRODUCTION

The first part of this book is concerned with normal aspects of ageing, including its biological, social and psychological parameters. It is important when seeking to understand the wealth of experiences of older people to acknowledge that for the vast majority of elderly people, growing old is not associated with pronounced problems of mental health although, as with other stages of life, there are significant challenges and hurdles to be overcome. Much of the literature in both sociology and psychology addresses the positive way in which elderly people face the transitions of this stage of their lives. However, for some elderly people the challenges can be great, and tremendous strain is placed on their capacity to cope effectively. As a consequence they experience increasing distress, anxiety, demoralisation and loneliness. In some instances, this increasing distress is the precursor of pronounced mental health problems in old age, and in others it represents a time of increased suffering but which, nonetheless, is finally dealt with constructively.

This chapter expands on the introduction to the material in Chapter 2, by exploring the interface between increasing distress and problems of mental health and the reasons why some elderly people are particularly vulnerable when confronting later life challenges that make them, as a consequence, increasingly prone to mental health problems. The vulnerabilities of elderly people relate to their increasing biological proneness to problems in cognitive functioning, to the social realities of many old people which make them more likely to experience loneliness, prejudice and isolation, and to the psychological transitions and stresses that demand a high level of resilience and resourcefulness.

Attention in this chapter focuses upon the

psychological transitions and stresses that pose problems for many elderly people. The material should be viewed as providing a link between the normal and the frankly pathological aspects of old age. By focusing on developmental problems, losses and vulnerabilities in old age, this chapter sets the scene for making sense of many of the more severe mental health problems witnessed in elderly people discussed in Part 3.

We begin with a discussion of the classic developmental psychology literature on old age and tackle in turn the views of the key authors Erikson, Butler, Coleman and Bromley, who have made a substantial contribution to the development of our main theme, that of late life transition or crisis, internal conflicts and problems of living that need to be confronted. The second part of the chapter focuses on stress and social support in old age and examines the impact of these factors on physical and mental health outcomes. A key issue here is a loss in old age which is examined in its manifold forms.

The emphasis in much of the classic developmental psychology literature on old age is on the notion of transition or crisis (see, for example, Erikson 1950), the internal conflicts and problems to be confronted. Erikson outlined developmental crises across the life cycle which were bipolar in nature and which provided a framework for understanding positive elements of growth in adulthood and old age, as well as negative and pathological aspects. The final transition in life he called 'integrity versus despair', illustrating his view that in old age there is the possibility of either health and wisdom or psychological suffering including misery, despair, depression, regret and disappointment.

Butler (1963) explored the same theme in his work on the life review. For him, the search for meaning and integration in old age is associated with either strength and wisdom or misery, depression and anxiety. These ideas are only sketchily explored by these authors although researchers have subjected them to further scrutiny. Evidence supports the view that many elderly people are immensely resourceful, lead positive and full lives in old age and continue to enjoy positive relationships and support. However, it is also clear that, for some, the more negative picture portrayed by both Erikson and Butler in their discussions of 'despair', and the pathological aspects of the life review, accurately portrays the miseries and unhappinesses of old age.

Furthermore, in the work of those authors particularly interested in health psychology (see, for example, Markides & Cooper 1989), it is clear that although, for the majority of elderly people, stresses such as retirement, ill health, relocation and widowhood do not pose real threats to their mental health status, for some elderly people these issues do represent real hurdles to enjoying and adapting to the challenges of old age. If the hurdles are not surmounted, mental ill health results.

An important question is how does one distinguish between those elderly people who adapt positively to the challenges of old age and those who do not? What are the variables that are important in determining healthy and constructive responses to the changes inherent in growing old? The answers to these questions are not straightforward; indeed, understanding resilience and resourcefulness at any stage of the human life cycle poses problems for the researcher. Why, for example, do some children cope positively with the impact of childhood deprivation and others not? These issues are increasingly being addressed by researchers in health psychology and developmental psychology, and attempts at teasing out the important variables are being made.

It is important to recognise that there are immense individual differences in response to stress, whether it is the stress of increased pain and ill health in old age or the stress of loss, such as loss of function, loss of purpose, loss of job, loss of friends or loss of a loved one. Factors which are known to be important in determining outcomes of coping with stress include:

- past experience and personality
- the way in which past stresses were dealt with
- resources available to the individual
- the amount of friendship, love and support available
- the meaning that current circumstances have for the individual.

Stresses that are associated with mental health problems among the elderly, that have been the focus of empirical study and critical review, include:

- widowhood
- other significant losses
- relocation
- retirement
- ill health.

Variables that are considered to be important in determining the impact of stress in old age include:

- the extent to which the individual enjoys close and intimate relationships and social support
- the financial and practical resources available
- the significance and personal meaning of past memories.

DEVELOPMENTAL CRISES AND MENTAL HEALTH PROBLEMS

In health psychology, where the work is dominated by cognitive–behavioural approaches to understanding the impact of stress, the emphasis of the work on old age is on environmental stressors commonly associated with this period of life. In developmental psychology on the other hand, much of the work has focused on the role in internal conflicts and predictable transitions, which are contingent upon the biological, psychological and social imperatives of growing old. For example, the work of Erikson (1950) and Butler (1963) on facing death and finding meaning in life at life's end highlights the significance of internal conflict and the way this can provoke feelings of anxiety and depression. Peck's (1968) work on finding personal meaning beyond work in retirement and on maintaining a sense of self in the face of declining health and physical decline, also illustrates this approach. Internal conflict and its relationship to increasing unhappiness and anxiety in old age can also be seen in many of the case studies described by Coleman (1986) in his research on the meaning and significance of reminiscence in elderly people.

THE WORK OF ERIKSON: INTEGRITY VERSUS DESPAIR

Erikson's (1950) understanding of personality development in old age is discussed at some length in Chapter 2. Here we reiterate his final stage of development and summarise what can go wrong. In Erikson's view, accepting the realities of life, including regrets and disappointments, and facing the closeness of death pose real problems for some elderly people. These things are particularly difficult to accept if there is the feeling that life was too short, or that it was wasted or that regrets are overwhelming. The fear of death in such instances can be great and can show itself in many forms. This feeling of despair is graphically described by Erikson. There is the sense that time is running out, that past opportunities were wasted. Indeed, there can be an overwhelming sense that life itself was wasted, and that at the end of life there is no opportunity to do things differently, to make good past regrets, losses and disappointments; that there are no other routes to gaining a sense of integrity. In Erikson's words:

The lack of this accrued ego integration is signified by fear of death; the one and only life cycle is not accepted as the ultimate of life. Despair expresses the feeling that the time is now short, too short for the attempt to start another life and

to try out alternate roads to integrity. Disgust hides despair, if often only in the form of 'a thousand little disgusts' which do not add up to one big remorse.   (Erikson 1950, p. 260)

In a severe form this may find expression through a deep depression and suicidal intent or through severe anxiety, obsessional ruminations, increased aggression and irritability or increased phobic reactions.

THE WORK OF BUTLER: THE LIFE REVIEW

Butler (1963) organised his ideas on the conflicts of old age within the framework of the concept of the life review. For him, the desire to make sense of life leads elderly people to review their life and it is this looking back over life that may provoke negative and pathological reactions. For example, in extreme cases the older person's preoccupation with the past may cause panic, terror, or even suicide. To quote from Butler (1963): 'I propose that this process (The Life Review) helps account for the increased reminiscence in the aged, *that it contributes to the occurrence of certain late-life disorders, particularly depression,* and that it participates in the evolution of such characteristics as candour, serenity, and wisdom among certain of the aged'. (Butler in Allman & Jaffe 1977, p. 329, my italics).

Butler suggests that the tasks of the life review are associated with both normal and healthy aspects as well as with distressing and pathological aspects of growing old. It is to the latter that we now turn in an attempt to unravel ways in which the challenges of growing old, in particular the challenges of facing death and decline and evaluating the significance of life, can lead to mild or severe mental health problems.

Butler, who was a psychiatrist, relied heavily on detailed case material in illuminating his discussion. He illustrates the themes of the fears about death, and what may come afterwards, in terms of judgements about the way in which one led one's life with reference to dream and nightmare material. He used dream material, derived from case studies, to illustrate the ways in which many elderly people fear death, and regret the way that they have led their lives. Many of the dreams cited in his work illuminate the fears of judgement and of death. The notion of judgement at the end of one's life is built into many religions, and appears to play an important role in the psychopathology of older people. For example, Butler (1963) cites the following dream to exemplify this point:

I dreamt that I had died and my soul was going up and when I reached the top I saw a great, huge statue – or living man – sitting there, and then a second man came over to me and asked, 'What do you want?' I answered, 'I want to get in here.' So the big man said, 'Let him in.' But then the second man asked, 'What did you do in the other world?' I told him a great deal about myself and was asked, 'What else?' I told of an occasion in which I helped an old lady. 'That's not enough. Take him away.' It was God judging me. I was very afraid and I woke up.   (Butler in Allman & Jaffe 1977, p. 330)

The significance of death, and the way in which facing it at the end of one's life may provoke high levels of anxiety and despair, tends to be underestimated and its significance is minimised by many health care workers working with elderly clients. Indeed, this may be a further manifestation of the tendency to deny the reality of death (see, for example, Kubler-Ross 1972). Butler argues that there are many reasons why death becomes increasingly an issue for concern among elderly people, partly because of the nearness of death, partly because during retirement there is more time for reflection and introspection and partly because the opportunity that work afforded to deny the reality of death has been removed.

The manifestation of the life review takes many forms, from a gradual and silent process of coming to terms with life and increasing recognition that life is coming to an end, to a more extreme form in which the struggle is apparent, and which may be accompanied by anxiety, guilt, despair and depression. Even in the mild form the work is active, though the process may be gradual, in which the content of one's life is allowed to slowly unfold. Under these circumstances there is often great pleasure accompanying the process as well as mild nostalgia and regret. In an extreme form, however, the anxieties associated with the task may be so great that it may involve an obsessive preoccupation with the past and may proceed to a state approximating terror and even result in suicide.

The life review may appear gradually in stray and apparently insignificant thoughts about the past and one's history. These thoughts may continue to appear in sudden spurts or may increasingly simply take over the person's inner world. They may undergo transformations as the past is progressively reintegrated and reorganised. Butler (1963) cites examples of the way in which elderly people have talked to him about the process. For example, a 76-year-old man said: 'My life is in the background of my mind much of the time; it cannot be any other way. Thoughts of the past play upon me; sometimes I play with them, encourage and savour them; at other times I dismiss them.' (Butler in Allman & Jaffe 1977, p. 331).

Butler relies not only on dream, day-dream and fantasy material, but also cites the way in which mirrors may be used by elderly people to look directly at themselves, as though issues that could normally be avoided or defended against force themselves to the fore when one is confronted with one's physical image. This point is also emphasised by Jaques (1965) in his work on the mid-life crisis. He suggests that the reality of growing old can no longer be denied, even in mid-life, when the physical manifestations are so apparent in mirror images of ourselves. Many people in mid-life find these manifestations, such as the sagging of the skin, the greying of one's hair and the age lines which mark the face, shocking. Butler illustrates the role of the mirror in prompting anxiety in the face of the recognition of being old in one elderly woman in the following way: 'I was passing by my mirror. I noticed how old I was. My appearance, well, it prompted me to think of death – and of my past – what I hadn't done, what I had done wrong' (cited in Allman & Jaffe 1977, p. 332).

Another patient was seen shouting angrily at herself in the mirror whilst in hospital. She explained to the nurse that she was really angry with herself because of things she had done in her life, then when she passed the mirror it felt like she was 'looking herself over'. She dealt with this eventually by avoiding all mirrors, because the pain of seeing herself became unbearable. It seems that concrete images of ourselves may undermine defensive manœuvres and leave us feeling psychologically naked, to face ourselves and our past lives, including the sources of guilt and regret.

Since the life review is associated with positive and normative elements as well as pathological ones, an important question is, what distinguishes those older people who gain some strength and pleasure from the process from those who appear to be undermined by it, and may thus suffer greatly in the face of the challenges it provokes?

Butler offers a number of reasons, which have a bearing on developmental issues of old age that go far beyond the process of the life review. First, he considers the current context to be important. Those who appear most severely affected tend to lead isolated lives in old age. They are people whose lives have been far more affected by an increasing contraction of life's attachments and have experienced significant psychosocial discontinuities, such as forced retirement or the death of a spouse. But equally important, in holding the key to understanding the impact of the process of reviewing life and why it is so painful for some individuals, is the life-long character of the individual and the way it developed at all stages of the life cycle.

With implicit reference to Erikson's (1950) work, Butler suggests that the life review is very painful if the older person has increasing insight but when this partial insight leads only to a sense of waste and futility. The painful insight at the end of one's life, that one never really lived, or that in viewing oneself realistically for the first time one feels completely inadequate or in some major way falls short of one's ideals, can lead to a sense of despair, misery and depression. It is often difficult to work therapeutically with such people because the losses are often not tangible; also the insights may be so unacceptable they are hard to communicate to a health care worker, or if they are communicated they may be very hard for both the elderly person and the carer to face. It is these more extreme examples that Butler feels may be associated with severe depression and suicide in later life (see Ch. 8 for further discussion of depression and Ch. 9 on suicide in later life).

A further group which may be vulnerable to psychological problems in later life are those who always place great store by the future, and tend to avoid the present. Those older people who fail to appreciate the things around them in the present and always hope for something that the future might bring, are also vulnerable to later-life depression. This view places great strain on old age, since this period of life may not be able to deliver all that is hoped for.

Finally, those who have lived their lives in such a way, either by cruelty or disregard of others, and there have genuine reasons for regret, may have real problems in looking at their past and accepting their lives in the face of death. Wicked and thoughtless acts in the past cannot be changed, they can only be lived with. For these people the guilt that they feel is real and there is no way of reversing the process. The only way they can conceptualise reparation is to wish they had lived their lives differently. The only way out of this dilemma is to think of forgiveness and redemption in a very different way, so that symbolic reparation can be achieved and their past lives accepted.

There are many ways that reparation can be achieved symbolically; for example, forgiveness for one's own past cruel or destructive deeds might be achieved by living life more generously in old age, and giving something back to the younger generations, such as grandchildren. Living life more selflessly in old age can help to repair cruelty and meanness in earlier phases of life. If the distress is facing the death of a loved person, then reparation is not in terms of bringing them, literally, back to life but rather giving, metaphorically, life to them in other ways. For example, living in a way that would have pleased the lost person, incorporating the positive aspects of the relationship into a new way of living; recognising that things are not the same after someone loved dies, but that character and future relationships can be enhanced by the experience.

Vulnerable old people may find the challenges described by Butler in the context of his work on the life review overwhelming, and distress and marked psychopathology may result (see also Ch. 2). The commonest manifestations include increased regret, anxiety, obsessional ruminations and depression. The depression may appear unrelated to current issues and thus, in terms of classic psychiatry, may be classified as 'endogenous'. However, the shifting of explanation in the direction of organic causes may reflect the failure of mental health workers to fully recognise the experience of deep despair and guilt among elderly people. The despair and guilt may not be related to obvious current circumstances, but rather to profound thinking about the nature and significance of life and death. The scope for skilled counselling and psychotherapy in this context becomes clear. But the more general plea, for greater understanding of the developmental tasks facing elderly people seeking meaning in life and ways to face death with some degree of equanimity, seems equally important.

The work of Butler raises many questions, and his reliance on case material makes it vulnerable to criticisms on the basis of methodological soundness. His ideas, although sketchily drawn out, have nonetheless led to an increased interest in qualitative research with the elderly (see, for example, the case material of Coleman (1986) and Knight (1992)), and to an interest in the meanings that older people ascribe to their circumstances and to their inner worlds. It is likely that this approach complements the emphasis on quantitative data and external stressors which characterises much of the work in health psychology.

THE WORK OF COLEMAN: REMINISCENCE

In his work on reminiscence, introduced briefly in Chapter 2, Coleman was struck by a minority of elderly people in his research sample who appeared anxious, demoralised and depressed by their circumstances. In his introduction to his work, Coleman (1986) commented that: 'a major characterising feature of the latter years of life is the relatively greater number and severity of losses individuals are faced with, both physically and socially'. He continues that, given the range and severity of challenges facing elderly people, 'a degree of resilience is needed to cope with the buffets of old age. Many not surprisingly find it difficult to keep going. *The high incidence of depression in later life has now been recorded by a number of authorities* (Gurland & Toner 1982) but is still inadequately recognised by the helping professions' (Coleman 1986, p. 22, my italics).

In his research sample, a number of the elderly subjects were clinically depressed and a third of the sample highly demoralised. The relationship between demoralisation, depression and loss was also clear to him from his research; for the men in the sample, being demoralised was associated with bereavement; for the women, if loss was conceived in more general terms – not simply the loss of a spouse – then it, too, was associated with depression in old age.

Coleman (1986) devotes one chapter in his book to a group within his sample who had negative attitudes to reminiscence and whose lives seemed to be overwhelmed by loss and depression. He discusses their case histories in some detail. The men in the sample had all been recently bereaved and could not come to terms with living alone. These men were miserable, lonely and often angry. Their current lives contrasted starkly with their past lives, but reminiscence was of no solace to them. It was associated with sinking into the depths of gloom and despair, and seemed hard to bear. The men were likely to idealise their wives, yet at the same time have many regrets about the past, and this made thinking about their personal histories painful and demoralising.

The women in the group had not experienced recent bereavements yet they, too, seemed to have experienced great loss, when loss was conceived in a broader sense. They also found the past hard to think about and seemed plagued by regrets and disappointments that were hard to bear. This work confirms the view that loneliness, isolation, guilt about the past and loss are linked with difficulties in accommodating the challenges and transitions of old age. The reader is referred to the work of Coleman for a more detailed description of these case studies. This empirical study chimes with the findings cited in the earlier work of Butler (1963).

THE WORK OF BROMLEY: PROBLEMS OF EMOTIONAL ADJUSTMENT IN LATER LIFE

The two main categories providing a framework for considering the problems of old age were those of developmental crises and the role of external stressors, emphasised in health psychology. Clearly there is much overlap between the two, and it is important not to construe them as mutually exclusive categories. One author whose work seems to straddle these categories is Bromley (1990) in his chapter on the problems of emotional adjustment in old age. He argues that some basic problems of emotional adjustment can be expected as part of the normal course of later life. He suggests that, with the onset of old age, individuals become increasingly prone to many psychological and physical problems. Elderly people experience increasing numbers of physical and psychological stresses, some of them severe, such as serious physical disease and injury, bereavement, relocation, social isolation and the process of dying.

Reappearance of basic emotions. In his recent review of the subject, Bromley (1990) argues that such stresses can be expected to elicit feelings and emotions at a level of intensity which the individual may not have experienced for many years. In particular, feelings of pain, grief, fear, loneliness and anger increasingly are seen to cause distress in old age. The reappearance of such strong, and often painful emotions (see Box 4.1), may come as something of a shock, with the individual ill-prepared for their intensity, and perhaps unable to cope effectively. It is likely that the hardest hit will be those elderly people who have a life-long history of not coping well with their own emotional life, or not communicating and sharing their feelings well with other people. Indeed, this may go some way in the direction of explaining some of the differences found as a function of gender (Pearlin et al 1981, Stroebe & Stroebe 1983, Bock & Webber 1972), since research has revealed that men have more difficulty in communicating strongly-felt and painful feelings.

Diminished coping. The process of adjustment in later life is partly that of coping with the irreversible effects of ageing, disability and disease. It relates, too, to social challenges and changes in the expectations that people have of older people. This range of potential stresses – biological, social and psychological – demands effective coping strategies if the elderly

---

Box 4.1 Adverse effects of ageing on emotional adjustment

1. Reappearance of basic emotional reactions
2. Diminished coping
3. Diminished emotional controls
4. Age-related stresses
5. Maladaptive temperaments
6. Maladaptive sentiments
7. Emotional exhaustion (shock)
(from Bromley 1990, p. 281)

person is not to feel overwhelmed and unable to weather the storms of old age. If there is an increasing sense that these challenges cannot be effectively dealt with, then diminished coping may lead to a sense of failure and strong, negative emotions such as resentment, irritation, anger, disappointment, ennui, anxiety, envy and unhappiness. This situation is described by Bromley (1990, p. 282) in the following way: 'It would not be surprising, therefore, to find that old age was accompanied by low chronic levels of anxiety and depression reflecting persisting stresses to which the person has partly habituated but nevertheless continues to anticipate in the interests of self-protection – consider, for example, moderate hypochondriasis, fear of strangers or crime, excessive dependence, worry over money'.

Diminished emotional controls. Bromley proposes that in old age there is, to some extent, evidence of diminished emotional controls. Clear evidence of the loss of control over emotional expression can be observed in certain pathological conditions of later life – in dementia and cerebral arteriosclerosis. Bromley goes one step further than this by suggesting that it is reasonable to suppose that even in 'normal' ageing these processes, associated with loss of normal control over the expression of emotions, are likely to occur, albeit in a mild form.

Age-related stresses. In considering age-related stresses, Bromley emphasises not only the profound impact that the stresses associated with old age are likely to have, but also the limited opportunity that many older people feel that they have available to them to escape or deal effectively and constructively with the challenges. The stresses which he cites that are typically associated with old age are:

- retirement
- disability
- bereavement
- isolation
- general infirmity
- loss of psychological capacities
- insecurity.

In addition, unlike the younger person, the older person does not have the same opportunity or ability to escape from, or compensate for, these unwanted circumstances. The overall effect of the age-related stresses is to aggravate the negative feelings and emotions already referred to.

Maladaptive temperaments. Of course, all this portrays an over-generalised and rather negative picture, and it is important to recognise the importance of individual differences and the role of mitigating factors. What is important in the context of this chapter is to seek to understand what it is about those older adults, who fail to cope with the challenges of old age, that leads them to fall foul of a vicious cycle of increased stress and the aggravation of negative emotions and counter-productive relationships. And to seek to understand why they, unlike other older people, seem unable to break free of this descending spiral of negative emotions, poor coping strategies and increased psychopathology and physical ill health. In seeking to answer these questions, Bromley looks to themes within the individual; he cites 'maladaptive temperaments; maladaptive sentiments; and emotional exhaustion' (see Box 4.1).

It is not possible to talk of a particular kind of personality structure that equips an individual to cope with the stresses and demands of old age. There are clearly many different ways and styles of dealing in a positive, constructive and fulfilling way with growing old. Like other writers in the field before him (for example Butler 1963), Bromley argues for broad personal resources such as flexibility, emotional stability and the ability to face challenges directly and develop positive coping mechanisms.

It is important, too, that individuals show some degree of self-awareness and self-perception that will enable them to fit their temperament to an appropriate environmental setting. Put simply, one would expect older individuals to move into the sorts of environments, and engage in the sorts of activities, best suited to their temperament and abilities (see, for example, Quattrochitubin & Jason 1983). Failure to find such a niche is likely to be associated with increased levels of dissatisfaction and frustration; this in turn could become associated with increased levels of depression and anxiety. We usually learn to live with environments we do not like but cannot change, such as living in an institution, although we often do so at some emotional cost.

Maladaptive sentiments. A further category in Box 4.1 is maladaptive sentiments: Bromley refers to 'enduring and complex systems of ideas and feelings about some object, person (including oneself), event or circumstance. ... Sentiments can endure and give satisfaction even when the object of the sentiment no longer exists. One can maintain an attitude towards an object or a friend even after there is no longer any contact' (Bromley 1990, pp. 287–288).

These attitudes can be very positive and colour important memories and indeed are part of one's sense of history and identity. However, there can be marked negative aspects to sentiments, and they can lead to problems in old age and a failure to deal positively with the challenges and changes that inevitably are associated with ageing. They can be maladaptive, for example, when they make it difficult for the older person to give up lost attachments, or activities that are no longer possible. A deep, sentimental attachment to former relationships, routines and lifestyles that have to be given up may lead to resistance, longing and a general sense of dissatisfaction with all alternatives. In this sense, for Bromley, it is not surprising that sentiments both represent an individual's past psychological ballast or capital accumulated over many years as well as major hurdles to flexibility and the capacity to change in later life.

Emotional exhaustion. The final category described by Bromley (Box 4.1), emotional exhaustion, is concerned with the behavioural and emotional consequences of chronic conflict and frustration. The behavioural manifestations take the form of apathy, depression, withdrawal and anger and can arise from two contrasting causes. First, there is the impact of long-term, low or moderate levels of stress associated with, for example, the cumulative effects of ageing and deprived living conditions. These could easily exceed the person's level of stress tolerance and capacity for coping. With these levels of stress the likelihood of 'emotional blocking' is increased. Jarvik and Russell (1979) argue that 'emotional blocking' as a strategy for coping with stress should not necessarily be viewed negatively, since it may be an effective way of coping with the numerous and often unpredictable losses and frustrations of later life.

Secondly, Bromley considers the impact of excessive levels of stress in the case, for example, of an environment which is actually unpleasant, disturbing or distressing. This might refer to the impact of poor quality institutional care (see, for example, Tobin 1989) where the environment is crowded, hostile, lacking in resources, controlled by unsympathetic, untrained people, which generates for the elderly person a classical 'no solution' situation in which apathetic withdrawal, punctuated by outbursts of rage and frustration is seen as the only way of coping.

The work of Bromley shifts between the significance of external events and the personal biography of the elderly person, including the resources that he has currently available to deal with the challenges of old age. In the next sections, focus is on a range of external stresses that are seen to be common in old age and are likely to present particularly difficult challenges for older people. In focusing upon the stressors, there is no intention to diminish the significance of the personal meanings of these events, rather to consider important themes that pervade the lives of many elderly people. In defending this line, I quote from Sheehy:

> We all have an aversion to generalities, thinking that they violate what is unique about ourselves. Yet the older we grow, the more we become aware of the commonality of our lives, as well as the essential aloneness as navigators through the human journey. ... I reread an observation by Willa Cather with a mixture of amusement and startled recognition: 'There are only two or three human stories, and they go on repeating themselves as fiercely as if they had never happened before'. (Sheehy 1977, p. 28)

STRESS, SOCIAL SUPPORT AND MENTAL HEALTH PROBLEMS IN OLD AGE: THE CONTRIBUTIONS FROM HEALTH PSYCHOLOGY

In seeking to understand stress and social support in old age as health-related phenomena, researchers have looked at both physical and mental health outcomes. Some of the strongest evidence available documenting the negative impact of stress on health and personal wellbeing, however, comes from the literature examining mental health outcomes. The effects of stress and social support seem to be greater for depression than for any other kind of psychiatric disorder (Wheaton 1983, Cronkite & Moos 1984, Kessler & McLeod 1985). Stress is likely to be of particular relevance to depression in old age because of the losses and deprivations often involved in the life events, which are common to elderly people, and the diminution in independence and control in old age. Conversely, social support is likely to have a particularly positive effect in mitigating the feelings of depression because of its power to promote feelings of control and self-worth, which are antagonistic to the feelings of despair, helplessness and worthlessness associated with depression.

In broadest terms, stress can be conceptualised as a condition which challenges or threatens personal wellbeing. There are three distinct types of stress which are typically discussed in the health psychology literature:

1. life events (such as bereavement)
2. chronic stress (such as living with chronic pain)
3. daily hassles (such as the daily problems associated with dealing with inadequate financial resources, difficult relationships and practical problems such as difficulties with mobility).

There are several well-known life event measures (e.g. the Schedule of Recent Events, Holmes & Rahe 1967; the Geriatric Social Readjustment Rating Scale,

Amster & Krauss 1974). Most life event measures enquire about events experienced during the recent past, both because stress is expected to be most relevant to current wellbeing and because memory problems threaten the reliability of reports of more distant events. The main research tool for measuring the impact of hassles is the Hassles Scale, developed by Lazarus and his associates (see, for example, DeLongis et al 1982). Hassles are expected to reflect relatively long-term or continual sources of stress, but they lack the intensity of life events and chronic stressors.

In considering the differential impact of life events, chronic stress and hassles as a function of age, some themes emerge. Elderly people tend to report fewer life events, but they experience greater unhappiness and more intrusion on their lives as a result of life events (Chiroboga & Dean 1978). With chronic stress, the impact of higher levels of pain and disability among elderly people is likely to be associated with higher levels of stress in these areas. Although there is little evidence to suggest that elderly people experience more daily hassles than younger people, older people report more hassles in the areas of health, social and environmental issues, and home maintenance.

Stress, support and depression

In looking at the relationship between stress, support and mental health status, in particular the presence of symptoms of depression, some interesting themes emerge with regard to the health of older people. Many more older people report depressive symptoms than qualify for a diagnosis of a clear depressive disorder. Furthermore, many more older adults report symptoms of depression than do their younger counterparts (Gurland et al 1980, Blazor & Williams 1980) although they are less likely, for a number of reasons, to meet the diagnostic criteria for a depressive illness. There is evidence to suggest that the realities of the lives of elderly people make them more prone to mild forms of depression, but not a full-blown clinical depression. The factors that are likely to play a role in this include the increased incidence of physical illness and pain among elderly people, the losses associated with retirement, the losses of friends and loved ones through death, and increased daily hassles associated with health, maintaining social contacts and the pressures of home maintenance. Gaining social support is often more difficult to enjoy because of increased isolation, which is a function of difficulties in mobility and transport and decreased social contacts because of illness and death.

Furthermore, research also indicates that elderly people, especially elderly women, are more likely to receive physical treatments for depression, such as ECT, and less likely to receive 'talking therapies' which, although more time-consuming, may be in the longer term more beneficial and appropriate. The significance of this work is that elderly people are likely to have to face more challenges and that there are greater demands made upon their coping strategies. It does not, however, provide an answer to the question why some elderly people are simply unable to cope effectively with these challenges and succumb to their deleterious effects.

THE DEATH OF A LOVED PERSON: PROBLEMS OF BEREAVEMENT IN OLD AGE

The death of a loved person is one of the most psychologically distressing and shocking events that most of us have to deal with. Grief refers to the powerful emotions of sadness and despair, even guilt and anger, that follow the loss of a loved one. The normal process of grieving is a painful process that lasts many months, or even years.

Freud (1917), in his seminal paper, *Mourning and Melancholia*, stressed the difficulty of coming to terms with loss and coined the phrase 'the work of mourning'. This 'work of mourning' is very difficult: the loss of a loved one provokes such anxiety that, to begin with, the individual cannot face, and so uses various means to resist, acceptance of a terrible truth. The earliest stage in response to the death of a loved person is characterised by high levels of anxiety, panic and shock. The painful reality of the loss takes some time to be accommodated. When this occurs, the next phase is associated with the painful sense of loss, dejection, hopelessness, despair and misery. Gradually the loss is accepted and the individual adapts to this new reality and begins slowly to reorientate himself to the changed environment and begins to adjust and form new relationships.

It is this last phase in response to loss, the phase of resolution, that defines healthy or normal adaptation to bereavement. In Freud's (1917) paper, it is characterised by an acceptance that the loved person is lost and that the individual gradually becomes 'emancipated from the ties to the lost loved person'. That is, the lost person is psychologically given up. More recent work suggests that healthy grief is achieved not by simply 'letting go', but by internalising an image of the lost person that is positive (see, for example, Klein 1940). In this way, the memories of the lost person in some way alter, and add to, the inner world of the person who is left behind. As a consequence, the bereaved person is changed by the experience but, overall, changed in a positive way. Thus, the dead person is not simply lost, nor given up, but the external reality that the person is no longer there is admitted, whilst at the same time something internally is changed and augmented.

In pathological forms of grief this process goes wrong. The stages of the resolution of grief cannot be managed, and the person is stuck with feelings of dejection, abandonment, misery, guilt, anger and self-reproach. What distinguishes this group from those who are able more successfully to navigate a course through loss has been the subject of much scrutiny. Among elderly people, failure to cope with the emotional challenges of grief can have disastrous consequences for wellbeing and healthy adaptation in old age. In a severe form, it can be linked to deep depression and suicide, and psychotic episodes including paranoia and delusional states; in less extreme forms it is associated with heightened states of anxiety, obsessional behaviour, increased hypochondriacal feelings, feelings of regret, guilt and milder forms of depression.

An important question in this context is, why are some elderly people more prone to pathological forms of grief? Worden (1983) provides five main categories in his discussion of the difficulties that some people have in grieving loss, and are thus vulnerable to developing pathological grief reactions. These are:

1. Relational factors. These refer to the nature and quality of the relationship between the bereaved person and the deceased.
2. Circumstantial factors. The circumstances surrounding the death of a loved person that may make it harder to grieve.
3. Historical factors. People who have had complicated grief reactions in the past will have a higher probability of having complicated grief reactions in the present. 'Past losses and separations have an impact on current losses and separations and attachments and all these factors bear on future loss and separation and capacity to make future attachments' (Simos 1979, p. 27).
4. Personality factors. Those people, for example, who are unable to tolerate extremes of emotional distress and withdraw in order to defend themselves against such strong feelings, are particularly vulnerable. Because of this inability to tolerate emotional distress, they short-circuit the process and often

develop a complicated grief reaction. Those who do not tolerate dependency feelings well will also have difficulty in grieving.

5. Social factors. Grief is a social process as well as an intensely personal one. It can therefore only be understood with reference to social factors. The three main kinds of social factors outlined by Lazare (1979), as influencing the grief response, are:
   a — when the circumstances surrounding the loss feel to be unspeakable (as in the case of suicide)
   b — when the loss is socially negated, that is when those around the bereaved person act as if the loss has not happened
   c — the absence of a social support network.

Certain contextual factors play an important role in determining the outcome of bereavement in old age. For example, the increased isolation experienced by many elderly people affords them less opportunity for support, intimacy and comfort, all factors which are known to militate against the more severe negative effects of loss, and increase their vulnerability to pathological outcomes. Many elderly people have lived a long time, often 30 or 40 years, with their spouse and so that making sense of life without their husband or wife is challenging. Their partner may have been the only really close source of physical affection, and the only one who saw worth and value in them. The need for a partner, and the resulting difficulties in dealing with loss, may be great even if there had been life long experiences of ambivalence in the relationship.

The likelihood of replacing a partner in old age is small. Cleveland and Giantureo (1976) suggest that, of widows aged over 65, fewer than 1% will remarry. Often, too, in old age the level of dependency upon partners increases, especially if there is mutual dependence because of ill health and so the relationship may be characterised by high levels of co-dependency, making the pain of loss hard to bear. Grief work can be complicated when co-dependence is associated with a mixture of feelings which are often quite ambivalent. Angry, hostile and resentful feelings towards the lost spouse can cloud the work of mourning, and lead to high levels of guilt and depression.

Pathologies of grief

The way in which ambivalent feelings are associated with pathologies of grief is discussed fully by Pincus (1974) and Parkes (1972). Pathologies of grief can take many forms; the commonest include delayed grief reaction, prolongation of the grief reaction and distortions of the grief reaction.

Delayed reaction refers to a postponement of the grief reaction. The delay may be some months or even some years. When the grief finally finds expression, it may be experienced in an acute and dramatic way. Prolongation of grief is another problem, especially when the fact of death has been denied. Loneliness and social isolation, with attendant separation anxiety, often heighten this problem. In her discussion of loneliness among elderly bereaved people, Sanders (1989) emphasises how frightening the experience of being alone can feel. As our culture becomes increasingly 'couple-companiate', single people have a difficult time fitting into places where they had been comfortable before the loss (Lopata 1969). For some, the situation can be very frightening indeed. One widow discussed her anxiety, in the following way:

When I thought my nephew was leaving and maybe I would be alone, I was desperate ... I was really desperate ... I was really afraid and I was desperate ... And I am not so much afraid of somebody coming in and hurting me or anything like that, as I am thinking, 'I am alone because there's nobody ever going to be with me again ... and going berserk.' That's my fear. It isn't a fear of somebody coming in, because that doesn't bother me. It's the other part of being alone – there's nobody.   (Sanders 1989, p. 194)

Lopata describes this as 'loneliness anxiety' (Lopata 1973, 1974), which often leads the bereaved person to undertake busy work as a means of avoiding loneliness, if this is possible.

Even if the work of mourning comes to a healthy resolution, whereby the loss is faced and accepted, the future may look more bleak to the elderly person than to the younger person. The younger person has a future ahead that facilitates a positive outlook on what life still has yet to bring. The brutal reality for many very old widows and widowers is one of increased loneliness and isolation, and little opportunity for comfort and support in the future. If the future is honestly faced it may feel like a rather bleak and barren landscape; the alternative is to avoid honest appraisal and to secretly, or even publicly, maintain the relationship in fantasy. This may be because the pain of complete acceptance simply cannot be borne.

Raphael (1984) comments that this may account for that fact that among very old widows and widowers there is a tendency to continue a style of life that is strongly governed by what the spouse would have done or wished. There may be private conversations with him; he may be asked for guidance. Moss and Moss (1979) have sensitively outlined the vital role this 'image' of the dead spouse plays in the life of elderly widows and widowers, including the effects it may have on remarriage. They note, too, how this tie to the image may be reinforced by personal and social expectations, by loyalty, and even by expectations of the children.

The helplessness of elderly bereaved people may frighten those who are charged with their care. In addition to this, anger about the death and its circumstances may find external expression through hostility towards potential carers. In this way, older bereaved people may make it all the more difficult to receive the help that they often desperately need.

Many elderly people, not used to showing their feelings, may express their grief indirectly through symptoms of ill health. There has been a proliferation of literature on pathological aspects of grief (see, for example, Speck 1978, Parkes 1972, Raphael 1984, Worden 1983, Sanders 1989). The commonest forms of pathological reactions to grief described in the literature are:

1. Excessive activity, with no apparent feelings of loss. This activity bears many similarities to the manic activity associated with manic-depressive psychosis, and can be understood as a means to deny or defend against the misery associated with the loss. As a defence it is precarious and leaves the elderly person vulnerable to mental health problems.

2. Development of symptoms similar to those of the deceased, often with related psychosomatic illness. This is linked to over-identification with the lost, loved person and represents, in part at least, an attempt to hold on to the image and deny the loss and separateness.

3. Alteration in relationships with friends and family. For example, all social contacts may be shunned and the person may become a recluse, or may need supervision because of giving away large sums of money. This is felt by the bereaved person to be a way of coping with the loss, although is unlikely to be an effective coping strategy for long. Social withdrawal is linked to increasing problems of mental health and cognitive deterioration.

4. Furious hostility against people associated with the way in which the death was handled, often leading to constant letters of complaint and constant resentment towards other people. This anger and resentment reflects a difficulty in feeling sadness and accepting the feelings of loss. This response is more likely to occur in ambivalent relationships, where there are feelings of guilt and regret which cannot be faced. The guilty feelings are pushed outside and the rest of the world is experienced as

irascible —

culpable; this seems preferable to the bereaved person than acknowledging difficult emotions within. It is as though the hostility is a defence against feelings of misery, guilt and personal regret, and leads the bereaved person often to appear highly irascible. This strategy may cut the individual off from social contacts and support, which makes the task of grieving all the more difficult.

5. Behaviour resembling a more psychotic pattern with a lack of any emotional expression, living in a daze, and acting in a 'wooden manner'. This is likely to occur in extreme cases when the grief is associated with internal chaos and disintegration.

6. Severe depression with insomnia, guilt, and bitter self-reproach. Because in some instances the bereaved elderly person may feel the need to punish himself for what has happened, there is an increased risk of suicide in these cases.

In seeking to make sense of why some older people experience such forms of pathological grief, it is important to refer to their social situation, in particular, the extent to which they can enjoy some degree of social support, kindness, understanding and companionship. It is also important to take account of their past history, including past losses and separations, and the way in which they were handled. Early losses and separations which were poorly handled make later losses more difficult to deal with. The nature of the relationship between the deceased and the spouse is also a critical component. The presence of ambivalent feelings and negative emotions make the work of mourning complicated. Higher levels of dependency and the length of time the couple had lived together before the bereavement are important variables.

Gender

Many people argue that, if there are pathologies of grief in old age, the repercussions in terms of the quality of life remaining can be particularly severe. This is not to say that elderly people are more prone to pathologies of grief than younger people; this appears not to be the case (see Ch. 2). However, for the reasons outlined, when there are pathologies in old age they are likely to have highly detrimental consequences. In addition, the research on bereavement suggests that elderly, isolated men are especially prone to pathologies of the grief response.

In a study that looked at the way in which doctors and nurses deal with bereaved relatives in general hospitals, we found that a persistent concern among

hospital staff was the lack of community support for recently bereaved elderly men in the community, many of whom lived isolated lives (Rentoul 1989). The work of many of the voluntary agencies (for example CRUSE) reveals that it is often elderly, isolated men who are in danger of being engulfed by a combination of grief, isolation and lack of comfort, intimacy and support. The impact can be so great that it increases mortality. There is a great deal of research evidence, which indicates that sex differences are important. Helsing & Szklo (1981), Helsing et al (1981), Rees & Lutkins (1967) and Ward (1976) all show that the mortality risk of widowhood is greater for men. A number of other writers have echoed the special problems of widowers (Bernardo 1970, Bock & Webber 1972, Durkheim 1951, Hyman 1983).

Health, mortality and morbidity

Many health psychologists, medical sociologists and social gerontologists note that older men, and especially older widowers, are less socially integrated than their female counterparts, and are thus more susceptible to a host of problems that range from loneliness to suicide. In contrast to these findings, one British study reports higher mortality rates due to widowhood for women (Jones & Goldblatt 1986). It is hard to reconcile the findings of this study with other research. It is likely that an important factor influencing mortality rates following bereavement is the social context, more specifically, social support which influences the individual's capacity to confront the stress of widowhood; and most of the literature points to men having more difficulty in avoiding the mortality risk of widowhood than women.

Not only does widowhood increase the mortality risk, it also, unsurprisingly, increases the morbidity risk. In the words of Ferraro (1989, p. 75): 'If widowhood can in some cases precipitate death for the bereaved, then it should come as no surprise that heightened morbidity accompanies the grieving process of widowed people. The major recent questions in the study of widowhood and threats to health are when, how severe, and upon whom are these effects most likely to occur'.

From his review of the literature on this subject, Ferraro (1989) concludes that the majority of empirical studies of widowhood do, in fact, show some sort of health decline (Hyman 1983, Maddison & Viola 1968, Owen et al 1982, Parkes 1970, 1975, Parkes & Brown 1972, Vachon et al 1982, Wan 1982, 1984). In considering the findings in more detail, for the majority of people the decline in health status is a short-term

ambivalence

effect, and most likely after the death of a spouse. The long-term effects tend to be modest or non-existent unless there are complicating conditions.

Increasing research attention is now being paid to understanding better the nature of these complicating conditions that make bereavement for a minority of elderly people so hard to bear. Some of these conditions were those observed on the mortality measures. For instance, the more isolated adults were more likely to show enduring signs of health decline (for example, Dimond et al 1987, Vachon et al 1982). This certainly accords with much of the research literature on social stress. It is important to note, however, as Ferraro (1989) reminds his reader, that often resources such as social support can act as both a cause of better health and also a product of it. Advantage accumulates. For many older people, increasing poor health can have a spiralling effect and lead increasingly in the direction of isolation, loneliness and despair.

One further factor which influences the impact of bereavement on health is the extent to which the death of the spouse was expected. When death is un-anticipated, the blow is often much greater and the impact upon health consequently more negative. For example, both Lundin (1984) and Parkes (1975) show that health decline is more likely when the death of a spouse is unexpected, or when the period of time the older person has to accommodate the reality that their spouse is likely to die is short. This 'shock' factor is important in influencing the eventual impact on the health of the bereaved.

To confound these findings, some researchers (for example Gerber et al 1975) have revealed that, among those widowed because of their spouse's long and chronic illness, a very lengthy preparation and care-giving time was associated with greater morbidity. It is difficult to draw clear conclusions from these findings; it may be that there is a curvilinear relationship between length of time anticipating death and increase in morbidity. Sudden and unexpected loss of a spouse creates special problems (see, for example, Rentoul 1989), but so may attempting to care for a chronically ill spouse for several years. This is the explanation suggested by Ferraro (1989), although other factors may also be influential, such as the nature of the relationship that characterised the marriage, and the feelings aroused in the care-giver by looking after a sick spouse for a long period of time, especially if it involves the arousal of highly ambivalent feelings. Pathological responses to bereavement have long been associated with difficulties in dealing with negative feelings towards the lost spouse (see, for example,

Pincus 1974, Parkes 1972), such as resentment and hostility, or a relationship that was characterised by longstanding feelings of ambivalence.

In concluding his review of the literature on widowhood and its impact on health status among the elderly, Ferraro (1989) draws the following conclusions:

- Mortality risk is greater for men during the first 6 months after the bereavement.
- The impact on women is less significant and is more likely to occur a couple of years after the death of a spouse.
- Widowhood does precipitate a decline in health, in particular, psychophysical health status. The decline is rapid for the first 2 years following the bereavement and then tails off.

There are, of course, many exceptions to this and also important countervailing forces, the most important of which seem to be the presence of social contact and support.

Social support

Many researchers and clinicians working in this field therefore argue in favour of social interventions for vulnerable elderly people in the form of increased social support. The stress literature emphasises over and over again the ways in which social support and close interpersonal relationships act as a buffer to the deleterious effects of stressful life events (Bernardo 1970, Parkes & Brown 1972, Vachon et al 1982, Stroebe & Stroebe 1983). Those studies which have focused specifically upon the impact on health status of social support following bereavement note its positive effect (Dimond et al 1987, Ferraro et al 1984, Parkes & Brown 1972, Vachon et al 1982). Intervention programmes are increasingly looking for ways of identifying vulnerable elderly people and providing support for them following bereavement. However, such programmes are often seen to be expensive (despite the fact that in the long term they may be highly cost effective) and it is often left to the voluntary sector to provide support for those who have at least enough resources to seek appropriate help (for example, the work of CRUSE is invaluable in this context).

Some studies (for example Rentoul 1989), have found that in many areas the support for isolated, bereaved elderly people is limited or non-existent. It is often left in the hands of already hard-pressed general practitioners. Health visitors, increasingly under pressure to work where need is seen to be greatest, are often encouraged to put their energies into working with children at risk, or elderly people with established problems such as Alzheimer's disease. An important opportunity for mental health promotion among bereaved elderly people is thus being lost.

THE GRIEFS OF GROWING OLD: OTHER LOSSES IN OLD AGE

Raphael (1984), in the context of her research on grief and bereavement, looked at the issue of loss and grief in old age. The losses that she considered went far beyond the losses of bereavement and included a wide range of situations which, she argued, nonetheless demanded recognition and grief. She used discursive interviews with elderly people in an attempt to get to grips with the losses that they were facing, and how they attempted to come to terms with them. For example, she cites the following quotation from her study: 'I longed for the days when I was young and fit – when I didn't need to carry anything around with me – just myself. Sometimes I would wonder if it was all worth it. I was just a walking pill factory, that was all' (Mary aged 65 years, in Raphael 1984, p. 283).

The griefs of growing old do not begin in old age but begin with the growing realisation that one cannot do, with ease, something that one was able to do at one time without thought; that one will not, now, achieve the fullness of one's hopes and dreams; that one's life is not limitless, but finite, and that the time remaining is not great. In her discussion Raphael (1984) considers the following losses in old age:

- loss of vision
- loss of hearing
- loss of sexual function
- losses of body function
- loss of health and wellbeing
- loss of brain function
- loss of work
- loss of relationships.

For Raphael, it is this accumulation of losses that distinguish elderly from younger people.

Perceptual losses

Loss of vision and hearing alters the experience of the physical and social world. Both losses potentially increase a sense of isolation and demand some adjustment. If the losses are not accommodated and adapted to, they may lead to a state of chronic anger and resentment, depression or denial of the impairment, with failure to readjust to an altered life-style and the consequent need for aids and additional care. As perceptual impairments become more of a problem, the sense of social isolation and the opportunities for misunderstandings increase; particularly worrying is the increased opportunity for paranoid misinterpretation of social interactions in vulnerable old people.

Loss of sexual function

Although there are vast individual differences in sexual functioning in old age, some common patterns emerge (George & Weiler 1981, Sadock et al 1976). Both men and women show some gradual diminution of sexual interest, arousal, and activity from their fifties onwards. Whilst many elderly people may maintain satisfactory and stable sexual activity, even into their eighties, the general trend is one of cessation or decline. Sadock et al (1976) suggest that ageing affects a man's capabilities more than a woman's. The realisation that sexuality does not now, and will not again, have the joyful thrust and urgency of youthful desire, brings sadness. If the loss of the sexuality of youth can be accepted and mourned many older couples settle into a pattern of altered but satisfying sexual intimacy.

In many instances, loss of sexual function is complicated by psychological conflict, so that these factors may interfere with the grief and mourning associated with relinquishing it. Some people may bitterly regret that they did not enjoy sex to the full when they had the chance, or their sense of missed opportunity may lead them to envy the sexual freedom of the youth of today. For others sexual activity was the main chance for physical intimacy and closeness and with the loss of sex, opportunities for other forms of physical closeness like cuddles and kissing are lost too. This may be a further cause of deep regret, with a growing sense of physical isolation.

Loss of bodily functions

Loss of bodily functions may not be sudden or lead to an acute sense of loss but, over longer periods of time, irritability, sadness and a difficulty in accepting that one can no longer do many of the things that were previously easy and pleasurable may reflect the reaction to loss. The patient who seems preoccupied with his body functions, what he can and cannot do, may in some ways be showing his chronic grief and mourning for what he cannot accept. When mobility and independence are severely hampered by such conditions as a stroke, there may be an extreme sense of loss which becomes associated with intense grief and mourning. If such issues are poorly resolved, the chronically angry, resentful, older person, demandingly dependent, may alienate the support of those whose care he desperately needs.

It is in the face of these kinds of challenges that the elderly person, who is not mentally ill but deeply distressed, would benefit from counselling or psychotherapy. It is often these services that are not seen as appropriate, either by medical or social services, because of the person's age or circumstances and they are not, therefore, offered as a treatment of choice. In many instances this distress, which is unacknowledged and unsupported, turns into chronic anxiety, aggressive or depressive states. Loss of function of bladder and bowel deserve special mention since they involve not only a sense of loss but are also sources of great distress and social embarrassment.

Loss of cognitive function

Loss of brain or cognitive function may be one of the greatest sadnesses for many people as they age. When there is loss of cerebral functioning, combined with awareness and insight, the grief may be very great. Angry and irritable feelings are common, followed by sadness and depression as the reality and finality of the loss are recognised. There are often, too, associated anxieties about the loss of control, particularly when there is emotional lability, as well as fear of dependence on others. This loss may be most acutely felt by those who have highly valued their mental functions, and have seen these as a key element of the self.

Loss of work: the impact of retirement

In a review of the literature on the psychological meanings of work, Singh (1982) considers the functions of work in a man's life (and increasingly in the life of women). For many people work provides an important source of self-esteem and achievement, or an outlet for creativity. It may be a key element of identity, in that major elements of the way in which self is defined and experienced is in terms of work. Furthermore, work may provide a structure within which the individual can identify himself within the hierarchy of an organisation. It may be seen as providing a system of interpersonal relationships which are rewarding in terms of friendship, or a source of conflict. Work may be a source of interesting activity, or an escape from unpalatable thoughts or difficult circumstances; it may be a source of pleasure or pride; or it may be seen as burdensome drudgery that is strongly resented.

Work may provide many things, which are not readily articulated because they relate to unconscious reasons for seeking a particular kind of work. For example, some people may be drawn to the helping professions because of an unconscious urge to take care of others, or to constantly make reparation in the lives of other people, in an attempt to deny damage in their own lives. When these opportunities are removed with the loss of work, the individual may be left to face the force of their need to take care of others, and the defensive value of those needs and how miserable they feel, without the outlet that work provided.

The hours and style of work may reflect certain personality features. The well-known type A personality (see, for example, Friedman & Rosenman 1974, Byrne & Rosenman 1986, Matthews 1982) may be lost without the opportunity that work offered to be driven to over-commitment, long hours and constant deadlines. Raphael (1984) points, too, to the way in which obsessional people may relish careful, detailed application to highly specific tasks. Those with strongly narcissistic or histrionic traits may only flourish in work situations that provide drama and narcissistic supplies. For some people, work may be the only place where they feel valued and fulfilled. Some people long to be at their place of work, and others feel that to escape from work is their only opportunity for freedom. For most people there are ambivalent feelings towards work, with loved and hated elements, which complicate the feeling towards its loss.

The impact of retirement in old age can only be understood with reference to the meaning of work to the person. For those who are financially impoverished by the loss of work, for those whose identity is completely bound up with work, for those whose life seems without meaning in the absence of work and for those without family or a social network, a future without work and all that it afforded seems grim. These people may be vulnerable to the pathological effects of the grief of the loss of work. It is not easy to anticipate exactly what the loss of work will mean; the retiring person may not realise this until close to the time of retirement or even after it. The comfortable familiarity of the place of work, the people at work, the tasks carried out at the place of work, all contribute to the fabric of the individual's existence. When these are first gone there is often a great sense of loss and a feeling of being bereft. The work, and all that it meant, will be gradually mourned. If the process of mourning is successful, then other things will gradually take the place of work: indeed, the individual may discover many other things that are more important than work, and discover enjoyment in many things that were previously neglected or avoided. The process of coming to terms with the loss of work, like that of facing other losses, may go wrong and end up in a spiral of despair and increasing loneliness.

Like many losses and life changes, retirement demands changes in self-image and the way in which individuals orientate themselves to the world. Some people respond to the changes with some degree of fear, resistance, even denial of the events and their implications. For these people, the full realisation of the impact only hits home on the first day of not working. For many, there is a 'honeymoon' period when the freedom of not working is enjoyed and feels like a long holiday. Only when the months of not working progress does the older person begin to feel a sense of emptiness, boredom and frustration. These feelings may lead the person to begin to long for work, to idealise the work situation, and to feel an increasing sense of anger, irritation and frustration with the world, in which he no longer feels important and valued. It may be difficult to communicate these feelings for many reasons; for example, the older person may not be used to talking about feelings, or it may be difficult to simply admit that he is unable to enjoy the freedom of not working, especially since other people may envy the position of the retired person.

A further difficulty for many elderly couples is adjusting to increased time together. For many couples, the chance for the first time in life to enjoy time together and follow the kind of leisure interests they did not previously have the opportunity to pursue, provides a great source of satisfaction in later life. However, for other couples increasing time together highlights previously avoided difficulties in the relationship. The adjustment may take many months, or may never be adequately resolved especially in marriages where there has been a history of marital disharmony and for whom the increased closeness and intimacy cannot be tolerated, and simply breeds unhappiness.

Loss of independence: relocation in old age

The work of Tobin (see, for example, Tobin 1989) has been influential in portraying a picture of the impact, especially the psychological repercussions, of relocation to long-term care settings. Institutionalisation is a special example of relocation that refers, for the elderly, to relocating from non-institutional to long-term institutional care settings. The process of institutionalisation when old begins before the actual relocation, and starts when the older person anticipates the impact of relocation and is aware of the impending event. The psychological effects during the anticipatory phase are likely to differ as a function of the meaning of the relocation to the elderly person but, for all older people, is likely to involve some sense of loss and abandonment and some need to redefine self in terms of someone who can only survive with the additional protection of institutional care.

The next significant phase is the first month following admission, when most newly admitted residents become disorientated, some become severely depressed, some manifest bizarre behaviours, and others deteriorate quite rapidly. Influenced by his clinical mentor, Jerome Grunes (Psychiatric Consultant at the Drexel Home for the Aged in Chicago), Tobin refers to this as the 'first month syndrome' (1989). This syndrome is brought about by many factors, including the conscious realisation of the stressfulness of living in a total institution, the less conscious inner experience of being more physically vulnerable and closer to death, and also the confusion brought about by the social relocation to a strange and unfamiliar environment.

After the first month some residents recover and re-establish their pre-admission health status, whereas others continue to deteriorate, and experience increasing problems of physical and mental health, and may have their death hastened. These issues are discussed fully in the seminal work of Tobin and Lieberman (1976), in their detailed longitudinal study on becoming institutionalised when old in nursing homes.

Adverse outcomes

In seeking to disentangle the variables that are associated with negative outcomes as opposed to positive ones, Tobin (1989) considers a variety of resources and strategies that can be drawn upon by the older person, and also considers the role of outside factors, such as the kind and quality of care provided. In terms of resources of elderly people and their capacity to master the situation, passivity is seen to increase vulnerability to the negative effects of relocation, and is associated with adverse outcomes.

There are a number of different measures of adverse outcomes, but the two commonest used are increases in mortality and morbidity rates. Tobin (1989) reports that in different conditions of relocation there was an increase in both mortality and morbidity in about half the sample studied. The kinds of adverse outcomes varied as a function of the relocation situation. Excessive mortality rates were observed when a group of elderly people were moved en masse from a state mental hospital to long-term care facilities. In the other relocation situations studied, adverse outcomes took the form of increased morbidity.

For most elderly people, adverse outcomes are associated with the negative meanings attributed to living in a long-term care setting for older people. In terms of personal meanings, those elderly people who viewed entering such a care setting as a 'calamity', or representing 'giving up everything', or thought of it as a place 'to die', were likely to respond to admission with feelings of depression, hopelessness and despair. Furthermore, in the words of Tobin (1989, p. 42): 'Also not surprising was that the deteriorating psychological portrait, a portrait usually attributed to living in a total institution, was accompanied by feelings of being abandoned by their family, as revealed, for example, by their reconstruction of earliest memories'.

Poor psychological status was associated with a redefinition of self as a person who had been abandoned, with no place to go but to a setting that had always been feared and dreaded. Feelings of abandonment can best be understood if institutionalisation is considered as a family process, in which members of the family are usually involved in the decision to admit an elderly person into long-term care, and also that the emotional reverberations of such a decision are likely to be felt by many family members, not simply by the elderly person. Although a disproportionate number of older people in long-term care settings may be without nuclear family relations, the majority of people in such settings do have close family members involved in the decision-making.

Most families go to great lengths to avoid admitting family members to long-term institutions, and usually do so as a last resort. Among those elderly who do have family members who are involved in the decision-making process, the situation evokes problems in family relationships that are persistent, but often veiled, and the family manifests, according to Brody (1977), 'internalised guilt-inducing injunctions against placing an elderly spouse or parent regardless of the most reality-based determinants of the placement' (cited in Markides & Cooper 1989, p. 115). More recently, Brody (1985) attributed the myth of how previous generations cared better for their elderly members to these kinds of feelings.

The most important personal characteristic that is associated with poor health outcomes (both increases in mortality and morbidity) following relocation was passivity. Absence of positive prognostic indicators was also seen to be significant; for example, absence of a strong sense of self, of hope, of aggression, of coping strategies and of interpersonal relationships were all seen to be associated with poor health outcomes.

Poor quality of care, in particular nursing care, was also associated with poor physical and mental health outcomes and low scores on measures of self-worth. The implications of this for caring for elderly people in long-terms settings is clear; efforts should be made to provide high quality care and to mobilise the resources of older people. Ways should be sought to increase healthy protest, effective coping strategies, the instilling of hope and the development of a sense of self-worth and a positive self-image. Increased levels of irritability and aggression should be tolerated and seen as having positive effects. Ways of, in Tobin's (1989, p. 151) words, 'Enhancing life in the institution by preservation of the self'. For more information on supporting elderly people in institutional settings, see Chapter 27.

CONCLUSION

Many of the authors cited in this review emphasise that the process of growing old provides challenges for all people (Bromley 1990, Coleman 1986, Tobin 1989, Erikson 1950, Butler 1963, Knight 1992). Most old people are able to rise to these challenges and overcome the hurdles, though they may experience heightened anxiety and mild depression in their efforts to do so. However, a minority of elderly people are vulnerable in the face of the common stresses and developmental crises of old age, and face more significant threats to their mental health status. This may find expression in mild depression, increased anxiety, regret and guilt, as well as in more severe mental health problems, including severe depression, suicide, obsessional disorders, hypochondriacal problems and psychosis.

The origins of these vulnerabilities are manifold, and relate to both the past history of the individual and current circumstances. The development of personality across the life cycle needs to be addressed in making sense of vulnerabilities in old age, in particular long-standing problems of attachment, separation and loss, feelings of dependency and insecurity that were never adequately resolved during earlier phases of life.

The capacities of resilience, the ability to respond constructively to changing circumstances, to be resourceful in the face of loss and suffering and to be able to give and receive support and comfort from other people, are all characteristics highlighted in the literature associated with positive coping in old age. The corollary of this is that the absence of these characteristics is associated with poorer coping and problems of mental health in old age.

The current situation, in which the elderly person finds him or herself, also plays a significant role in influencing the way in which old age is experienced and coped with. The important role of environmental stress, of social isolation and lack of support, intimacy and companionship are all important variables in understanding why some elderly people seem unable to cope with the problems of old age. The role, too, of sensitive professional care, either nursing care in an institution (Tobin 1989), or psychotherapeutic care in the community (Knight 1992), should not be underestimated in understanding the ways in which elderly people learn, or fail to learn, to deal with the challenges and losses confronting them.

Although the experience of old age is unique to each individual, some themes do emerge in the literature that suggest some commonality of experience. All people have to face death, and the majority have to face waning health and increasing physical disability. Many have to confront the loss of work and the loss of friends and loved persons at the end of life. Some, too, have to face loss of independence and learn to give up independent living and relocate to some kind of sheltered housing or institutional care.

In addition to this, society may not be kind to older people and increased social isolation, prejudice and poverty may further add to the psychological challenges of old age. Issues of class are also important, and should be accommodated when seeking to make sense of vulnerabilities among elderly people. In the majority of studies that have considered social status as a variable, the findings are unequivocal; those with more education and income are likely to cope better in overcoming the challenges and hurdles of old age. Being higher up the socioeconomic ladder seems to offer many advantages, including better health, larger social networks, and more coping resources (see, for example, Ferraro 1989).

The discussion in this chapter is not meant to suggest that old age is a stressful time for all people, but rather to state that there are many potentially stressful circumstances which may have to be faced. Many old people face them with tremendous resourcefulness and wisdom; indeed with greater understanding and equanimity than at any other point in life. However, some elderly people, especially those who are vulnerable in terms of their past lives and current circumstances, find the tasks and transitions of old age hard to bear, and suffer emotionally as a consequence. This suffering may fall within the gamut of normal psychological functioning, or it may fall outside it and be expressed clinically as a pronounced mental health problem. The increased distress may also be an early warning sign that the elderly person is struggling and in danger of succumbing to more pronounced mental health problems. These early signs offer social and medical services an opportunity for early intervention and positive mental health promotion. Ignoring the warning signs may result in healthy, but struggling elderly people, descending into a spiral of increased mental health problems.

REFERENCES

Allman L R, Jaffe D T (eds) 1977 Readings in adult psychology: contemporary perspectives. Harper Row, New York

Amster L E, Krauss H H 1974 The relationship between life crises, and mental deterioration in old age. International Journal of Aging and Human Development 5: 51–55

Bernardo F M 1970 Survivorship and social isolation: the case of the aged widower. The Family Coordinator 19: 11–25

Blazor D, Williams C D 1980 Epidemiology of dysphoria and depression in an elderly population. American Journal of Psychiatry 137: 439–444

Bock E W, Webber I L 1972 Suicide among the elderly: isolating widowhood and other mitigating alternatives. Journal of Marriage and the Family 34: 24–31

Brody E M 1977 Long term care of older people. Human Science Press, New York

Brody E M 1985 Parent care as normative stress. The Gerontologist 25: 19–29

Bromley D B 1990 Behavioural gerontology: central issues in the psychology of ageing. John Wiley, Chichester

Butler R N 1963 The life review: an interpretation of reminiscence in the aged. Psychiatry 26: 65–76. Reprinted in: Allman L R, Jaffe D T (eds) 1977 Readings in adult psychology: contemporary perspectives. Harper Row, New York

Byrne D G, Rosenman R H 1986 The type of A behaviour patterns as a precursor to stressful life events: a confluence of coronary risks. British Journal of Medical Psychology 59: 75–82

Chiroboga D A, Dean H 1978 Dimensions of stress: perspectives from a longitudinal study. Journal of Psychosomatic Research 23: 47–55

Cleveland W P, Giantureo D T 1976 Remarriage probability after widowhood: a retrospective method. Journal of Gerontology 31: 99–103

Coleman P G 1986 Ageing and reminscence processes. John Wiley, Chichester

Cronkite R C, Moos R H 1984 The role of predisposing and moderating factors in the stress–illness relationship. Journal of Health and Social Behavior 25: 372–393

DeLongis A, Coyne J, Dakof G, Folkman S, Lazarus R S 1982 Relationship of daily hassles, uplifts, and major life events to health status. Health Psychology 1: 119–136

Dimond M, Lund D A, Caserta M S 1987 The role of social support in the first two years after bereavement in an elderly sample. The Gerontologist 27: 599–604

Durkheim E 1951 Suicide: a study in sociology. Free Press, Glencoe, IL

Erikson E 1950 Childhood and society. Norton, New York. Republished 1965 Penguin, Harmondsworth, London

Ferraro K F 1989 Widowhood and health. In: Markides K S, Cooper C L (eds) Aging, stress and health. Wiley, Chichester

Ferraro K F, Mutran E, Barres C M 1984 Widowhood, health and friendship support in later life. Journal of Health and Social Behaviour 25: 245–259

Freud S 1917 Mourning and melancholia. In: Sigmund Freud Collected papers, vol 4. New York, Basic Books

Friedman M, Rosenman R H 1974 Type A behaviour and your heart. New York, Knopf

George L K, Weiler S J 1981 Sexuality in middle and later life. Archives of General Psychiatry 38: 919–923

Gerber, I Rusalem R, Hannon N, Battin D, Arkin A 1975 Anticipatory grief and aged widows and widowers. Journal of Gerontology 30: 225–229

Gurland B J, Toner J A 1982 Depression in the elderly: a review of recently published studies. In: Eisdorfer C (ed) Annual review of Gerontology and Geriatrics 3: 228–265

Gurland B J, Dean L, Cross P, Golden R 1980 The epidemiology of depression and dementia in the elderly: the use of multiple indicators of these conditions. In: Cole J O, Barrett J E (eds) Psychopathology of the aged. Raven Press, New York

Helsing K J, Szklo M 1981 Mortality after bereavement. American Journal of Epidemiology 114: 41–52

Helsing K J, Szklo M, Comstock G W 1981 Factors associated with mortality after widowhood. American Journal of Public Health 71: 802–809

Holmes T, Rahe R 1967 The social readjustment rating scales. Journal of Psychosomatic Research 11: 213–218

Hyman H H 1983 Of time and widowhood. Duke University, Durham, NC

Jaques E 1965 Death and the mid-life crisis. International Journal of Psychoanalysis October 1965

Jarvick L F, Russell D 1979 Anxiety, ageing and the third emergency reaction. Journal of Gerontology 34: 197–200

Jones D R, Goldblatt P O 1986 Cancer mortality following widow(er)hood: some further results from the office of population censuses surveys longitudinal study. Stress Medicine 2: 129–140

Kessler R C, McLeod J D 1985 Social support and mental health in community samples. In: Cohen S, Syme S L (eds) Social support and health. Academic, New York

Klein M 1940 Mourning and its relation to manic-depressive states. Reprinted in: Klein M (1988) Love, guilt and reparation and other works 1921–1945. Virago, London

Knight B G 1992 Older adults in psychotherapy. Sage, London

Kubler-Ross E 1972 On death and dying. Journal of the American Medical Association February 1972

Lazare A 1979 Unresolved grief. In: Lazare A (ed) Out-patient psychiatry: diagnosis and treatment. Williams and Wilkins, Baltimore

Lopata H 1969 Social psychological aspects of role involvement. Sociology and Social Research 58 (April): 285–298

Lopata H 1973 Self-identity in marriage and widowhood. The Sociological Quarterly 14: 407–418

Lopata H 1974 Loneliness: forms and components. In: Weiss R S (ed) Loneliness: the experience of emotional and social isolation. MIT Press, Cambridge, MA

Lundin T 1984 Morbidity following sudden and unexpected bereavement. British Journal of Psychiatry 144: 88–84

Maddison D, Viola A 1968 The health of widows in the year following bereavement. Journal of Psychosomatic Research 12: 297–306

Markides K S, Cooper C L (eds) 1989 Aging, stress and health. Wiley, Chichester

Matthews K A 1982 Psychological perspectives on type A behaviour pattern. Psychological Bulletin 91: 293–323

Moss M S, Moss S Z 1979 The image of the dead spouse in the remarriage of elderly widow(er)s. Paper read at the 32nd Annual Meeting of the Gerontological Society, November 1979, Washington, DC

Owen G, Fulton R, Markusen E 1982 Death at a distance: a study of family survivors. Omega 13: 191–225

Parkes C M 1970 The first year of bereavement. Psychiatry 33: 444–467

Parkes C M 1972 Bereavement: studies of grief in adult life. Tavistock, London

Parkes C M 1975 Determinants of outcome following bereavement. Psychosomatic Medicine 34: 449–461

Parkes C M, Brown R J 1972 Health after bereavement. Psychosomatic Medicine 34: 449–461

Pearlin L I, Leiberman M A, Menaghan E G, Mullan J T 1981 The stress process. Journal of Health and Social Behaviour 22: 337–356

Peck R C 1968 Psychological development in the second half of life. In: Neugarten B L (ed) Middle age and aging. University of Chicago Press, Chicago

Pincus L 1974 Death in the family. Random House, New York

Quattrochititubin S, Jason L A 1983 The influence of introversion–extroversion on activity choice and satisfaction among the elderly. Personality and Individual Differences 4: 17–22

Raphael B 1984 The anatomy of bereavement: a handbook for the caring professions. Hutchinson, London

Rees W D, Lutkins S G 1967 Mortality after bereavement. British Medical Journal 4: 13–16

Rentoul L 1989 Communicating with bereaved relatives in a large hospital: problems and possibilities. Paper presented to the annual conference of the McMillan Society, King's College, London

Sadock B J, Kaplan H I, Freedman A M 1976 Frigidity, dyspareunia, and vaginismus. In: Marmor J (ed) The sexual experience. Williams and Wilkins, Baltimore

Sanders C M 1989 Grief: the mourning after. John Wiley, Chichester

Sheehy G 1977 Passages. Bantam Books, Toronto

Simos B G 1979 A time to grieve. New York, Family Service Association

Singh B S 1982 Work and wellbeing. Paper presented at the annual Royal Australian and New Zealand College of Psychiatry section: social and cultural meeting. Salamander Bay, New South Wales, Australia 1–4 April 1982

Speck P 1978 Loss and grief in medicine. Ballière Tindall, London

Stroebe M S, Stroebe W 1983 Who suffers more? Sex differences in health risks of the widowed. Psychological Bulletin 93: 279–301

Tobin S S 1989 The effects of institutionalization. In: Markides K S, Cooper C L (eds) Aging, stress and health. John Wiley, Chichester

Tobin S S, Lieberman M A 1976 Last home for the aged: critical implications of institutionalization. Jossey-Bass, San Francisco

Vachon M L S, Sheldon A R, Lancee W J, Lyall W A, Rogers J, Freeman S J J 1982 Correlates of enduring stress patterns following bereavement: social network, life situation and personality. Psychological Medicine 12: 783–788

Wan T T H 1982 Stressful life events, social support networks, and gerontological health. Lexington, Lexington, MA

Wan T T H 1984 The health consequences of major role losses in later life: a panel study. Research on Ageing 6: 469–489

Ward A W M 1976 Mortality of bereavement. British Medical Journal 1: 700–702

Wheaton B 1983 Stress, personal coping resources, and psychiatric symptoms: an investigation of interactive models. Journal of Health and Social Behavior 24: 208–229

Worden J W 1983 Grief counselling and grief therapy. Tavistock Publications, London

RECOMMENDED READING

Bromley D B 1990 Behavioural gerontology: central issues in the psychology of ageing. John Wiley, Chichester. *This is a highly accessible and up-to-date book on a wide range of themes relating to old age. The chapter on emotional and adjustment problems in old age provides a helpful link in understanding the pressures of old age and the ways in which vulnerable elderly people may face increasing difficulty in coping. The framework he provides for organising and integrating the material on these issues is particularly useful.*

Coleman P G 1986 Ageing and reminiscence processes: social and clinical implications. Wiley, Chichester. *This book provides an excellent introduction to the clinical and theoretical implications of reminiscence in old age. In particular it considers the ways in which, in some elderly people, the tasks and transition of old age are linked to distress and depression. The case studies of those elderly people, who, although not suffering from pronounced mental illnesses, are nonetheless clearly unhappy, guilt-ridden, angry and anxious, are helpful in understanding the interface between vulnerability and mental health problems in old age.*

Markides K S, Cooper C L (eds) 1989 Aging, stress and health. Wiley, Chichester. *This book covers a range of potentially stressful situations of particular relevance to old age, and considers, with reference to empirical data, the relationship between stress, health and illness among elderly people. Although it looks at morbidity in terms of both physical and mental health indicators, there is plenty of material on mental health. The chapters on institutionalisation and the elderly, widowhood, and depression and the elderly are very helpful in seeking to understand the links between stress and subsequent mental health problems in later life.*

Erikson E H, Erikson J M, Kivnick H Q 1986 Vital involvement in old age: the experience of old age in our time. Norton, New York. *Important update of Erikson's psychoanalytic ideas on the experience of old age.*

Tobin S S 1991 Personhood in advanced old age: implications for practice. Springer, New York. *Tobin's contributions to understanding the experience of old age from the point of view of elderly people have been enormous. His work on institutionalisation and the impact on the emotional lives of old people has been particularly influential. This book represents an up-to-date account of some of his ideas on the experience of growing old.*

Knight B G 1992 Older adults in psychotherapy. Sage, London. *This is one of the few published books on psychotherapy with older people. It presents a number of case studies and looks at the implications for clinical practice of a range of distresses experienced by elderly clients.*

Allman L R, Jaffe D T (eds) 1977 Readings in adult psychology: contemporary perspectives. Harper Row, New York. *This is a collection of papers that have been influential in the development of ideas in the psychology of old age. Although many of the papers were written over 20 years ago, their contribution to the development of ideas in the field of gerontology is significant. The methods of research and the types of data obtained (such as conversations and dream material) are viewed increasingly as important sources of data, in complementing the emphasis on quantitative approaches to research, that characterised work in subsequent years.*

Raphael B 1984 The anatomy of bereavement: a handbook for the caring professions. Hutchinson, London. *An excellent review of the literature on bereavement. There is a particularly interesting section on losses in old age, which looks at the literature on grief, which pertains to significant loss, though not that of simply facing the death of a loved person. It covers the losses of retirement, of function, of sexuality and of perceptual abilities. The clinical implications of the material is discussed with great sensitivity.*

Sanders C M 1989 Grief: the mourning after. John Wiley, Chichester. *Another book which looks at the literature on bereavement. It covers similar ground to the book of Beverly Raphael (1984), and is rich in clinical case material and empirical research evidence. An excellent introduction to the theoretical issues of death, dying and bereavement.*

5

Learning disability in later life

John Brown

Learning disability has long been one of the 'Cinderella' services when it comes to the allocation of resources. Those resources that have been provided have, through their scarcity, been selectively focused. The result is that in a general area of neglect there are pockets of greater neglect. The topic of learning disability in later life is one such pocket. To some extent this is understandable as it is only in recent years that demographic profiles have changed significantly for this to become a potential issue. Yet at the same time, the lack of a focus is a product of the way that services and policies have evolved over the years. This chapter attempts to outline this evolution to provide an appreciation of the policy dynamic in learning disabilities that provides the context for developing what is, at present, a still embryonic recognition of the importance of later life for this group of service users.

Early in 1995 the Department of Health as part of its 'Health of the Nation' initiative published a document that outlined a strategy for people with learning disabilities (Department of Health 1995a). When originally published in 1992, *The Health of the Nation* White Paper had identified five key areas:

- coronary heart disease and stroke
- cancer
- HIV/AIDS and sexual health
- accidents
- mental health (Department of Health 1992a).

These areas provided the basis for the discussion in the strategy for learning disabilities. This was clear recognition that people with a learning disability shared common health problems with the rest of the population. Yet there is a crucial difference between the two documents.

Whereas the original White Paper had identified particular targets to achieve in each of the areas, the document on learning disabilities was much more circumspect. A broad view of the particular needs of the user group is presented rather than a detailed and considered analysis. This is partly due to the long-standing problem of definition and aetiology (Race 1995a, b), but also partly to the relative lack of information available for this particular group of users when compared to others. This is especially the case with regards to mental health problems in learning disabilities, with the one possible exception of challenging behaviour (Department of Health 1993), and the problems faced by the individual with learning disabilities in later life. The reasons for this are very much a legacy of the history of perception of learning disabilities and the policies that have been designed on the basis of this perception.

Although learning disabilities has been a government priority since 1976 (Department of Health and Social Security 1976) other groups have been seen as having a more urgent priority when allocating scarce resources. The result is that other groups are often better catered for when compared to learning disabilities. This is reflected not only in the development of service provision and patterns of support and care (Audit Commission 1992b) but also in the amount of information available from surveys and research upon which to base policy decisions and practice interventions. One result is that there is little certainty on the numbers of people surviving to late life with a learning disability. In 1992 the Department of Health stated:

There is no precise information available nationally about the number of people with learning disabilities, or the degree of those difficulties. The number *may* be growing, as advances in health care mean people with particular forms of disability have a greater life expectancy. This will result in a higher proportion of people with more profound or multiple handicaps and consequently higher levels of dependency. Also people with learning disabilities may manifest at an earlier age health problems associated with old age.   (Their emphasis, Department of Health 1992b, p. 2)

The implications are profound not only for the individuals with a learning disability but also for any family that they may have. While it is not possible to be precise, the 1995 *Health of the Nation* strategy document identifies what is seen as a discernible trend ' ... with the rise in life expectancy, more parents continue as carers into old age and more people with learning disabilities are outliving their parents' (Department of Health 1995a, p. 8). The scale of the contribution and the critical role that parents and families play as informal carers is indicated when government figures, allowing for the fact that there is no precise information, are considered.

In England, the Department of Health estimates for guidance purposes that there are between 120 000 and 160 000 adults with severe or profound learning disabilities (Department of Health 1992c, p. 2). The number living in NHS institutions in 1993 was 16 000 with social services providing residential places for a further 11 400 and the independent sector another 24 100 (Department of Health 1995a, p. 8). The total of some 52 100 is less than half the lower guidance figure of 120 000 if it is assumed that all those in residential care are the most severely or profoundly disabled. Such a comparison cannot be made with any degree of statistical confidence. It is meant only, in the absence of reliable and alternative figures, as a rough illustration to indicate the crucial contribution that parents and families play in providing support for some of the most demanding individuals. It is not unexpected that this is the case.

In 1973, a study was published based on work in Sheffield that showed that those with the most severe and profound learning disability were not to be found in institutions but in their parents' homes (Bayley 1973). Earlier research had indicated that those who were to be found in local authority residential care for the elderly were those where there was little or no family support rather than the residents being the most frail among the elderly (Townsend 1962). A more recent collection of readings on informal carers for different client groups has repeated this general finding (Twigg 1992). Yet in spite of the long-standing evidence for the importance of parents and families and the clear implications for them as more people with a learning disability live longer, and which the Department of Health recognises in the extract above, the policy agenda is still very much influenced by a history coloured by debates over residential care. Again, this is a legacy of the history of perception of learning disability and the policies that reflect this perception.

PERCEPTIONS AND POLICIES

It was not until the Mental Deficiency Act of 1913 that the specific needs of those with what is now referred to as learning disabilities were officially recognised as distinct from those with mental health problems. Until that time the two groups had been treated as very similar in government legislation (Jones 1972). While the 1913 legislation has to be seen as a landmark, the way that learning disabilities was classified displays the negative connotation associated with this group of users. The terms used – 'idiot', 'imbecile', 'feeble-minded' and 'moral defective' – graphically display, no matter how distasteful, the stigma that this group experienced. Subsequent changes in terminology, while indicating changes in philosophy and understanding, have not eliminated this stigma. This has meant that in policy terms people with a learning disability, whether through ignorance, fear or guilt, are all too often marginalised and their difficulties placed behind those of other groups when it comes to allocating scarce resources. Current policies of community care differ little in this respect compared to earlier policies of institutionalisation where the emphasis was very much out of sight out of mind.

The Mental Health Act of 1959 provided the foundation upon which current policies of community care can trace their origin. The legislation was based upon the findings of a Royal Commission established in 1954 to review mental health services. The Commission had a clear remit to include learning disabilities. Establishment of the National Health Service in 1948 meant that learning disabilities followed the example of mental health with Poor Law institutions formerly run by local authorities, and where the bulk of residential care was provided, becoming classified as NHS hospitals (Jones 1972). Both groups were now seen as sharing similar experiences – large anonymous, alienating institutions, all too often dominated by a medical model that saw problems in terms of a disease to be treated by medical techniques and technology. Little attempt was being made, except in a few pioneer schemes (Tizard 1964), to address, let alone recognise, the impact of the social environment and the interpersonal element underlying behaviour and its interpretation. The 1959 legislation attempted to change this by arguing that community care was not only an appropriate but also essential part of responding to the needs of some of the most vulnerable people in society.

Yet while the proposals were adopted in principle by the then Conservative government, the full import for those with a learning disability was again compromised by terminology. The terms of the 1913 Act were to be replaced by two legal categories 'mental subnormality' and 'severe mental subnormality'. Again, it is hard to escape negative connotations. Publication in 1969 of a national study of hospitals for people with a learning disability cogently captured the challenge faced by policy-makers at that time and subsequently with its title, *Put Away* (Morris 1969). Progress was still slow in gaining acceptance and understanding for those with a learning disability.

In the same year that *Put Away* was published, the government released a report on Ely Hospital in South Wales that catalogued incidents of abuse of resident rights and the depersonalised way in which some staff approached their duties (Department of Health and Social Security 1969). It was increasingly difficult to ignore the inappropriate setting that many hospitals provided for those with a learning disability and the deleterious effect that this had not only upon the personal development of the residents, but also upon the morale of staff. The coincidence of publication of an academic study and report of a committee of enquiry both of which were to agree on the problems faced by residents living in long-stay hospitals for those with a learning disability was to galvanise the government into action. The White Paper *Better Services for the Mentally Handicapped* was published 2 years later (Department of Health and Social Security 1971a) and was to remain government policy through successive administrations until 1991 (Dorrell 1991).

The symbolic shift in official policy that the White Paper signified was captured on the title page with the use of the term 'mental handicap'. This did not replace the legal use of the term 'mental subnormality' and 'severe mental subnormality' which remained in force until the 1983 Mental Health Amendment Act and the introduction of the replacement terms of 'mental impairment' and 'severe mental impairment' respectively. At no time did the use of mental handicap have the force of law behind it and although its use was criticised (Campaign for the Mentally Handicapped 1973), in the context of the early 1970s the term marked a decided attempt to move away from the negative connotations evoked by the terms used for people with a learning disability in previous legislation. The White Paper also encapsulated current thinking on community care.

Hospital places were to be reduced by almost half over the next 20 years, from 52 000 beds to 27 000 beds. Local facilities were to be built up to compensate for this reduction and services were to be based upon the principle that ' ... each handicapped person needs stimulation, social training and education in order to develop to his maximum capacity and to exercise all the skills he acquires, however limited they be' (Department of Health and Social Security 1971a, p. 9). Some proposals have not stood the test of time. Arguments for hostel places of up to 20–25 beds in the community to house those rehabilitated from long-stay hospital care now appear inappropriate. But at a time when long-stay hospitals regularly accommodated 1500 beds, and occasionally exceeded 2000 beds, such a proposal was a considerable advance on previous thinking. Progress, however, was slow in taking the proposals in the White Paper forward. Reviewing the decade of the 1970s, the Department of Health and Social Security (it was not to be called the Department of Health until 1988) commented that it appeared the 20 year target for hospital bed reduction would not be achieved as the hoped for rate of closure had not been attained (Department of Health and Social Security 1980). This had also been apparent to a number of voluntary organisations and pressure groups.

In 1978 MENCAP, MIND, the Spastics Society (now called SCOPE) and the Campaign for Mentally Handicapped People (which was subsequently to become Values in Action) joined together to form a campaign under the title 'Exodus'. This was brought about by a sense of despair that the large long-stay hospital would ever disappear. Hospital enquiries were still continuing (Department of Health and Social Security 1971b, House of Commons 1974, Department of Health and Social Security 1978) and there was a prevailing sense that the only way that hospital places would run down was by preventing children with learning disabilities being referred there in the first place. Support came from the National Development Group which argued that those already in hospital had no realistic possibility of ever leaving and resources should focus upon making their life as comfortable as possible while preventing the admission of children (National Development Group 1978). Reports on child health services (Committee on Child Health Services 1976) and special educational needs (Department of Education & Science 1978) provided added weight.

The result was that the emphasis in policy became one of very much concentrating upon children with the government providing extra resources in the early/mid 1980s in an attempt to get the remaining children out of long-stay hospitals for those with a learning disability (Leonard 1991). Services for adults were not neglected but they did not have the prominence given to those for children. The momentum of enquiry and focus of energy could not be said to be the same at that time between children and adults, and attention upon the issues associated with later life in learning disabilities was very much a marginal interest for policy makers and academics alike. However, the emphasis upon the personal development of children and the design of appropriate patterns of service assisted the widespread adoption of a philosophy of 'normalisation' (Wolfensberger 1972). This has made a profound impact upon the provision provided for all people with a learning disability.

Throughout the 1970s and 1980s, normalisation has informed debates about the way in which people with a learning disability should be encouraged to become integrated members of society. This impact can be found in broad-based policy statements encapsulated in the phrase 'an ordinary life' (King's Fund 1983)

through to specific guidance on standards of care and quality residential homes (Department of Health/Social Services Inspectorate 1989) and checklists for the inspection of day services (Department of Health/Social Services Inspectorate 1992). Normalisation is a phrase that can provide the vehicle for a range of approaches (Towell 1991). Different authors stress different aspects but all recognise a series of values as underlying the approach (Centre for Policy on Ageing 1984):

- dignity
- privacy
- independence
- choice
- rights
- fulfilment.

They are values that everyone can subscribe to in Western culture. Yet each of these values could be taken as the antithesis of the experience of many people with a learning disability, irrespective of their age and the setting that they find themselves. Further discussion on normalisation can be found in Chapter 27.

In the atmosphere of the debates around learning disabilities over the last 2 decades, the failure often to realise these values in the residential hospital setting has been taken as indictment of that provision. In particular, the point has been made that not only have these values failed to inform some hospital practice but that as people with a learning disability are not ill in a medical sense then the hospital is an inappropriate place for them to live (Ryan & Thomas 1995). If they require hospital treatment then they should have access to the same services that everyone else in the community has – they should be treated as no different. This has been a powerful argument. It has been persuasive across all areas of disability, and not just learning disabilities (Swain et al 1993, Oliver 1990). It has provided a strong base for the development of moves towards both advocacy and empowerment (Hersov 1992). Yet it is not necessarily that clear cut and such an interpretation of normalisation is overly simplistic. The 1995 *Health of the Nation* strategy is explicit that access to general community facilities can pose problems (Department of Health 1995a, p. 8): 'The needs for health care of people with learning disabilities are mostly similar to other people's; but there are some differences and complexities which may require additional attention. People with learning disabilities often find it difficult to use health services open to the population as a whole, and sometimes they find barriers put in their way'.

At the same time, it is also only a short step away from denying that people with a learning disability should have specialist facilities to denying that they have any needs that require specialist treatment.

Recent research has shown that difficulties in evaluating the impact of community care in learning disabilities can obscure the fact that 'normal' outcomes often require an extraordinary input built upon a base of specialist skills (Wright et al 1994). In a national review of services for people with learning disabilities and associated mental health problems the point was made that: ' ... Life for people with major disabilities in good services will often look quite ordinary but this ordinariness will be the product of a great deal of careful planning and management' (Department of Health 1993, p. 10).

Such planning and management requires the recognition that there are specialist roles built upon specialist knowledge. What this specialist knowledge and associated skills should be is again coloured by a history of perceptions, this time the perception of the relevance of skills associated with particular professions.

SPECIALIST SKILLS

In 1991 the Minister of Health announced at the MENCAP annual conference that 'mental handicap' as a term was no longer to be used by government and would be replaced by 'learning disability' (Dorrell 1991). This adoption of yet another term to refer to the user group could be seen as potentially bringing to a close a long-standing debate, and at times acrimonious controversy, between nursing and social work, the two main groups working with people with a learning disability. With nursing predominately based within the hospital setting, the criticisms levelled at long-stay hospitals were, by extension, criticisms of the nursing staff who worked there. A major review of the nurse's role in learning disabilities showed that this was too simplistic (Department of Health and Social Security 1979). The review also presented in its report a series of principles (see Box 5.1) based on lessons derived from the impetus provided by the insights of normalisation. These still provide the most succinct summary of a philosophical and moral initiative that informs much current debate about service provision (Department of Health and Social Security 1979, pp. 35–37).

Support was forthcoming for the principles outlined in the report. The reception of the report, nonetheless, was less than enthusiastic from some nursing staff. While agreeing with the principles outlined, exception

was taken over the model of care that the report outlined which proposed the transfer of staff to local authority responsibility. This opposition was symbolised by nursing doggedly adhering to the use of the term 'mental handicap' while others, including social work, began to adopt the term 'learning difficulties'. While the nursing validation body still uses the term 'mental handicap' in its awards, in spite of the Dorrell statement, the debate was in many ways false. As debates raged during the 1980s significant developments were taking place in nurse training and in the development of links between the different professional bodies.

In 1982 the nurse validating body for England introduced a new training for nurses preparing to work with people with learning disabilities (English National Board 1983). This was a radical departure from previous training in that the emphasis was very much upon working in community and domiciliary settings rather than in the hospital. The principles of normalisation were prominent. At the same time, the first initial steps towards joint and shared training were beginning to be made between nursing and social work (Brown 1992). The result has been that what has currently come to be called shared learning between professionals has made greatest headway in learning disabilities rather than in the more high profile groups (Brown 1994). This is not to say that this is a development universally accepted by all professional practitioners involved with learning disabilities.

In 1993, old anxieties among some nurses surfaced again with the prospect that learning disabilities would be removed from pre-registration nurse training. The resulting furore led the Department of Health to establish, after making a commitment to maintain this level of specialist training, a small project team to identify the specific contribution of the nurse to the support and care of people with a learning disability. The resulting report, published in 1995, consisted of three documents under the title *Continuing the Commitment* (Kay et al 1995a, Kay et al 1995b, Department of Health 1995b). Here, specific knowledge and skills of the learning disability nurse are identified.

In particular, emphasis is placed upon eight areas (Kay et al 1995a, pp. 18–36):

1). Assessment of need;
2). Health surveillance and health promotion;
3). Developing personal competence;
4). Use of enhanced therapeutic skills;
5). Managing and leading teams of staff;
6). Enhancing the quality of support;
7). Enablement and empowerment; and
8). Co-ordinating services.

Box 5.1   The principles presented in the *Report of the Committee of Enquiry into Mental Handicap Nursing and Care* (DHSS 1979)

Broad Principles:
(a) mentally handicapped people have a right to enjoy normal patterns of life within the community;
(b) mentally handicapped people have a right to be treated as individuals; and
(c) mentally handicapped people will require additional help from the communities in which they live and from professional services if they are to develop to their maximum potential as individuals.

Living Like Others Within the Community:
(a) mentally handicapped children should be able to live with a family ...
(b) any mentally handicapped adult who wishes to leave his or her parental home should have the opportunity to do so.
(c) any accommodation provided for adults or children should allow the individual to live as a member of a small group.
(d) if they wish so, mentally handicapped people should be able to live with their peers who are not mentally handicapped ...
(e) staffed accommodation should wherever possible be provided in suitably adapted houses which are physically integrated with the community.
(f) these homes should be as local as possible to help the handicapped person to retain contact with his own family and community ...
(g) mentally handicapped people should be able to live in a mixed sex environment ...
(h) mentally handicapped people should be able to develop a daily routine like other people.
(i) there should be a proper separation of home, work and recreation.

Individuality:
(a) the right of an individual to live, learn and work in the least restrictive environment appropriate to that particular person.
(b) the right to make or be involved in decisions that affect oneself.
(c) acceptance that individual needs differ not only between different individuals, but within the same individual over time.
(d) the right of parents to be involved in decisions about their children.

Service Principles:
(a) mentally handicapped people should use normal services wherever possible.
(b) existing networks of community support should be strengthened by professional services rather than supplanted by them.
(c) 'specialised' services or organisations for mentally handicapped people should be provided only to the extent that they demonstrably meet or are likely to meet additional needs that cannot be met by the general services.
(d) if we are to meet the many and diverse needs of mentally handicapped people we need maximum co-ordination both within and between agencies and at all levels. The concept of a life-plan seems essential if co-ordination and continuity of care is to be achieved.
(e) finally, if we are to establish and maintain high quality services for a group of people who cannot easily articulate and press their just claims, we need someone to intercede on behalf of mentally handicapped people in obtaining services.
(Source: Department of Health and Social Security 1979, pp. 35–37)

These areas are seen as reflecting activities in a ' ... rapidly changing environment in which nurses and others work demands that new roles emerge as needs and priorities change' (Kay et al 1995a, p. 35). These new roles mean that the debate between nursing and social work about skills and services no longer has the resonance it had until very recently. What is at issue is not who has the specialist skills but is the case for specialist skills accepted by those now responsible for services in a 'rapidly changing environment'?

The introduction of an internal market for both health and social care has created new requirements for the organisation and administration of services. This has profound implications for all those involved in the support and care of those with a learning disability. It is a development that offers potential gains for the individual with the emphasis upon services being determined by needs assessment. But it also highlights the problem faced by all those in

learning disabilities convincing those who now determine the allocation of resources, the purchasers, that the support and care of those with a learning disability requires specialist skill. There is no guarantee that this will be the case. The new purchasers of services are not necessarily immune from the problems of perception, prejudice and ignorance that the earlier discussion on the negative connotations of terminology underlined. The importance of this is highlighted in the *Health of the Nation* strategy document (Department of Health 1995a).

THE INTERNAL MARKET AND LEARNING DISABILITIES

Current policy on the internal market is encapsulated in the NHS and Community Care Act 1990, that embodies the main points from a series of White Papers: *Promoting Better Health* (Department of Health and Social Security 1987), *Working for Patients* (Department of Health 1989a) and *Caring for People* (Department of Health, 1989b). The subsequent publication of *The Health of the Nation* (Department of Health 1992a) can also be viewed as part of this sequence. Collectively, these documents have led to the introduction of services that have transformed the design, delivery and responsibility for services for all those with a learning disability as well as the whole population. These changes fall into eight main areas:

1. The internal market – where a distinction is made between the purchasers, or commissioners, of services, such as District Health Authorities, and the providers of services, such as hospitals.
2. The creation of self-governing trusts – where hospitals are largely responsible for their own fund-raising and income generation and compete with other hospitals for contracts from purchasers.
3. The introduction of new General Practitioner contracts related, in part, to attaining various performance targets.
4. The promotion of General Practitioner Fundholders who administer their own budget and are purchasers of services direct from hospitals on behalf of their patients.
5. The distinction between health and social care in the organisation and delivery of services in the community.
6. The design of services on the basis of a comprehensive assessment of individual need.
7. The development of care management to provide an integrated pattern of services to the individual user.
8. The re-focusing of the role of social service departments away from being a provider of care to a role where they are a purchaser, especially for residential care and the acquisition of a responsibility for registration and inspection of care homes.

These changes have been introduced throughout the early part of the 1990s. In learning disabilities, the situation to which they applied was dramatically different from the one that had existed only a decade earlier. Then, as already referred to, the Department of Health had expressed concerns that the 1971 target for the reduction in hospital beds would not be attained (Department of Health and Social Security 1980). By the time the internal market was about to be introduced not only had the target been attained, it had been exceeded (Department of Health 1992b). The reason for this has been given as the ideological drive of the government that favoured the private sector over statutory provision. This provided the momen-

tum that meant that the problems faced by the local authorities in funding community care were bypassed by placing former hospital residents directly into private care with the costs being covered by social security payments (Korman & Glennerster 1990). With fewer people with a learning disability in long-stay hospital provision than ever before, the traditional focus upon the relevance of that accommodation became one where concerns have been reported over the speed of the closure programmes (Wright et al 1994). Issues have also emerged around ensuring the attainment and maintenance of standards and quality of residential provision in the community (Sinclair & Brown 1995).

Although the debate over hospital provision has moved on, this has done little to alter the fact that the bulk of care is still provided by informal carers. The introduction of an internal market with the emphasis upon individual needs assessment held out the prospect, for the first time, of constructing packages of that care directly addressed to the situation that each person with a learning disability and their carers found themselves in. This has not proved to be the case on any significant scale.

In 1992 the Audit Commission published a series of documents that provided a preliminary assessment of the progress being made with the reforms. Two of these reports outlined a picture where the hoped for re-direction and improvements in services were not being realised (Audit Commission 1992a, Audit Commission 1992b). Too much was being sought in too short a time. The reforms did not necessarily have the full support of managers responsible for implementing them and there was little local organisational support to provide guidance and direction. The unmistakeable message that comes through is that the reforms were politically led with little appreciation of the complexity of delivering them on the ground. The opportunity for a new individual-based needs assessed service, with potential clear benefits for those with a learning disability, was beginning to falter. Subsequent progress reports from the Audit Commission showed that this was indeed the case.

Over 2 consecutive years the financial problems faced in providing health and social care were highlighted (Audit Commission 1993, Audit Commission 1994). Traditional problems of under-resourcing persisted and were being exacerbated with the additional costs of meeting new responsibilities. The casualty was introducing an individual needs-led service for all users. Assessment had to take into account what an authority could afford. As a needs assessment carried the force of law for its recommendations to be implemented, pressure emerged to ensure that only those services that could be offered were to be identified in the assessment (Audit Commission 1993). All user groups, and not just learning disabilities, have experienced this problem. But if previous experience is drawn upon, the expectation must be that learning disability, with its low profile and low prestige, will suffer disproportionately compared to other groups. Again, perceptions and attitudes come to the fore. Here the most significant development with the introduction of the internal market has been the pivotal contribution made by purchasers. Among these, the role played by the general practitioner is now paramount.

Moves to a primary-led health service marks one of the most significant developments in recent years in the National Health Service (Department of Health 1992d). At the same time, the general practitioner has begun to have an increasing involvement in community care with a subsequent blurring of the distinction between primary and community care. This was signalled in the *Caring for People* where the role of the general practitioner was taken as embracing ' ... ill health and social handicap' (Department of Health 1989b, para 4.12). Such a comprehensive remit promotes the general practitioner to a prominence in service provision that cannot be ignored by those involved in learning disabilities.

There is little reason to expect that the attitudes of general practitioners, and their possible lack of awareness and appreciation, are any different from the rest of the community when it comes to an understanding of learning disabilities. Here the *Health of the Nation* strategy document comes to the fore (Department of Health 1995a). It is written very much in a style that is designed to inform and educate those responsible for services, such as general practitioners, who may have little understanding of learning disabilities but whose future purchasing decisions may well have considerable impact upon the quality of life of the user with a learning disability. This is an approach that the Department of Health has also adopted in one of its *Continuing the Commitment* documents where a series of case studies are presented for purchasers to begin to develop an appreciation of the heterogeneous nature of learning disability and the specialist skills required of practitioners (Department of Health 1995b). Both documents present examples of the skills that are likely to be called upon. For example, the following issues are identified when diagnosing possible mental health problems (Department of Health 1995a, p. 34):

Diagnosis may depend on symptoms described by the patient:
— some obvious features may be non-specific (such as agitation, or other behavioural change), while other features may be hard to elicit (such as suicidal ideas);
— symptoms may be described in an unfamiliar way. For example, 'loss of interest' may be described in terms of reduced time spent in an activity at a day centre;
— changes in behaviour may be described in a way which misleads a doctor. For example, a doctor may not think to ask whether 'Self-injurious Behaviour' could represent an attempt at suicide, or whether 'Challenging Behaviour' could be a response to pain or emotional distress; and
— doctors may not know what to expect from a person with learning disabilities, and make mistaken assumptions.

What is notable is that nowhere in the document is specific consideration given to the problems presented by the older person with a learning disability. Reference is made to the fact that among those who need additional attention are those ' ... becoming old ... (and who) have parents or carers who are elderly, sick or, for other reasons, no longer able to provide care and support' (Department of Health 1995a, p. 8). Comment is also made that 'there is a strong association between early onset of Alzheimer's disease (a cause of dementia) and Down's Syndrome' (Department of Health 1995a, p. 34), but this is not developed. Similarly, among the 14 vignettes in *Continuing the Commitment*, not one relates to the many potential problems faced by those with a learning disability who are facing the challenge of becoming old. This is not altogether unexpected. The emphasis upon children, and to a lesser extent young adults, has dominated the literature in learning disabilities, as has already been described. Other reports that have presented examples have also ignored this particular group (Department of Health and Social Security 1979). As more people with a learning disability live longer it can be expected that this area will enter the policy arena.

It is an arena that is still changing rapidly. The problems associated with diagnosis mentioned above are not especially daunting to overcome. As was commented in another document that presented similar examples, ' ... none of these raises complex issues, but some prior consideration is needed if people with learning disabilities ... are to be satisfactorily treated' (Department of Health 1992b, p. 5). The challenge is to ensure, at a time of considerable change in service provision, that recognition of issues in later life are accompanied by appropriate resources to enable 'prior consideration' that prevents them becoming problems to the detriment of the quality of life of individuals and their families and carers.

REFERENCES

Audit Commission 1992a Community care: managing the cascade of change. HMSO, London

Audit Commission 1992b The community revolution: personal social services and community care. HMSO, London

Audit Commission 1993 Taking care: progress with care in the community. Health and Personal Social Services Bulletin No 1. HMSO, London

Audit Commission 1994 Taking stock: progress with community care. Community Care Bulletin No 2. HMSO, London

Bayley M 1973 Mental handicap and community care. Routledge and Kegan Paul, London

Brown J 1992 Professional boundaries in mental handicap: a policy analysis of joint training. In: Thompson T, Mathias P (eds) Standards and mental handicap: keys to competence. Baillière Tindall, London

Brown J 1994 Demarcation and the public sector: the impact of the contract agenda upon mental health practice. In: Thompson T, Mathias P (eds) Lyttle's mental health and disorder, 2nd edn. Baillière Tindall, London

Campaign for the Mentally Handicapped 1973 The action needed now. Campaign for the Mentally Handicapped, London

Centre for Policy on Ageing 1984 A home life: a code of practice for residential care. Centre for Policy on Ageing, London

Committee on Child Health Services 1976 Fit for the future. The Court Report. Cmnd 6684. HMSO, London

Department of Education and Science 1978 Special educational needs. The Warnock Report. Cmnd 7212. HMSO, London

Department of Health 1989a Working for patients. Cm 555. HMSO, London

Department of Health 1989b Caring for people. Cm 849. HMSO, London

Department of Health 1992a The health of the nation. Cm 1986. HMSO, London

Department of Health 1992b Health services for people with learning disabilities (mental handicap) HSG(92) 42. Department of Health, London

Department of Health 1992c Social care for adults with learning disabilities (mental handicap) LAc (92) 15. Department of Health, London

Department of Health 1992d Report of the inquiry into London's health service medical education and research. Tomlinson Report. HMSO, London

Department of Health 1993 Services for people with learning disabilities and challenging behaviour or mental health needs. Mansell Report. HMSO, London

Department of Health 1995a The health of the nation: a strategy for people with learning disabilities. Department of Health, London

Department of Health 1995b Learning disability: meeting needs through targeting skills. Department of Health, London

Department of Health and Social Security 1969 Report of the committee of inquiry into allegations of ill-treatment and other irregularities at the Ely Hospital Cardiff. Cmnd 3975. HMSO, London

Department of Health and Social Security 1971a Better services for the mentally handicapped. Cmnd 4683. HMSO, London

Department of Health and Social Security 1971b Report of the Farleigh committee of inquiry. Cmnd 4557. HMSO, London

Department of Health and Social Security 1976 Priorities for health and personal social services in England. HMSO, London

Department of Health and Social Security 1978 Report of the committee of inquiry into Normansfield Hospital. Cmnd 7357. HMSO, London

Department of Health and Social Security 1979 Report of the committe of enquiry into mental handicap nursing and care. The Jay Report. Cmnd 7468. HMSO, London

Department of Health and Social Security 1980 Mental handicap: progress, problems and priorities. HMSO, London

Department of Health and Social Security 1987 Promoting better health. Cm 249. HMSO, London

Department of Health/Social Services Inspectorate 1989 Guidance on standards for the residential care needs of people with learning disabilities. HMSO, London

Department of Health/Social Services Inspectorate 1992 Caring for quality: day services. HMSO, London

Dorrell S 1991 Address to the annual conference for MENCAP. Unpublished paper, Department of Health

English National Board for Nursing, Midwifery and Health Visiting 1983 Syllabus of training professional register, part 5: Registered Nurse for the Mentally Handicapped. ENB, London

Hersov J 1992 Advocacy – issues for the 1990s. In: Thompson T, Mathias P (eds) Standards and mental handicap: keys to competence. Baillière Tindall, London

House of Commons 1974 Return to an order: report of the committee of inquiry into South Ockendon Hospital. HMSO, London

Jones K 1972 A history of the mental health services. Routledge and Kegan Paul, London

Kay B, Rose S, Turnbull J 1995a Continuing the commitment: the report of the learning disability project. Department of Health, London

Kay B, Rose S, Turnbull J 1995b Learning disability nursing project: resource package. Department of Health, London

King's Fund 1983 An ordinary life. King's Fund Centre, London

Korman N, Glennerster H 1990 Hospital closure: a political and economic study. Open University Press, Buckingham

Leonard A 1991 A home of their own. Gower, Aldershot

Malin N (ed) 1995 Services for people with learning disabilities. Routledge, London

Morris P 1969 Put away. Routledge and Kegan Paul, London

National Development Group 1978 Helping mentally handicapped people in hospital. Department of Health and Social Security, London

National Health Service and Community Care Act 1990. HMSO, London

Oliver M 1990 The politics of disablement. Macmillan, Basingstoke

Race D 1995a Classification of people with learning disabilities. In: Malin N (ed) Services for people with learning disabilities. Routledge, London

Race D 1995b Causes of learning disabilities. In: Malin N (ed) Services for people with learning disabilities. Routledge, London

Ryan J, Thomas F 1995 The politics of mental handicap, 2nd edn. Penguin, Harmondsworth

Sinclair I, Brown J 1995 Quality assurance and inspection. In: Malin N (ed) Services for people with learning disabilities. Routledge, London

Swain J, Finkelstein V, French S, Oliver M (eds) 1993 Disabling barriers – enabling environments. Sage Publications, London

Thompson T, Mathias P (eds) 1992 Standards and mental handicap: keys to competence. Baillière Tindall, London

Thompson T, Mathias P (eds) 1994 Lyttle's mental health and disorder, 2nd edn. Baillière Tindall, London

Tizard J 1964 Community services for the mentally handicapped. Oxford University Press, Oxford

Towell D (ed) 1991 Normalisation: an ordinary life in practice. King's Fund Centre, London

Townsend P 1962 The last refuge. Routledge and Kegan Paul, London

Twigg J (ed) 1992 Carers research and practice. HMSO, London

Wolfensberger W 1972 The principle of normalisation in human services. National Institute for Mental Retardation, Toronto

Wright K, Haycox A, Leedham I 1994 Evaluating community care: services for people with learning disabilities. Open University Press, Buckingham

RECOMMENDED READING

Malin N (ed) 1995 Services for people with learning disabilities. Routledge, London. *An up-to-date collection that covers a wide range of topics on learning disability. A useful source for figures on incidence and statistics on different settings.*

Thompson T, Mathias P (eds) 1992 Standards and mental handicap: keys to competence. Baillière Tindall, London.

Thompson T, Mathias P (eds) 1994 Lyttle's mental health and disorder. 2nd edn. Baillière Tindall, London.
Both of these provide a wide range of material. The quality is generally strong.

Wright K, Haycox A, Leedham I 1994 Evaluating community care: services for people with learning disabilities. Open University Press, Buckingham. *An excellent book with a very comprehensive bibliography.*

Department of Health 1995 The health of the nation: a strategy for people with learning disabilities. Department of Health, London. *Short but essential reading on the priorities for policy in learning disabilities.*

Ryan J, Thomas F 1995 The politics of mental handicap, 2nd edn. Penguin, Harmondsworth. *Written in a swingeing style this conveys the passion that many felt about the inadequacies of long-stay hospitals.*

Audit Commission 1992a Community care: managing the cascade of change. HMSO, London.

Audit Commission 1992b The community revolution: personal social services and community care. HMSO, London.
Both provide detailed, but largely accessible, accounts of issues surrounding the introduction of the internal market.

6

Assessment of older people

Susan Ritter
Mary Watkins

INTRODUCTION

This chapter focuses on elucidating the needs and problems of the individual user of health and social services. It does not deal directly with questions of priority of care nor with questions of quality of life. We look at the challenges of need and risk assessment and identify aspects of elderly people that concern the assessor. We discuss aetiological and vulnerability factors, instrumental behaviours, psychological assessment and assessment of organic changes. Later sections give an overview of assessment principles and procedures.

Normative and ipsative assessment

There is general agreement that assessment of older people needs to be comprehensive (Lishman 1987, Battcock & Castleden 1990). Ipsative assessment, in which people are assessed in relation to themselves, relies also on elements like information from third parties and a history in order to make sense of phenomena here and now. Normative assessment, in which people are assessed in relation to other people (compare normative reference groups Hyman & Singer 1968), relies also on in-depth knowledge of the individuals to be confident that the norms of a measure fit them.

Description of phenomena

Descriptive psychopathology is defined as the attribution by an observer of symptoms to behaviour of a patient. It began as a way of organising knowledge about mental events that were seen either as continuous or discontinuous with usual experience (Berrios 1984). Information about mental events was derived from introspection – from people's accounts of their subjective experience – and from observation of behaviour. The grouping and classification of mental events have resulted in the two distinct disciplines of psychology and psychiatry, the first concerned with the study of internal states and processes and observable behaviours, the second concerned with the study of abnormal variants of the same phenomena.

An important transition was marked by the observation that psychological terms such as thought disorder are at least at one step removed from internal states and processes for which terms like thinking and feeling are used (Grounds 1987). Grounds (1987) also notes that to talk about disorders of thinking (cognition) and of mood (affect) is to imply the presence of lesions in a person's mind. This has a number of consequences. First, the subjective experience of people who feel that their thinking is being interfered with by an outside force is poorly described by the term 'thought disorder'. Secondly, there is potential for confusion when a person reports a mental event such as hearing a voice when no one else is present. To describe this report as an auditory hallucination implies that the reported voice falls into a category of psychopathological symptoms and that it is the same kind of symptom as other reports of hearing a voice. The Present State Examination questions the respondent minutely about perceptual anomalies in order to be able to reduce the information to categories of symptoms (Wing et al 1974). Sims (1995) provides useful guidelines for working out with people what they are perceiving when they describe perceptual experiences such as 'voices'.

Another problem occurs with a term like 'insight' which at first appears analogous with 'delusion'. To have insight into a delusional system implies that individuals have learned to control or compensate for the lesion in their mind that the delusion represents. David (1990, p. 803) suggests that the predisposition to 'form inferences in an idiosyncratic way is a key element of delusional experience'. Clearly this predisposition cannot be described as a 'lesion'.

McWalter et al (1994) argue that commonly used scales such as the Clifton Assessment Procedure for the Elderly (Pattie & Gilliard 1979) or the Mini Mental State Examination (Folstein et al 1975) rely on methods of operationalising abstract concepts to score items. When clinicians infer from these measures other abstract concepts such as 'dependency, impairment, burden or stress' (McWalter et al 1994, p. 214), they begin to strain the confines of reliability and validity. When assessment purports to describe people's behaviour, direct observation is essential to supplement self-report or report by carer or other caregiver.

The construct 'loss of appetite' is an inference from a number of behaviours that together may be described as not eating, but a person may not eat for reasons ranging from badly-fitting false teeth to being unable to feed the electricity meter. In these circumstances Schutte and Malouff (1995, p. 5) recommend that 'by treating a scale score as a piece of evidence rather than as a conclusion in itself, clinicians can minimise assessment errors'.

The implication for assessors of this conceptual minefield is to gather many pieces of evidence from many sources before coming to conclusions about what is wrong.

ASSESSMENT OF NEED AND RISK

Whatever explanatory model is used, the initial collection of information needs to be as objective and as value-neutral as possible. In this section we discuss the issues involved in assessing need and risk.

Measurement of need

Needs assessment originated as an epidemiological technique that was in its early days informed by a 'sense that whatever is possible for any should be available for all' (Vickers 1958, p. 599). This idea lies behind much of the current debate about whether an identified need is an objective analogue of an individual's entitlement to professional services. Marshall (1994) argues that at least one approach to needs assessment, that of the Medical Research Council (see below), is defective because having identified a need it does not indicate whether it must be acted upon. Rabkin's (1986) observation that, by the 1960s, mental health needs assessment had developed in the USA as an ad hoc means of monitoring the use of federal funding for community mental health centres, shows that meeting needs is not simply a question of resources but of management of service delivery.

Defining the term 'need' is complicated by two essentially different uses to which it is put. On the one hand, identifying need is meaningless unless opportunities are also identified for an individual to meet those needs but, on the other hand, the resources available to meet the needs of different groups within the population are limited by what society is prepared to provide. In social policy, 'need' is one of the bases for plans for allocating resources. In this context, the term 'need' is a construct derived from aggregated and cross-sectional data concerning population characteristics. Census data, such as the number of people aged

65 and over, are often combined with prevalence data, such as the number of people who are diagnosed as having Alzheimer's disease. It is here that this use of the term 'need' overlaps with another use, which is based on an appraisal of the individual within his environment, and is directed to identifying deficits or lacks that, if remedied, would restore him to one or more states:

- improved social functioning
- improved psychological functioning
- improved standard of living
- increased personal autonomy
- improved quality of life.

These terms rely for their definition not only on inferences from aggregated data but also on implicit values. Statistical summaries of mortality and morbidity provide an index of public health, but not of the health of individuals, nor of the causes of ill health. There are a number of other serious problems with the notion of needs assessment. Richman and Barry (1985) argue that a needs-based approach to health care weighs against the maintenance of personal autonomy and against recovery from ill health. Rabkin (1986) observes that 'need' and 'problem' are terms that are used as if they are interchangeable. To some extent the concept of needs-based assessment militates against technically efficient health care because a diagnosis names an observable disease process while a need for mental health care may be identified independently of observable phenomena that are amenable to explanation and intervention (Hamid et al 1995).

Needs assessment may often involve determining whether people are suitable for available services. Dill (1993) critically analyses systems for defining needs. Like Marshall (1994), she argues that instrumental definitions, especially, fail to take account of lay perspectives, whether of the service users or their caregivers or carers. She suggests that service users, caregivers and carers ought to be involved in the preparation of clinical and social service practice guidelines. McWalter et al (1994) also make the point that a person may have some needs that are currently being met and other needs that are not currently being met. For example, a person with arthritis may need help with opening food containers to be able to continue preparing meals independently. The study by Williamson et al (1964) showed that the majority of older people living at home in Scotland had a range of impairments unknown to their general practitioners (Perkins 1991).

Mangen and Brewin (1991) discuss many of these issues that resulted in the development of the Medical Research Council (MRC) Needs for Care Assessment (Wing & Hailey 1972, Brewin et al 1987). They follow Miller (1976) in using a 'harm principle' to distinguish between instrumental need, functional need and intrinsic need. A person is harmed when he lacks the means (instrument) to achieve an end. This definition of instrumental need overlaps with the process of defining a problem in that it implies that the person may be unaware of or unwilling to acknowledge the need. Mangen and Brewin (1991) cite the example of people with alcoholism who define their need in terms of continued alcohol consumption but who, if harm is to be avoided, 'need' to stop drinking. An example of a functional need is the harm that people suffer if they are unable to perform a function. Examples of functions include getting up and down stairs (to do the shopping), heating the home (to avoid hypothermia) and eating healthy food (to avoid malnutrition). Housing, access to public transport and income are examples of intrinsic needs which, if not met, cause harm to people.

Brewin et al (1987) equate 'problems in functioning' with needs for treatment or care. 'Social disablement' is the term that encompasses 'lowered physical, psychological and social functioning' (p. 972). Accordingly, the MRC Needs for Care Assessment identifies needs for which effective interventions can be deployed. Unfortunately it is not validated for use with older people. More recently, Phelan et al (1995) have developed a measure (the Camberwell Assessment of Need) designed to meet the statutory requirement for comprehensive needs assessments of people with severe mental illness. Again this is not validated for an older population. Consequently, Hamid et al (1995) observe, needs for care, needs for psychiatric interventions and mental health needs are inferred haphazardly from various diagnostic procedures and measures of social functioning.

In measuring need, therefore, assessors should be aware of:

- the difference between problems and needs
- the importance of incorporating the user's and caregiver's perspectives
- the value of distinguishing between instrumental, functional and intrinsic needs.

By including these issues in the assessment, the measurement of need will be comprehensive.

Measurement of risk

The Department of Health (1994) is unequivocal about the requirement for risk assessment to be a multidisciplinary activity. The Department names the components of a risk assessment as those listed in Box 6.1. These components of risk assessment highlight the importance of consultation with key informants, which is essential for accurate assessment of legal and safety issues such as the ability of people to manage their own affairs, vulnerability to attack or exploitation, or consequences of untreated disease. Hamid et al (1995) have included carers' perspectives in developing an elderly persons' assessment schedule.

Co-morbidity, one of the Department of Health's components of risk assessment, refers to the presence of concurrent disease, risky health behaviours, psychosocial difficulties and other factors that increase the vulnerability of the other person. For example, Kennedy et al (1989) found that concurrent physical illness strongly predicted depressive symptoms in a sample of older people living in New York.

ASSESSMENT OF AETIOLOGICAL AND VULNERABILITY FACTORS

Possible aetiological and vulnerability factors may be considered by the professional with most skills in the relevant areas. These factors include:

- organic factors
- psychosocial factors
- hereditary factors.

This chapter deals in detail with organic and psychosocial factors that increase vulnerability and risk in older people. Hereditary factors are especially relevant to the assessment of cognitive impairment.

In Chapter 3 Herbert and Thomson consider age-related changes in bodily systems. Here we highlight aspects of these systems which feature in assessment, and also the assessment of age-related changes and substance use disorder which can have a very damaging impact on physical health and social functioning. Later sections discuss the assessment of instrumental behaviours, psychological function, organic changes, coping and health behaviours.

Cardiovascular system

Although heart disease is the major cause of mortality in people aged 60 and over (Beaglehole 1990), it should not be assumed to be a cause of presenting problems in older people (Lueckenotte 1994). Lueckenotte (1994) provides a systematic guide to assessing: peripheral circulation, pulses, venous sufficiency, blood pressure, jugular venous pressure, and heart sounds. Weight, the presence of concurrent disease like emphysema, diabetes or hypertension, and health behaviours including diet, exercise and substance use all need to be scrutinised when assessing the cardiovascular system.

Respiratory system

Lueckenotte (1994) also provides a systematic guide to assessing respiratory rate and rhythm, peripheral circulation, thoracic expansion, resonance of lung fields and breath sounds. A person with confirmed lung

---

Box 6.1 Components of a risk assessment

The Department of Health (1994) names the following components of a risk assessment:
- Documentation of past history of self-harm or violence, because a previous occurrence best predicts a future occurrence.
- Description of the specific risky behaviours.
- The patient's self-report.
- Suicidal ideation.
- Hostility to others.
- Statement of intent to harm self or others.
- Reports of key informants
  —family, carers, significant others
  —professional caregivers
  —other professionals
  —police
  —social services
  —housing departments
  —residence managers
  —concerned individuals
  —neighbours.
- Observations by professional caregivers
  —nurses
  —psychologists
  —occupational therapists
  —psychiatrists
  —general practitioners.
- Results of formal examination
  —by psychologists
  —by psychiatrists.
- Assessment of the possibility that the patient could mislead observers.
- Co-morbidity
  —substance use disorder
  —relationship difficulties
  —experience of physical or sexual abuse or both
  —perpetration of physical or sexual abuse or both
  —vulnerability to stress.
- Actuarial and statistical calculation based on research evidence.
- Estimate of the overall likelihood that the assessed risky behaviours could occur.
  (Department of Health 1994)

disease should already be subject to respiratory disease monitoring by the general practitioner who will have a system for providing influenza immunisation, for regular assessment, and for supply of preventive medication and other treatment. Respiratory infection can precipitate delirium even in the cognitively unimpaired older person, and should always be considered if psychotic symptoms or behavioural dyscontrol appear suddenly; delirium is discussed in detail in Chapter 10. Hoch et al (1992) report a prevalence of 25–33% of sleep-disordered breathing (for example, sleep apnoea) among older people, although its effect on mortality and morbidity is not clear.

Endocrine system

Premature assumptions must be avoided in the assessment of endocrine regulations because of the interplay between the many factors involved, for example those implicated in diabetes.

Genitourinary system

A thorough assessment is necessary to ensure that apparent 'incontinence' cannot be treated by methods like timed or prompted voiding schedules, or that remediable genitourinary problems are not falsely attributed to ageing. An acute urinary tract infection can precipitate delirium, while chronic infection can lead to inappropriate attempts to void the bladder because of difficulties getting to a lavatory. Mandelstam (1985) and Lueckenotte (1994) provide detailed guidance for assessing involuntary urination, and for identifying its many causes.

Gastrointestinal system

Perkins (1991) argues that problems with teeth are very common in older people, and that they go untreated because of a belief that degeneration is inevitable with age. In fact, gum disease, ulcers, caries and general dental deterioration require prompt treatment and ongoing preventive management. Age-related changes in gastric and intestinal motility may result in symptoms ranging from heartburn to constipation that in turn lead to behaviours, such as avoiding food or exercise, that can damage health. Weight loss and malnutrition, especially protein-energy undernutrition, predict mortality and morbidity of older people (Sullivan et al 1991, Sullivan 1992). Obesity is

associated with mortality from cardiovascular disease. Burns et al (1989) did not find that clinical malnutrition correlated with cognitive impairment, but they did find that hospitalisation predicted significantly lower weight in people with dementia. In a community survey of people aged 75 and over, Jagger et al (1986) found that complaints of faecal incontinence were associated with complaints of difficulty in getting to the lavatory (see also Mandelstam 1985).

Musculoskeletal system

Bone density and mass decrease with ageing, the reduction accelerated by poor nutrition, hormonal changes, immobility and medication such as steroids. The quality of weight-bearing joints deteriorates, accelerated by disease, history of over-use or injury, and immobility. Muscle wasting results from disuse and immobility as well as from disease and injury. Conditions such as cervical spondylosis exemplify a positive feedback mechanism whereby decreased use and strength aggravate the deforming process. Paradoxically, however, greater physical mobility among elderly people in countries with a rising life expectancy is associated with a higher risk of fracturing the hip (Finsen 1988). Physical deconditioning is a particular risk. It contributes to diminishing strength and power in muscles, delayed reactions, decreased flexibility, postural changes and loss of confidence, all of which amplify deconditioning. These are vulnerability factors that also amplify the adverse effects of unmet intrinsic needs like appropriate housing or available transport. Colantonio et al (1992) suggest that immobility is also a risk factor for stroke. Less generalised dysfunction such as difficulties in using the hands can also adversely affect a person's mobility and independence.

Pain

Conditions like post-herpetic neuralgia may not correlate directly with measures of affect (Helme et al 1989), but may contribute to a state of mind that begins to restrict a person's sense of self-efficacy and control. Ferrell et al (1990) found that 34% of residents in a nursing home complained of constant pain, mostly in the lower back and joints. Pain correlated with less socialisation with other residents. Although many cancers progress more slowly in older than younger people, they do metastasise and a secondary lesion, such as spinal metastases, may cause the presenting symptom such as back pain.

Substance use disorder

Despite a shortage of longitudinal data, older people are thought to be especially at risk of misusing alcohol, prescribed and non-prescribed drugs (Rosenberg 1995). Feinstein (1993) identifies substance use disorders as key variables for explaining differences in life span and access to health care. For example, as well as damaging every organ system, sustained heavy drinking exacerbates other conditions, disrupts relationships and is associated with social decline. Folstein et al (1985, p. 813) discuss the difficulties in 'penetrating the alcoholic's tendency to minimise his or her problem'. Rosenberg (1995) observes that, although in the USA the proportion of illegal drug users among people aged over 50 may be less than 2%, this represents a sizeable number. There is some evidence that as some drug addicts get older they give up their drug habits, but there is also evidence that others change to substances like alcohol. Strang & Gurling (1989) found little evidence of excess harm from high doses of heroin in a small sample of older heroin users. Rosenberg (1995) suggests that although so little is known about drug use in people aged over 55, older people who have drug use disorders are likely to be discriminated against by health care agencies, especially if they need long-term care. Substance use disorder in old age is discussed in detail in Chapter 12.

ASSESSMENT OF INSTRUMENTAL BEHAVIOURS

'Functional' and 'instrumental' needs overlap with each other as well as with 'problems'. As might be expected, the ways of operationalising these needs to measure them also overlap. 'Functional assessment' is used for this process of measuring instrumental needs and behaviours. Katz (1983, p. 721) refers to 'functional health' measured by 'self-maintenance activities'. In this section we consider assessment of social performance and activities of daily living.

Social performance

Instrumental behaviours which are required for performance of social roles (Wing 1978, Wykes et al 1992) may be measured in terms of social attainment or social skills. Measures of social attainment are often culture – and gender – specific; for example the behaviours required for fulfilling the social roles of widow, wife, husband or friend. Measures of social skills can be applied to instrumental behaviours such

as self-care, cooking, budgeting and shopping (Spector et al 1987). For instance, self-care may include components such as hygiene, which in turn includes such behavioural units as wearing underwear, washing underwear unprompted, washing underwear if prompted, washing underwear if helped, not washing underwear at all.

Wykes & Hurry (1991) note that social performance is often defined in research with elderly people in terms of instrumental behaviour; for example the categories used in the Clifton Assessment Procedures for the Elderly (Pattie & Gilleard 1979). Little et al (1986, p. 58) define the ability to carry out instrumental activities of daily living as 'social competence'. They provide a brief self-completion behaviour scale which, when scored, rates social competence and which they used in conjunction with informant and observed performance ratings to evaluate the judgement of people living in residential care. They confirm that findings from older people living in institutions should be applied cautiously to those living in the community. Lawton & Brody (1969) developed a measure of instrumental activities of daily living but this suffers from a 'floor effect', discussed later in this chapter.

Activities of daily living

The Index of Activities of Daily Living (Katz et al 1963) has undergone many developments. It was designed to measure independence, using ratings of performance of bathing, dressing, going to the toilet, transfer (mobility), continence, and feeding. Part of its rationale was its supposed analogue with the development of children and of 'primitive' peoples, combining measures of 'vegetative' (biological) and culturally defined (psychosocial) activities. Lazarides et al (1994) criticise the Katz Index for its inability to discriminate between the different profiles of disability caused by different disorders, for example stroke or arthritis. Measures of activities of daily living are used extensively to evaluate functional status, especially in the area of health insurance (Stewart et al 1981).

Locomotion

Assessment of mobility needs to be practically oriented to the provision of appliances and to adaptations in the home which positively improve a person's ability to function independently. Getting about is an important aspect of locomotion because it is usually purposeful (Volicer et al 1994). Roberts (1990) discusses the assessment of functional walking: for example, walking to the lavatory, using it and walking back to one's chair. McKeith et al (1992) suggest that falling and unsteadiness are more characteristic of people with senile dementia of Lewy body type, and are contraindications to the use of neuroleptics. Impaired muscle tone (spasticity, contractures, flaccidity) following stroke or other head injury also impairs a person's abilities to get about unaided and so to manage his home (Nydevik & Asberg 1992).

The condition of a person's feet depends on genetic (e.g. bunions), developmental (e.g. the effect of dropped or high arches on hammer toes or callouses) and environmental factors (for example, the role of high heels in shortening the Achilles tendon). In turn, people's mobility depends partly on the condition of their feet. Perkins (1991) notes that poor quality foot care is associated with the false belief that problems are inevitable with increasing age.

Dysfunction

Molloy et al (1991, p. 103) define dysfunctional behaviour as 'an inappropriate action or response, other than an activity of daily living (ADL) in a given social milieu, that is a problem for the caregiver'. Accordingly they have developed a checklist for completion by caregivers that measures problem behaviours. The Sickness Impact Profile (Bergner et al 1981) also measures behavioural dysfunction across 12 dimensions, and has been further developed for use in different settings (for example, Gerety et al 1994). The reader is referred to Bowling 1995 for more measures of dysfunction.

Dyscontrol. Behavioural dyscontrol in advanced dementia presents particular problems for caregivers, and may result in activities like repetitive questioning, excessive walking behaviour, day and night reversal, hitting, shouting, taking off clothes, binge-eating, inappropriate urination and defaecation, getting lost in the home, and using gas or electricity inappropriately (Pruchno & Resch 1989, Burns et al 1990, Burns 1992). It is important to assess fully each of these behaviours because someone who, say, does not replace his clothes after visiting the lavatory, may be severely demented but equally may have a more circumscribed brain lesion that does not cause generalised cognitive impairment. Conversely, a person may have little or no cognitive impairment, and behavioural dyscontrol may be a sign of what has been termed 'social breakdown in the elderly' which may be amenable to behaviour therapy (Ungvari & Hantz 1991a, b). Lesions in the frontal lobe appear to alter sexual behaviour, either disinhibiting the usual controls or reducing sexual interest depending on the

site of the lesion (Pruchno & Resch 1989, Kolb & Whishaw 1990).

Because behavioural dyscontrol is a feature of advanced dementia, of delirium and of social breakdown, it is essential that caregivers who describe it are asked to give a history of its onset and recent course. A person who has dementia can develop acute toxic reactions to neuroleptics or infection that are reversible (Burns et al 1990, McKeith et al 1992). Someone who suddenly becomes aggressive, disinhibited or more incoherent than usual must be thoroughly assessed physically as soon as possible after onset of the disturbed behaviour because psychogenic causes are most unlikely. A neurological examination may be difficult because of the problem behaviour, but should be attempted. Molloy et al (1991) have developed a checklist for completion by caregivers which measures problem behaviours.

Dyspraxia

Dyspraxia implies inability to carry out willed, purposeful movements and results from brain lesions that may be focal or diffuse. This inability may also be termed apraxia which itself contains a number of categories, all discussed by Lishman (1987). Disruption of willed movement appears to occur at the level of planning the action, as well as at the level of executing it. Assessment ranges from asking the person to perform a number of actions, like raising his hand, using a comb, buttoning a jacket or cardigan, pouring fluid into a cup or glass, to more formal testing of actions like finger-tapping, building blocks, or demonstration of object use (for example keys) (Lishman 1987).

Impairment of such motor behaviours can be localised by these tests to lesions in different areas of the brain, but the complex nature of apraxia means that the tests themselves must be carried out stringently, and the clinician must ensure that results cannot be attributed to more simple explanations such as recalcitrance, fatigue, anxiety or an acute infection. Paresis and paralysis must also be excluded. The person may be able to carry out the same actions spontaneously. The main sign is that the person cannot perform the movement on request. Each test must therefore be standardised and be identical on each testing occasion. The response must be quantified in the same way on each occasion. Each impaired and each unimpaired response must be itemised (Kolb & Whishaw 1990). Other tests examine, for example, lateralisation of any deficit and these are outlined in the section on sensory impairment.

Adaptation

Behavioural adaptation comprises communication, activities of daily living and social interaction (Ward et al 1991). It implies that people manage themselves and their environment more or less effectively. It has a strong cognitive component in that individuals' expectations and disposition materially affect how they adapt to their environment. Expectations and mood interact as in 'learned helplessness' (Abramson et al 1978, Brewin 1985). For example, feelings of anxiety might restrict a person moving about freely. It is well known that delusions and hallucinations impede people's ability freely to interact with their environment but, more generally, dispositional style may affect attributions about everyday experiences and social interaction. Schonfield (1983) argues that sensory impairment and mental illness are the likeliest causes of diminished social skills in older people. Social ties can insidiously disintegrate as a result.

Purposive interaction by people with their environment may be affected by the interaction of internal vulnerability and external hazards. People's self-appraisal may be adversely affected by social expectations of their adaptation: for example, the commonly stated notion that older people are an increasing burden on society may both deter people from seeking help when needed, and confirm a depressive view of themselves as worthless.

The estimation of behavioural adaptation to current life circumstances lies at the heart of any plan to maximise autonomy and to place the least restriction on a person's environment. Some people adapt even to quite severe cognitive impairment, and decompensate only when physically ill or when there is a change in their social circumstances. Such decompensation is quite predictable, so that caregivers can make contingency plans before imposing changes on the older cognitively impaired person.

Adaptation by people to their environment is sometimes reciprocal, sometimes not, but achieving a permanent balance is not possible even if the environment is apparently static (Dubos 1965). Brewin & Furnham (1986) argue that interpersonal relationships perhaps exemplify the pressures and hazards of adaptation. Hostility and criticism by caregivers may contribute to decompensation by an individual. Self-critical attributions can lead to social avoidance and to a discrediting of a person's sense of self (Goffman 1968). It is therefore essential that the interaction between an individual's cognition, social interaction and social support is fully explored (Brewin 1988).

Many factors that contribute to the development of depression are modifiable (Backer 1985). Kennedy et al (1989) argue that older people are more likely to retain their independence if the factors of response to illness and impairment, feelings of isolation, response to bereavement, and socioeconomic conditions are addressed in programmes of care.

Attributional style

Since Kanfer and Saslow's (1965) review of behavioural approaches to management of psychiatric treatment, it has become routine to explore the effect of people's perceptions of themselves and their environment on their problems of daily living, and to develop attributional explanations of behaviour. Ingram (1990) discusses the distorting effect of what he calls heightened 'self-focused attention' on vulnerability of people with impulse-control disorders as well as those with psychotic disorders. Attributional style is an important factor in the maintenance of depressive symptoms. Beck et al (1979) argue that some individuals respond to events like stress, illness and bereavement idiosyncratically. People can hold a set of mistaken beliefs about themselves and the world that Beck et al (1979, p. 11) classify into the 'cognitive triad'. Whether an episode of depression activates these beliefs, or whether they exist as a relatively permanent background to the person's life, they appear to prolong and maintain the duration of the episode. These issues are discussed further in Chapter 19.

Teasdale (1988) argues that empirical evidence for Beck's (1978) cognitive model of vulnerability to depression is inconsistent. He asks: 'What underlies the vulnerability of some people to become clinically depressed following environmental events, and what determines whether depression will be transient or more persistent?' (p. 248), and suggests that vulnerability to onset of depression and vulnerability to persistence of depressive symptoms are distinct phenomena. He argues that it is relatively easy to assess the presence of negative automatic thoughts using a measure such as the Dysfunctional Attitude Scale (Silverman et al 1984), but much less easy to measure Beck at al's (1979) negative schema within which automatic thoughts operate and which they are said to maintain.

Teasdale (1988) also cites evidence that negative automatic thoughts are present in people diagnosed as having bipolar disorders for which a biological basis is fairly well-accepted (DSM-IV). He proposes that a psychological phenomenon that he terms 'differential activation' (p. 251) is responsible for persistent depression, and that onset of depression is triggered by a range of factors, including life events and biological variables. This means that assessment needs to distinguish between individuals who are vulnerable to acute but self-limiting depressive symptoms, and those who, once depressed, will remain so because they develop persistently dysfunctional cognitive structures such as ruminations and interpretive bias, often based on previous experiences while depressed. Teasdale (1988) argues further that 'depressogenic cognitive processes' (p. 262) that are still present when a person has recovered from a depressive episode predict relapse. He identifies global self-description in terms such as 'worthless', 'pathetic' and 'stupid' as a powerful predictor of persistent depression.

Assessment of attributional style

Brewin (1985) disagrees with Teasdale's conclusions about onset of and vulnerability to depression, arguing that the relationship between attributions and coping is crucial. Power et al (1995) used the Dysfunctional Attitudes Scale (Silverman et al 1984) to assess cognitive vulnerability in the series of depressed individuals followed up by Duggan et al (1991). Anderson et al (1983) emphasise the importance of developing measures of attribution within the situations that potential respondents live. Otherwise people's experience may be further distorted and mistakenly directed treatment offered. Depression in old age is discussed in detail in Chapter 8.

PSYCHOMETRY

Psychometry assumes that 'any behaviour is a function, essentially, of a subject's ability, personality, motivation, state, mood and situation' (Kline 1993, p. 329). The stability of measures of these constructs over the lifespan is debatable (for example, Finn 1986), and non-specialist assessors need to bear in mind the shortcomings of non-validated measures and the use of validated measures with previously untested populations. Woods (1994) discusses in detail the main psychological tests used for assessing older people. Tests of cognitive function such as the revised Wechsler Adult Intelligence Scale (Wechsler 1981) or National Adult Reading Test (Nelson 1991) may be used only by appropriately qualified psychologists. Other tests of cognitive function such as the Mill Hill Vocabulary Scale (Raven 1994) and the Raven's Progressive Matrices (Raven 1992) must be carried out under the supervision of a psychologist.

Measurement of cognitive function

Plomin & Thompson (1993) suggest that cognitive ability through the lifespan is partly predicted by genetic factors, and partly by scholastic achievement (which is also subject to genetic effects). Fratiglioni et al (1993), in a multi-centre study, found that the effect of education on results on the Mini Mental State Examination (Folstein et al 1975) varied between countries. Studies that show that the Mini Mental State Examination is affected by educational achievement have been carried out among black American samples (e.g. Fillenbaum et al 1990). Previously high educational achievement may result in false negatives on testing for dementia, and previously low educational achievement may result in false positives, especially if the subject is depressed (Orrell et al 1992). Scherr et al (1988) found, in a large survey in New England, that apparently diminished cognitive function in people aged over 65 was predicted by lower educational achievement and lower socioeconomic status, as well as by physical impairment. These findings mean that any assessment of an elderly person's cognitive ability must include independent information about family patterns as well as about his educational achievement so that individual measures are interpreted within their true social context.

Stereotypes of declining cognitive function among the elderly are held by elderly people themselves as well as society as a whole. Camp & Pignatiello (1988) found that elderly people were likely to judge their memory as defective even in the face of testing that showed their ability to retrieve facts was unimpaired by age. This finding means that self-report is not a reliable way of estimating changes in cognitive function, and that mood and self-esteem are important factors to consider when measuring performance. Roth et al (1986) warn that self-report of memory problems is more likely to be associated with depressed mood than a dementing process. Mechanic (1979) reminds us that it is not so much a psychiatric observation as a social one that psychological distress, such as low mood, leads to an unfavourable subjective perception of health which in turn leads to increased morbidity. Ott & Fogel (1992) also point out that the presence of dementia may lead to false negatives on a self-rating depression scale, even one validated for use with older people, such as the Geriatric Depression Scale (Yesavage et al 1983).

Orrell et al (1992) suggest that many tests of cognitive ability are biased for age. That is, much older people may score as demented because a number of questions were designed and tested with younger samples. They also found that four measures discriminated poorly between organic and so-called 'functional' disorders in a hospitalised sample aged between 60 and 94, nearly two-thirds of whom were women.

Response to cognitive demands

Cognitive demands may be categorised and tested in a number of ways. Abstract thinking, decision-making, problem-solving and reasoning ability may require testing with psychometrically valid measures, although observation of activities, like budgeting and shopping, provides good evidence for referral for more detailed investigations. Judgement is difficult to assess, and is noted in our later discussion of frontal lesions of the brain. Assessment of judgement also relies on observation and reports of informants who know the person well.

Acquisition of new knowledge and skills may be tested in a simplistic way, as when a person is asked to memorise and retrieve from memory a piece of information such as a name and address (Institute of Psychiatry 1978), but really requires specialist assessment. Wykes et al (1990, 1992) have used measures of reaction time in younger people with schizophrenia as an analogue of response-processing to find out if poor response-processing predicts dependence on psychiatric care. The authors conclude that good response-processing, measured as rapid reaction-time, strongly predicts independence. Kail & Salthouse (1994) suggest that response-processing predicts cognitive performance over the life span.

Quite simple articles can be used to help test constructional ability. People can be asked to use matchsticks to construct geometric shapes like a square or triangle, or to copy more complicated shapes, or to do a jigsaw puzzle (Institute of Psychiatry 1978). Connelly & Jamieson (1991) provide a diagram that the assessor asks the respondent to copy and that can be scored.

Memory

The role of 'benign senescent forgetfulness' (Kral 1962) is controversial (McEntee & Crook 1991, O'Brien & Levy 1992). Mayes (1988) summarises approaches to assessing memory, emphasising the importance of distinguishing between so-called 'functional' memory impairment (for example, the loss of autobiographical memory in people who disappear from family homes and reappear in hospital), and organic memory impairment.

A number of studies show that age is not in itself a predictor of memory loss. For instance, although recall of public events seems to decrease with increasing age, recall of autobiographical events seems to remain intact (Howes & Katz 1992). Kausler et al (1988) show that education is an important variable to consider when examining memory proficiency. Rose (1992) reasons that perceptual filtering, a mechanism that allows adults to select from their environment the aspects they perceive to be relevant or important to them, is one of the ways in which maturity occurs. The neuronal loss that is observed in normal adults has been posited as a cause of memory disorders in old age because it is also observed to a much greater extent in disorders like Alzheimer's disease. Rose (1992, p. 113) argues against this proposal, asking, 'Is the life of the elderly person so impoverished that it ceases to be of interest to learn or remember?'

Christensen (1991), however, found that although her sample of 'memory complainers' was not as impaired as a comparison group of demented respondents, their subjective estimate of failing memory correlated with their performance on objective assessment. She concludes that memory complaints should not be ignored and that, if tests confirm a recent deterioration, individuals should be followed up and their memory regularly reassessed (always in the context of other factors including social and environmental ones). Beardsall & Huppert (1990, p. 305) emphasise that 'it is extremely unlikely' that the same memory assessment techniques would be suitable for basic research, diagnosis, and assessment of response to treatment.

ORGANIC CHANGES

An assessor must attend to organic as well as to psychosocial and behavioural factors in the daily life of the individual being assessed. Organic changes may be acute or chronic, focal or diffuse and a programme of care will depend to a large extent on these differences. 'Cognitive impairment leads to functional impairment' (Volicer et al 1994, p. M223), and it is absolutely essential that the causes of observed cognitive impairment are correctly identified because of the potentially lethal consequences of, say, treating someone who has Lewy body dementia with neuroleptics (McKeith et al 1992). Readers are referred to Chapter 11 and to Lishman (1987, p. vii) for the necessary background to 'the psychological pheno-mena associated with the various organic disorders of the nervous system, and ... of those numerous extracerebral diseases, toxic, metabolic and endocrine, which affect the brain indirectly'. Testing of cerebral function 'must not be hurried; the patient may tire easily and several sessions may be needed for complete examination' (Institute of Psychiatry 1978, p. 14).

Sensory impairment

In this section we introduce aspects of sensory assessment, some of which are discussed further in Chapter 17.

Visual impairment

Visual function is affected by localised changes in the eye, and by changes in the brain. Localised functional changes may result from disease (for example, glaucoma) or from age-related processes (for example, cataracts, presbyopia, diminished production of tears), some of which may be related to lifestyle (for example, exposure to sunlight), and some to general health (for example, diabetes). Lueckenotte (1994) provides a step-by-step guide for assessing the eyes and visual function, including visual fields. Some of the steps depend on the person who is being assessed understanding and following the instructions of the assessor. If there is any doubt about the presence of functional deficits that place the individual at risk (for example, glaucoma or visual field impairment) referral for specialist assessment is essential. A practical point during assessment of visual function is that deficits may affect part but not all of the visual field. Someone who has a loss of one quadrant of the visual field will appear to be 'blind' to objects located in that quadrant. The assessor needs to sit in different positions in order to check that measurement of visual function is not distorted by the presence of a partial loss of field of vision.

Visual perceptual deficits occurring as a result of specific brain lesions include lack of eye–hand coordination and inability to follow visually a moving object (Kolb & Whishaw 1990). Lack of eye–hand coordination can be assessed by placing an everyday object such as a paperback book in front of the person and asking him to pick it up. He may fumble for the book and on repeated trials will pick it up only inadvertently. Ability to follow a moving object can be assessed by holding up a forefinger about 45 cm in front of a person's face and asking them to touch their nose and your finger alternately while you move your finger. This exercise can be repeated several times with the person using the same finger before changing to the other hand and repeating the exercise.

Auditory impairment

Auditory function is affected by localised changes in the ear, and by changes in the brain. Older people who complain of problems with their hearing should have their ears visually inspected with an auroscope to exclude causes such as infection or impacted ear wax. Acuity of hearing can be tested crudely using a ticking watch and a tuning fork (Lueckenotte 1994). The assessor needs to be properly trained in the use of the auroscope and tuning fork, to ensure safety and to know when there is need for specialist referral.

Neurological impairment results in a variety of auditory perceptual deficits depending on the site of the lesion. Failure to recognise sounds is the important sign, and may be mistaken for a functional impairment of hearing. People with an auditory perceptual deficit do not know what they are hearing or fail to recognise familiar music (Lishman 1987).

Olfactory impairment

Olfactory perception is incompletely understood. Deficits are usually inferred from a person's response to strong smells, tested with bottles containing preparations such as peppermint, eucalyptus oils or acetone. Battcock & Castleden (1990) suggest that at home orange zest can be used. It is extremely difficult to make inferences about affective responses to smell that, nevertheless, are an important component of olfaction.

Somasthetic impairment

Like impaired sense of space, somasthetic impairment includes 'neglect' or even denial of existence by people of parts of their body. It also includes what is commonly called distortion of body-image. Asking people to sketch a human body or asking them to perform movements or point to and name parts of their own body may reveal an inability to identify parts of it (Lishman 1987). Neglect results from organic impairment, but the extent to which other forms of somasthetic impairment also have an organic cause is debatable. Dysmorphophobia, a belief that parts of one's body are deformed, can result in extreme social avoidance. Affective disorders may be associated with misperceptions of bodily function that lead to delusions, for example, of cessation of bowel function. Failure to eat and the ensuing constipation confirm such beliefs. Although some people may explain perceived ill health in somatic terms, or may believe they have a serious illness in ways that do not respond to disconfirmatory evidence, Barsky et al (1991) did not find that increasing age amplified these tendencies. Factitious disorder appears to characterise younger people, but needs to be borne in mind when, for example, cutaneous lesions fail to heal in otherwise optimum conditions.

Impaired sense of space

Impaired sense of space includes a number of phenomena which entwine with other impairments, especially visual ones, to result in lack of visuospatial awareness. Impaired sense of space often appears as 'neglect' of objects within the visual field, or of objects described from memory. For example, contralateral visuospatial neglect might show up when a person is asked to copy a clockface with numbers and hands pointing to quarter-past nine. A right hemisphere lesion might result in neglect of the left visual field with the person omitting the digits from 7 to 11, the left side of the clockface's circumference, and the hand pointing to the figure 9. People's ability to find their way about might be unimpaired even though they are unable to draw from memory a map that includes the western side of a given area (Cutting 1990, Rosenfield 1992).

Deficits in reaching can occur in people with bilateral parietal lesions and may result, for example, in an inability successfully to pick up, light and place a cigarette in the mouth (Kolb & Whishaw 1990). If tests like drawing a clockface, or carrying out a sequence of purposeful actions suggest unilateral or bilateral parietal lesions then detailed neuropsychological testing is indicated, using a battery of measures (see Flicker et al 1991, for a standard battery of general measures). A set of tasks designed to screen for visuospatial and other organic impairment is contained in a small handbook for psychiatrists in training (Institute of Psychiatry 1978).

Impaired sense of time

Sims (1995) discusses impaired sense of time in detail. When assessing people who appear to have such an impairment it is important to give them an unhurried opportunity to describe what they experience. Affective and anxiety disorders can distort perception of the passage of time. Organic impairment results in inability to remember past events, or to grasp the passage of time. A disrupted sleep–wake cycle is a common result of impaired sense of time, but it is not clear to what extent this is a perceptual disorder of memory and cognition, or a disorder of circadian rhythms. Sense of time can be tested by asking the person to state the day of the week, month and year. Other typical questions include, 'What time is it now?', 'How long have we been talking?', 'When did you marry?', 'When did you give up work?'

Impaired sense of self

'Depersonalisation' and 'derealisation' are vague terms for unpleasant occurrences when a person feels estranged from himself or from the environment. Sims (1995) discusses these phenomena in detail. It is important to attend carefully to people who appear to have such experiences because variants of these feelings characterise psychosis (more common in older women) and organic brain impairment (Lishman 1987, Rosenfield 1992, Sims 1995).

Other neurological signs

Lishman (1987) emphasises the need particularly in the neurological examination to interpret abnormal findings in relation to all the clinical features. Organic factors affecting mental and physical health may include infection, neoplasm and neurodegeneration. Neurological signs are prominent in people with dementia syndromes and have different kinds of significance. Once current symptoms have been identified a physical, neuropsychological and neuropsychiatric assessment can determine whether organic factors are reversible and, if so, what would be the appropriate treatment options.

Primitive reflexes. Primitive reflexes such as snout and grasp reflexes predict earlier onset and higher mortality in people with Alzheimer's disease, and are associated with specific cerebral abnormalities such as enlarged lateral ventricles or frontal lobe atrophy and with severe cognitive impairment (Burns et al 1991, Forstl et al 1992). A grasp reflex is elicited by stroking the palm of a person's hand. A snout reflex is elicited by lightly touching the lips. When the lips are touched they protrude as if in an exaggerated pout. Other abnormal reflexes may appear before severe cognitive impairment is apparent. These are described by Lishman (1987) and include the palmo-mental and the glabella-tap reflexes. The palmo-mental reflex is elicited by stroking the muscle at the base of the thumb. If the palmo-mental reflex is present the muscles on the ipsilateral side of the person's chin twitch. The glabella-tap reflex is elicited by tapping the forehead just above the nose. The person will blink each time. The abnormality consists of failure of the blink response to habituate to the tapping stimulus. These reflexes can appear after heart surgery.

Ataxia. Ataxia, or broad-based gait, can indicate neurological problems before cognitive impairment has become very obvious (Lishman 1987). Extrapyramidal signs such as resting tremor, akinesia, cogwheel rigidity and akathisia are associated with Parkinson's disease. They may also be associated with neuroleptic medication even at small doses. They have also been found to be associated with calcified basal ganglia and diffuse cerebral atrophy, both of which predict earlier mortality in people with Alzheimer's disease (Burns et al 1991). Atypical Parkinsonian movement disorders have been associated with diffuse Lewy body pathology (Gibb 1989).

Abnormal frontal lobe function. Signs of abnormal frontal lobe function include impaired olfaction, impaired planning of motor behaviours, increased risk-taking or impulsivity but, most of all, a changed pattern of conforming to social mores and a general disinhibition of social behaviour (Lishman 1987, Kolb & Whishaw 1990). If detected they require detailed neuropsychological testing to distinguish between focal and diffuse abnormalities, and to assist with planning the programme of care.

Praxis

Praxis is defined as purposeful motor activity. We separate it from activities of daily living because elements of praxis are key areas for assessment of organic impairment, so estimating the extent of cognitive deficits. Basic elements of praxis include speech and locomotion.

Speech

Speech can be disorganised in mood disorders, in a variety of psychotic disorders and in organic disorders. Sims (1995) emphasises that the relationship between thinking and speaking is extremely complex, and that inferences about thought processes that are drawn from speech are unreliable. Thomas (1995) discusses various approaches to language disorder. Put very simply, two components of speech are vocalisation and language. Vocalisation includes the motor aspects of speech, while language includes communication and understanding of speech. Reading and writing comprise both aspects and are important areas for assessment. It is essential to remember that focal lesions might cause quite severe speech impairment while other cognitive functions remain intact, but that

the speech difficulties may adversely affect performance, causing the assessor to identify dyspraxia by mistake (Institute of Psychiatry 1978). Speech, language and communication assessment is discussed in detail in Chapter 17.

Dysarthria. Dysarthria results from disruption of motor aspects of speech which may be slurred, nonfluent, faint or at worst, incoherent (Lishman 1987).

Dysphasia. Dysphasia is a term that comprises many aspects of speech disturbance including comprehension (as in receptive dysphasia), as well as speech production. Lishman (1987) and Kolb & Whishaw (1990) discuss in detail the classification of dysphasia and aphasia. Developments in scanning techniques mean that inferences from clinical and neuropsychological assessment can be confirmed and located fairly precisely. Absence of dysarthria does not mean that language function may not be substantially impaired, as in nominal aphasia when the person is unable to name objects, often while retaining the ability to describe what they are used for.

Language

Andreasen's (1979) Thought, Language and Communication Scale measures verbal behaviour, but it has not been validated with older people. However, it does enable an interviewer to categorise unusual use of language and so point the way to more detailed neuropsychological assessment. Generally the interview itself will give the assessor a good idea of any difficulties and will indicate what further testing is necessary.

Reading and writing. Some people with language deficits may be able to speak fluently but be unable to understand what they read. Others may be able to write spontaneously while their ability to read is preserved.

Communication. Communication breaks down when a person's use of language becomes highly idiosyncratic, becomes highly restricted as in perseverative repetition of phrases and questions, or when a person shouts or cries out regardless of the circumstances. It is essential to disentangle the causes of communication disorders because of the very different prognoses and treatments for depression, dementia syndromes or psychosis of old age.

COPING

Park and Smith (1991, p. 79) argue that 'many of the problems associated with ageing are essentially behavioural problems which can be prevented through behavioural change in the early as well as later years of the lifespan'. Bandura (1989) developed the idea that coping is an element of self-agency, also discussed by a number of other writers in the context of social cognitive theory (Rosenstock et al 1988). However, Hawkins (1992) argues that the later elaboration of social learning theory into social cognitive theory weakens its explanatory power. Terry and O'Leary (1995) studied undergraduates to assess whether the constructs self-efficacy and perceived behavioural control modified actual behaviour as opposed to intended behaviour. They found that measures of self-efficacy did not predict actual behaviour, but that measures of perceived behavioural control did predict actual behaviour. Although the sample for this study was drawn from a young population, the concepts of self-efficacy and perceived behavioural control are relevant to assessment of coping skills and instrumental behaviours, and may predict help-seeking behaviours in older people. Lauver (1992) discusses in detail what she calls 'care-seeking behaviour' in the context of the health belief model (Rosenstock 1966) and the theory of reasoned action (Ajzen & Fishbein 1980), in order to find variables that predict the likelihood of individuals taking preventive action on behalf of their own health. Caserta (1995) draws these themes together in a review of health education with older people, arguing that cognition, environment and social settings are key variables to take into account when using health promotion methods that have been tested with younger samples with specific disorders such as cancer and heart disease.

Croake et al (1988) report that older women are significantly more likely than younger people and older men to express fearfulness. A commonly reported crime against older people is fraud, ranging from the confidence trickster who poses as an official from a utility company to firms that assess non-existent needs for house or garden repairs and then extort excessive payments for work carried out. McGhee (1983) suggests that adverse life events and social isolation increase vulnerability to fraud, and that coping skills can be enhanced when education and a questioning disposition do not already protect the individual. Kennedy & Silverman (1984–1985) confirm that women are more fearful of crime than men, reporting that older people who socialise with their neighbours are less fearful than more isolated individuals. Krause (1991) explains why practice of social skills might diminish with increasing age. His survey of more than 1000 older people found that financial problems and fear of crime predicted social

isolation and mistrust of others. Lower social class also predicted depressive symptoms and isolation.

Coping presents a paradox because hypothesised components of coping such as self-efficacy and response-efficacy are in themselves adaptive behaviours, whereas the concept of coping includes maladaptive behaviours. For instance, expectation of failure leads to social avoidance (Kafer & Davies 1984). Rippetoe and Rogers (1987) suggest that a highly maladaptive coping strategy is avoidant thinking, which greatly reduces the efficacy of self-care and self-protective behaviours (Leary et al 1986). Within the category of self-protection is health-protective behaviour, discussed next.

HEALTH BEHAVIOUR

Modifying health behaviours is thought to be an important way of reducing avoidable mortality and morbidity. A number of ways of approaching this topic appeared from the 1960s onwards, developing themes such as 'health is a dynamic balance' (Vickers 1958, p. 602), or Dowie's (1975) argument that people can be defined as the producers of their own health rather than as consumers of health services. The notion of 'successful' ageing implies that people exercise considerable control over their health. For instance, Dustman et al (1990) found that men aged between 50 and 62 who were physically fit and had better aerobic performance also performed better on neurocognitive testing than less fit men of the same age, suggesting that disability-free life expectancy is a distinct phenomenon.

There are now at least eight so-called models of health behaviour, four of which are reviewed by Weinstein (1993). Kasl & Cobb (1966a, p. 246) provide a conceptual framework for considering health, illness and sick-role behaviours, defining health behaviour as 'any activity undertaken by a person believing himself to be healthy, for the purpose of preventing disease or detecting it in an asymptomatic form'. Harris and Guten (1979) emphasise that this includes self-defined self-protective behaviour, and should not be restricted to people who are currently symptom-free. Rosenstock (1966) formulated the health belief model used in many subsequent studies. A number of more recent studies have used various frameworks to look at risk-reduction behaviours of gay men, self-surveillance behaviours of women at risk of breast cancer and exercise behaviours. Risk-taking behaviours have also been studied, but there is a dearth of studies of older people (Rippetoe & Rogers 1987, Rosenstock et al 1988, Bandura 1989, Hawkins 1992, Lauver 1992, Ronis 1992,

Weinstein 1993, Frisch & Clemen 1994, Caserta 1995, Terry & O'Leary 1995).

Ransford (1986) emphasises that populations apparently underserved by health services, such as, in the USA, black North Americans of lower socioeconomic status, are no less likely to engage in health protective behaviours. This evidence of agency and, perhaps, of self-efficacy is accompanied by evidence of confidence in the health services. Among the outcome variables that Kruse et al (1993) identify as leading to 'successful' ageing, subjective factors such as self-efficacy exert a strong influence.

Effect of isolation/restriction

Strom & Strom (1989) surveyed 400 grandparents to identify topics for a programme of education aimed at helping families to develop as their numbers and generations increase. The identified topics provide a helpful checklist of the areas to look at when assessing the person in the family context. They include specific behaviours that can be observed during the average home visit:

- sharing feelings and ideas with peers
- listening to the views of younger people
- intergenerational communication skills (Strom & Strom 1989).

Social isolation is often seen as a 'cause' of depression, but from the perspective of Krause's (1991) survey it will be seen that low mood itself may inhibit confiding approaches to other people, may distort the magnitude of perceived financial problems and may delay requests for help in crises such as crime victimisation or bereavement. Teasdale (1988, p. 256) argues that 'negatively biased information processing' and inhibition of people's sense of control over their environment become a positive feedback mechanism that amplifies the depressed mood which in turn feeds cognitive bias.

Revenson & Johnson (1984) found in a survey that recency of loss, especially of an intimate attachment, more strongly predicted feelings of loneliness than did isolation (for example, living alone). Chappell & Badger (1989) list some indicators of social isolation that they tested in another large survey of older people. However, Thompson & Heller (1990) illustrate the difficulty of using survey methods to attribute the direction of effect of factors such as social support and psychological wellbeing on perceived social isolation. Creecy et al (1985) also tested the causal effect of a number of factors on feelings of loneliness, finding that

age itself was not a predictor. Brewin (1988) reviews research into couples and marital problems that indicates that loneliness, depression and lack of exposure to new experiences strongly bias distressed individuals towards restricted interpretation of and communication about themselves in relation to their environment. Lumpkin & Johnson (1987) have developed a measure of social engagement intended to distinguish between voluntary and involuntary social isolation.

In the previous sections we have covered a lot of material relevant to the assessment of elderly people with possible mental health problems. Assessment can be carried out at a number of different levels and requires knowledge and expertise which is only available within coordinated multidisciplinary teams. We turn now to consider the process of assessment.

PRINCIPLES OF ASSESSMENT

Collaboration by health care and social services agencies in formulating and implementing procedures for assessing older people is essential, for there is evidence that where they do so, practice improves (SSI & DH 1995). The principles of social services support for National Health Service patients include the following:

- provision by health authorities of health service support to local authorities
- provision by local authorities of social work support to the National Health Service
- joint agreements between local and health authorities concerning community care. National Health Service and Community Care Act.

Key components of effective service delivery are linked information systems that can move data vertically and horizontally between all levels of the health care and social services systems, so that individual agencies can act on information without waiting for data to move to the centre and out again to the periphery of the system. In the absence of regularly updated and reliable information, agencies have to provide for unpredicted events or demands in planning their resource allocation (Richman & Barry 1985, Abel-Smith 1994, SSI & DH 1995). There is evidence that multidisciplinary psychogeriatric teams that work on an outreach basis, preferably in people's homes, achieve reliable diagnoses and safely manage effective and efficient programmes of care (Collighan et al 1993). Other service models, however, remain comparatively fragmented with various consequences.

Harwin (1973, p. 269) evaluated district nurses' assessment of older patients to find whether what he called 'alternative medical personnel' reliably detected mental disorder in physically impaired older people. He found that district nurses successfully identified the high rates of psychiatric morbidity present in this group, but failed to exploit their knowledge except in crises. That is, they took psychological distress in physically impaired older people for granted and did not refer patients for help that would have alleviated this distress.

A more recent study examined the sensitivity of practice nurses to psychological distress in patients attending their clinics, finding that their ratings of patients' psychological wellbeing reached no more than chance agreement with the ratings of the patients themselves (Plummer 1995). However, Herzberg (1995, p. 174) reviewed a number of studies of assessment of older people which indicate that 'professions other than doctors are capable of making safe and comprehensive first assessments'. It is essential that assessors at least refer appropriately on the basis of their encounters with patients and clients (Wilkinson et al 1993) and that all staff are provided with the necessary training in assessment methods. According to Herzberg (1995) the decisive factor in psychogeriatric assessment is teamworking, in which the team uses its range of professional viewpoints to consider each referral, and so provides depth of knowledge and support for the person making the initial assessment.

ASSESSMENT PROCEDURES

This chapter has discussed environmental, psychological, social and organic perspectives on the assessment of older people. It has also looked at the effect of people's sense of control over their problems of daily living. These perspectives need to be brought together for the purposes of a structured assessment.

The Department of Health suggested that assessment methods and implementation strategies should be developed locally (Department of Health 1990). However, the Royal College of Physicians (1992) observed that the development of separate measures would inhibit comparison of outcomes and quality indicators and make communication and coordination between health and social care providers difficult. They have therefore funded eight different centres to test the feasibility of using a set of assessment measures for seven areas (Ross & Bower 1995), listed in Box 6.2.

Ross and Bower (1995) tested the use of standardised measures for use by district nurses with older people and found some positive advantages.

Box 6.2 Set of assessment measures for feasibility study (Ross & Bower 1995)

1. Activities of daily living (ADL)
- physical ADL
- mobility
- instrumental ADL.

2. Mental health functioning
- cognitive
- presence of psychiatric symptoms.

3. Psychosocial functioning
- emotional wellbeing in a social and cultural context.

4. Physical health functioning
- self-perceived health status
- physical symptoms and diagnosed conditions
- health service utilisation
- activity levels and measures of incapacity.

5. Social resources
- accessibility of family, friends and a familiar/professional, voluntary helper
- availability of these resources where needed.

6. Economic resources
- income compared to an external standard.

7. Environmental resources
- adequate and affordable housing
- siting of housing in relation to transport, shopping and public services.

They found that the mean time to complete an assessment was 39 minutes, which was similar to the time district nurses usually spent on a first assessment visit. The authors suggest that priorities and collaborative care planning can be defined more successfully using these measures than when different health and social care workers use a variety of assessment strategies and tools.

Measures

Normative assessment procedures need valid and reliable measures. At minimum, measures must have been widely tested, be internally consistent, have test–retest consistency and be both sensitive and specific to the constructs being measured (Streiner & Norman 1991, Schutte & Malouff 1995). A few commonly used measures are mentioned to highlight the issues involved when selecting a means of rating various attributes that might characterise an older person.

Kline (1993) discusses five different methods of constructing psychological tests. He argues that factor analytic tests based on empirically derived variables yield reliable and meaningful data. As noted previously, if assessors use schedules that have not been validated on a population similar to that being assessed they cannot assume that a measure that has been tested on a different population will yield valid and reliable information. Orrell et al (1992) point out that different versions of measures of cognitive function have the same name. Many of the available measures do not meet psychometric criteria. Culture-dependent measures are clearly unsuitable for use with people from ethnic groups other than those used for validation. For example, the Bedford Alzheimer Nursing Severity Scale has been validated with a North American sample that was predominantly white (Volicer et al 1994); it needs to be validated with other populations.

Educational achievement and poverty also interfere with reliable performance on measures such as the Mini Mental State Examination (Folstein et al 1975) which predominantly taps verbal abilities (O'Connor et al 1989, Mitrushina & Satz 1991). However, Jorm et al (1988) argue that, on more specific testing, the apparent bias of the Mini Mental State Examination disappears. They warn that 'all too often it is assumed that differences found between groups on some scale represent true differences on the attribute the scale purports to measure, when they could be due to test bias' (p. 730). Schutte and Malouff (1995) recommend that, before using the Mini Mental State Examination, the interviewer needs information about the respondent's educational achievement, physical impairment, and whether English is the first language. Kua & Ko (1992) provide an example of a screening measure of cognitive impairment designed for use in developing countries, and available in Chinese and Malay. Park and Kwon (1990) have developed a Korean version of the Mini Mental State Examination.

The British Geriatrics Society and the Research Unit of the Royal College of Physicians recommend four standardised assessment measures. The Barthel Activities of Daily Living Index (Mahoney & Barthel 1965) estimates disability by measuring functional activities of daily living. The Abbreviated Mental Test (AMTS) (Hodkinson 1972) assesses cognitive function. The Geriatric Depression Scale (Brink et al 1982, Yesavage et al 1983) assesses mood. The Philadelphia Geriatric Centre Morale Scale (Lawton 1975, McCulloch 1991) assesses subjective wellbeing.

Screening measures of cognitive function include the Gresham Ward Questionnaires (Institute of Psychiatry 1978) which assess general orientation and memory for past personal events, recent personal events and general events. Although the Cambridge Mental Disorders of the Elderly Examination (CAMDEX) takes 90 minutes to administer, it does not necessarily need a psychiatrist to use it (although training is required) and it provides robust data about mental state, functional behaviour, mood and health status (Roth et al 1986, O'Connor et al 1991). The Information-Memory-Concentration Test (IMC) (Blessed et al 1968) tests cognitive function, and correlates this with severity of dementia. The National Adult Reading Test (Nelson 1991) estimates premorbid intelligence of people with cognitive impairment. For research purposes, Wing et al (1990) developed the Schedules for Clinical Assessment in Neuropsychiatry (SCAN) from the Present State Examination (Wing et al 1974) which is included in the SCAN. SCAN is designed for experienced clinicians, for whom training in its use takes 1 week. The data collected during an interview provide profiles of clinical phenomena, clinical and differential diagnoses which are gathered into a 'formulation' of a person's needs and problems (see below). The World Health Organization is also developing schedules for the clinical examination of dementia (Copeland et al 1994, Levy 1994).

Multidimensionality

Magnusson (1993) discusses the 'principle of dynamic interaction' between perception, cognition and biological factors in the day-to-day functioning of an individual. Schonfield (1983) emphasises that inferences about social skills should not be drawn from assessment of perceptual and motor skills. For example, assessment of dementia comprises three complementary approaches:

- diagnosis
- measure of severity and extent of cognitive impairment
- measure of behavioural dysfunction (Roth et al 1986).

The Clifton Assessment Procedures for the Elderly (CAPE) (Pattie & Gilleard 1979) comprise measures of various areas such as behaviour and cognition. Idler & Kasl (1991) list the areas to be covered by a multidimensional assessment of health:

- self-report
- use of medical care
- social networks
- internal resources including religious beliefs and attributional style
- family health
- exposure to environmental hazards.

Mrazek and Haggerty (1994) identify cultural competence as a key element of research into preventive interventions. They provide a concise summary of the skills comprised in cultural sensitivity. Rodenburg et al (1991) argue that their assessment schedule is both culturally sensitive and, despite its brevity, multidimensional. Marshall (1994, p. 27) discusses his model of 'need decision making ... which incorporates the perspectives of patients and relevant caregivers'. He identifies three criteria for acting upon identified needs:

- the cooperation criterion
- the caregiver stress criterion
- the severity criterion (Marshall 1994, p. 33).

Ensuring that these criteria are included in an assessment should also ensure that it is multidimensional.

Measurement of change

Change is measured from screening (that is, baseline) to review. If change is to be measured accurately over time and a number of different workers are likely to observe the older person in different settings, it follows that repeated measures must have good inter-rater reliability as well as be easy to use. It is always necessary to use a combination of measures, including a screening test such as the Mini Mental State Examination, a behavioural scale that measures activities of daily living, and a measure of intellectual decline (Blessed et al 1968, Folstein et al 1974). Little et al (1987) found that an unreliable measure used for baseline assessment compounded its errors when repeated in order to estimate change. They emphasise the 'importance of tailoring assessments to the ability of subjects when monitoring change' (p. 139). Problems with reliability of measures over time also result from the use of scales whose potential scores depend on the language ability of the respondent (Volicer et al 1994).

Morgan & Hatsukami (1986) found a 'floor effect' – most scores congregating at the negative end of the scale – in a subscale of the Shipley Institute of Living Scale (Shipley 1940) similar to that found by Little et al (1987) who assessed severely cognitively impaired respondents with the Psychogeriatric Assessment Schedule (Bergmann et al 1975). Morgan & Hatsukami caution against using such measures for screening purposes. Volicer et al (1994) have developed a scale that they argue does not suffer from a floor effect and is designed for use with people who have severe cognitive impairment. They append the seven-item four-point (score 7 to 28) Bedford Alzheimer Nursing

Severity Scale. A score of 7 indicates no impairment, and a score of 28 indicates complete impairment. Another nursing scale, the Nurses' Observation Scale for Geriatric Patients, is in the process of development (Tremmel & Spiegel 1993).

The assessment interview

The aim of interviewing people is to gain their individual perceptions of their current problems in their own words. The interview can also serve as an analogue of day-to-day functioning, and is preferably conducted in the person's home. The length of an interview will be entirely dependent on the state of the patient and the urgency of conducting a comprehensive initial assessment or a fast assessment that relates to the person's immediate acute care needs. Bird & Cohen-Cole (1990, p. 69) identify three functions of a 'medical interview':

- gathering biological and psychosocial data
- responding to the interviewee's emotions
- influencing interviewees to change their behaviour.

An interview may make it clear that the person being assessed does not answer some questions, appears to make up answers or is confused by the questions. Such responses generally indicate that a rapid initial evaluation of the person's safety and of immediate problems of daily living is needed: focusing on the person's ability to breathe, eliminate and maintain a safe environment. Even in a short interview the assessor must be sensitive to the individual's perspective and priorities, to maximise the chance of collaboration between caregivers and the person being assessed (Perkins 1991).

Diagnosis

Diagnosis alone is inadequate for planning care because the presentation, severity and natural history of any disorder vary from person to person (Richman & Barry 1985). One of the main benefits of accurate diagnosis is the prompt and assertive treatment of acute illness, but the prompt and assertive provision of health and social services depends on many factors other than diagnostic category. ICD-10 (World Health Organization 1992) and DSM-IV (American Psychiatric Association 1993) provide operational criteria on which a reliable diagnosis may be based, but these criteria do not tell the whole story about people within their social setting. Nevertheless, the distinction between psychosocial and organic determinants of a person's current situation is central to a programme of care that promptly and assertively treats acute ill health (Miller et al 1991).

Lishman (1987, p. 577) argues that 'investigations are ... principally directed at detecting remediable conditions, or uncovering systemic disorders which may be worsening the clinical picture'. Accurate diagnosis thus helps to determine whether health care is necessary, and acts as the 'first step in management' (Lishman 1987, p. 584). Orrell et al (1992) found that diagnosis by a consultant was more reliable than standardised measures in discriminating between organic and so-called 'functional' disorders in a hospitalised sample of older people. Marks & Toole (1995, p. 1) argue that, although a diagnosis 'broadly maps out someone's likely problem now and/or in the future', it does not specify the 'main remediable problems'.

History

Onset

An accurate history of the onset of current problems makes a powerful difference to whether the programme of care is directed to control of disability and impairment or to treatment of acute disease. Delirium, which is often very treatable, must crucially be distinguished from dementia, and sudden onset is one of the key features of delirium (Corrigan & Bogner 1994, Schutte & Malouff 1995). The dementia syndromes begin and progress insidiously so that people can be quite impaired by the time they come to the attention of health or social services. Information from at least one third party is essential. Delirium is discussed in Chapter 10, and dementia in Chapter 11.

Chronicity

Duggan et al's (1991) follow-up study of a series of depressed individuals is especially relevant to assessment of older people because it suggests that depression follows a much less benign course over the lifespan than had previously been supposed. Their findings support Teasdale's (1988) hypothesis that the personality trait 'neuroticism' predicts a poor outcome for someone who has been hospitalised for a depressive episode. Conley (1984) argues that traits such as neuroticism are relatively stable over the life span.

Documentation

Schogt & Sadevoy (1987, p. 179) provide general guidelines for preparing reports on 'protective service

needs of the impaired elderly living in the community', but each service provider should have its own guidelines and standards (Wing et al 1995).

The life chart and genogram

To identify psychosocial factors that may have contributed to the service user's current problems, it may be useful to compile a life chart, a genogram and a sociogram of the person's family and friends. These devices enable the assessor to outline the social context and environment of the person being assessed, to identify whether the person is socially isolated and whether any family members or friends are providing significant levels of informal care. Because they are graphical they act as concise summaries of complex and detailed data that often get lost in narrative accounts of the same material.

Production of a life chart involves examining with the person important life events. Seemingly remote events may be extremely important in terms of contributing factors to mental state. For example, experiences that occurred during military service or during combat or as a civilian during hostilities form a substrate for later development of depressive illnesses in people as they get older. More recent events such as the death of a spouse or sibling, or retirement, are also frequently contributory factors to depressive illnesses. Financial issues should also be considered. Inadequate income may contribute to poor diet, cold and ultimately to people being physically ill with accompanying psychological symptoms and problems.

A genogram may be used to identify any hereditary factors that may contribute to illnesses, such as cerebral-vascular dementia or manic depressive psychosis. The genogram is a useful way of opening a discussion about a person's family network, including long-ago losses, bereavements, estrangement and their effects currently. Life charts and genograms are valuable teaching aids and we have reported their use with student nurses (Ritter et al, in press).

Involving the carers

Zarit et al (1985) have devised a stress adaptation framework for involving caregivers in assessment of older people. This approach has been described and used successfully with people with Alzheimer's disease. Zarit et al (1985) argue that, although a trained health or social worker can rapidly assess a service user's health and social needs, to do so in isolation from the informal caregiver or family unit would be insensitive or irresponsible. The stress adaptation framework focuses on identifying the areas of care that carers find most difficult to cope with, and on examining ways of augmenting coping skills, and of reducing tension within family units.

Watkins (1984, 1987) applied a combination of an activities of living approach and Zarit et al's (1985) stress management approach to both in-patient and community oriented settings for people with dementia syndromes (Watkins 1984, 1987). Watkins argues that it is necessary to describe the effectiveness of carers' strategies for coping with clients' problems and whether they cause any stress within the family unit and/or to the caregiver. There are two stages. First the named nurse or key worker gives information to the service user and carer, family or significant others. Second, a problem-solving cycle is used to help resolve problems associated with the dementing person. The named nurse or key worker helps the carer to reveal behaviours that cause them most distress. Most carers report finding certain problems more difficult to cope with than others. For example, most carers can tolerate a person's inability to dress and walk unaided, but most find it difficult to cope with inappropriate urination or aggressive behaviour.

Self-assessment

Fillenbaum (1979) compared the self-assessments of their health by older people with objective ratings by unspecified workers and found that they correlated for respondents living in the community, but not in institutions. Women were more likely to be rated as being in poorer health than they assessed themselves. Fillenbaum (1979) interprets this as indicating that women in the study were able to tolerate objectively poorer levels of impaired health, implying that extra care must be taken when assessing women's health needs.

Dowrick (1993) found that members of a primary health care team were likely to be unaware of older people's problems with social isolation, memory and bereavement even if a person was currently being seen by a member of the team. Reubenstein et al (1984) indicate that a three-way assessment may be more reliable, incorporating self-assessment, report by a significant other, and a report by, for example, a nurse.

Reuben et al (1992) suggest that self-report must be supplemented by systematic observation and rating of performance. Ott and Fogel (1992) found that cognitively impaired respondents assessed themselves as not depressed, whereas observers rated them as

depressed. Dean et al (1993) have developed an observation schedule for assessing the quality of interaction by severely cognitively impaired older people with their caregivers that compensates for unreliable self-assessment. Another scale (MOSES, Helmes et al 1987, Pruchno et al 1994) rates caregivers' accounts of their observations of nursing home residents.

The formulation of needs and problems

An assessment moves towards a formulation of a person's needs and problems. The formulation must include an account of the psychosocial aspects of the person's situation and be tailored to the individual's predicament. Formulation by professionals of their clients' difficulties can be subject to many biases, including the notion of 'deservedness'. An older person who is perceived to be a 'burden' may attract a covertly hostile response disguised in the jargon of helping. The formulation therefore encompasses information from all aspects of the assessment regardless of the disciplines of the people who conduct the various parts of it. Sims (1995) provides one example of how to write a clinical formulation. It begins with a description of the person together with the current social circumstances, followed by a summary of the 'presenting complaint' (not at this stage in terms of any explanatory model). An account of how the referral came about comes next, together with the person's current status (e.g. supervision register, section of the Mental Health Act 1983, Court of Protection). A summary of the history of the presenting complaint leads to the diagnosis and differential diagnoses if appropriate. Aetiological factors are presented together with a summary of the supporting evidence derived from investigations (social, psychological, clinical). Prognosis is an essential component partly because of the requirement to assess and manage risk. Finally the formulation outlines the short and long term goals of the programme of care.

Public policy and assessment

We turn now to consider the impact of public policy on the process and procedures for assessing the elderly people. At their most basic, the resources to be allocated to health and social care are financial. The National Health Service reforms that began with the Griffiths report (Department of Health and Social Security 1983) aimed to put in hand health care that:

- is necessary
- is technically efficient
- costs as little as possible (Abel-Smith 1994).

Technically efficient health care includes:

- 'rational prescribing' of essential drugs (Abel-Smith 1994)
- performing only those investigations that are relevant both to the likely diagnosis and the treatment entailed by the diagnosis
- matching through-put of patients and availability of staff.

At the time of writing, the Conservative Government model of health care is 'managed competition'. That is, health care providers have to compete for contracts from health authorities and GP fund-holders. The idea is to use resources more efficiently by:

- identifying existing resources and services
- expanding the services provided by existing resources
- restricting extra funding to specific improvements that reflect changes in the behaviour of health care providers (whether organisations or individuals).

The nature of assessment depends partly on the individual professional's definition of mental health, partly on the limits to what can be provided by the health and social services, and partly on the standards and criteria of individual service providers (Vickers 1958, Richman & Barry 1985). Current policy concerning health care for older people is dominated by the concept of needs-led assessment, comprising:

- collaboration between health care and social services agencies
- screening
- identification of a single person who is responsible for an assessment
- comprehensive assessment within a stated timespan
- matching of services to identified needs (SSI & DH 1995).

Problems with a philosophy of needs-led assessment have been discussed earlier in this chapter.

The care programme approach (CPA)

All individuals who come into contact with the specialist or secondary level mental health services have been subject to the Care Programme Approach (CPA) since 1990 (HC[89]5 1989). Most people with serious and enduring mental health problems are also subject to care management by social services. Although this chapter has focused on assessment in relation to mental health care, an underlying assumption is always that of coordinated social and health care from the first stages of assessment to systematic evaluation of the programme of care.

The number of professionals involved in care programming will be related to the severity and intensity of an individual's problems. Some service users will only require a minimal CPA. Department of Health (1994) guidelines suggest that when a patient needs the attention of one member of the health care team, the CPA requirements are simple:

- The consultant will probably do the assessment, perhaps with some input from a social worker and mental health nurse.
- The member of the team who will be carrying out care interventions will be the key worker.
- The care plan will be very short, indicating the regular interventions planned, on which the service user and carer should be consulted (Department of Health 1994, p. 125).

In the minimal care plan approach, changes in the patient's condition will be monitored by the key worker who will inform other appropriate members of the team about changes in the patient.

The more complex care programme approach is required for individuals with severe mental illness where coordinated multidisciplinary teamwork is essential. Complex needs assessment will require several members of the health care team's involvement including a psychiatrist, social worker and mental health nurse. In the more complex care programme approach there are four stages:

1. Systematic assessment of the health and social care needs of the patient with particular regard as to whether the patient has a severe and enduring (i.e. chronic) mental illness.
2. Drawing up of a package of care agreed with members of the multi-disciplinary team, local authority care manager, general practitioner, service users and their carers.
3. Nomination of a key worker to keep in close contact with the patient.
4. Regular review and systematic monitoring of the patient's needs and progress, and of the delivery of the care programme (Department of Health 1994, p. 126).

The CPA implies therefore, among other things, that

individuals have a right to rapid and flexible access to services. To ensure such access each discipline must be capable of carrying out at least an initial evaluation and of referring appropriately for a full assessment if necessary.

OUTCOME EVALUATION

Assessment alone will not improve outcomes for older people (McVey et al 1984, Katz et al 1985). A programme of care must not be directed only to the needs and problems identified at assessment, but also be evaluated by repeating of the same measures that were used at baseline. Techniques such as 'goal attainment scaling' enable specific review of care plans (Rockwood et al 1993). Functional status, for example in the dimensions of mobility, physical activities, role activities, self-care activities and general limitations, is often used as the basis for assessing response to treatment (Stewart et al 1981). The Sickness Impact Profile (Bergner et al 1981) can be self-administered or completed by an interviewer. Katz et al (1992) discuss the reliability and validity of a range of measures of health status designed to rate outcomes of medical care.

MANAGEMENT OF CARE

Management of care comprises:

- the prevention or control of disability
- measurement of infirmity and impairment
- prompt and assertive rehabilitation of people recovering from acute episodes of ill health
- prompt and assertive provision of health or social services, or both.

Managing care means maintaining people in the least restrictive environment as is compatible with their safety or the safety of other people, and maintaining maximum personal autonomy that is compatible with personal safety or safety of other people.

Although systematic and sensitive assessment is an essential requirement of community care and the care programme approach, it has been argued that the full and comprehensive assessment of individuals is rarely fulfilled (HC[89]5 1989, Dickinson & Young 1990). Ideally the health care team allocates responsibility between team members for assessing the presenting problems: whether new or long-term, their precipitants and the reasons why they have occurred at this time. Immediate and future management issues will be identified. This is particularly important when a person is at home and considered by the referrer to be at risk,

whether through self-neglect, actively suicidal behaviour, or abuse by a family member or caregiver. Liaison with the source of referral can be done by someone of the same discipline. In some instances it may be necessary to invoke a guardianship order or use a section of the Mental Health Act to protect the person from harm. In the event of coercive treatment, it is essential that a psychiatrist and social worker are involved at an early stage of assessment. For a detailed discussion of legal issues see Chapter 28.

Ethical issues

Perhaps the most difficult ethical issue concerning the care and treatment of older people is to ensure that they are involved in decisions relating to active medical and nursing intervention in case of terminal illness. For example, people in the final stages of Alzheimer's disease may be unable to state their preferences but a relation may make it clear that they would not have chosen to have their life prolonged in these circumstances. Full discussion is also necessary before interventions such as flu vaccination are offered.

Whenever possible, the health care assessor identifies the person's feelings concerning active intervention and also consults families and significant others. When complex decisions relating to whether active treatment should be undertaken to prolong life, the health care team, other professional caregivers, service users, their families, carers and significant others are involved in the process of decision making. For example, when a person with Alzheimer's disease is no longer able to eat or drink but could be fed through a nasogastric tube, the decision to tube-feed must be made plainly observable so that records concerning the decision-making process are explicit and an audit trail can be followed. See Chapter 28 for further discussion of ethical issues.

Provision of appropriate support

Care options usually require consideration of whether older people with mental health problems are willing to have in-patient treatment or whether they would rather stay at home with maximum treatment and support. People with dementia can and should be involved in deciding whether they use long term community care at home or enter residential care.

Older people may wish to stay at home in relative independence while younger family members including daughters and sons may prefer that their parents are supported in residential facilities. It is important that the care team identifies these kinds of conflicts and ensures that the older person's preferences are met whenever possible. In some circumstances, when an old person is being cared for at home by one person alone, it is necessary to identify the level of stress caused to the caregiver (Levin et al 1989, Watkins 1994). If carers are too stressed it is more likely that the caregiving relationship will falter. Following a comprehensive assessment, the care team will have to weigh up whether the needs of the carer or the patient are most important. In some instances the care options will relate very closely to the carer's perceived needs as well as those of the patient. If carers feel sufficiently supported, cognitively and physically impaired older people are more likely to be able to stay in their family environments.

CONCLUSION

The overriding purpose of assessment is to confirm the extent to which a referral warrants intervention by a service provider. This purpose encompasses three categories of activities (clinical investigation, social enquiry and functional assessment) that, when completed, provide a description and explanation of observed phenomena, and measure the needs, risk status and health status of the individual who has been referred. An assessment fulfils two further goals. The first is that the programme of care focuses specifically on the needs and problems identified during the assessment. We have summarised our guidelines for assessing older people in Table 6.1.

Table 6.1 Guidelines for assessing older people

Guideline	Rationale
Only carry out tests you have been formally trained to use – i.e. at minimum you have received a comprehensive explanation of their use and purpose; you have observed them in use; you have carried them out while being observed by a supervisor; and you have practised their use independently but under supervision.	(a) Standardised tests are rendered worthless if used inconsistently or without regard for inter-rater or inter-observer reliability. (b) Many psychological tests are copyrighted for use by qualified psychologists only. (c) Many psychological tests depend for their validity on being kept confidential within the professional group responsible for using them.
Adhere strictly to the conditions stated by each test for its use, ensuring that wording is not varied, that prompts are given only as instructed, and that instructions to the person being tested are identical to the wording of the test.	(a) To maintain consistency of test conditions. (b) To avoid introducing test bias when using an otherwise reliable measure.
Where possible, assess a person in an environment or situation with which he or she is familiar.	So that you see the person, so far as possible, as he or she is in everyday circumstances.
Be prepared to split an assessment into a number of sessions, ensuring that the conditions for each session are as far as possible identical each time.	(a) Fatigue or distractibility are likely to distort findings from assessment activities. (b) Unless sessions are as like each other as possible, it will be difficult to argue that results are consistent or comparable.
When possible, negotiate the timing and duration of sessions with the person being assessed, or with his or her caregiver(s) or both.	So that your work fits in with their routine of activities such as mealtimes, or occupational therapy, or shopping.
Ensure that if sessions are split, you have divided the test material appropriately.	So that you don't waste time by, say, scheduling a short test in an afternoon; or that you don't try to cram too much into a session.
Take with you to assessments one or two pairs of over the counter reading spectacles.	A common reason for not filling in self-report questionnaires is, 'I haven't got my reading glasses'. Even cognitively unimpaired people have been known to place their spectacles in the egg box in the fridge.
Ensure that the location where assessment will be carried out is private, undisturbed and free from interruptions.	Even when somebody is being assessed at home, there may be distractions such as family, pets or the television.

Table 6.1   Guidelines for assessing older people *(contd)*

Guideline	Rationale
Ensure that both you and the person being assessed can be comfortably seated, that there are at least two light sources, neither of which is over-bright, and that you can move to either side of the person without being intrusive.	Testing of sensory impairment may be distorted by lateral or functional deficits that give the impression of being a global or cognitive deficit. For example, sitting on the side of someone's 'bad' ear; or sitting at an angle where someone with visual field impairment can't see you.
Especially on first meeting the person to be assessed, introduce yourself and outline in lay language the purpose of your visit.	(a) A person's social skills may remain relatively intact even in the presence of severe cognitive impairment. (b) The usual courtesies should have the effect of helping to allay anxiety.
Explain why you have come to see the person being assessed, ensuring that you do not use words or phrases like 'test', 'how well you perform', 'difficult/easy'.	(a) You want to see people functioning as they do day-to-day. (b) Many people become flustered when they are being tested, especially if they think their living situation might improve or deteriorate significantly as a result of their performance on testing.
Ask the person being assessed whether he or she would like a familiar person such as a carer or other caregiver to be present during assessment sessions.	As long as the caregiver does not try to assist or otherwise interfere with the assessment, she may provide a reassuring presence, and can offer to do things like making refreshments.
Offer guidance or praise only as indicated by the test materials.	It's probably acceptable to say 'Yes, use a pen if you want'. But it is not acceptable to say 'Well done' or 'That's right' or 'Yes' when a person answers a question that forms part of a measure.
Observe people carrying out assessment tasks with, as well as without, items like spectacles, hearing aid, walking aids or any other appliance that they use in activities of daily living.	The confidence that comes, say, from using a stick may make a difference to a person's performance that needs to be observed.

The second goal is that, when the programme of care is reviewed, the repetition of the same procedures and measures carried out during the assessment ensures that the effectiveness of the care is measured against the baseline measures. This means that assessment is a dynamic activity that changes in response to the changes in the service user's needs and problems. In addition, the person responsible for the assessment must bear in mind the Department of Health's (1994) guidance on risk assessment. For instance, when Bruce & Hoff (1994) use an epidemiological survey to argue for vigorous prevention and early intervention in major depression this is an example of actuarial and statistical calculation based on research evidence. And when the assessor is asked to estimate the overall likelihood of risky behaviour, intellectual decline is an important example. 'The cardinal symptom of senile dementia is progressive cognitive impairment' (Little et al 1987, p. 135) that leads in turn to observable functional impairment (Volicer et al 1994).

Interventions that affect the health status and disability-free life expectancy of older people may be grouped under the following headings:

- health behaviour
- early detection and assertive treatment of illness, including mental illness
- alleviation of socioeconomic hardship.

This implies that assessment is meaningless unless it is directed towards an effective intervention.

In summary, assessment aims to:

- prevent disability
- treat illness promptly and assertively
- provide services promptly and assertively
- maintain people in their own home for as long as possible
- provide prompt and assertive rehabilitation to people recovering from acute illness or decompensation
- help individuals to maintain personal autonomy compatible with personal safety.

REFERENCES

Abel-Smith B 1994 An introduction to health. Longman, London

Abramson L Y, Seligman M E P, Teasdale J 1978 Learned helplessness in humans: critique and reformulation. Journal of Abnormal Psychology 87: 49–74

Ajzen I, Fishbein M 1980 Understanding attitudes and predicting social behaviour. Prentice Hall, Englewood Cliffs NJ

Alexopolous C, Abrams R, Young R, Shamoian C 1988 Cornell scale for depression in dementia. Biological Psychiatry 23: 271–284

American Psychiatric Association 1993 Diagnostic and statistical manual of mental disorders, 4th edn. American Psychiatric Association, Washington DC

Anderson C A, Horowitz L M, French R de S 1983 Attributional style of lonely and depressed people. Journal of Personality and Social Psychology 45(1): 127–136

Andreasen N C 1979 Thought, language and communication disorders. Archives of General Psychiatry 36: 1315–1330

Backer G 1985 Social group work in a group practice: group work with the retired elderly in Copenhagen Scandinavian Journal of Primary Health Care 3(1): 45–48

Baker D, Illsley R 1990 Trends in inequality in health in Europe. International Journal of Health Sciences 1(2): 89–111

Bandura A 1989 Human agency in social cognitive theory. American Psychologist 44(9): 1175–1184

Barsky A J, Frank C B, Cleary P D, Wyshak G et al 1991 The relation between hypochondriasis and age. American Journal of Psychiatry 148(7): 923–928

Battcock T, Castleden M 1990 Assessment of the nervous system. In: Beech J R, Harding L (eds) Assessment of the elderly. NFER-Nelson, Windsor

Beaglehole R 1990 International trends in coronary heart disease mortality, morbidity and risk factors. Epidemiological Review 12: 1–15

Beardsall L, Brayne C 1990 Estimation of verbal intelligence in an elderly community: a prediction analysis using the shortened NART. British Journal of Clinical Psychology 29: 83–90

Beardsall L, Huppert F A 1991 A comparison of clinical, psychometric and behavioural memory tests: findings from a community study of the detection of dementia. International Journal of Geriatric Psychiatry 6: 295–306

Beck A T, Rush A J, Shaw B F, Emery G 1979 Cognitive therapy of depression. Guilford Press, New York

Bergner M, Bobbitt R A, Carter W B, Gilson B S 1981 The sickness impact profile: development and final revision of a health status measure. Medical Care 19(8): 787–805

Berrios G E 1984 Descriptive psychopathology: conceptual and historical aspects. Psychological Medicine 14: 303–313

Bird J, Cohen-Cole S A 1990 The three-function model of the medical interview. In: Hale M S (ed) Methods in teaching consultation-liaison psychiatry. Karger, Basel

Blessed G, Tomlinson B E, Roth M 1968 The association between quantitative measures of dementia and of senile change in the cerebral grey matter of elderly subjects. British Journal of Psychiatry 114: 797–811

Bowling A 1995 Measuring health. Open University Press, Buckingham

Branch L G, Guralnik J M, Foley D J et al 1991 Active life expectancy for 10 000 caucasian men and women in three communities. Journal of Gerontology 46(4): M145–M150

Brewin C R 1985 Depression and causal attributions: what is their relation? Psychological Bulletin 98(2): 297–309

Brewin C R 1988 Cognitive foundations of clinical psychology. Lawrence Erlbaum Associates, Hove and London

Brewin C R, Furnham A 1986 Attributional versus preattributional variables in self-esteem and depression. Journal of Personality and Social Psychology 50(5): 1013–1020

Brewin C, Wing J K, Mangen S P, Brugha T S, MacCarthy B 1987 Principles and practice of measuring needs in the long-term mentally ill: the Medical Research Council needs for assessment. Psychological Medicine 17: 971–981

Brink T L, Yesavage J A, Lum O, Heersema P, Adey M, Rose T L 1982 Screening tests for geriatric depression. Clinical Gerontologist 1(1): 37–43

Brown G W, Harris T 1978 Social origins of depression. Tavistock, London

Bruce M L, Hoff R A 1994 Social and physical health risk factors for first-onset major depressive disorder in a community sample. Social Psychiatry and Psychiatric Epidemiology 29(4): 165–171

Burns A 1992 Psychiatric phenomena in dementia of the Alzheimer's type. International Psychogeriatrics 4(Supplement 1): 43–54

Burns A, Marsh A, Bender D A 1989 Dietary intake and clinical, anthropometric and biochemical indices of malnutrition in elderly demented patients and non-demented subjects. Psychological Medicine 19: 383–391

Burns A, Jacoby R, Levy R 1990 Behavioural abnormalities and psychiatric symptoms in Alzheimer's disease: preliminary findings. International Psychogeriatrics 2(1): 25–36

Burns A, Jacoby R, Levy R 1991 Computed tomography in Alzheimer's disease: a longitudinal study. Biological Psychiatry 29(4): 383–390

Camp C J, Pignatiello M F 1988 Beliefs about fact retrieval and inferential reasoning across the adult lifespan. Experimental Aging Research 14(2): 89–97

Carr-Hill R A 1991 Allocating resources to health care: is the QALY (Quality Adjusted Life Year) a technical solution to a political problem? International Journal of Health Services 21(2): 351–363

Carr-Hill R A, Morris J 1991 Current practice in obtaining the 'Q' in QALYs: a cautionary note. British Medical Journal 303(6810): 1136–1137

Caserta M S 1995 Health promotion and the older population: expanding our theoretical horizons. Journal of Community Health 20(3): 283–292

Chappell N L, Badger M 1989 Social isolation and well-being. Journal of Gerontology 44(5): S169–S176

Christensen H 1991 The validity of memory complaints by elderly persons. International Journal of Geriatric Psychiatry 6: 307–312

Colantonio A, Kasl S V, Ostfeld A M 1992 Level of function predicts first stroke in the elderly. Stroke 23(9): 1355–1357

Collighan G, MacDonald A, Herzberg J, Philpot M, Lindesay Journal of 1993 An evaluation of the multidisciplinary approach to psychiatric diagnosis in elderly people. British Medical Journal 306: 821–824

Collins L M 1994 Comment on 'how many causes are there of aging-related decrements in cognitive function?' Developmental Review 14(4): 438–443

Conley J J 1984 Longitudinal consistency of adult personality: self-reported psychological characteristics across 45 years. Journal of Personality and Social Psychology 47(6): 1325–1333

Connelly P J, Jamieson F E 1991 Objective assessment of praxis – the OAP digram: simply testing for dementia. International Journal of Geriatric Psychiatry 6: 667–672

Copeland J R M, Kelleher M J, Kelliet J M et al 1976 A semi-structured clinical interview for the assessment of diagnosis and mental state in the elderly: the Geriatric Mental State Schedule I: development and reliability. Psychological Medicine 6: 439–449

Copeland J R M, Dewey M R E, Henderson A S et al 1988 The Geriatric Mental State Schedule used in the community: replication studies of the computerized diagnosis AGECAT. Psychological Medicine 18: 219–223

Copeland J R, Prilipko L, Sartorius N 1992 The WHO collaborative study: development of evaluation instruments for the assessment of dementia. Clinical Neuropharmacology 15(Supplement 1, Part A): 491A–492A

Corrigan J D 1989 Development of a scale for assessment of agitation folowing traumatic brain injury. Journal of Clinical and Experimental Neuropsychology 11: 261–277

Corrigan J D, Bogner J A 1994 Factor structure of the Agitated Behaviour Scale. Journal of Clinical and Experimental Neuropsychology 16: 386–392

Creecy R F, Berg W E, Wright R Jr 1985 Loneliness among the elderly: a causal approach. Journal of Gerontology 40(4): 487–493

Croake J W, Myers K M, Singh A 1988 The fears expressed by elderly men and women: a lifespan approach. International Journal of Aging and Human Development 26(2): 139–146

David A S 1990 Insight and psychosis. British Journal of Psychiatry 156: 798–808

Davies K J A (ed) 1991 Oxidative damage and repair: chemical, biological and medical aspects. Pergamon, Oxford

Davis D L, Bradlow H L 1995 Can environmental estrogens cause breast cancer? Scientific American 273(4): 144–149

Davis P B, Morris J C, Grant E G 1990 Brief screening tests versus clinical staging in senile dementia of the Alzheimer's type. Journal of the American Geriatrics Society 38: 129–135

Dean R, Proudfoot R, Lindsay J 1993 The Quality of Interactions Schedule (QUIS): development, reliability and use in the evaluation of two domus units. International Journal of Geriatric Psychiatry 8: 819–826

Department of Health and Social Services Inspectorate 1994 Mental Illness (The Health of the Nation Key Area Handbook) 2nd edn. HMSO, London

Department of Health 1990 The NHS and Community Care Act. HMSO, London

Department of Health and Social Security 1983 National Health Service Management Inquiry. Department of Health and Social Security, London

Department of Health and Welsh Office 1989 General practice in the National Health Service. HMSO, London

Dickinson E, Young A 1990 Framework for medical assessment of functional performance. The Lancet 335: 778–779

counter reading spectacles.

Dickson D W, Crystal H A, Mattiace L A et al 1991 Identification of normal and pathological ageing in prospectively studied nondemented elderly humans. Neurobiology of Ageing 13: 179–189

Dill A 1993 Defining needs, defining systems: a critical analysis. The Gerontologist 33(4): 453–460

Dowie J 1975 The portfolio approach to health behaviour. Social Science and Medicine 9: 619–631

Doyal L, Gough I 1984 A theory of human needs. Critical Social Policy 10: 6–38

Dubos R 1965 Man adapting. Yale University Press, New Haven

Duggan C, Lee A S, Murray R M 1991 Do different subtypes of hospitalized depressives have different long-term outcomes? Archives of General Psychiatry 48(4): 308–312

Dustman R E, Emmerson R Y, Ruhling R O et al 1990 Age and fitness effects on EEG, ERP, visual sensitivity and cognition. Neurobiology of Ageing 11: 193–200

Eagger S A, Levy R, Sahakian B J 1992 Tacrine in Alzheimer's Disease. Acta Neurologica Scandinavica 85: 75–80

Eggert E G M et al 1977 Caring for the patient with long-term disability. Geriatrics 32: 102

Ellis A 1962 Reason and emotion in psychotherapy. Lyle Stuart, New York

Feinstein J S 1993 The relationship between socioeconomic status and health: a review of the literature. Milbank Memorial Fund Quarterly 71(3): 279–322

Ferrell B A, Ferrell B R, Osterweil D 1990 Pain in the nursing home. Journal of the American Geriatric Society 38(4): 409–414

Fichera S, Zielinski R, Tremont G , Mittenberg W 1994 Psychometric properties of the Agitated Behaviour Scale. Journal of Clinical and Experimental Neuropsychology 16: 386–392

Fillenbaum G 1980 Comparison of two brief tests of organic brain impairment: the MSQ and the Short Portable MSQ. Journal of the American Geriatric Society 28(8): 381–384

Fillenbaum G G, Smyer M A 1981 The development, validity and reliability of the OARS multidimensional functional assessment questions. Journal of Gerontology 36(4): 428–434

Fillenbaum G, Heyman A, Williams K, Prosnitz B, Burchett B 1990 Sensitivity and specificity of standardized screens of cognitive impairment and dementia among elderly black and white community residents. Journal of Clinical Epidemiology 43: 651–660

Finn S E 1986 Stability of personality self-ratings over 30 years: evidence of an age/cohort interaction. Journal of Personality and Social Psychology 50(4): 813–818

Finsen V 1988 Improvements in general health among the elderly: a factor in the rising incidence of hip fractures? Journal of Epidemiology and Community Health 42(2): 200–203

Flicker C, Ferris S H, Reisberg B 1991 Mild cognitive impairment in the elderly. Neurology 41: 1006–1009

Folstein M F, Folstein S E, McHugh P R 1975 Mini mental state: a practical method for grading the cognitive state of patients for the clinician. Journal of Psychiatric Research 12: 189–198

Folstein M, Anthony J, Parhead J, Duffy B, Gruenberg E 1985a The meaning of cognitive impairment in the elderly. Journal of the American Geriatrics Society 33: 228–235

Folstein M F, Romanoski A J, Nestadt G et al 1985b Brief report on the clinical reappraisal of the Diagnostic

Interview Schedule carried out at the Johns Hopkins site of the Epidemiological Catchment Area Programme of the NIMH. Psychological Medicine 15: 809–814

Forstl H, Burns A, Levy R, Cairns N, Luthert P, Lantos P 1992 Neurologic signs in Alzheimer's disease. Archives of Neurology 49(10): 1038–1042

Fortinsky R H, Granger C V, Seltzer G B 1981 The use of functional assessment in understanding home care needs. Medical Care 19(5): 489–497

Fratiglioni L, Jorm A F, Grut M, Vittanen M, Holmen K, Ahlbom A, Winblad B 1993 Predicting dementia from the Mini Mental State Examination in an elderly population: the role of education. Journal of Clinical Epidemiology 46(3): 281–287

Frisch D, Clemen R T 1994 Beyond expected utility: rethinking behavioural decision research. Psychological Bulletin 116(1): 46–54

Gerety M B, Cornell J E, Mulrow C D 1994 The Sickness Impact Profile for Nursing Homes (SIP-NH). Journal of Gerontology 49(1): M2–M8

Gibb W R 1989 Neuropathology in movement disorders. Journal of Neurology, Neurosurgery and Psychiatry Supplement: 55–67

Goffman E 1968 Stigma. Penguin, Harmondsworth

Grounds A 1987 On describing mental states. British Journal of Medical Psychology 60: 305–311

Grundy C T et al 1994 The Hamilton Rating Scale for Depression: one scale or many? Clinical Psychology: Science and Practice 1: 197–205

Hamid W A, Howard R, Silverman M 1995 Needs assess ment in old age psychiatry: a need for standardization. International Journal of Geriatric Psychiatry 10: 533–540

Harris D M, Guten S 1979 Health protective behaviour: an exploratory study. Journal of Health and Social Behaviour 20(1): 17–29

Harrison P J 1991 Are mental states a useful concept. Journal of Nervous and Mental Disease 179(6): 309–316

Harwin B 1973 Psychiatric morbidity among the physically impaired elderly in the community. In: Wing J K, Häfner H (eds) Roots of evaluation. Oxford University Press, London

Hawkins R M 1992 Self-efficacy: a predictor but not a cause of behaviour. Journal of Behaviour Therapy and Experimental Psychiatry 23(4): 251–256

Heath H 1995 Health assessment of people over 75. Nursing Standard 9(37): 30–37

Helme R D, Katz E, Gibson S, Corran T 1989 Can psychometric tools be used to analyse pain in a geriatric population. Clinical and Experimental Neurology 26: 113–117

Helmes E, Csapo K G, Short J A 1987 Standardization and validation of the Multidimensional Observation Scale for Elderly Subjects. Journal of Gerontology 42: 395–405

Herzberg J 1995 Can multidisciplinary teams carry out competent and safe psychogeriatric assessments in the community. International Journal of Geriatric Psychiatry 10: 173–177

Hoch C C, Reynolds C F III, Buysse D J et al 1992 Sleep-disordered breathing in healthy and spousally bereaved elderly. Neurobiology of Ageing 13: 741–746

Hodkinson H M 1972 Evaluation of a mental test score for assessment of mental impairment in the elderly. Age and Ageing 1: 233–238

Hopkins A 1993 Clinical neurology. Oxford University Press, Oxford

Howard R, Castle D, Wessely S, Murray R 1994 A comparative study of 470 cases of early-onset and late-onset schizophrenia. British Journal of Psychiatry 163: 352–357

Howes J L, Katz A N 1992 Remote memory: recalling autobiographical events from across the lifespan. Canadian Journal of Psychology 46(1): 92–116

Hyman H H, Singer E (eds) 1968 Readings in reference group theory and research. Free Press, New York

Idler E L, Kasl S 1991 Health perceptions and survival: do global evaluations of health status really predict mortality? Journal of Gerontology 46(2): S55–S65

Illsley R, Baker D 1991 Contextual variations in the meaning of health inequality. Social Science and Medicine 32(4): 359–365

Institute of Psychiatry 1978 Notes on eliciting and recording clinical information. Oxford University Press, Oxford

Jagger C, Clarke M, Davies R 1986 The elderly at home: indices of disability. Journal of Epidemiology and Community Health 40: 139–142

Jorm A F, Scott R, Henderson A S, Kay D W K 1988 Educational level differences on the mini mental state: the role of the test bias. Psychological Medicine 18: 727–731

Kafer N F, Davies N F 1984 Vulnerability of self and interpersonal strategies: a study of the aged. Journal of Psychology 116: 203–206

Kahn R L, Goldfarb A I, Pollack M, Peck A 1960 Brief objective measures for the determination of mental status in the aged. American Journal of Psychiatry 117: 326–329

Kail R, Salthouse T A 1994 Processing speed as a mental capacity. Acta Psychologica 86: 199–225

Kanfer F H, Saslow G 1965 Behavioural analysis: an alternative to diagnostic classification. Archives of General Psychiatry 12: 529–538

Kasl S V, Cobb S 1966a Health behaviour, illness behaviour and sick-role behaviour I. Archives of Environmental Health 12: 246–266

Kasl S V, Cobb S 1966b Health behaviour, illness behaviour and sick-role behaviour II. Archives of Environmental Health 12: 531–541

Katz J N, Larson M G, Phillips C B, Fossel A H, Liang M H 1992 Comparative measurement sensitivity of short and longer health status questionnaires. Medical Care 30(10): 917–925

Katz P R, Dube D H, Calkins E 1985 Use of a structured functional assessment format in a geriatric consultative service. Journal of the American Geriatrics Society 33(10): 681–686

Katz S 1983 Assessing self-maintenance: activities of daily living, mobility, and instrumental activities of daily living. Journal of the American Geriatric Society 31(12): 721–727

Katz S, Stroud M W 1989 Functional assessment in geriatrics: a review of progress and direction. Journal of the American Geriatric Society 37(3): 267–271

Katz S, Ford A B, Moskowitz R W, Jackson B A, Jaffe M W 1963 The Index of ADL: a standardized measure of biological and psychosocial function. Journal of the American Medical Association 183(12): 914–919

Katz S, Branch L G, Branson M H, Papsidero J A, Beck J C, Greer D S 1983 Active life expectancy New England. Journal of Medicine 309(20): 1218–1224

Katzman R, Brown T, Fuld P, Peck A, Schecter R, Schimmel H 1987 Validation of a short orientation-memory-concentration test of memory impairment. American Journal of Psychiatry 140: 734–739

Kausler D H, Salthouse T A, Saults J, Scott 1988 Temporal memory over the adult lifespan. American Journal of Psychology 101(2): 207–215

Kennedy G J, Kelman H R, Thomas C, Wisniewski W, Metz H, Bijur P E 1989 Hierarchy of characteristics associated with depressive symptoms in an urban elderly sample. American Journal of Psychiatry 146(2): 220–225

Kennedy L W, Silverman R A 1984–1985 Significant others and fear of crime among the elderly. International Journal of Aging and Human Development 20(4): 241–246

Kline P 1993 Handbook of psychological testing. Routledge, London

Kolb B, Whishaw I Q 1990 Fundamentals of human neuropsychology. W H Freeman and Co., New York

Kral V A 1962 Senescent forgetfulness: benign and malignant. Canadian Medical Association Journal 86: 257–260

Krause N 1991 Stress and isolation from close ties in later life. Journal of Gerontology 46(4): S183–S194

Kruse A, Lindenberger U, Baltes P B 1993 Longitudinal research on ageing: the power of combining real-time, microgenetic and simulation approaches. In: Magnusson D, Casaer P (eds) Longitudinal research on individual development. Cambridge University Press, Cambridge

Kua E H, Ko S M 1992 A questionnaire to screen for cognitive impairment among elderly people in developing countries. Acta Psychiatrica Scandinavica 85: 119–122

Lauver D 1992 A theory of care-seeking behaviour. Image 24(4): 281–287

Lawton M, Brody E 1969 Assessment of older people: self-maintaining and instrumental activities of daily living. Gerontologist 9: 179–186

Lawton M P 1975 The Philadelphia Geriatric Centre Morale Scale: a revision. Journal of Gerontology 30(1): 85–89

Lazaridis E N, Rudberg M A, Furner S E, Cassel C K 1994 Do activities of daily living have a hierarchical structure? An analysis using the longitudinal study of ageing. Journal of Gerontology 49(2): M47–M51

Leary M R, Atherton S C, Hill S, Hur C 1986 Attributional mediators of social inhibition and avoidance. Journal of Personality 54(4): 704–715

Levin E, Sinclair I, Gorbach P 1989 Families, services and confusion in old age. Avebury Gower Publishing, Aldershot

Levy R 1994 Ageing-associated cognitive decline. International Psychogeriatrics 6(1): 63–68

Lishman A W 1987 Organic psychiatry. Blackwell, Oxford

Little A, Hemsley D, Volans P, Bergmann K 1986 The relationship between alternative assessments of self-care ability in the elderly. British Journal of Clinical Psychology 25: 51–59

Little A, Hemsley D, Volans J 1987 Comparison of current levels of performance and scores based on change as diagnostic discriminators among the elderly. British Journal of Clinical Psychology 26: 135–140

Lueckenotte 1994 Pocket guide to gerontologic assessment, 2nd edn. C V Mosby, St Louis

Lumpkin J R, Johnson B 1987 An empirical test of the relationship between isolation and disengagement of elderly persons. Psychological Reports 60: 823–830

McCulloch B J 1991 A longitudinal investigation of the factor structure of subjective wellbeing: the case of the Philadelphia Geriatric Centre Morale Scale. Journal of Gerontology 46(5): P251–P258

MacDonald A J D, Mann A H, Jenkins R, Richard L, Godlove C, Rodwell G 1982 An attempt to determine the impact of four types of care upon the elderly in London by the study of matched groups. Psychological Medicine 12: 193–200

McEntee W J, Crook T H 1991 Serotonin, memory and the ageing brain. Psychopharmacology 103: 143–149

McGhee J L 1983 The vulnerability of elderly consumers. International Journal of Aging and Human Development 17(3): 223–246

McKeith I, Fairbairn A, Perry R, Thompson P, Perry E 1992a Neuroleptic sensitivity in patients with senile dementia of Lewy body type. British Medical Journal 305(6855): 673–678

McKeith I G, Perry R H, Fairbairn A F, Jabeen S, Berry E K 1992b Operational criteria for senile dementia of Lewy body type (SDLT). Psychological Medicine 22(4): 911–922

McKeown T, Lowe C R 1950 Survey of patients in Western Road Infirmary. British Medical Journal 1(4649): 323–327

MacLennan W J 1988 The ageing society. British Journal of Hospital Medicine 39(2): 112–118

McVey L J, Becker P M, Saltz C C, Feussner J R, Cohen H J 1989 Effects of a geriatric consultation team on functional status of elderly hospitalized patients. Annals of Internal Medicine 110(1): 79–84

McWalter G, Toner H, Corser A, Eastwood J, Marshall M, Turvey T 1994 Needs and needs assessment: their components and definitions with reference to dementia. Health and Social Care 2: 213–219

Magnusson D 1993 Human ontogeny: a longitudinal perspective. In: Magnusson D, Casaer P (eds) Longitudinal research on individual development. Cambridge University Press, Cambridge

Mahoney F I, Barthel D W 1965 Functional evaluation: the Barthel index. Maryland Medical Journal 14: 61–65

Mandelstam D (ed) 1985 Incontinence and its management. Croom Helm, Beckenham

Mangen S, Brewin C 1991 Needs and needs assessment. In: Bebbington P (ed) Social Psychiatry. Transaction, London

Marks I, Toole S 1995 Problem-centred care planning: a primer for mental health care. Section of experimental psychopathology, Institute of Psychiatry, London

Marshall M 1994 How should we measure need? Philosophy, Psychiatry and Psychology 1(1): 27–40

Mayes A R 1988 Human organic memory disorders. Cambridge University Press, Cambridge

Mechanic D 1979 Correlates of physician utilization: why do major multivariate studies of physician utilization find trivial psychosocial and organizational effects. Journal of Health and Social Behaviour 20: 387–396

Medawar P B 1985 The future of life expectancy. Clinical Orthopedics 201: 2–8

Mental Health Act, 1983. HMSO, London

Miller B L, Lesser I M, Boone K B, Hill E, Mehringer C M, Wong 1991 Brain lesions and cognitive function in late-life psychosis. British Journal of Psychiatry 158: 76–82

Miller D 1976 Social justice. Clarendon Press, Oxford

Mitrushina M, Satz P 1991 Effect of repeated administration of a neuropsychological battery in the elderly. Journal of Clinical Psychology 47(6): 790–801

Molloy D W, McIlroy W E, Guyatt G H, Lever J A 1991 Validity and reliability of the Dysfunctional Behaviour Rating Instrument. Acta Psychiatrica Scandinavica 84: 103–106

Morgan S F, Hatsukami D K 1986 Use of the Shipley Institute of Living Scale for neuropsychological screening of the elderly: is it an appropriate measure for this population? Journal of Clinical Psychology 42(5): 796–798

Mrazek P J, Haggerty R J (eds) 1994 Reducing risks for mental disorders. National Academy Press, Washington DC

National Health Service and Community Care Act 1990. HMSO, London

Nelson H E 1991 The National Adult Reading Test (NART), 2nd edn. NFER-Nelson, Windsor

Nolan-Hoeksema S 1987 Sex differences in unipolar depression: evidence and theory. Psychological Bulletin 101: 259–282

Nunnally J 1978 Psychometric theory. McGraw Hill, New York

Nydevik I, Asberg K H 1992 Sickness impact after stroke: a 3 year follow-up. Scandinavian Journal of Primary Health Care 10(4): 284–289

O'Brien J, Levy R 1992 Age-associated memory impairment. British Medical Journal 304: 5–6

O'Connor D W, Pollitt P A, Treasure F P, Brook C P B, Reiss B B 1989 The influence of education, social class and sex on Mini-Mental State scores. Psychological Medicine 19: 771–776

O'Connor D W, Pollitt P A, Jones B J, Hyde J B, Fellowes J L, Miller N D 1991 Continued clinical validation of dementia diagnosed in the community using the Cambridge Mental Disorders of the Elderly Examination. Acta Psychiatrica Scandinavica 83(1): 41–45

Orrell M, Howard R, Payne A, Bergmann K, Woods R, Everitt B S, Levy R 1992 Differentiation between organic and functional psychiatric illness in the elderly: an evaluation of four cognitive tests. International Journal of Geriatric Psychiatry 7: 263–275

Orrenius S 1995 Apoptosis: molecular mechanisms and implications for human disease. Journal of Internal Medicine 237(6): 529–536

Ott B, Fogel B 1992 Measurement of depression in dementia: self versus clinician rating. International Journal of Geriatric Psychiatry 7: 899–904

Park J-H, Kwon Y C 1990 Modification of the Mini Mental State Examination for use in the elderly in a non-Western society. International Journal of Geriatric Psychiatry 5: 381–387

Park D C, Smith A D 1991 Importance of basic applied research from the viewpoints of investigators in the psychology of ageing. Experimental Ageing Research 17(2): 79

Pathy M S J, Bayer A, Harding K, Dibble A 1992 Randomized trial of case finding and surveillance of elderly people at home. The Lancet: 890–893

Patrick D L, Bush J W, Chen M M 1973 Toward an operational definition of health. Journal of Health and Social Behaviour 14: 6

Pattie A H, Gilleard G J 1979 Manual of the Clifton Assessment Procedures for the elderly. Hodder & Stoughton, Sevenoaks

Perkins E R 1991 Screening elderly people: a review of the literature in the light of the new general practitioner contract. British Journal of General Practice 41(350): 382–385

Perry E K, McKeith I, Thompson P et al 1991 Topography, extent and clinical relevance of neurochemical deficits of Lewy body type, Parkinson's disease and Alzheimer's disease. Annals of the New York Academy of Science 640: 197–202

Pfeiffer E 1975 Multidimensional functional assessment: the OARS [Older Americans Resources and Services] methodology. Duke University, Durham, NC

Phelan M, Slade M, Thornicroft G et al 1995 The Camberwell assessment of need: the validity and reliability of an instrument to assess the needs of people with severe mental illness. British Journal of Psychiatry 167: 589–595

Plomin R, Thompson L A 1993 Genetics and high cognitive ability. Ciba Foundation Symposia 178: 67–84

Plummer S 1995 A study of the ability of practice nurses to detect psychological distress in patients attending their clinics. Unpublished MSc dissertation. Institute of Psychiatry, London

Power M J, Duggan C F, Lee A S, Murray R M 1995 Dysfunctional attitudes in depressed and recovered depressed patients and their first-degree relatives. Psychological Medicine 25: 87–93

Pruchno R A, Resch N L 1989 Aberrant behaviour and Alzheimer's disease: mental health effects on spouse caregivers. Journal of Gerontology 44(5): S171–S181

Pruchno R A, Kleban M H, Resch N L 1994 Psychometric assessment of the Multidimensional Observation Scale for Elderly Subjects (MOSES). Journal of Gerontology 43(6): 164–169

Qureshi K N, Hodgkinson H M 1974 Evaluation of a ten-question mental test in the institutionalized elderly. Age and Ageing 3: 152–157

Rabkin J G 1986 Mental health needs assessment: a review of methods. Medical Care 24(12): 1093–1109

Ransford H E 1986 Race, heart disease, worry and health protective behaviour. Social Science and Medicine 22(12): 1355–1362

Raven J C 1992 Standard progressive matrices. Oxford Psychologists' Press, Oxford

Raven J C 1994 Mill Hill vocabulary scale. Oxford Psychologists' Press, Oxford

Reuben D B, Siu A L, Kimpau S 1992 The predictive validity of self-report and performance-based measures of function and health. Journal of Gerontology 47(4): M106–M110

Reubenstein L Z, Schairer C, Wieland G D, Kane R 1984 Systematic biases in functional status assessment of elderly adults: effects of different data sources. Journal of Gerontology 39(6): 686–691

Revenson T A, Johnson J L 1984 Social and demographic correlates of loneliness in late life. American Journal of Community Psychology 12(1): 71–85

Reynolds W J, Rushing W A, Miles D L 1974 The validation of a function status index. Journal of Health and Social Behaviour 15: 271

Rice-Evans C A, Burdon R H 1994 Free radical damage and its control. Elsevier, London

Richman A, Barry A 1985 More and more is less and less: the myth of massive psychiatric need. British Journal of Psychiatry 146: 164–168

Rippetoe P A, Rogers R W 1987 Effects of components of protection-motivation theory on adaptive and maladaptive coping with a health threat. Journal of Personality and Social Psychology 52(3): 596–604

Ritter S, Norman I J, Rentoul L, Bodley D E 1996 A model of clinical supervision for nurses undertaking short placements in mental health care settings. Journal of Clinical Nursing 5: 149–158

Roberts P 1990 Assessing mobility. In: Beech J R, Harding L (eds) Assessment of the elderly. NFER-Nelson, Windsor

Robine J M, Ritchie K 1991 Healthy life expectancy: evaluation of global indicators of change in population health. British Medical Journal 302(6774): 457–460

Rockwood K, Stolee P, Fox R A 1993 Use of goal attainment scaling in measuring clinically important change in the frail elderly. Journal of Clinical Epidemiology 46(10): 1113–1118

Rodenburg M, Hopkins R W, Hamilton P F, Ginsburg L, Nashed Y, Minde N 1991 The Kingston standardized cognitive assessment. International Journal of Geriatric Psychiatry 6: 867–874

Ronis D L 1992 Conditional health threats: health beliefs, decisions and behaviours among adults. Health Psychology 11(2): 127–134

Rose S 1992 The making of memory. Bantam Press, London

Rosenberg H 1995 The elderly and the use of ilicit drugs: sociological and epidemiological considerations. International Journal of the Addictions 30(13, 14): 1925–1951

Rosenfield I 1992 The strange, familiar and forgotten. Picador, London

Rosenstock I M 1966 Why people use health services. Milbank Memorial Fund Quarterly 44(2): 94–127

Rosenstock I M, Strecher V J, Becker M H 1988 Social learning theory and the Health Belief Model. Health Education Quarterly 15(2): 175–183

Ross F M, Bower P 1995 Standardised assessment for elderly people (SAFE) – a feasibility study in district nursing. Journal of Clinical Nursing 4: 303–310

Roth M, Tym E, Mountjoy C Q et al 1986 CAMDEX: a standardized instrument for the diagnosis of mental disorder in the elderly with special reference to the early detection of dementia. British Journal of Psychiatry 149: 698–709

Royal College of Physicians and British Geriatric Society 1992 Standardised assessment scales for elderly people: a report of the joint workshops. Research Unit of the Royal College of Physicians and the British Geriatrics Society, London

Scherr P A, Albert M S, Funkenstein H H et al 1988 Correlates of cognitive function in an elderly community population. American Journal of Epidemiology 128(5): 1084–1101

Schogt B, Sadevoy J 1987 Assessing the protective needs of the impaired elderly living in the community. Canadian Journal of Psychiatry 32: 179–184

Schonfield D 1983 The variety of social skills. International Journal of Aging and Human Development 17(1): 39–42

Schutte N S, Malouff J M 1995 Sourcebook of adult assessment strategies. Plenum, New York

Shipley W C 1940 A self-administering scale for measuring intellectual impairment and deterioration. Journal of Psychology 9: 371–377

Silverman J S, Silverman J A, Eardley D A 1984 Do maladaptive attitudes cause depression? Archives of General Psychiatry 41: 28–30

Sims A C P 1993 Schizophrenia and permeability of self. Neurology, Psychiatry and Brain Research 1: 133–135

Sims A C P 1995a Symptoms in the mind, 2nd edn. W B Saunders, London

Sims A C P (ed)1995b Speech and language disorders in psychiatry. Gaskell, London

Social Services Inspectorate, Department of Health 1995 Moving on: report of the National Inspection of Social Services Department arrangements for the discharge of older people to residential or nursing home care. Department of Health, London

Spector W D, Katz S, Murphy J B, Fulton J P 1987 The hierarchical relationship between activities of daily living and instrumental activites of daily living. Journal of Chronic Disease 40(6): 481–489

Spiegelhalter D J, Gore S M, Fitzpatrick R, Fletcher A E, Jones D R, Cox D R 1992 Quality of life measures in health care III: resource allocation. British Medical Journal 305(6863): 1205–1209

Starr J M, Whalley L J, Inch S, Shering P A 1992 The quantification of the relative effects of age and NART-predicted IQ on cognitive function in healthy old people. International Journal of Geriatric Psychiatry 7: 153–157

Steel K, Maggi S 1993 Commentary: ageing as a global issue. Age and Ageing 22: 237–239

Stewart A L, Ware J E, Brook R H 1981 Advances in the measurement of functional status: construction of aggegate indexes. Medical Care 19(5): 473–488

Strang J, Gurling H 1989 Computerized tomography and neuropsychological assessment of long-term high-dose heroin addicts. Bristish Journal of Addiction 84: 1011–1019

Streiner G R, Norman D L 1991 Health measurement scales. Oxford University Press, Oxford

Strom R, Strom S 1989 Grandparents and learning. International Journal of Ageing and Human Development 29(3): 163–169

Sullivan D H 1992 Risk factors for early hospital readmission in a select population of geriatric rehabilitation patients. Journal of the American Geriatrics Society 40(8): 792–798

Sullivan D H, Walls R C, Lipschitz D A 1991 Protein-energy undernutrition and the risk of mortality in a select population of geriatric rehabilitation patients. American Journal of Clinical Nutrition 53(3): 599–605

Swaab D F 1991 Brain ageing and Alzheimer's disease: 'wear and tear' versus 'use or lose it'. Neurobiology of Ageing 12: 317–324

Teasdale J 1988 Cognitive vulnerability to persistent depression. Cognition and Emotion 2(3): 247–274

Terry D J, O'Leary J E 1995 The theory of planned behaviour: the effects of perceived behavioural control and self-efficacy. British Journal of Social Psychology 34(2): 199–220

Thomas P 1995 Thought disorder and communication disorder. British Journal of Psychiatry 166: 287–290

Thomas P, Fraser W 1994 Linguistics, human communication and psychiatry. British Journal of Psychiatry 165: 585–592

Thompson C (ed) 1994 The instruments of psychiatric research. Wiley, Chichester

Thompson M G, Heller K 1990 Facets of support related to well-being. Psychology and Aging 5(4): 535–544

Tombaugh T N, McIntyre N J 1992 The mini mental state examination: a comprehensive review. Journal of the American Geriatrics Society 40: 922–935

Townsend P, Davidson N, Whitehead M (eds) 1988 The Black Report and the health divide. Penguin, Harmondsworth

Tremmel L, Spiegel R 1993 Clinical experience with the NOSGER (Nurses' Observation Scale for Geriatric Patients): tentative normative data and sensitivity to change. International Journal of Geriatric Psychiatry 8: 311–317

Ungvari G S, Hantz P M 1991a Social breakdown in the elderly I. Comprehensive Psychiatry 32(5): 440–444

Ungvari G S, Hantz P M 1991b Social breakdown in the elderly II. Comprehensive Psychiatry 32(5): 445–449

Vetter N J, Jones D A, Victor C R 1984 Effects of health visitors working with elderly patients in general practice: a prospective controlled trial. British Medical Journal 288: 369–372

Vetter N J, Lewis P A, Ford D 1992 Can health visitors prevent fractures in elderly people? British Medical Journal 304: 888–990

Vickers G 1958 What sets the goals of public health? The Lancet 1(7021): 599–604

Volicer L, Crino P B 1989 Involvement of free radicals in dementia of the Alzheimer type: a hypothesis. Neurobiology of Ageing 11: 567–571

Volicer L, Hurley A C, Lathi D C, Kowall N W 1994 Measurement of severity in advanced Alzheimer's disease. Journal of Gerontology 49(5): M223–M226

Wapner S, Craig-Bray L 1992 Person-in-environment transitions: theoretical and methodological approaches. Environment and Behaviour 24(2): 161–188

Ward T, Murphy E, Procter A 1991 Functional assessment in severely demented patients. Age and Ageing 20: 212–214

Watkins M 1988 Lifting the burden. Geriatric Nursing and Home Care 8(9): 18–20

Watkins M 1987 The problem of confusion: an examination of Roper's Activities of Living model. In: Easterbrook J (ed) Elderly care towards holistic nursing. Edward Arnold

Watkins M 1994 An evaluation of CREST, a night hospital for elderly people suffering from dementia. Unpublished PhD Thesis, King's College, London

Wechsler D 1981 Manual for the Wechsler Intelligence Scale for Adults – Revised. Psychological Corporation/ Harcourt Brace Jovanovich, New York

Weinstein N D 1993 Testing four competing theories of health-protective behaviour. Health Psychology 12(4): 324–333

Whitehead A 1973 Verbal learning and memory in elderly depressives. British Journal of Psychiatry 123: 203–208

Wilkinson G, Allen P, Marshall E, Walker J, Browne W, Mann A H 1993 The role of the practice nurse in the management of depression in general practice: treatment adherence to antidepressant medication. Psychological Medicine 23: 229–237

Wilkinson R G 1992 Income distribution and life expectancy. British Medical Journal 304(6820): 165–168

Williams M E 1984 Implications of an aging physiology. American Journal of Medicine 76(6): 1049–1054

Williamson J, Stokoe J H, Gray S 1964 Old people at home: their unreported needs. The Lancet 1: 602–604

Winblad I 1993 Comparison of the prevalence of disability in two birth cohorts at the age of 75 years and over. Journal of Clinical Epidemiology 46(3): 303–308

Wing J K 1978 Reasoning about madness. Oxford University Press, London

Wing J K 1989 The measurement of social disablement: the MRC social behaviour and social role performance schedules. Social Psychiatry and Psychiatric Epidemiology 24: 173–178

Wing J K 1990 Meeting the needs of people with psychiatric disorders schedules. Social Psychiatry and Psychiatric Epidemiology 25: 2–8

Wing J K, Hailey A M (eds) 1972 Evaluating a community psychiatric service. Oxford University Press, London

Wing J K, Cooper J E, Sartorius N 1974 Measurement and classification of psychiatric symptoms. Cambridge University Press, Cambridge

Wing J, Rix S, Curtis R 1995 Report of a Clinical Standards Advisory Group Committee on schizophrenia, vol. 2: protocol for assessing services for people with severe mental illness. HMSO, London

Wolfe B L 1986 Health status and medical expenditure: is there a link? Social Science and Medicine 22(10): 993–999

Woods R T 1994 Problems in the elderly: investigation. In: Lindsay S J E, Powell G E (eds) The handbook of clinical psychology, 2nd edn. Routledge, London

World Health Organization 1992 The ICD-10 classification of mental and behavioural disorders. WHO, Geneva

Wykes T, Hurry J 1991 Social behaviour in psychiatric disorders. In: Bebbington P (ed) Social psychiatry. Transaction, London

Wykes T, Sturt E 1986 The measurement of social behaviour in psychiatric patients: an assessment of reliability and validity of the SBS schedule. British Journal of Psychiatry 148: 1–11

Wykes T, Sturt E, Katz R 1990 The prediction of rehabilitative success after three years: the use of social, symptom and cognitive variables. British Journal of Psychiatry 157: 865–870

Wykes T, Katz R, Sturt E, Hemsley D 1992 Abnormalities of response-processing in a chronic psychiatric group. British Journal of Psychiatry 160: 244–252

Yesavage J A, Brink T L, Rose T L et al 1983 Development and validation of a geriatric depression screening scale. Journal of Psychiatric Research 22: 165–170

Zarit S H, Orr N K, Zarit S M 1985 The hidden victims of Alzheimer's disease: families under stress. New York University Press, New York

RECOMMENDED READING

American Psychiatric Association 1993 Diagnostic and statistical manual of mental disorders, 4th edn. American Psychiatric Association Washington DC. *DSM-IV is, along with ICD-10, essential for clinicians who are seriously interested in distinguishing between mental disorders and other kinds of functional impairments. The important thing to note about this manual is that it classifies mental disorders rather than being a classification of people. The use of multiaxial diagnostic systems, such as those comprised by DSM-IV, ensures that the aim of holistic assessment may be a realistic* one. *DSM-IV is therefore not restricted to psychiatrists, but can be profitably used by all other health care professionals along with social work colleagues.*

Beech J R, Harding L 1990 Assessment of the elderly. NFER-Nelson, Windsor. *The size of this slim textbook belies the comprehensive coverage of approaches to assessment of older people. It provides a good overview of the area, including enough information to make it both interesting and useful as a resource for a range of health care professionals.*

Duggan C, Lee A S, Murray R M 1991 Do hospitalised depressives have different long term outcomes? Archives of General Psychiatry 48,4: 308–312. *This paper is an important contribution to epidemiological knowledge of the natural history of psychiatric disorders. Most forms of depression are eminently treatable, and it is essential that people who have suffered a serious depressive illness are not lost to follow-up and monitoring.*

Herzberg J 1995 Can multidisciplinary teams carry out competent and safe psychogeriatric assessments in the community. International Journal of Geriatric Psychiatry 10: 173–177. *This is an important paper describing a well evaluated model of psychogeriatric care. It does indeed show that multidisciplinary teams can carry out competent and safe assessments. It also discusses the conditions necessary for effective multi-professional teamwork. The role of non medical members of the team is also discussed.*

Kolb B, Whishaw I Q 1990 Fundamentals of human neuropsychology, 3rd edn. W. H. Freeman and Company, New York. *This textbook provides an overview of comparative approaches to human brain function. It is intended for undergraduate students, but the authors suggest that a range of other readers will find the information contained within it relevant to their practice. Of particular interest to clinicians are the clinical vignettes that illustrate the sometimes complex theories and principles of brain organisation. This book provides a sound basis for approaches to assessing disorders of function.*

Lishman A W 1987 Organic psychiatry: the psychological consequences of cerebral disorder, 2nd edn. Blackwell Scientific. *This highly respected standard textbook systematically and comprehensively reviews the material on brain dysfunction. It therefore complements Kolb and Whishaw (see above). Although originally designed for physicians and psychiatrists, the widening scope of responsibility of other health professionals for health status assessment makes this textbook indispensable for guiding practice.*

Lueckenotte A G 1994 Pocket guide to gerontologic assessment, 2nd Edn. C V Mosby, St Louis. *This pocket book is designed to help nurses (and other health workers) to assess the health status of older people in various settings. It has guidelines for taking a history and carrying out a physical and mental state assessment. It also provides guidelines for assessing all the main organ systems. The appendices contain laboratory values and detailed information on urinary incontinence and prevention of pressure ulcers in adults.*

Marks I, Toole S 1985 Problem centred care planning: a primer for mental health care. *Although this short booklet does not specifically deal with planning care for older people, it is an essential resource for anyone wanting to use problem-oriented approaches to case management.*

McKeith I G, Perry I H, Fairbairn A F, Jabeen S, Berry E K 1992 Operational criteria for senile dementia of Lewy body type (SDLT). Psychological Medicine 22,4: 911–922. *The evidence for sub types of the dementia syndromes is accumulating more and more rapidly. McKeith and his colleagues at the University of Newcastle have elucidated the differential characteristics of neuronal damage. Because of the potential health risks of using neuroleptic medication all health care professionals have a responsibility to know about the implications of different symptoms in people with dementia.*

Rosenberg H 1995 The elderly and the use of illicit drugs: sociological and epidemiological considerations. International Journal of the Addictions 30, 13 and 14: 1925–1951. *The lack of data regarding substance use disorders in older people does not mean that there is no problem. This review is a key introduction to the area.*

Sims A 1995 Symptoms in the mind: An introduction to descriptive psychopathology. W B Saunders Company, London. *This textbook is also aimed at undergraduates, and is a thoroughly up to date overview of the foundations of psychiatry. While it is written by a psychiatrist for psychiatrists it is recommended for nurses, social workers, occupational therapists and clinical psychologists.*

Teasdale J 1988 Cognitive vulnerability to persistent depression. Cognition and Emotion 2,3: 247–274. *Teasdale's work on the causes of depression is central to our current understanding of the mechanisms of lowered mood.*

Ungvari G S, Hantz P M 1991 Social breakdown in the elderly I. Comprehensive Psychiatry 32(5): 440–444 and social breakdown in the elderly II. Comprehensive Psychiatry 32(5): 445–449. *These two papers provide a good basis for approaching isolated and hostile older clients. Indications that behaviour therapy may help such people support arguments for a systematic approach to management of care, so that problems can be appropriately targeted and treated assertively.*

Rockwood K, Stolee P, Fox R A 1993 Use of goal attainment scaling and measuring clinically important change in the frail elderly. Journal of Clinical Epidemiology 46(10): 113–118. *Review is a key stage in the care programme approach. It is immensely facilitated by a problem-oriented approach (see Marks and Toole). It is also facilitated by a quantification of targets and progress towards them. This paper is one example of such quantification.*

World Health Organization 1992 The ICD-10 Classification of mental and behavioural disorders. World Health Organization, Geneva. *ICD-10 is more commonly used for classifying disorders in order to identify diagnostic groups. Clinicians need to be familiar both with DSM-IV (see American Psychiatric Association above) and ICD-10, in order to assess for themselves and contribute to discussions of diagnosis, treatment and therefore potential evaluation of quality of life of older service users.*

7

Anxiety in later life

Marcus Richards

INTRODUCTION

It is clear that the nature of anxiety changes across the life span. Fears that are almost universal in infancy, such as those evoked by strange objects, sudden noise or loss of support, give way to childhood anxieties associated with previously neutral phenomena such as darkness and animals (Jersild & Holmes 1935). As adulthood is approached, concrete fears come and go, and abstract fears, including fear of ridicule, disease and death, begin to develop. Some of these fears, particularly fears associated with loss of physical ability, significant others and financial independence, become prominent during later life.

Many fears experienced by older people are regarded as normal and appropriate to daily living. Yet for some, anxiety reaches pathological severity during later life, as it sometimes does during the earlier years. This chapter explores the nature of fear and anxiety in later life and addresses the diagnosis, prevalence and clinical management of anxiety disorders experienced by older people.

ANXIETY IN NORMAL AGEING

Later life brings a host of stressors, particularly those associated with illness and dependency, institutionalisation, crime and financial status. Since these often are genuine threats, responses to these stressors in older people tend to blur the lines between 'normal' and 'pathological' anxiety. As Bienfeld aptly comments, 'the clinician walks a fine line between pathologising a healthy response and failing to recognise neurotic dysfunction' (Bienfeld 1994, p. 711).

Nevertheless, studies suggest that anxiety in normal elderly people tends to be practical in nature, governed by judgements about the consequences of aversive events as much as by reactions to the event itself

131

(Fattah & Sacco 1989). In this regard, Sato (1983) found that older people were more anxious about economic hardship than about criticism or failure of friendship. Fear of violent crime among the elderly has been widely publicised by the media although the nature of this fear is complex. On one hand, such fear is out of proportion to the actual danger; older people are most likely to be anxious about violence yet the least likely to be its victim (Clarke & Lewis 1982, Kay 1988). On the other hand, degree of anxiety about violence is more likely to be determined by appraisal of its consequences than by determination of its likelihood. This is particularly true of older people with physical disabilities, who fear the consequences of an attack (e.g. falling).

An important focus for normal anxiety in later life concerns loss and threat of loss, particularly of physical ability, health, opportunities for valued action and significant others (Verwoerdt 1981). It might therefore seem surprising that fear of death is not especially prominent among older people (Bascue & Lawrence 1977, Kalish 1985), although attitudes to death can vary widely, even within the same group (Fiefel 1956). To some extent, these can be predicted from psychometric measures of anxiety (Rhudick & Dibner 1962) and life satisfaction (Tate 1982). Situational factors are also important. For example, older people living by themselves are more fearful of death than older people living within institutions (Swenson 1962).

CLASSIFICATION OF ANXIETY DISORDERS

There has been considerable debate as to whether pathological anxiety is best conceived as the extreme end of a homogeneous trait which is normally distributed in the population, or whether it is more useful to maintain the distinction between specific anxiety disorders, each with its own aetiology, clinical characteristics and optimal therapeutic strategy (Marks 1979, Eysenck 1979). A detailed consideration of this debate is beyond the scope of the present chapter and its clinical significance remains unclear. Nevertheless, the majority of published studies on anxiety disorders adhere to the formal system of classification set forth by either the Diagnostic and Statistical Manual of Mental Disorders (DSM III-R; American Psychiatric Association 1987) or the mental and behavioural section of the International Classification of Diseases (ICD-10; WHO 1992). A working knowledge of these systems is therefore important. Some of the major categories of anxiety disorder within the ICD system are described below.

Categories of anxiety disorder

Phobic anxiety disorders (ICD-10 F40)

Diagnostic criteria for the phobic anxiety disorders are listed in Box 7.1.

Box 7.1 ICD-10 diagnostic criteria for phobic anxiety disorders (F40)

Classification
F40.0 Agoraphobia
F40.00 Agoraphobia without panic
F40.01 Agoraphobia with panic
F40.1 Social phobias
F40.2 Specific (isolated) phobias
F40.8 Other phobic anxiety disorders
F40.9 Phobic anxiety disorders, unspecified.

Characteristics
- The anxiety is evoked mainly by certain well defined situations or objects (external to the individual) which are not currently dangerous
- The objects and situations are characteristically avoided
- The anxiety varies in severity from mild unease to terror
- The anxiety is not relieved by the knowledge that other people do not regard the situations as dangerous or threatening
- There is a focus on somatic symptoms and an association with secondary fears, e.g. of dying, losing control or going mad.

Diagnostic guidelines
- All psychological or autonomic symptoms must be primarily manifestations of anxiety and not secondary to other symptoms, e.g. delusions or obsessional thoughts
- The anxiety must be restricted to or predominate in the defined situation or object
- Avoidance of the phobic situation must be a characteristic feature.

Box 7.1 shows that ICD-10 distinguishes agoraphobia without panic (corresponding to the DSM III-R code of 300.22), agoraphobia with panic (DSM III-R 300.21; panic with agoraphobia), social phobias (DSM III-R 300.23), from specific (isolated) phobias (DSM III-R 300.29) and unspecified phobic disorders; diagnostic criteria listed in Box 7.1 are common to all phobias. Two important criteria for phobic disorder are that the fear is evoked by objects or situations that are not in themselves dangerous and that the object of the fear is external to the individual (fear of bodily processes are classified as somatiform disorder).

Panic disorder (ICD-10 F41.0)

Diagnostic criteria for panic disorder are listed in Box 7.2.

That corresponding to DSM III-R code is 300.01 (panic without agoraphobia). As with phobic disorders, there is no source of real danger associated with the onset of symptoms.

Box 7.2   ICD-10 diagnostic criteria for panic disorder (F41.0)

Characteristics
- Recurrent attacks of severe anxiety (panic), not restricted to any particular situation or set of circumstances (and therefore unpredictable)
- There are multiple autonomic symptoms and depersonalisation
- There is a secondary fear of dying, losing control or going mad
- Associated with escape from the situation and subsequent avoidance of that situation
- Unpredictable and frequent attacks associated with fear of being alone or being in public, and fear of having another attack.

Diagnostic guidelines
- Phobias must be ruled out
- Several attacks of autonomic anxiety should have occurred within a period of about 1 month, in circumstances where there is no danger and without being confined to known or predictable situations
- There is comparative freedom from anxiety symptoms between attacks (although anticipatory anxiety is common)
- Not secondary to depressive disorders (especially for men).

Box 7.3   ICD-10 diagnostic criteria for generalised anxiety disorder (F41.1)

Characteristics
- Generalised and persistent anxiety, not restricted to any particular environmental circumstances (i.e. 'free floating')
- Associated with fear of death or illness
- More common in women
- Often related to chronic environmental stress
- Fluctuating, chronic course.

Diagnostic guidelines
- Primary symptoms of anxiety most days for at least several weeks at a time, and usually for several months
- Involves apprehension, motor tension (restless fidgeting, trembling, tension headaches, inability to relax, etc.) and autonomic reactivity (light headaches, sweating, tachycardia, dizziness, dry mouth, etc.)

Box 7.4   ICD-10 diagnostic criteria for mixed anxiety and depressive disorder (F41.2)

- Used when the symptoms of both anxiety and depression are present but neither set of symptoms, considered separately, is sufficient to justify a diagnosis
- If both are present and severe enough to justify individual diagnoses, both disorders should be recorded. But if, for practical reasons, only one diagnosis can be made, depression should be given precedence
- Rule out adjustment disorders (F43.2; symptoms occurring in close association with significant life changes or stressful life events)
- Rule out persistent anxiety depression (F34.1; dysthymia).

Generalised anxiety disorder (ICD-10 F41.1)

Diagnostic criteria for generalised anxiety disorder are listed in Box 7.3. That corresponding to DSM III-R code is 300.02.

Mixed anxiety and depression disorder (ICD-10 F41.2)

Diagnostic criteria for mixed anxiety and depression disorder are listed in Box 7.4. This category has no corresponding code in DSM III-R although it is useful when both disorders are present with a mild degree of severity. Note that depression is given priority if there is only limited opportunity to record clinical information.

Other anxiety disorders

Other major classes of anxiety disorders listed within ICD-10 are obsessive–compulsive disorder (F42), adjustment disorder (F43), dissociative and conversion disorder (F44) and somatiform disorder (F45). All these have corresponding codes within DSM III-R.

DIFFERENTIAL DIAGNOSIS

Accurate clinical diagnosis of anxiety, whether to enable estimates of disease prevalence or to plan therapeutic intervention, depends on the criteria used to distinguish a target disease from other diseases. While this may seem a truism, it should be emphasised that the diagnostic systems described above tend to be hierarchical, with anxiety located low down the hierarchy. This section outlines some of the important differential diagnoses associated with the assessment of anxiety.

Depression

Depression frequently occurs in association with anxiety (Gersh & Fowles 1979, Hamilton 1983) and may be masked by it (Barraclough 1971). The relationship between these two disorders in later life is complex and only careful history taking will reveal the nature of the depression (e.g. endogenous or reactive) and whether anxiety is primary or secondary to depression (Lader 1982, Kay 1988). Yet depressive illnesses are generally assumed to be more serious than anxiety disorders and are traditionally given greater weight within classification systems (Clare & Blacker 1986). One important reason for this is risk of suicide in patients with anxiety and endogenous depression (Kay 1988).

Dementia

Patients with anxiety can experience symptoms of memory loss, even when cognitive impairment is not confirmed by formal testing (Philpot & Levy 1987). Conversely, the early stages of dementia can present as symptoms of anxiety (Lader 1982, Lindesay 1991a). Lader (1982) has suggested that the dementing process can impair the ability of older people to adapt to changing conditions and this can lead to a severe neurosis. Progressive dementias reveal themselves over time and careful follow-up will enable these to be documented.

Other psychiatric disorders

Functional psychoses, such as paranoid states and schizophrenia, can sometimes present as simple anxiety (Lindesay 1991a). In addition, although panic attacks are rare in older people, delirium may resemble panic at this stage, particularly when the sufferer is frightened by hallucinations or imagined persecutions (Lindesay 1991a). Differential diagnosis is achieved through careful history taking.

Other organic conditions

Several acute brain syndromes can be associated with anxiety. According to Lader (1982), these include subacute delirious states secondary to covert infection (especially pneumonia), drug-induced toxic states, electrolyte or hormonal imbalance and dehydration. In most cases, these conditions reveal themselves over short periods of time (Lader 1982).

EPIDEMIOLOGY OF ANXIETY DISORDERS

Prevalence estimates of anxiety depend on the classification system used and the location of anxiety within hierarchical diagnostic systems means that prevalence estimates may be underestimates of the true rate of anxiety disorders (Lindesay 1991a). For example, if anxiety occurs in the presence of depression, it may be labelled as depressive neurosis or atypical depression.

Prevalence estimates of anxiety in later life also depend on where the investigator looks for the disorder. The most straightforward method to investigate the prevalence of any medical condition is through scrutiny of clinical records. In the case of anxiety disorders, relevant sources include general practice clinics, general hospital services and the specialist psychiatric services (in-patient wards, out-patient clinics and mental health community centres). In all cases, however, the manner in which anxiety comes to the attention of these different clinicians profoundly affects estimates of prevalence at each service. The main alternative to record review is to assess directly people in the general population by sampling households within a defined geographical area.

Anxiety in primary care settings

Shepherd et al (1964) found that neurosis was the most common psychiatric complaint among general practice patients. However, in spite of an accumulation of chronic psychiatric cases with increasing age, these authors noted a steady decline in consulting rates for all psychiatric disorders (particularly for new cases) after the middle years of life. A similar trend was shown for anxiety disorders in two OPCS studies (OPCS 1979, 1986).

In a survey of approximately 9000 general practice patients, anxiety disorders were identified in 10% of patients aged 65 and older, in contrast to 21% for all ages (Watts et al 1964). This was the case even though the elderly consult their doctors more frequently than younger people (Kay 1988). There are several possible reasons for this decline. First, there are important differences in subjective and somatic symptoms of anxiety between older and younger people and these differences may affect diagnostic and referral practices. For example, physical illness, financial matters and violent crime are of particular concern to older people. Anxiety surrounding these topics is more likely therefore to be dismissed as reasonable (and therefore not morbid) in an older person than in a younger person. In addition, somatic symptoms play a complex role in the labelling of anxiety in general practice. Although the somatic symptoms of anxiety in older people are similar to those in younger people, they are more likely to be regarded by the GP as manifestations of physical illness (Lindesay 1991a). However, the true extent to which the elderly somatise their anxiety remains controversial; although some studies have reported a high somatising tendency among the elderly (MacDonald 1973, Weyerer 1983), Lindesay (1991a) suggests that this may be the result of subtle encouragement by medical services, who are particularly likely to pay attention to physical symptoms.

Anxiety in specialist medical services

Older people rarely seek psychiatric consultation for anxiety within a general hospital setting (Folks & Ford 1985, Popkin et al 1981). Yet anxiety is found to occur in up to 10% of hospital patients when these patients are independently assessed (Bergmann & Eastham 1974, Kay et al 1987). It should be noted that a complex relationship exists between anxiety states and physical illness in elderly people. This was demonstrated in older people randomly assessed at home by Kay and Bergmann (1966), who showed an association between functional psychiatric disorders (mainly neurosis) and physical disability at the time of assessment and between the former and increased mortality on follow-up.

Nowhere, however, is the relationship between anxiety and physical illness more evident than in a general hospital setting. Anxiety can be evoked by physical disorders, some of which increase in frequency with ageing. According to Lindesay (1991a), the most important physical causes are cardiovascular (e.g. myocardial infarction, orthostatic hypotension), respiratory (e.g. asthma, chronic obstructive airway disease), endocrine (e.g. hyperthyroidism, hypoglycaemia) and neurological (e.g. epilepsy, head injury). In addition, anxiety states occur in those who suffer chronic disabling conditions such as arthritis, sensory impairment and abnormal postural mechanisms (Marks 1981, Lindesay 1990). Surgery is also associated with anxiety, although there is some evidence that older hospital patients are less anxious about disfiguring procedures than younger people (Frank et al 1984, Hughson et al 1986). In this regard, it is important to recall Fattah and Sacco's (1989) observation that the severity of situational anxiety is determined by the perceived consequences of a threatening event. This is consistent with the earlier finding of Peach and Pathy (1979) that older people feel more anxious about inability to perform activities of daily living following myocardial infarction than about the symptoms of the disease itself.

It should be noted in the present context that psychosocial problems among elderly people can be associated with chronic use of over the counter (OTC) medications (Shader & Greenblatt 1982) and many of these medications can cause symptoms of anxiety. These effects have been summarised by Gardner & Hall (1982). Many OTC preparations, particularly certain analgesics, sedative-hypnotics and cold allergy preparations evoke CNS excitation or depression, agitation and autonomic symptoms that accompany anxiety states. This is the case when correct or even low doses are used (Gardner & Hall 1982). It is therefore particularly important to document OTC drug use, especially since this is often concealed by patients (Gardner & Hall 1982).

Anxiety in psychiatric services

As might be expected, only patients with severe anxiety disorders tend to be admitted to in-patient psychiatric services. Furthermore, GP referral rates to psychiatric services decline with age, with a lower likelihood of referral for neurotic patients compared to psychotic patients (Shepherd et al 1981). Consequently, anxiety states account for only 5% of psychiatric admissions after the age of 65 (OPCS 1983). Referral rates for outpatient psychiatric services are also low (Shepherd et al 1981).

This trend is in marked contrast to that for depressive disorders, which increase in proportion after this age (MacDonald 1973, Spicer et al 1973). In fact, the presence of depression may be the crucial factor in determining psychiatric referral for older people with anxiety disorders (MacDonald 1973). As noted earlier, this will lead to the underestimation of anxiety disorders among elderly people in psychiatric wards since depression tends to take priority in diagnostic classification. It should be noted, however, that referral rates are not exclusively a matter of GP discretion; Shepherd et al (1981) found that patients or their relatives were often unable to accept a suggestion that they should be seen by a psychiatrist.

Anxiety in the community

So far, judgements about the occurrence of anxiety in later life have been based on medical record reviews. We have seen that each type of medical service acts as a filter, progressively reducing the numbers of people who present with diagnosed anxiety disorders. Thus anxiety is frequently encountered in general practice, although elderly people are vulnerable to having certain complaints dismissed as preoccupations natural for an older person. In both general practice and hospital medical services, somatic symptoms of anxiety are likely to be misinterpreted as manifestations of physical illness in older people. Finally, few elderly people with anxiety disorders are referred to specialist psychiatric services by general practitioners. Those who do attend these services tend to have problems of a quite serious nature and therefore are unrepresentative of the elderly community as a whole.

One way to circumvent this filtering process is to sample the general population by randomly assessing people at home within a defined geographical area. However, difficulties of this approach can be overpowering. In particular, anxiety states are relatively infrequent so large numbers of people have to be sampled, often at great expense. Nevertheless, population-based studies provide the most accurate and unbiased estimates of prevalence.

The largest of these studies is the multi-site Epidemiological Catchment Area (ECA) programme in the USA (e.g. Regier et al 1988, Weissman et al 1985). The ECA study interviewed people aged 18 and older from randomly selected households, using the National Institute of Mental Health Diagnostic Interview Schedule (DIS; Robins et al 1981). This instrument enables selected DSM-III diagnoses to be

derived while suspending the diagnostic hierarchy of the standard DSM system (see above). ECA prevalence estimates for phobic disorders and panic disorder are shown in Table 7.1. Based on extrapolation performed by Kay (1988), there is a clear fall in the prevalence of phobias and panic disorder after age 65. Within the diagnostic categories used by the ECA programme, phobic disorders were the most common type of anxiety in later life.

Recent studies in the UK have favoured the Geriatric Mental State (GMS, Copeland et al 1986), a semi-structured interview and its associated computer algorithm AGECAT, which generates psychiatric diagnoses at five levels of confidence, based on prevailing clinical practice. Using this system, Copeland et al (1987) assessed 1070 people aged 65 and older randomly drawn from 360 GP patient lists. These authors reported a prevalence rate of 2.4% for all neurosis, with 1.1% for non-phobic anxiety and 0.7% for phobias. These prevalence estimates are clearly lower than those reported by the ECA studies. It should be noted, however, that the GMS requests raters to exclude fears that they consider reasonable for an older person, such as fear of going out because of crime.

Lindesay et al (1989) also suggested that the GMS utilises more severe diagnostic criteria than DSM-III. These authors randomly sampled 890 older people within the Lewisham and North Southwark Health District of South East London, using the electoral register. Anxiety was measured by a schedule that incorporated items from several scales, including the GMS. They reported that 3.7% of their total sample had general anxiety and 10% had a phobic disorder.

An important question concerns the extent to which anxiety disorders identified in the community are

Table 7.1 Prevalence rates for anxiety disorders in subjects aged 65 and older based on recent community studies

Study	Location	Survey period	N	Diagnostic criteria	% General anxiety	% Phobic disorder	% Panic disorder
Myers et al 1984	New Haven, USA (ECA)	1980–1981	611	DIS/DSM-III	–	3.3	0.2
	Baltimore, USA (ECA)	1981	923	DIS/DSM-III	–	11.7	0.1
	St Louis, USA (ECA)	1981–1982	576	DIS/DSM-III	–	2.2	0.05
Regier et al 1988	5 USA sites (ECA)	1980–1985	5702	DIS/DSM-III	–	4.8	0.1
Weissman et al 1985	New Haven, USA (ECA)	1980–1981	2588	DIS/DSM-III	–	3.9	0.1
Copeland et al 1987	Liverpool, UK	–	1070	GMS/AGECAT	1.1	0.7	–
Lindesay et 1989	London, UK	1986	890	GA scale[1]	3.7	10.0	0

Footnote
[1] Generalised anxiety scale (author devised scale incorporating GMS items).

longstanding or emerge during later life. Unfortunately, the proportion of anxiety disorders that can be classified as late onset (with no previous history of the disorder) has ranged from 5% (Kay et al 1964) to 50% (Bergmann 1971), with an intermediate estimation of 30% (Lindesay 1991b). In Lindesay's study, agoraphobia tended to be of late onset whereas specific phobias tended to be longstanding.

MANAGEMENT OF ANXIETY DISORDERS IN LATER LIFE

It is salutary to begin with Shader and Greenblatt's statement that treating an older person for anxiety requires a 'thoughtful, comprehensive evaluation of psychiatric, social and medical status' (Shader & Greenblatt 1982, p. 8). As Lindesay (1991a) points out, the continuing care of an older person with anxiety is the responsibility of the primary care team, although specialist psychogeriatric services provide expertise in assessment and acute treatment, as well as advice to general practitioners, nurses, other clinicians and carers.

Treatment of anxiety in the elderly falls into two broad categories, pharmacological and psychological. Since most older people are treated for anxiety within a primary care setting, the first of these is more commonly adopted. As Lindesay (1991a) comments, this is not an ideal state of affairs, since other management strategies can be safer and can provide longer term benefits. Nevertheless, a knowledge of pharmacotherapy techniques is important for understanding treatment of anxiety in elderly people.

Pharmacological treatment

As discussed in Chapter 23, drug disposition in the elderly differs from that in younger adults and optimal therapeutic doses may be lower for older people (Shader & Greenblatt 1982). Age-related changes responsible for this include changes in the gastrointestinal tract (affecting absorption), a higher proportion of adipose tissue (which increases the distribution of lipid soluble compounds such as diazepam), increased sensitivity of certain drug receptor sites and decreased renal and hepatic function (which reduce the rate of drug clearance).

Other important considerations when prescribing psychotropic medication to the elderly are noted by Lindesay (1991a). Certain drugs may be contraindicated by physical illnesses that are common among old people. For example, benzodiazepines depress the respiratory system and some antidepressants have cardiovascular actions. Some compounds may also interact with other drugs. It is therefore important to obtain thorough drug histories from patients, especially since many older people practice polypharmacy (Shader & Greenblatt 1982). Finally, judgements must be made about the likelihood of compliance with the prescribed drug regime and about the possibility and consequences of its abuse, including suicide.

The major class of drug used to treat anxiety in the elderly is the benzodiazepines, particularly oxazepam. Antidepressants, neuroleptics and monoamine oxidase inhibitors, other sedative hypnotics (e.g. chloral hydrate) and new agents such as buspirone, are sometimes used. Advantages and disadvantages of these drugs are discussed in Chapter 23 and also reviewed by Shader and Greenblatt (1982) and by Lindesay (1991a). There is general agreement that barbiturates, antihistamines, beta adrenergic blocking agents and propanediols are not recommended for elderly people.

Psychological treatment

As Sheikh & Swales (1994) note, a combination of breathing and muscle relaxation training, guided imagery, systematic desensitisation, relabelling of anxiety reactions, insight into irrational beliefs and systematic homework assignments provide useful therapeutic regimes for a variety of anxiety disorders in the elderly. As these authors point out, however, older patients can be particularly fearful during an acute anxiety disorder and may need a greater amount of reassurance and clinical contact time than younger patients.

Data from large scale studies of cognitive–behaviour therapy for anxiety in older people are not yet available. However, individual case studies reveal successful outcomes using desensitisation therapy, imaginal exposure, relaxation techniques and stress inoculation training in the case of phobic anxiety (Hussian 1981, Thyer 1981, Leng 1985, Woods & Britton 1985). Some of these techniques are discussed in Chapter 19. Sheikh & Swales (1994) also suggest that patient education about the disorder and its treatment can be particularly beneficial to older patients with anxiety. Such education constitutes an important part of stress management programmes (Garisson 1978). Regardless of the particular regime chosen, however, we should note Lindesay's (1991a) comment that prolonged clinical benefit will only be achieved by gradually withdrawing unnecessary domiciliary support provided by family and social services.

CONCLUSION

We began this chapter by emphasising that the nature of anxiety changes across the life span. We saw that anxiety in normal ageing tends to be concerned with practical issues, older people often being more anxious about the consequences of an aversive event than about the event itself. There is, in addition, considerable evidence that the prevalence of anxiety declines across the life span. This is the case regardless of whether the investigator examines medical records or randomly surveys people in the population. When considering these findings, however, it should be borne in mind that anxiety in older people may easily be overlooked. Certain fears, such as fear of crime, are easily dismissed as feelings natural to an older person. Somatic symptoms of anxiety are likely to be misinterpreted as manifestations of physical illness in older people. Finally, there is a tendency for anxiety to take second place to depression within the major formal classification systems for psychiatric disorders. Since the proportion of depressive disorders tends to rise in later life, this results in cases of anxiety being missed.

Treatment for anxiety in older people falls into two categories – pharmacological and psychological: since anxiety in older people is mostly treated by general practitioners, the former is more commonly used. In this regard, the benzodiazepines, particularly oxazepam, is the agent of choice. There is, however, evidence that psychological treatments, including relaxation, behavioural and cognitive techniques, can be used with success.

ACKNOWLEDGEMENT

Support during the preparation of this chapter was provided by an Alzheimer's Disease Society Research Fellowship to the author.

REFERENCES

American Psychiatric Association 1987 Diagnostic and statistical manual of mental disorders, 3rd edn. revised (DSM-III-R). American Psychiatric Association, Washington DC

Barraclough B 1971 Suicide in the elderly. In: Kay D W K, Walk A (eds) Recent developments in psychogeriatrics. Headly Bros, Kent

Bascue L O, Lawrence R E 1977 A study of subjective time and death anxiety in the elderly. Omega 8: 81

Bergmann K 1971 The neuroses of old age. In: Kay D W K, Walk A (eds) Recent developments in psychogeriatrics. Headly Bros, Kent

Bergmann K, Eastham E J 1974 Psychogeriatric ascertainment and assessment for treatment in an acute medical ward setting. Age and Ageing 3: 174–178

Bienfeld D 1994 Nosology and classification. In: Copeland J R M, Abou-Saleh M T, Blazer D G (eds) Principles and practice of geriatric psychiatry, part H: neuroses. John Wiley, Chichester

Clare A W, Blacker R 1986 Some problems affecting the diagnosis and classification of depressive disorders in primary care. In: Shepherd M, Wilkinson G, Williams P (eds) Mental illness in primary care settings. Tavistock Publications, London

Clarke A H, Lewis M J 1982 Fear of crime among the elderly. British Journal of Criminology 22: 49–62

Copeland J R M, Dewey M E, Griffiths-Jones H M 1986 Computerised psychiatric diagnostic system and case nomenclature for elderly subjects: GMS and AGECAT. Psychological Medicine 16: 89–99

Copeland J R M, Dewey M E, Wood N, Searle R, Davidson I A, McWilliam C 1987 Range of mental illness among the elderly in the community: prevalence in Liverpool using the GMS–AGECAT package. British Journal of Psychiatry 150: 815–823

Eysenck H J 1979 The conditioning model of neurosis: criticisms considered. The Behavioral and Brain Sciences 2: 188–199

Fattah E A, Sacco V F 1989 Crime and victimization in the elderly. New York, Springer Verlag

Fiefel H 1956 Older persons look at death. Geriatrics 11: 127–130

Folks D G, Ford C V 1985 Psychiatric disorders in geriatric medical/surgical patients, part 1: report of 195 consecutive consultations. Southern Medical Journal 78: 739

Frank R G, Kashani J H, Kashani S R, Wonderlich S A, Umlauf R L, Ashkanazi G S 1984 Psychological response to amputation as a function of age and time since amputation. British Journal of Psychiatry 144: 493–497

Gardner E R, Hall R C W 1982 Psychiatric symptoms produced by over the counter drugs. Psychosomatics 23: 186–190

Garrison J E 1978 Stress management training for the elderly: a psychoeducational approach. Journal of the American Geriatrics Society 26: 397–403

Gersh F S, Fowles D C 1979 Neurotic depression: the concept of anxious depression. In: Depue R A (ed) Psychobiology of depressive disorders. Academic Press, New York

Hamilton M 1983 That clinical distinction between anxiety and depression. British Journal of Pharmacology 15: 165S–169S

Hughson A V M, Cooper A F, McArdle C S, Smith D C 1986 Psychological impact of adjuvant chemotherapy in the first two years after mastectomy. British Medical Journal 293: 1268–1271

Hussian R A 1981 Geriatric psychology: a behavioural perspective. New York, Van Nostrand Reinhold

Jersild A T, Holmes F B 1935 Children's fears. Teachers College Bureau of Publications, New York

Kalish R A 1985 Death, grief, and caring relationships, 2nd edn. Brooks-Cole, Monterey, CA

Kay D W K 1988 Anxiety in the elderly. In: Noyers R, Roth M, Burrows G D (eds) Handbook of anxiety, vol 2: classification, etiological factors and associated disturbances. Elsevier, Amsterdam

Kay D W K, Bergmann K 1966 Physical disability and mental health in old age: a follow up of a random sample of people seen at home. Journal of Psychosomatic Research 10: 3–12

Kay D W K, Beamish P, Roth M 1964 Old age mental disorders in Newcastle upon Tyne, part 1: a study of prevalence. British Journal of Psychiatry 110: 146–158

Kay D W K, Holding T A, Jones B, Littler S 1987 Psychiatric morbidity in Hobart's dependent aged. Australian and New Zealand Journal of Psychiatry 21: 463–468

Lader M 1982 Differential diagnosis of anxiety in the elderly. Journal of Clinical Psychiatry 43: 4–7

Leng N 1985 A brief review of cognitive–behavioural treatments in old age. Age and Ageing 14: 257–263

Lindesay J 1990 The Guy's/Age Concern Survey: physical health and psychiatric disorder in an urban elderly community. International Journal of Geriatric Psychiatry 5: 171–178

Lindesay J 1991a Anxiety disorders in the elderly. In: Jacoby R, Oppenheimer C (eds) Psychiatry in the elderly. Oxford University Press, Oxford

Lindesay J 1991b Phobic disorders in the elderly. British Journal of Psychiatry 159: 531–541

Lindesay J, Briggs C, Murphy E 1989 The Guy's/Age Concern Survey: prevalence rates of cognitive impairment, depression and anxiety in an urban elderly community. British Journal of Psychiatry 155: 317–329

MacDonald C 1973 An age specific analysis of the neuroses. British Journal of Psychiatry 122: 477–480

Marks I 1979 Conditioning models for clinical syndromes are out of date. The Behavioural and Brain Sciences 2: 175–177

Marks I 1981 Space phobia: syndrome or agoraphobic variant. Journal of Neurology, Neurosurgery and Psychiatry 44: 387–391

Myers J K, Weissman M M, Tischler G L et al 1984 Six-month prevalence of psychiatric disorders in three communities: 1980–1982. Archives of General Psychiatry 41: 959–967

OPCS (Office of Population Censuses and Surveys) 1979 Morbidity statistics from general practice: second national survey 1971–1972. HMSO, London

OPCS (Office of Population Censuses and Surveys) 1983 Mental health statistics for England. HMSO, London

OPCS (Office of Population Censuses and Surveys) 1986 Morbidity statistics from general practice: third national survey 1981–1982. HMSO, London

Peach H, Pathy J 1979 Disability in the elderly after myocardial infarction. Journal of the Royal College of Physicians 13: 154–157

Philpot M, Levy R 1987 A memory clinic for the early diagnosis of dementia. International Journal of Geriatric Psychiatry 2: 195–200

Popkin M K, Mackenzie T B, Callies A L 1981 Psychiatric consultation to geriatric medically ill inpatients in a university hospital. Archives of General Psychiatry 41: 703–707

Regier D A, Boyd J H, Burke J D et al 1988 One-month prevalence of mental disorders in the United States. Archives of General Psychiatry 45: 977–986

Rhudick P J, Dibner A S 1962 Age, personality, and health correlates of death concerns in normal aged individuals. In: Tibbits C, Donahue W (eds) Social and psychological aspects of aging. Columbia University Press, New York

Robins L N, Helzer J E, Crougham J, Ratcliffe K S 1981 National Institute of Mental Health Diagnostic Interview Schedule: its history, characteristics, and validity. Archives of General Psychiatry 38: 381–389

Sato S 1983 An investigation of anxiety-provoking situations among the aged. Journal of Child Development 19: 5

Shader R I, Greenblatt D J 1982 Management of anxiety in the elderly: the balance between therapeutic and adverse effects. Journal of Clinical Psychiatry 43(9:2): 8–18

Sheikh J I, Swales P J 1994 Acute management of anxiety and phobias. In: Copeland J R M, Abou-Saleh M T, Blazer D G (eds) Principles and practice of geriatric psychiatry, part H: neuroses. John Wiley, Chichester

Shepherd M, Cooper B, Brown A C, Kalton G W 1964 Minor mental illness in London: some aspects of a general practice survey. British Medical Journal 2: 1359–1363

Shepherd M, Cooper B, Brown A C, Kalton G W 1981 Psychiatric illness in general practice, 2nd edn. Oxford University Press, Oxford

Spicer C C, Hare E H, Slater E 1973 Neurotic and psychotic forms of depressive illness: evidence from age-incidence in a national sample. British Journal of Psychiatry 123: 535–541

Swenson W M 1962 Attitudes towards death in an aged population. In: Tibbits C and Donahue W (eds) Social and psychological aspects of aging. Columbia University Press, New York

Tate L A 1982 Life satisfaction and death anxiety in aged women. International Journal of Aging and Human Development 15: 299

Thyer B A 1981 Prolonged in-vivo exposure with a 70-year-old woman. Journal of Behaviour Therapy and Experimental Psychiatry 12: 69

Verwoerdt A 1981 Clinical geropsychiatry, 2nd edn. Williams and Wilkins, Baltimore

Watts C A H, Cawte E C, Kuenssberg E V 1964 Survey of mental illness in general practice. British Medical Journal 2: 1351–1359

Weissman M M, Myers J K, Tischler G L et al 1985 Psychiatric disorders (DSM-III) and cognitive impairment among the elderly in a US urban community. Acta Psychiatrica Scandinavica 71: 366–379

Weyerer S 1983 Mental disorders among the elderly: true prevalence and use of medical services. Archives of Gerontology and Geriatrics 2: 11

Woods R T, Britton P G 1985 Clinical psychology with the elderly. Croom Helm, London

World Health Organization 1992 Tenth revision of the international classification of diseases, chapter V (F): mental and behavioural disorders. WHO, Geneva

RECOMMENDED READING

Kay D W K 1988 Anxiety in the elderly. In: Noyers R, Roth M, Burrows G D (eds) Handbook of anxiety, vol. 2: classification, etiological factors and associated disturbances. Elsevier, Amsterdam

Lindesay J 1991 Anxiety disorders in the elderly. In: Jacoby R, Oppenheimer C (eds) Psychiatry in the elderly. Oxford University Press, Oxford

Copeland J R M, Abou-Saleh M T, Blazer D G (eds) 1994 Principles and practice of geriatric psychiatry, part H: neuroses (100–109). John Wiley, Chichester. *These three chapters provide good general overviews of anxiety in later life.*

Shepherd M, Cooper B, Brown A C, Kalton G W 1981 Psychiatric illness in general practice, 2nd edn. Oxford University Press, Oxford. *This book provides an interesting insight into anxiety and other psychiatric illnesses as they occur in primary care settings.*

Shader R I, Greenblatt D J 1982 Management of anxiety in the elderly: the balance between therapeutic and adverse effects. Journal of Clinical Psychiatry 43: 8–16

Woods R T, Britton P G 1985 Clinical psychology with the elderly. Croom Helm, London. *These two sources provide detailed information about therapeutic intervention for anxiety in older people. The former concentrates on pharmacotherapy and the latter describes psychological treatments.*

8

Depression and mania in later life

Colin Hughes

INTRODUCTION

This chapter is concerned with depression and mania in late life. Mania is far less common than depression in elderly people and presents far fewer age-related implications for care and treatment. Thus emphasis is given here to depression and consideration of mania is confined to those aspects which are of particular note for elderly people. For both disorders, however, the chapter emphasises the need for a positive approach to detection and assessment, and to care, treatment and follow-up. This should be based on a thorough knowledge of main presenting features and effective treatment approaches.

PRESENTATION OF DEPRESSION IN LATE LIFE

Most elderly people experience the same range of normal emotions, depending on circumstances and events, as they have done during other periods in their lives. Most elderly people are as satisfied with their lives as at any other age and enjoy their retirement, their interests, their families and their friends. Despite the increased likelihood of losing a loved one or of physical illness and disability, old age is not necessarily a time of sadness and depression. Unfortunately, a minority of elderly people do suffer from depression severe enough to interfere with their daily lives.

CASE EXAMPLES

The case examples given in Boxes 8.1–8.3 illustrate the main presentations of depression in elderly people.

Mr Smith (Box 8.1) suffers from a severe depressive episode. His mood is depressed but he also has a number of other key symptoms which, together, are characteristic of a depressive episode. A good

---

Box 8.1 George Smith

Mr Smith, aged 85, lives in a comfortable rented council house, a quarter of a mile from the village shops. His wife died 5 years ago. He has two daughters and a son who all live in nearby villages. Another son died 9 months ago. Mr Smith has become increasingly depressed over the past 2 months. He feels miserable and no longer enjoys the TV and radio or the company of his family. He feels irritated and restless in company. He also feels tired all the time and has no interest in household chores, although he normally prided himself on keeping a tidy house. Mr Smith no longer walks into the village for shopping, relying on his neighbours to do this for him. He spends most of the day just sitting on the settee, glancing at the newspaper, but not being able to concentrate on it for long, or looking out of the window pondering over and over about the hopelessness of the situation. He has little appetite for food and sleeps fitfully at night. He does not like getting up in the morning because he feels that it is going to be a long lonely day. He cannot see anything to look forward to in the future and cannot see himself getting better. Mr Smith does wonder sometimes if life is worth living. He has no active physical illness, although his deteriorating eyesight worries him. He has felt depressed like this before, after his wife died. At the request of his family he was seen by his general practitioner (GP) who prescribed an antidepressant and referred him to the community mental health team for further assessment.

---

description of these symptoms in an elderly person, or a person of any age, is given in the 10th edition of the WHO International Classification of Diseases, known as ICD-10 (World Health Organization 1992). It describes the following symptoms:

1 Depressed mood

The mood is depressed to a degree that is abnormal for the person and mainly uninfluenced by circumstances. The person may feel depressed, sad or 'down in the dumps' and may appear depressed. The mood can vary somewhat during the day and, in more severe depression, is often worse in the morning.

2 Loss of interest and enjoyment

The depressed person describes not being as interested in previous usual activities, 'not caring anymore', or not being able to experience pleasure. They may withdraw from family and friends and neglect activities which were previously a source of pleasure.

3 Reduced energy leading to increased fatigue and diminished activity

This is experienced as sustained fatigue even in the absence of physical exertion. The smallest tasks seem impossible to complete and motivation and drive are lowered. Psychomotor retardation may result, with slowed monotonous speech, increased pauses before answering, slow body movements, and decreased amount of speech (poverty of speech) or muteness. In the most severe cases depressive stupor may develop.

4 Reduced concentration and attention

The person may complain of memory problems and indecision and may appear distracted.

5 Reduced self-esteem and self-confidence

The person has negative thoughts about themselves saying, for example, 'I am not as good as other people' or, 'I am not a very interesting person anymore'.

6 Ideas of guilt and unworthiness

The person has distorted beliefs about current or past failings or blames himself for some untoward event or for his illness. The person may believe that they do not deserve the attention of their family or the concern of the doctor or nurse. Ideas of guilt and worthlessness can be delusional in intensity.

7 Bleak and pessimistic views of the future

The person believes that the future will be unpleasant, that something bad will happen or there is no future. He may believe that the treatment will not help, and that he will not recover. The person experiences feelings of hopelessness and helplessness.

8 Ideas or acts of self-harm or suicide

Often, the person thinks that they would be better off dead. They may have thoughts of self-harm, with or without a specific plan, or may have attempted suicide.

9 Disturbed sleep

The problem can be in getting to sleep, waking in the middle of the night or waking early in the morning. Waking early, 2 hours or more before the usual time, is especially characteristic of severe depression.

(10) *Diminished appetite*

The person no longer enjoys food so eats less and often loses weight.

In addition, psychomotor agitation may be prominent instead of diminished activity with the person not being able to sit still, pacing about, wringing their hands or pulling at their hair or clothes.

Anxiety is a common feature. The person may have some obsessional or hypochondriacal symptoms.

In isolation some of these symptoms could clearly be part of a normal reaction to the losses sometimes associated with older age. It would not be unusual for an elderly person to feel some sadness or pessimism as health deteriorates and some interests have to be given up. Normal biological ageing might result in reduced vitality and diminished activity. Physical illness might disturb sleep and reduce appetite.

In clinical practice a person is diagnosed as suffering from a depressive disorder on the basis of a psychiatric examination. This takes account of many factors such as previous psychiatric problems, family history and the absence of symptoms of other psychiatric disorder. However, the person will usually be considered to be suffering from a depressive disorder only when a number of the above symptoms are experienced, that is, when the depressive syndrome is present. In consequence, the person will usually have difficulty continuing with usual activities, and relationships are likely to be affected.

The International Classification of Diseases, ICD-10, describes several types of depressive disorder. George Smith (Box 8.1) suffers from what is known as a depressive episode. For research and audit purposes, as well as for general clinical use, ICD-10 gives diagnostic guidelines for describing depressive episodes as mild, moderate or severe. The first three symptoms above, depressed mood, loss of interest and enjoyment, and reduced energy, are regarded as particularly important. For a mild depressive episode there should be present at least two of these three symptoms plus at least two of the others. For a moderate depressive episode there should be present at least five (preferably six) symptoms in total, again with two of the first three present. For a severe depressive episode at least seven should be present including all of the first three. Symptoms should have been present for about 2 weeks. By examining the case example of George Smith we can see how his depressive episode would be classed as severe.

A severe depressive episode is equivalent to 'major depression' in the influential US classification system which is published in the 4th edition of the Diagnostic

---

Box 8.2   Marjorie Jones

Mrs Jones, aged 71, believed that her husband was poisoning her food. She also believed that she had cancer of the bowel. Such thoughts occupied her mind constantly, causing her enormous anxiety, and she would pace about the house wringing her hands. She was eating and drinking very little and had lost weight. Her mood was very depressed and she had lost interest in all her usual activities. She said that she was not getting on with her husband and believed that he was too good for her. These problems had developed in the previous 5 weeks. She was seen by a psychiatrist at home and admitted to the mental health unit of the district general hospital.

---

and Statistical Manual of Mental Disorders known as DSM-IV (American Psychiatric Association 1994). It is mentioned here because much recent research has used the DSM system.

One of the first important tasks in providing effective mental health care for elderly people with depression is to recognise the presence of the key symptoms described above which help to define the presence of a depressive disorder.

A severe depressive episode can present with psychotic symptoms, with hallucinations or delusions as illustrated by the case of Marjorie Jones (Box 8.2). Mrs Jones had a severe depressive episode with psychotic symptoms. She had delusions concerned with her having cancer (a hypochondriacal delusion), with no longer being deserving of her husband (a delusion of unworthiness) and with her husband poisoning her (a paranoid delusion). In addition to these types of delusion, a severely depressed person may believe that their body is rotting away or indeed that they are dead (a nihilistic delusion). They may experience hallucinations, such as hearing voices saying derogatory things about them or accusing them of doing evil things (auditory hallucinations). They may perceive an unpleasant smell (an olfactory hallucination) especially if they believe that they are also physically ill.

Depressive episodes usually occur as either a single first episode or in the context of previous depressive episodes (recurrent depressive disorder), with the latter sometimes described as unipolar depression. However, as we shall see, if a person has experienced one or more manic episodes too, then they would be classified as having bipolar affective disorder.

Mrs Watson (Box 8.3) has a milder depressive disorder.

> **Box 8.3** Betty Watson
>
> Mrs Watson is 75 years old. Her husband died 9 years ago. She has arthritis in her back, knees and ankles and has angina. Her mood has been somewhat depressed since her grandson, aged 21, with whom she had always had a very close relationship, moved away to another job 18 months ago. She gets tearful sometimes, although her mood is brighter for a few days at a time especially when in company or when expecting a visit from her grandson. She no longer enjoys the garden and greenhouse, partly through loss of interest and partly through the pain from the arthritis in her lower back. She has become particularly anxious about her angina and grumbles that the doctor does not visit often enough. Mrs Watson has also become very disgruntled that she has a home help visit only once a fortnight when she knows that there are people without the problems she has who have a weekly visit. About 8 weeks ago she stopped going to the local voluntary day centre which she usually attended 1 day a week and enjoyed. She still walks to the shops several times a week. Her appetite has remained good and her sleep pattern has not changed. Mrs Watson is being seen by a social worker at home for counselling.

In this case the mood disturbance is chronic and variable. Mrs Watson feels well for periods but most of the time she feels depressed with everything being an effort. She tends to brood and complain. She does not fulfil the criteria for a mild depressive episode and under ICD-10 she would be classed as suffering from dysthymia (a classification which has largely replaced the term neurotic depression).

When depressed mood occurs as part of a period of adjustment to some significant life change, such as moving into a residential home for example, but few other symptoms occur, it is described in ICD-10 as a brief or prolonged depressive reaction. This has largely replaced the term reactive depression. Its counterpart, endogenous depression, should only be used

---

> **Box 8.4** Main ICD-10 categories for mood (affective) disorders
>
> F30 Manic episode
> F31 Bipolar affective disorder
> F32 Depressive episode
> F33 Recurrent depressive disorder
> F34 Persistent mood (affective) disorders (including dysthymia)
> F43 Reaction to severe stress, and adjustment disorders.

descriptively to refer to a depressive episode which does not appear to have been caused by an external psychosocial event.

Box 8.4 summarises the main ICD-10 categories for mood disorders and gives their numeric codes (F30–F43).

Differences in presentation between elderly people and younger adults

Some differences have been reported in the presentation of depression in elderly people compared to younger adults. In a study of in-patients Brown et al (1984) found that elderly patients had more sleep disturbance, agitation and bodily complaints (with no clear physical cause) than the younger ones. They also had less suicidal ideas and loss of libido. Another study, again predominantly of in-patients, found elderly patients to be more psychotic and agitated (Brodaty et al 1991). However, when Musetti et al (1989) studied physically well, predominantly out-patient elderly, they found few important differences when compared with the younger patients. The elderly patients were more retarded, less hostile, less self-blaming and had fewer suicidal ideas but had greater weight loss. It has been suggested therefore that the stereotype of the 'elderly depressive' as being agitated and hypochondriacal may just be a reflection of the more severe illness of in-patient samples (Baldwin 1991b). In general, the clinical presentation of depression in elderly people is much the same as in any other age group. The similarities in presentation are far more important than any differences.

PREVALENCE AND INCIDENCE OF DEPRESSION IN ELDERLY PEOPLE

Prevalence

Prevalence, expressed as a percentage, refers to the number of people with a particular disorder within a given population. Actual estimates of prevalence of depression in elderly people vary due to a number of factors. Different samples have been studied and there may have been real differences in separate populations. Different instruments have been used to detect depressive symptoms and these then have been interpreted in different ways to define a 'case' of depression (Livingston & Hinchliffe 1993). Nevertheless, a pattern does emerge from the many studies undertaken over recent years. A prevalence of between 10% and 15% is found in community samples of over 65s for depressions severe enough to merit clinical intervention. For example, two recent studies in London reported rates of 13.5% and 15.9% respectively (Lindesay et al 1989, Livingston et al 1990). When stricter definitions are used, rates of severe depression are found up to around 3% (Blazer & Williams 1980, Copeland et al 1987).

With this information, a health or social service could estimate the number of elderly people suffering from depression within the population served. For instance:

Total population of service area = 200 000
If 15% are over 65 years, number of those over 65 =
   15% of 200 000 = 30 000
Number estimated to be suffering from significant
   depression = 10% (say) of 30 000 = 3000

Appropriate caution is needed in interpreting the results for your own area – for example, some studies suggest that depression may be less common in rural areas (O'Hara et al 1985, Wade 1993).

When samples other than community samples have been studied, especially high prevalence rates have been found. Rates have been reported at 26% among the clients receiving home care services from a local authority social services department (Banerjee 1993), at 23% in elderly medical in-patients (Burn et al 1993), at 31% in elderly people attending their GP (MacDonald 1986), at up to 40% in UK social services residential homes (Ames 1991), at 23% in Alzheimer's disease sufferers (Burns et al 1990), and at 23% in the carers of dementia sufferers (Dura et al 1990). Anyone working with these populations or in these settings should therefore have a particularly high index of suspicion for depression.

Incidence

Incidence, expressed as a percentage, refers to the number of new cases that arise within a given population in a given time period. Two recent community studies have found rates of incidence of 2–3% per year (Copeland et al 1992, Blanchard et al 1994). We might reasonably expect therefore to find around two to three new cases of depression a year for each 100 elderly people in our service area. Again, for an elderly population of 30 000, we might expect up to around 900 new cases of depression each year.

Such information on prevalence and incidence can help health and social service planners to ensure that appropriate resources are allocated to this important client group. This applies both at present, and especially in the future, as the size of the elderly population increases in the early decades of the next century.

CAUSES OF DEPRESSION IN LATE LIFE

The pathway into a depressive disorder in elderly people is usually the result of some combination of physical, psychological and social factors and comprehensive assessment will often reveal the significance of some of these factors for a particular individual.

Factors found to be associated with depression in elderly people, and which can best be regarded as predisposing factors, include:

- female sex
- past history of depression
- family history of depression
- widow(er)hood
- poverty
- living in an institution
- poor physical health
- lack of social support
- personality
- brain changes (subtle and coarse).

Precipitating factors include:

- severe life events (including physical illness and bereavement)
- retirement
- major social difficulties
- medications.

Some evidence for the role of these factors is described here. For a more detailed discussion refer to the excellent review by Katona (1993).

Predisposing factors

Depression in elderly people, as at all other ages, tends to be more common in females. In a Liverpool study, for instance, 13.6% of females had a depressive disorder compared to 7.6% of males (Copeland et al 1987). The reasons for this remain unclear, although interactions of other predisposing factors are likely to be involved. High proportions of depressed elderly people have had previous episodes of depression; for example Musetti et al (1989) found that 67% of depressed patients had had previous episodes. Although it is common to find a positive family history of depression in the depressed elderly, it is generally thought that genetic factors are less important as age of onset increases (Hopkinson 1964). Depression is associated with widowhood and divorce (Pahkala 1990). As we shall see, bereavement can precipitate a depressive disorder, but the social support of being married may act as a buffer to other stressful events.

Low income has been shown to be associated with the onset of new depression (Kennedy et al 1990). Given that depression has been found to occur at very high rates in residential and nursing homes (Ames 1991), living in an institution must be regarded as a possible predisposing factor. Although this is likely to be linked to high levels of disability in some homes, the psychosocial environment has an important impact if choice and control are restricted and there is limited opportunity for meaningful interaction and activity.

In the classic paper by Murphy (1982) the onset of depression was found to be associated with chronic poor health. It seems that the irritation and frustration of chronic pain or disability can predispose to depression in the presence of other events, the latter being 'the last straw' as it were. Important chronic conditions are severe arthritis, cardiac disease, stroke, dementia and Parkinson's disease (Ouslander 1982). Having hearing difficulties also has been found to be associated with depression (Evans et al 1991). Murphy (1982) found that elderly people who lacked the social support of a confiding relationship were more vulnerable to depression when experiencing a severe life event. However, Henderson et al (1986) found that reduced availability of more diffuse relationships, such as with friends and neighbours, was associated with depression, and that close relationships made no difference. Clearly, individuals will find support in their own individual pattern of relationships depending on the meaning of the relationships to their current situation. Interestingly, Evans et al (1991) found that having a home help was associated with the absence of depression, and suggested that such a service may be important in meeting the emotional as well as the physical needs of clients.

Certain personality traits may make an individual more vulnerable to depression. Post (1972) found that obsessional traits were common in his sample. More recently Abrams et al (1991) found an association between 'neuroticism' and depression. By neuroticism they meant being emotionally overactive and labile, and having frequent vague somatic complaints and multiple worries over apparently minor matters.

A range of brain changes may act as predisposing factors. These include subtle neurochemical and neuroanatomical changes. The levels of the neurotransmitters, noradrenaline and serotonin, are reduced in normal ageing, and these neurotransmitters are also probably underactive in depression. The level of monoamine oxidase, which reduces the concentration of neurotransmitters in the synapse, have been reported as increased in normal ageing. One suggestion, therefore, is that such normal neurochemi-

cal changes may act as a vulnerability factor in some individuals (Ferrier & McKeith 1991). This is an expanding area of research and it is likely that other neurotransmitters are also involved and interactions will undoubtedly be complex. Jacoby et al (1981) found a sub-group of depressed elderly people who had significantly increased size of ventricles, found on computerised tomography (CT) scan, but without signs of dementia. They formed a distinct sub-group, having a distinct clinical picture and a higher death rate from extracerebral causes at follow-up. It is suggested, therefore, that some subtle neuroanatomical changes may be a vulnerability factor for some elderly people. What the possible brain changes might be remains to be seen although there is already much interest in the association of lesions in subcortical white matter with depression in elderly people (Baldwin 1993).

Finally, the coarse brain damage of a stroke may be a vulnerability factor. An association has been found between depression in long-term stroke survivors (up to 5 years) and size of lesion after controlling for functional impairment (Sharpe et al 1994). Also, some evidence suggests that lesion location is also important (Robinson et al 1984), although the methodology of the latter study has been criticised (House 1987).

Precipitating factors

The experience of severe life events is associated with the onset of depression in elderly people (Murphy 1982, Emmerson et al 1989). Such events included:

- separations and deaths
- major negative revelations or life-threatening illness to someone close
- financial or material loss
- enforced change of residence
- physical illness.

Murphy (1982) found that 48% of depressed patients had experienced at least one severe life event in the year prior to onset compared with 23% of normal subjects. Also, 28% of depressed patients had experienced a severe physical illness compared with only 6% of normal subjects. Illnesses such as myocardial infarction or stroke can be interpreted as signs of approaching death, and loss of mobility can mean loss of independence, loss of social interaction and loss of self-esteem.

Murphy (1982) found that bereavement preceded depression in 9% of cases. This is confirmed as a trigger factor by Green et al (1992), who found bereavement of a close figure within the previous 6 months in 14% of new cases of depression in the community. Pahkala

(1990) found that retirement was associated with depression in men, although retirement due to illness was associated with depression in both sexes.

Major social difficulties are also associated with depression in elderly people (Murphy 1982, Pahkala 1990). These difficulties can be concerned with work, housing, the health of others, children, marriage and finances. Murphy (1982) found that 42% of patients, compared to 19% of normal subjects, had a major social difficulty in the 2 years before onset of depression.

Depressive symptoms or a depressive disorder have been reported to be associated with many different drugs, although often a strict causal relationship does not stand up to scrutiny (Bayer & Pathy 1989). The following drugs are particularly likely to precipitate depression, especially in people with a history of depressive disorder or a family history of depressive disorder:

- reserpine
- clonidine
- methyldopa
- diuretics
- betablockers
- benzodiazepines
- levodopa
- corticosteroids
- cimetidine
- digoxin
- indomethacin.

Psychological mechanisms

Some psychological models of depression provide possible explanations of how some life events (such as ill health or bereavement) are associated with depression in elderly people. Seligman (1975) described a state of 'learned helplessness' through work with animals. This developed when animals were not allowed to control their environment. For example, an animal might make appropriate responses to escape from a situation but because of the experimental design was unable to escape. Thus the animal had no control over the outcome and tended to develop learned helplessness, an apathetic, non-responding state. This was seen as analogous to depression in humans. Clearly, many elderly people experience unpleasant events over which they may have little control, such as deteriorating health or bereavement, so the concept of learned helplessness offers some explanation for their association with depression in elderly people.

The learned helplessness concept was developed by

Abramson et al (1978) to explain why events might cause depression in some individuals only. They suggested that style of thinking about the situation is crucial. People with a tendency to believe that lack of control over one event (e.g. deteriorating health) means that they will necessarily have little control over other situations, are more likely to develop depression as a consequence of interpreting the initial event in that global manner. This 'attributional style', as it is called, is therefore a possible cognitive variable mediating between some events and depression (see Hanley & Baikie 1984 for a more detailed discussion).

Beck developed a cognitive theory of depression (Beck et al 1979) which is discussed in detail in Chapter 19. This theory suggests that some individuals develop a tendency to evaluate certain events in negative ways because of certain beliefs that they have come to hold through childhood experiences, for example. Deteriorating health in an elderly person may activate a belief such as 'in order to be happy, I must always be physically fit', which is a very rigid and potentially dysfunctional belief to hold. As a result, poor health may be accompanied by negative thoughts such as 'I can't cope with this', or 'I'll never be happy again'. Such thoughts are considered to have important influences on mood and so the dysfunctional beliefs and such negative automatic thoughts are also possible cognitive factors in the development and maintenance of depression in some individuals.

DETECTION OF DEPRESSION IN ELDERLY PEOPLE

Community surveys have consistently found only small proportions of depressed elderly people to be receiving treatment. Livingston et al (1990) found that only 13% of their London sample of depressed elderly were prescribed antidepressants. Copeland et al (1992) found just 4% of their Liverpool sample receiving antidepressants. More recently, Blanchard et al (1994) found that 14% of their London sample were prescribed antidepressants with a further 5% receiving counselling or supportive therapy. It is certainly not being suggested here that all depressed elderly people should be taking an antidepressant but these findings do suggest that depression in many elderly people may go undetected or be under-treated.

It certainly seems that depression in elderly people is not always readily detected. A number of studies have found that GPs often under-diagnose the problem, and since they are often the gate-keepers to other key services this is serious. Iliffe et al (1991) surveyed a sample of GP patients in London and found 52 to be mild to severely depressed, yet depression was recorded in the notes of only three and only six had been prescribed an antidepressant. Also, Jack et al (1988) found that a GP, on interviewing specifically for depression, missed what were considered to be 32 out of 50 cases in a Newcastle GP practice sample. Similarly, a study of GPs in Australia found that they missed 12 out of 15 cases of depression in elderly surgery attenders when they had been specifically instructed to assess for its presence (Bowers et al 1990). Junior doctors and general nurses also have been found to be poor in detecting depression in elderly medical patients (Rapp et al 1988, Jackson & Baldwin 1993).

Community care officers and community care workers (none with social work qualifications) from a local authority social services department had low recognition rates of depression amongst their elderly clients (Banerjee 1993).

The separate problem of under-treatment is highlighted by Macdonald (1986). He found that GPs had no difficulty in recognising depression in elderly patients who attended surgery, again when specifically instructed to assess for its presence. However, this tended not to be followed by treatment or referral to psychiatric services. It seems possible that the GPs had generally negative views about the effectiveness of treatments (physical or otherwise) for elderly people.

There are a number of reasons why depression in elderly people may go undetected. Elderly people come from a generation that conceives psychological and physical processes in a different way to younger generations. Consequently, complaints tend to be of physical illness and physical aspects of depression rather than depressed mood and other psychological problems. Elderly people especially may also not be aware that depression is a distinct disorder which is treatable. Only 38% of depressed elderly people found in one community survey said that they had discussed their psychiatric symptoms with their GPs (Blanchard et al 1994). A depression may be overlooked by the professional when physical illness is also present, with any depressive symptoms being considered 'understandable' in terms of the person's physical state. Depressive symptoms may be also considered understandable in terms of the person's psychosocial background, thereby mistaking depressive disorder for disadvantage or demoralisation. Some depressive symptoms may be regarded as part of the normal ageing process, with an ageist attitude accepting this process as one of decline. The presence of dementia with symptoms overlapping those of depression may distract attention from the underlying depression. The depressive disorder may be expressed in an unusual way, as hypochondriasis, complaints of pain or loneliness, or as a behaviour problem such as incontinence or food refusal. Finally, many professionals may lack adequate knowledge of the key symptoms of depressive disorder. Bowers et al (1990) found that GPs generally knew to look for depressed appearance, sleep disturbance and loss of appetite in their elderly patients but few mentioned other key symptoms. Similarly, Jackson & Baldwin (1993) found that general nurses could detect the symptom of depressed mood in medical patients but not the syndrome of a depressive disorder.

Given these problems, it is clear that many of the issues that arise in the detection of depression in elderly people are educational. These are issues being addressed by the Defeat Depression Campaign, an initiative of the Royal College of Psychiatrists and the Royal College of General Practitioners launched in 1992 (Priest 1994). One of its objectives is to reduce the stigma associated with depression and to increase the public's awareness of its nature and treatment. Another is to increase the knowledge of GPs and other health care professionals in the recognition of depressive disorders. A further important objective, in the light of possible under-treatment, is to increase professionals' knowledge of the effective treatment of depression.

How then can we ensure that a possible depression in an elderly person is detected? Bear in mind the following:

- Always remember to check for the presence of all the key symptoms of a depressive disorder (as described at the beginning of this chapter) if depression is suspected.
- Remember that a person can suffer from depression and a physical disorder or dementia at the same time.
- Do not make the mistake of attributing a number of depressive symptoms to psychosocial circumstances and so do nothing further about them.
- Use one of the screening instruments (described below) that have been developed specifically for depression in elderly people.

Screening instruments

GDS

The Geriatric Depression Scale (GDS) consists of 30 questions which focus on the thoughts (cognitive aspects) and feelings (affective aspects) of depression experienced over the past week (Yesavage et al 1983). It therefore avoids the possible problem of over-estimating depression in elderly people by asking about physical symptoms which, as we have seen, may be more ready complaints. Its simple yes/no answer format is easy to complete and can also be administered by interview if eyesight or manual dexterity is poor. Clearly, what is needed in a useful screening instrument is one that detects most cases of depression (has high sensitivity) without finding too many people scoring as probably depressed who turn out not to be (has high specificity). At a cut-off score of 10 (i.e. 11 or more indicates probable depression) the GDS performs well on these characteristics. It adequately detects depression in medically ill in-patients, both in the acute setting (Ramsay et al 1991, Jackson and Baldwin 1993) and in the continuing care setting (Shah et al 1992). The original validation study was with psychiatric out-patients and in-patients (Yesavage et al 1983) and, more recently, it has been found to be effective in primary care (Katona & Katona 1993). It can also be used with people with dementia of a mild to moderate severity if, obviously, they can understand the questions and memory impairment is not too severe (Burke et al 1992). The Royal College of Physicians and the British Geriatrics Society support the use of the GDS to screen for depression in elderly people in hospital (Royal College of Physicians 1992).

GDS – short form

A short form of the GDS has also been developed with just 15 questions (Yesavage 1988). This instrument, an adaptation of which is shown in Box 8.5, is especially useful when fatigue and poor concentration are problems, with physically ill patients, for example. Scores of six or more indicate probable depression. Although it has not been studied as intensively as the original long form, results so far are very promising (Sheikh & Yesavage 1986, Bayer & Pathy 1989, Jackson & Baldwin 1993). The Royal College of General Practitioners has recommended its use as part of the health check to be offered annually to all over 75s under the GP contract (Williams & Wallace 1993) and more recently, Katona and Katona (1993) have found that just four items of the instrument (questions 1, 3, 6 and 7) will identify most primary care patients with significant depression.

BASDEC

An alternative screening instrument is the Brief Assessment Schedule Depression Cards (BASDEC).

Box 8.5 The Geriatric Depression Scale (short form) (Adapted from Sheikh & Yesavage 1986) with permission from the Haworth Press Inc.

1. Are you basically satisfied with your life?	Yes/No
2. Have you dropped many of your activities and interests?	Yes/No
3. Do you feel that your life is empty?	Yes/No
4. Do you often get bored?	Yes/No
5. Are you in good spirits most of the time?	Yes/No
6. Are you afraid that something bad is going to happen to you?	Yes/No
7. Do you feel happy most of the time?	Yes/No
8. Do you often feel helpless?	Yes/No
9. Do you prefer to stay at home, rather than going out and doing new things?	Yes/No
10. Do you feel you have more problems with memory than most?	Yes/No
11. Do you think it is wonderful to be alive?	Yes/No
12. Do you feel pretty worthless the way you are now?	Yes/No
13. Do you feel full of energy?	Yes/No
14. Do you feel that your situation is hopeless?	Yes/No
15. Do you think that most people are better off than you are?	Yes/No

The following answers score 1 point:
No to 1, 5, 7, 11, 13
Yes to 2, 3, 4, 6, 8, 9, 10, 12, 14, 15

This consists of 19 statements in large bold type on cards which are handed to the person to be sorted one at a time into piles indicated by a 'true' and a 'false' card. So far BASDEC has only been validated on elderly medical in-patients, when it performed as well as the GDS and was highly acceptable to the patients (Adshead et al 1992). Pitt (1992) suggests that it should be a useful assessment and screening tool in primary care.

Selfcare (D)

Finally, the Selfcare (D) is a self-administered test of 12 items requiring the ticking of one of four or five boxes for each item. It has been found to be effective in detecting depression in elderly patients attending their GP surgery (Bird et al 1987) and in the community (Blanchard et al 1994).

ASSESSMENT OF THE ELDERLY DEPRESSED PERSON

A comprehensive assessment of an elderly person with depression is essential for an effective plan of care and treatment to be formulated. Wherever the assessment is taking place, in hospital, at home or in a residential or nursing home, it will often need to involve more than one discipline. Effective multidisciplinary working is therefore essential to the process. The following list summarises the main areas that the assessment should cover:

- severity of current episode (mild, moderate, severe)
- duration and development (vulnerability factors, precipitants, course)
- maintaining factors (e.g. avoidance, alcohol abuse, family dynamics)
- past history of depression (and mania) and treatment response
- previous personality and family history of mood disorder
- current symptom profile (e.g. as described in ICD-10). Note:
  —suicidal ideas
  —anhedonia *inability to experience pleasure*
  —negative thinking
- factors affecting symptoms (situations and events)
- effect on usual psychosocial functioning. Note:
  —neglect of food and fluids
  —effect of extreme agitation
- main problem areas as seen by the client
- social network (family, friends, local resources)
- current and past physical problems
- current medication (and compliance).

Severity can be judged on ICD-10 diagnostic guidelines or on the severity of particular problems such as suicidal ideas or neglect of food and fluids. Vulnerability and precipitating factors should be noted as these may require specific intervention (in the case of deteriorating physical health or bereavement, for example), to maintain recovery and prevent relapse. Maintaining factors such as not going out or alcohol abuse should also be investigated as they are likely to need intervention for full recovery to be achieved. Enquiries should be made about previous personality, any previous depressive or manic episodes and family history of such problems. Family dynamics should be assessed, as inappropriate interactions may have developed during the progress of the illness which will now work against the plan of treatment and impede recovery. For instance, a carer might have become frustrated and irritated with the lack of interest and motivation of the sufferer. As a result the carer may have withdrawn somewhat, thereby unwittingly intensifying the lack of motivation and withdrawal of the sufferer.

When checking for the presence of all the key symptoms of a depressive disorder it is particularly

important to assess for anhedonia (the inability to experience pleasure) and psychological symptoms, since an elderly person may not complain of depressed mood as such. This is especially important for clients with physical illness when physical symptoms of sleep disturbance, appetite change, fatigue, and psychomotor retardation may equally be due to a depression or the physical illness. It is important to ask about what activities the person usually engages in and enjoys, and whether such activities have been dropped, and for what reasons, so as to assess for the presence of anhedonia. Psychological symptoms include how the person feels about themselves, about the world and about how they see the future (Beck's cognitive triad). Such negative thinking can be an important indication of mental state – 'I'm a burden', 'I've no nice clothes to wear to the day centre', 'It's too late to help me, I'm finished'. Negative thoughts about themselves may be concerned with being worthless – 'Don't bother with me, you must have more needy people to visit' – or with guilt and self-blame – 'We should not have moved here, it's all my fault'.

It is essential to ask about thoughts of suicide in the assessment of depression. 'Do you ever think that life is not worth living?' is a useful initial question. Increasing levels of severity of suicidal ideas are indicated by the following thoughts:

- 'Life is not worth living' (without any thoughts of self-harm).
- 'I think I would be better off dead.'
- With the most serious – 'I can't go on, I'm going to end it all' – the means of self-harm is likely to have been considered.

Many elderly people will talk about death, saying, for example, that they are ready to go when their time comes. This acceptance of death is different to the desperate talk of wanting an end to their present torment and considering suicide. Asking about suicidal thoughts does not encourage suicidal acts. Indeed, on asking about suicidal ideas, I have often found that the person has been reassured and impressed by the thoroughness of the interview. It has sometimes had a positive therapeutic effect in that the person has seen that their situation is being taken seriously, and so the questioning has been a first step in countering their hopelessness and helplessness.

Often we are faced with assessing someone with a number of clear depressive symptoms, who has been bereaved in recent months. Depressed mood, loss of interest, poor concentration, poor sleep, poor appetite, weight loss and agitation are all common features of normal grieving in elderly people. Clearly this is usually a personal matter for the bereaved, their family and friends. Grief can, however, become complicated by a depressive disorder, thereby warranting further professional involvement (Worden 1991). How can we tell when this might be the case? Jacobs and Lieberman (1987) suggest a number of useful pointers. Clear psychotic symptoms may be present, not just disbelief about the loss or the common hallucinations of normal grief. The presence of any of the following symptoms suggest a bereavement complicated by a depressive disorder:

- a pervasive loss of self-esteem
- marked psychomotor retardation
- suicidal ideas.

However, when the common features are present without the three above, but when they have persisted for many months (e.g. 6–12 months), or are experienced as totally overwhelming, or there is severe impairment of social and occupational functioning, then again, a depressive disorder may be present.

As discussed in Chapter 4, an elderly person with a severe depressive disorder can sometimes appear to have dementia, thereby having what has been called 'pseudodementia'. There may be evidence of self-neglect and withdrawal, with scoring on the Mini-Mental State Examination suggesting significant cognitive impairment. However, careful assessment is likely to reveal a number of important depressive symptoms (e.g. negative thinking), a shorter history of problems, with clearer onset, actual complaints of memory problems, and 'don't know' answers to orientation questions. This is in contrast to someone with dementia, whose problems are likely to be of a longer duration with an insidious onset and who is likely to be unconcerned about forgetfulness and to answer orientation questions keenly but incorrectly.

Areas of risk are clearly important to assess as they have implications as to whether the person may need to be treated urgently in hospital, or whether an intensive supportive package needs to be arranged urgently to maintain the person safely in the community. We have considered the area of suicidal thoughts. Neglect of food, and particularly fluids, can soon put an elderly person in danger. Extreme agitation can exhaust an elderly person, precipitate falls, and add to neglect of self care.

Assessing the client's view of the situation and the main problem areas as seen by them will be important in planning care and treatment, as their perceptions will be important starting points. They may be able to describe situations (e.g. spending time in the garden) and events (e.g. visits from grandchildren) that affect symptoms, such as mood and interest, positively though only briefly.

The person's social network should be carefully assessed. This includes family relationships, friends, and participation in meetings or luncheon clubs. Particularly supportive relationships should be noted as these can be used to help in treatment. A change in overall pattern of network may be needed to prevent relapse. The effect of the current problems on family and other carers should be assessed as they may require support themselves.

Many physical illnesses can present with symptoms of depression such as fatigue, loss of appetite, psychomotor retardation or depressed mood. Examples are disorders of thyroid function, electrolyte disturbances, anaemia, vitamin deficiencies and malignancy (Ouslander 1982). It is important therefore that medical examination and indicated investigations are carried out in all persons being assessed for depression. Also, the disabling effects of illnesses such as arthritis or stroke should be assessed, as supportive measures to maximise understanding and independence will have a bearing on effectiveness of other areas of treatment for depression.

The person may be taking medication that can contribute to depressive symptoms (refer back to section on causes). An antidepressant may be being taken at the prescribed, but sub-therapeutic, dose. Level of compliance with current medication will guide planning of care and treatment of the depressive disorder.

PRINCIPLES OF CARE AND TREATMENT OF DEPRESSION

Just as the pathway into a depressive disorder is usually the result of some combination of physical, psychological and social factors, the pathway out of depression is also multifaceted. Most elderly people with a depressive disorder will therefore require some combination of physical, psychological and social interventions to achieve the best recovery and, just as important, to maintain that recovery and prevent relapse. Such multidimensional care and treatment often dictates that the most effective approach will involve the efforts of a number of different disciplines. As with assessment, this applies whatever the care setting.

An important initial decision is whether the person can be treated at home or needs to be admitted to hospital. This will depend not only on the severity of the depression but also on social circumstances, such as level of family and social services support, and risk

---

Box 8.6 Edna Roberts

Miss Roberts, aged 72, became severely depressed following a burglary at her flat. She became very agitated and could not enjoy or concentrate on her main interests of sewing and embroidery. She was sleeping poorly and had lost her appetite. At times she felt like 'ending it all' by taking all the tablets that she had. Prior to the burglary she had stopped walking to the shops because of the increased pain from her arthritic knees. The home help, who had weekly contact with her, reported her concerns to her senior who contacted the GP.

The GP and a community psychiatric nurse (CPN) made an urgent joint visit. Miss Roberts was clearly suffering from a severe depressive episode, but as the suicide risk was assessed to be low and intense input from the home help ensured adequate food and fluid intake, the decision was made to manage her at home. The GP prescribed an antidepressant and referred her for physiotherapy for her arthritic knees which had been restricting her social life as walking out was so painful. Counselling by the CPN allowed her to express her feelings of anger at being burgled and talk about her health concerns. The CPN also used cognitive-behavioural interventions to encourage her gradually to resume previously enjoyable activities and to challenge negative thoughts such as: 'I can't cope by myself any

more', 'I'll have to go into a home'. Unfortunately, because of her reluctance to go out, a niece who normally visited each month and took her out in the car, had stopped visiting. The CPN contacted her and explained the current approach. The niece began visiting again, initially to spend some time talking at home, but with a view to resuming the car trips.

The GP and CPN monitored Miss Roberts' mental state closely and the effects and side-effects of the antidepressant. After 4 weeks she had improved considerably. The intensity of home help visiting was gradually decreased to encourage previous independence. At this stage she was seen by a social worker who discussed the social restrictions imposed by her arthritic knees. The social worker subsequently introduced her to a local authority day centre where she met some old friends whom she had not been able to see for several years. Her mood improved further. It was only possible to discuss her social restrictions and possible solutions to this after her mood had improved and she could concentrate and look forward to the future. The physiotherapy and a change of analgesic medication eased the pain in her knees and she found that she could manage to visit some of the shops again. She was followed up by the social worker.

---

of suicide. Most people with depression, at any age, are treated at home in the primary care setting (Paykel & Priest 1992).

We now turn to the case of Edna Roberts (Box 8.6), which illustrates a number of important principles of care and treatment of an elderly person with depression:

- It is a problem-solving exercise based on a thorough assessment.
- A multidimensional approach is usually needed with some combination of physical, psychological and social interventions.
- A multidisciplinary approach is often needed.
- Physical problems should always be treated.
- The timing of interventions is important.
- Involvement of family members is important.
- Careful monitoring of fluid and dietary intake is essential.

Miss Roberts could be treated at home. As she suffered from a severe depressive episode she was prescribed an antidepressant which she was willing to take. This was combined at an early stage with psychological therapy by the community psychiatric nurse (CPN). Resuming activities was also facilitated by attention to her physical problem. Since she could

not walk as far as previously, thus restricting her social network, the intervention of the social worker in introducing her to a day centre adequately compensated for this. This was also seen as an important part of relapse prevention.

Marjorie Jones (Box 8.2) had a severe depressive episode with psychotic symptoms and was eating and drinking very little. She was admitted to hospital and received electroconvulsive therapy. She made an excellent recovery.

Betty Watson (Box 8.3) had a mild depressive disorder, dysthymia. She was helped at home by a number of interventions. Counselling by a social worker helped with her worries of living alone without her grandson and gave her confidence to attend the day centre again. Her domestic needs we re-reviewed and home help visits were increased to twice weekly. The GP reviewed her physical state. A change of medication helped considerably with her back pain and she was reassured that her angina was well controlled. Her dysthymia improved significantly. She still has occasional days of sadness but these seem to pass more readily now.

These three cases illustrate that an effective plan of care and treatment for a particular individual will consist of the appropriate balance of physical, psychological and social interventions. This balance will be determined by a problem-solving approach based on a thorough assessment. Components of this multidimensional approach are discussed in detail in other chapters, in particular pharmacological and electroconvulsive therapy (Ch. 23), counselling (Ch. 16) and cognitive therapy (Ch. 19), and so only brief summaries of therapeutic approaches are presented here.

Antidepressant drugs

Up to around 60% of patients suffering from moderate to severe depression improve significantly with antidepressant drugs (Benbow 1992, Menon & Jacoby 1993). Tricyclic antidepressants such as lofepramine and dothiepin are commonly prescribed. The additional sedative effect of dothiepin is useful when agitation or poor sleep is a problem. The newer SSRIs (selective serotonin re-uptake inhibitors), fluoxetine, paroxetine, sertraline and fluvoxamine, are as effective and generally have fewer side-effects. They are safer in overdose, although their prescription is no substitute for proper management of suicide risk. The need to avoid certain foods and cough and cold medicines has probably deterred some doctors from using MAOIs (monoamine oxidase inhibitors) such as phenelzine, but the introduction of a new class of MAOIs relatively free of such interactions, such as moclobemide, may change this. All antidepressants can take up to 4–6 weeks to produce the desired effect. To prevent relapse it has been suggested that antidepressant drugs should be continued for at least 2 years after recovery (Old Age Depression Interest Group 1993). When hallucinations or delusions are present, an antipsychotic drug such as haloperidol or trifluoperazine will usually be needed alongside the antidepressant (Baldwin 1991b).

Lithium

If a person has not responded to initial treatment with an antidepressant, the addition of lithium can often be beneficial (Finch & Katona 1989). Continuing lithium is effective in preventing relapse in patients who have had recurrent depressive episodes (Ghose & Coppen 1989). Blood serum levels of lithium need monitoring to ensure they stay within therapeutic limits. Patients should be warned about the risk of toxicity and told to stop taking the lithium if they become unwell – particularly with diarrhoea, nausea or vomiting – and inform their doctor. Thyroid function should be monitored as lithium can cause hypothyroidism and possibly hyperthyroidism (Lazarus 1989). Because lithium is excreted mainly by the kidneys, renal function should also be monitored since any impairment will contribute to toxicity. Lithium can also cause renal impairment.

Electroconvulsive therapy (ECT)

ECT can be effective in severe depression when antidepressants have failed. It may be the treatment of choice for patients whose lives are threatened by high suicide risk, refusal of food and fluids, marked psychomotor retardation or when delusions are present (Benbow 1989).

Psychosocial interventions

Although many people improve with physical treatments when they are indicated, significant numbers recover slowly, have partial recoveries, or do not respond at all. Psychosocial interventions are also needed, as an adjunct or alternative (Woods 1993). They may contribute to a faster recovery and, most importantly, are likely to be crucial in helping to maintain improvement and prevent relapse. Where social isolation, poor housing or bereavement, for example, have contributed to the development of the depression, a complete and lasting recovery is unlikely unless these psychosocial factors are dealt with in their own right. In the milder depressive disorders, where physical treatments may not be indicated, treatment will be by psychosocial interventions alone.

Cognitive behaviour therapy and brief dynamic psychotherapy appear to be equally effective in treating depression in elderly people, either on an individual or group basis (Hughes 1993). Evidence so far relates to elderly out-patients with non-psychotic, unipolar depression of mild to moderate severity. Cognitive behavioural interventions can also be used to help with anxiety when this accompanies the depression, as it often does. The use of interpersonal psychotherapy deserves consideration (Sholomskas et al 1983) as it has been found to be as effective as cognitive therapy in younger adults (Elkin et al 1989).

Counselling is an important intervention when a client needs help to resolve conflict or needs help with problem-solving and decision-making. Also, effective counselling skills are integral to offering care and support to a distressed person when the main therapeutic thrust is from medication or a social intervention. As issues of loss are often associated with depression, bereavement counselling or grief therapy may be needed. Family issues commonly arise in treatment and although some can be straightforward to resolve, others may require formal family therapy (Benbow et al 1990).

In the problem-solving approach to depression described here, other psychosocial interventions will have important influences. These include:

- a check on welfare benefit entitlement
- referral to a day centre, luncheon club or support group
- referral for home help and meals on wheels
- help with re-housing.

I have often been pleasantly surprised how such interventions, which at the time perhaps seemed to be relatively minor parts of the overall plan of care and treatment, seem to have made the greatest impact on the depressive disorder. Also, it is likely that clients will have their own interests and resources to draw on which they feel can be used to supplement other treatment approaches. Music, art, exercise, food, relaxation and meditation, for example, can all be a focus of therapeutic activity.

PROGNOSIS OF DEPRESSION

Most studies of prognosis are of hospital in-patients or out-patients treated mainly with antidepressants and/ or ECT and therefore, on the whole, deal with more severe depression. On the basis of earlier studies (Post 1972, Murphy 1983) looking at outcome following treatment, Millard (1983) suggested: 'Possibly in old age a new "rule of three" should be constructed for the hospital treatment of depression: no matter what is done, a third get better, a third stay the same, and a third get worse' (Millard 1983, p. 375).

Recent studies, however, point to a brighter prospect with at least three-quarters of patients initially recovering or improving significantly (Baldwin 1988). Nonetheless, there still remains a tendency for relapse

and incomplete recovery. For instance, Baldwin and Jolley (1986) report the outcome of 98 elderly in-patients admitted with 'severe non-neurotic depressive states', 44 of whom had psychotic symptoms. At 1 year follow-up 47% had been well throughout the year, 11% had relapses which had been detected and treated successfully so were again well at 1 year, 15% were in relapse, 18% had continued to have some symptoms, and 8% had died.

Another significant finding of outcome studies is that the death rate in elderly people who have become depressed is often higher than normally expected at that age (Murphy et al 1988). This is not completely accounted for by suicides or by poorer physical health. Cardiovascular disease and pneumonia are the commonest causes of death amongst this group but the reasons for this are not clear. It is possible that stressful severe life events contribute to heart disease and depression and that depression has an effect on the immune system.

Little is known about the prognosis following treatment by GPs in the community. However, one study gives an indication of the prognosis of depression in elderly people in the community if left untreated. Copeland et al (1992) followed up the majority of depressed elderly people found in an earlier community survey. Table 8.1 shows the outcome at 3 year follow-up. Nearly one-third of all cases were still depressed after 3 years with only around one-fifth completely recovered. The outcome for the more severe cases, those with 'depressive psychosis', is particularly poor considering that these are also possibly the most treatable cases. Again, the death rate for the depressed cases was significantly higher than for the well subjects. These findings can be considered to be the untreated prognosis in the community, since only 4% of cases were prescribed antidepressants and there was no evidence of any other treatments being offered. This generally poor prognosis emphasises the importance of detecting depression and treating it appropriately.

Table 8.1 Three year outcome (expressed as %) of depression in elderly people in a Liverpool community sample

	Recovered	Depressed	Died	Other cases	Sub-case of depression
All cases (n = 107)	22.4	30.8	23.4	10.3	13.1
DP (n = 25)	8.0	36.0	24.0	12.0	20.0
DN (n = 82)	26.8	29.3	23.2	9.8	11.0

Note: DP = 'depressive psychosis'
DN = 'depressive neurosis'
Sub-case = some depressive symptoms present but below case threshold
(Adapted from Copeland et al 1992)

Returning to the outcome of the hospital cases, a number of factors seem to be associated with a poorer prognosis (Baldwin 1991a). These include:

- initial and supervening serious physical ill health
- ensuing severe life events
- more severe depression
- duration of onset exceeding 2 years.

Bearing these factors in mind, and considering that there does appear to be room for improvement in prognosis, especially in preventing relapse, the following points should be considered:

- The initial episode of depression should be adequately treated, whether in hospital or in primary care, with attention given to psychological and social interventions as well as adequate treatment with antidepressant medication or ECT.
- When antidepressants are used, compliance should be carefully monitored as initial side-effects may deter an elderly person from continuing with an adequate trial. Baldwin (1991b) stresses the importance of drug prophylaxis, that is, continuing with antidepressants after initial recovery to help prevent relapse, as well as the preventive effects of support groups.
- There needs to be careful follow-up to detect possible relapse. This will usually involve regular psychiatric out-patient or GP appointments, or contact with a CPN or social worker (Hughes 1992). A day hospital can be an effective bridge between in-patient treatment and discharge to a local support group or day centre.
- When clients have regular home help, it is useful that the home help knows to report changes in mood and behaviour. As with assessment and with care and treatment, a multidisciplinary effort is likely to be most effective in preventing relapse.
- New physical problems need prompt attention.
- The impact of life events, such as bereavement or moving into a residential home, should be monitored and appropriate help offered.

The case example of Mrs Holmes (Box 8.7) illustrates how careful follow-up and, in this case, social and practical interventions prevented a relapse of depression.

PREVENTING DEPRESSION IN LATE LIFE

Primary prevention

We have seen that depression in elderly people is often associated with social and economic difficulties and

---

Box 8.7 Constance Holmes

Mrs Holmes, aged 80, was being seen in the psychiatric out-patient clinic following successful in-patient treatment for severe depression. Around 18 months following the initial episode she was noted by the psychiatrist to be more depressed in mood compared to the previous appointment although there were no other depressive symptoms. She admitted this was because a good neighbour had moved away and that she was having increasing difficulties because of deteriorating eyesight, due to a degenerative condition. She was referred to a social worker in the community mental health team who arranged attendance at a local day centre where she made some new friends. The social worker also arranged an assessment at home for low vision aids to help with reading and supplied her with a number of kitchen aids which helped with some domestic tasks. Her mood improved and a possible relapse was prevented.

---

poor health. Any measures, therefore, that can improve the general welfare and standard of living of elderly people will, arguably, help to prevent the occurrence of depression. Clearly, societal attitudes and social policy are important here. Social policy can potentially be influenced through local and national political processes.

Prevention of physical illness and alleviation of accompanying disability are likely to be especially important in preventing the onset of depression (Murphy 1985). Elderly people should be encouraged to consult their GP about physical problems at an early stage. The annual health check to be offered to all over 75s under the GP contract should be an effective screening exercise. Important too is the provision of aids and adaptations at home to minimise practical difficulties that might accompany illness. Carers need to be helped by the provision of a full range of services to maximise their morale and to help the patient not to feel a burden. Clear explanations should be given to patients and carers on the implications of problems such as heart disease or stroke to allow necessary adaptation.

Improving the financial status of elderly people should improve general morale and maintain hope for the future by giving more control and independence over day-to-day decisions. Retirement pensions should be adjusted in proportion to the cost of living. Any professional working with a client should think to check entitlement to welfare benefits if circumstances suggest a need. Referral to a social worker or a welfare rights officer might be appropriate. Help with form filling will often be needed.

Murphy (1985) suggests that the overall social environment of a neighbourhood is also important in preventing the occurrence of depression. For elderly people to meet and form and maintain relationships there is the need for convenient transport in an area. There should be local shopping facilities and architectural schemes which encourage neighbours to meet. The social support derived from a network of relationships should help to buffer against the stresses of old age.

We have seen that bereavement is a common precipitant of depression in elderly people. Every elderly person who might be vulnerable and lacks social support should be able to receive bereavement counselling. This could be offered by volunteer counsellors or by professionals. It is important that the usefulness of such an intervention is explained to a reluctant elderly person and encouragement and help offered to access such services. When a possible severe mental health problem is suspected, then referral for specialist assessment is required.

Secondary prevention

Early case detection and treatment should minimise suffering and more serious illness, and prevent complications. There are two ways in which more disorders will be detected and treated earlier. Firstly, the public themselves need to be more aware of the nature of depression. This would reduce associated stigma and so people may more readily go to their doctor or nurse for advice and help. Secondly, professionals themselves need to be more aware of the problem and more skilled at detecting depression. All mental health workers have a responsibility for public education. Teaching and training of other professionals should also be a specific part of their job. All workers with elderly people should have the opportunity to become familiar with the key symptoms of a depressive disorder. Routine use of one of the screening instruments discussed earlier would be useful, especially in primary care and in residential and nursing homes. The annual over 75s health check has a mental health component and education of primary care workers who carry out these assessments is essential. Again, the basic armoury is a knowledge of the key symptoms of depression and familiarity with a screening instrument such as the Geriatric Depression Scale (Yesavage et al 1983).

Early case detection needs to be followed by prompt and appropriate intervention or by referral for further specialist assessment and care. The public and professionals alike need to be made aware of the range of treatment options for depression in elderly people. Again, specialist mental health workers have a responsibility for education. As we have seen, many of these issues are the concern of the Defeat Depression Campaign of the Royal College of Psychiatrists and the Royal College of General Practitioners (Priest 1994).

Tertiary prevention

This involves minimising the effects of established and continuing problems on the sufferer and carers. Planned and continuing follow-up is essential and care plans and treatment regimes should be kept under review. Practical help should be tailored to minimise further problems. This might involve ensuring entitlement to welfare benefits or continuing participation in a day centre. Carers need support. They may need counselling to help them work through any anger or guilt and may need advice on managing particular behaviour problems such as withdrawal or agitation.

MANIA IN LATE LIFE

Mania is much less common than depression in elderly people and presents far fewer specific implications for care and treatment in elderly people. It can occur for the first time in old age with no history of mood disorders. It usually occurs, however, in the context of previous episodes of either depression or mania, that is, in bipolar affective disorder. It is unusual for there to be a history of mania only, although a recent study found 12% of a sample of elderly manic in-patients to have unipolar mania (Shulman & Tohen 1994). A more usual finding is that around 60% of elderly people with bipolar affective disorder will have had a depressive episode as the first mood disorder (Snowdon 1991). Broadhead and Jacoby (1990) found the mean age of this first depressive episode to be 44 years, and that 10 of their 35 manic patients had three or more depressive episodes before developing mania. The mean age for the first manic episode was 59 years, with peak at 37 years and the other at 73 years. The case of Mr Dawson (Box 8.8) illustrates a common presentation of mania in elderly people.

ICD-10 describes three degrees of severity of mania. Each is characterised by elevated mood and increased activity and energy. The least severe form, hypomania, is characterised by:

- persistent mild elevated mood, for at least several days
- increased energy and activity

Box 8.8 John Dawson

Mr Dawson's problems started shortly after his wife had come home from a short stay in hospital for repair of a fractured hip. The GP thought that he had become confused as he had started to wander. Mr Dawson wanted to go out for walks day and night. He felt that he had so much energy. He was not sleeping at night and was irritable. His wife was still using a walking frame following her operation but he would push her away and verbally threaten her when she tried to persuade him to stay indoors. Because of a back problem he walked unsteadily with two walking sticks and so was in danger of falling if walking out alone. He said he felt 'on top of the world', and that they were the 'healthiest couple in the area'. He said that he owned several Rolls Royce cars. He talked continuously and in a circular manner, all the time finding amusement in his own comments. He was self-caring and was fully orientated with no evidence of memory problems. He was seen at home by the psychiatrist who diagnosed hypomania. Because of the risks at home, to himself and his wife, he was admitted to hospital. With nursing and the prescription of haloperidol, his mental state improved.

Box 8.9 Edith Jackson

Mrs Jackson had lived in the residential home for 3 years where she had been very happy. Following a recent fall, bumping her head, she had started 'talking rubbish' and had been admitted to hospital for physical investigations but no abnormalities had been found. She was now calling the home staff 'witches', and would only reluctantly allow them into her room. At times she threatened them with her walking stick. She talked constantly and would switch the content from topic to topic. There was a suspicious content to most of her thoughts. She believed that the home staff could listen into her conversations, that they were trying to get rid of her by 'feeding her up' so that she would have a heart attack. She said that she had an 'excellent brain, the best in the district' and could see through their tricks. She could not rest and spent long periods of time cutting up newspapers to 'make cushion filling'. She said that she felt depressed at times because of what was happening to her, but would then laugh out loud. Mrs Jackson could not sleep at night and was becoming exhausted. She was fully orientated. She was admitted to the mental health unit of the district general hospital under a section of the Mental Health Act (1983). Her mania settled quickly with zuclopenthixol. On follow-up, she had settled back into the residential home, being appreciative of the staff's attentions and enjoying being the centre of attention in the communal lounge with her good humour and joking.

- marked feelings of physical and mental wellbeing and efficiency
- increased sociability, talkativeness, overfamiliarity
- increased sexual energy
- decreased need for sleep.

Irritability can be a substitute for the euphoric sociability that is usually seen. Attention and concentration may be affected, thereby interfering with usual activities. Mr Dawson (Box 8.8) clearly showed many of the these features of hypomania. The irritability was an important feature which contributed to his behaviour problems and these became the pressing reasons for his admission to hospital.

More severe than hypomania is mania, but without psychotic symptoms. Most features of hypomania are likely to be present but with greater intensity. Excited mood, overactivity and pressure of speech with poor attention and loss of inhibitions usually results in the complete disruption of usual activities and interests. The person will usually have inflated self-esteem and grandiose ideas. As in hypomania, the mood disturbance can be one of irritability or suspiciousness rather than elation.

The most severe form of mania is mania accompanied by psychotic symptoms, delusions or hallucinations. Suspiciousness can lead to delusions of persecution and inflated self-esteem and grandiose ideas can be of delusional intensity. Extreme overactivity and little need for sleep can lead to near exhaustion and physical violence, with neglect of eating and drinking and personal hygiene. This is illustrated by the case of Edith Jackson (Box 8.9).

Mrs Jackson had mania with psychotic symptoms. She had delusions of persecution and her overactivity spilled into physical aggression. Mixed in with this, at times, was depressed mood. Her condition might have been mistaken for depression with agitation or a paranoid state. The overactivity and talkativeness (pressure of speech) were important distinguishing features. It is also important to note that she, and Mr Dawson (Box 8.8), were fully orientated with no confusion: mania can often look like an acute confusional state in an elderly person.

As with depression, mania in elderly people presents much the same as at any other age (Broadhead & Jacoby 1990). Some subtle differences have been noted, such as the mixture of depressive symptoms with the manic symptoms (as in the case of Mrs Jackson) but, generally, it is important to remember to assess for presence of the features described above.

Prevalence

Studies of prevalence in the community have not examined mania by itself, but have reported bipolar disorder. Weissman et al (1985) report a 6-month prevalence of 0.1% in a USA sample. Yassa et al (1988) found only 9.3% of patients admitted to a psycho-geriatric unit with a mood disorder suffered from mania. Snowdon (1991) estimates that at least 0.03% of elderly residents in his catchment area in Sydney, Australia, are admitted to hospital once or more per year because of bipolar affective disorder.

Causes

A number of factors have been found to be associated with the onset of mania in elderly people.

Family history

As with depression, although a family history of mood disorder is not unusual in elderly with mania, it appears that the possible genetic contribution is less with later onset of disorder (Stone 1989).

Brain changes

These appear to have an important role in precipitating mania in some elderly people. Broadhead and Jacoby (1990) found that 15 out of their 35 elderly patients with mania had some signs of cerebro-organic impairment. This was shown by CT scan abnormalities, history of stroke, or a dementia rating scale scoring within the demented range.

Life events

Ambelas (1987) has reported an association between life events and the onset of first mania in a mixed-age sample up to 76 years. It has also been suggested that, in late life, less stressful life events are necessary to precipitate mania (Shulman 1989).

Principles of care and treatment

Depending on the severity of the manic episode, the associated problems and the level of family support, an elderly person with acute mania can be treated at home, perhaps attending a day hospital. However, most elderly people in the acute phase of mania need admission to hospital, often compulsorily (under the Mental Health Act 1983 in the UK, or the equivalent legislation elsewhere). The main aims of nursing interventions then are to:

- ensure a safe and quiet non-stimulating environment
- re-channel overactivity into less harmful areas, shaping behaviour in appropriate directions
- ensure an adequate food and fluid intake
- ensure compliance with prescribed medication (Lyttle 1986).

Treatment in the acute phase usually consists of a neuroleptic such as haloperidol or zuclopenthixol to help control behaviour. If there is concern about sedation or extrapyramidal side-effects and the possibility of falls, then lithium might be used instead. However, the response is slower than with neuroleptics. The majority of elderly patients respond well to these treatments (Jacoby 1991).

Follow-up is essential, usually at a psychiatric out-patient clinic and by community psychiatric nurse or social worker. The neuroleptic will usually be continued into the recovery phase, perhaps for several months. If there is a history of mood disorder with more than one episode every few years then lithium is likely to be prescribed on a continuing basis to help prevent relapse. Serum levels of lithium and thyroid and renal function should be monitored. The client and family should be educated about early signs of relapse.

CONCLUSION

Depression and mania account for considerable distress in many elderly people. This chapter demonstrates that, given the right approaches, the majority of sufferers can be helped significantly, and emphasises that a positive multidimensional, multidisciplinary approach to detection, care, treatment, and follow-up is needed. Especially in relation to depression, it is possible that changes in societal attitudes and further development in health and social service provision may also contribute to prevention.

REFERENCES

Abrams R C, Young R C, Alexopoulos G S 1991 Neuroticism may be associated with history of depression in the elderly. International Journal of Geriatric Psychiatry 6: 483–488

Abramson L Y, Seligman M E, Teesdale J D 1978 Learned helplessness in humans: critique and formulation. Journal of Abnormal Psychology 87: 49–74

Adshead F, Cody D D, Pitt B 1992 BASDEC: a novel screening instrument for depression in elderly medical in-patients. British Medical Journal 305: 397

Ambelas A 1987 Life events and mania: a special relationship? British Journal of Psychiatry 150: 235–240

American Psychiatric Association 1994 Diagnostic and statistical manual of mental disorders, 4th revised edn. American Psychiatric Association, Washington

Ames D 1991 Epidemiological studies of depression among the elderly in residential and nursing homes. International Journal of Geriatric Psychiatry 6: 347–354

Baldwin B 1988 Late life depression: undertreated? British Medical Journal 296: 519

Baldwin B 1991a The outcome of depression in old age. International Journal of Geriatric Psychiatry 6: 395–400

Baldwin R C 1991b Depressive illness. In: Jacoby R, Oppenheimer C (eds) Psychiatry in the elderly. Oxford University Press, Oxford

Baldwin R C 1993 Late life depression and structural brain changes: a review of recent magnetic resonance imaging research. International Journal of Geriatric Psychiatry 8: 115–123

Baldwin R C, Jolley D J 1986 The prognosis of depression in old age. British Journal of Psychiatry 149: 574–583

Banerjee S 1993 Prevalence and recognition rates of psychiatric disorder in the elderly clients of a community care service. International Journal of Geriatric Psychiatry 8: 125–131

Bayer A J, Pathy M S J 1989 Identification of depression in geriatric medical patients. In: Ghose K (ed) Antidepressants for elderly people. Chapman and Hall, London

Beck A T, Rush A J, Shaw B F, Emery G 1979 Cognitive therapy of depression. Guilford, New York

Benbow S M 1989 The role of electroconvulsive therapy in the treatment of depressive illness in old age. British Journal of Psychiatry 155: 147–152

Benbow S M 1992 Management of depression in the elderly. British Journal of Hospital Medicine 48(11): 726–731

Benbow S M, Egan G, Marriott et al 1990 Using the family life cycle with later life families. Journal of Family Therapy 12: 321–340

Bird A S, MacDonald A J D, Mann A H, Philpott M P 1987 Preliminary experience with the Selfcare (D): a self-rating depression questionnaire for use in elderly non-institutionalized subjects. International Journal of Geriatric Psychiatry 2: 31–38

Blanchard M R, Waterreus A, Mann A H 1994 The nature of depression among older people in inner London, and the contact with primary care. British Journal of Psychiatry 164: 396–402

Blazer D, Willliams C D 1980 Epidemiology of dysphoria and depression in an elderly population. American Journal of Psychiatry 137(4): 439–444

Bowers J, Jorm A F, Henderson S, Harris P 1990 General practitioners' detection of depression and dementia in elderly patients. The Medical Journal of Australia 153: 192–196

Broadhead J, Jacoby R 1990 Mania in old age: a first prospective study. International Journal of Geriatric Psychiatry 5: 215–222

Brodaty H, Peters K, Boyce P et al 1991 Age and depression. Journal of Affective Disorders 23: 137–149

Brown R P, Sweeney J, Loutsch E, Kocsis J, Frances A 1984 Involutional melancholia revisited. American Journal of Psychiatry 141(1): 24–28

Burke W J, Nitcher R L, Roccaforte W H, Wengel S P 1992 A prospective evaluation of the Geriatric Depression Scale in an outpatient geriatric assessment centre. Journal of the American Geriatrics Society 40: 1227–1230

Burn W K, Davies K N, McKenzie F R, Brothwell J 1993 The prevalence of psychiatric illness in acute geriatric admissions. International Journal of Geriatric Psychiatry 8: 171–174

Burns A, Jacoby R, Levy R 1990 Psychiatric phenomena in Alzheimer's disease, III: disorders of mood. British Journal of Psychiatry 157: 81–86

Copeland J R M, Dewey M E, Wood M, Searle R, Davidson I A, McWilliam C 1987 Range of mental illness among the elderly in the community: prevalence in Liverpool using the GMS–AGECAT package. British Journal of Psychiatry 150: 815–823

Copeland J R M, Davidson I A, Dewey M E et al 1992 Alzheimer's disease, other dementias, depression and pseudodementia: prevalence, incidence, and three-year outcome in Liverpool. British Journal of Psychiatry 161: 230–239

Dura J R, Stukenberg K W, Kiecolt-Glaser J K 1990 Chronic stress and depressive disorders in older adults. Journal of Abnormal Psychology 99(3): 284–290

Elkin I, Shea M T, Watkins J T et al 1989 National Institute of Mental Health treatment of depression collaborative research programme: general effectiveness of treatments. Archives of General Psychiatry 46: 971–982

Emmerson J P, Burvill R W, Finlay-Jones R, Hall W 1989 Life events, life difficulties and confiding relationships in the depressed elderly. British Journal of Psychiatry 155: 787–792

Evans M E, Copeland J R M, Dewey M E 1991 Depression in the elderly in the community: effect of physical illness and selected social factors. International Journal of Geriatric Psychiatry 6: 787–795

Ferrier I N, McKeith I G 1991 Neuroanatomical and neurochemical changes in affective disorders in old age. International Journal of Geriatric Psychiatry 6: 445–451

Finch E J L, Katona C L E 1989 Lithium augmentation in the treatment of refractory depression in old age. International Journal of Geriatric Psychiatry 4: 41–46

Ghose K, Coppen A 1989 Lithium in the prophylaxis of depressive illness in late life. In: Ghose K (ed) Anti-depressants for elderly people. Chapman and Hall, London

Green B H, Copeland J R M, Dewey M E et al 1992 Risk factors for depression in elderly people: a prospective study. Acta Psychiatrica Scandinavica 886: 213–217

Hanley I, Baikie E 1984 Understanding and treating depression in the elderly. In: Hanley I, Hodge J (eds) Psychological approaches to the care of the elderly. Croom Helm, London

Henderson A S, Grayson D A, Scott R, Wilson J, Rickwood D, Kay D W K 1986 Social support, dementia and depression among the elderly living in the Hobart community. Psychological Medicine 16: 379–390

Hopkinson G 1964 A genetic study of affective illness in patients over 50. British Journal of Psychiatry 110: 244–254

House A 1987 Mood disorders after stroke: a review of the evidence. International Journal of Geriatric Psychiatry 2: 211–221

Hughes C P 1992 Community psychiatric nursing and depression in elderly people. Journal of Advanced Nursing 17: 34–42

Hughes C P 1993 A review of a psychological intervention for depression in elderly people. In: Brooker C, White E (eds) Community psychiatric nursing: a research perspective, volume 2. Chapman and Hall, London

Iliffe S, Haines A, Gallivan S, Booroff A, Goldenberg E, Morgan P 1991 Assessment of elderly people in general practice, 1: social circumstances and mental state. British Journal of General Practice 41: 9–12

Jack M A, Stobo S A, Scott L A, Sahgal A, Jachuck S J 1988 Prevalence of depression in general practice patients over 75 years of age. Journal of the Royal College of General Practitioners 38: 20–21

Jackson R, Baldwin B 1993 Detecting depression in elderly medically ill patients: the use of the Geriatric Depression Scale compared with medical and nursing observations. Age and Ageing 22: 349–353

Jacobs S, Lieberman P 1987 Bereavement and depression. In: Cameron O G (ed) Presentations of depression: depressive symptoms in medical and other psychiatric disorders. John Wiley, New York

Jacoby R 1991 Manic illness. In: Jacoby R, Oppenheimer C (eds) Psychiatry in the elderly. Oxford University Press, Oxford

Jacoby R J, Levy R, Bird J M 1981 Computed tomography and the outcome of affective disorder: a follow-up of elderly patients. British Journal of Psychiatry 139: 288–292

Katona C 1993 The aetiology of depression in old age. International Review of Psychiatry 5: 407–416

Katona C, Katona P 1993 Approaches to depression in old age. Psychiatry in Practice 12(4): 13–15

Kennedy G J, Kelman H R, Thomas C 1990 The emergence of depressive symptoms in late life: the importance of declining health and increasing disability. Journal of Community Health 15(2): 93–104

Lazarus J H 1989 Metabolic and endocrine effects of lithium. In: Ghose K (ed) Antidepressants for elderly people. Chapman and Hall, London

Lindesay J, Briggs K, Murphy E 1989 The Guy's/Age Concern Survey: prevalence rates of cognitive impairment, depression and anxiety in an urban elderly population. British Journal of Psychiatry 15: 317–329

Livingston G, Hinchliffe A C 1993 The epidemiology of psychiatric disorders in the elderly. International Review of Psychiatry 5: 317–326

Livingston G, Hawkins A, Graham N, Blizard B, Mann A 1990 The Gospel Oak study: prevalence rates of dementia, depression and activity limitation among elderly residents in inner London. Psychological Medicine 20: 137–146

Lyttle J 1986 Mental disorder: its care and treatment. Baillière Tindall, London

MacDonald A J D 1986 Do general practitioners 'miss' depression in elderly patients? British Medical Journal 292: 1365–1368

Menon R R, Jacoby R J 1993 Physical management of depression in the elderly. International Review of Psychiatry 5: 417–426

Mental Health Act 1983. HMSO, London

Millard P H 1983 Depression in old age. British Medical Journal 287: 375–376

Murphy E 1982 Social origins of depression in old age. British Journal of Psychiatry 141: 135–142

Murphy E 1983 The prognosis of depression in old age. British Journal of Psychiatry 142: 111–119

Murphy E 1985 Prevention of depression and suicide. In: Gray J A M (ed) Prevention of diseases in the elderly. Churchill Livingstone, Edinburgh

Murphy E, Smith R, Lindesay J, Slattery J 1988 Increased mortality rates in late-life depression. British Journal of Psychiatry 152: 347–353

Musetti L, Perugi G, Soriani A, Rossi V M, Cassano G B, Akiskal H S 1989 Depression before and after age 65: a re-examination. British Journal of Psychiatry 155: 330–336

O'Hara M W, Kohout F J, Wallace R B 1985 Depression among the rural elderly: a study of prevalence and correlates. The Journal of Nervous and Mental Disease 173(10): 582–589

Old Age Depression Interest Group 1993 How long should the elderly take antidepressants? A double-blind placebo-controlled study of continuation/prophylaxis therapy. British Journal of Psychiatry 162: 175–182

Ouslander J G 1982 Physical illness aand depression in the elderly. Journal of the American Geriatrics Society 30(9): 593–599

Pahkala K 1990 Social and environmental factors and depression in old age. International Journal of Geriatric Psychiatry 5: 99–113

Paykel E S, Priest R G 1992 Recognition and management of depression in general practice: consensus statement. British Medical Journal 305: 1198–1202

Pitt B 1992 BASDEC: effective screening for depression. Geriatric Medicine 22(11): 49–53

Post F 1972 The management and nature of depressive illnesses in late life: a follow-through study. British Journal of Psychiatry 121: 393–404

Priest R G 1994 Improving the management and knowledge of depression: marketing 'Defeat Depression Action Week' for the Defeat Depression Campaign. British Journal of Psychiatry 164: 285–287

Ramsay R, Wright P, Katz A, Bielawska C, Katona C 1991 The detection of psychiatric morbidity and its effects on outcome in acute elderly medical admissions. International Journal of Geriatric Psychiatry 6: 861–866

Rapp S R, Parisi S P, Walsh D A, Wallace C E 1988 Detecting depression in elderly medical inpatients. Journal of Consulting and Clinical Psychology 56: 509–513

Robinson R G, Kubos K L, Starr L B, Rao K, Price T R 1984 Mood disorders in stroke patients: importance of location of lesion. Brain 107: 81–93

Royal College of Physicians 1992 Standardised assessment scales for elderly people: report of the joint workshops of the Research Unit of the Royal College of Physicians and the British Geriatrics Society. Royal College of Physicians, London

Seligman M E 1975 Helplessness: on depression, development and death. Freeman, San Francisco

Shah A, Phongsathorn V, George C, Bielawska C, Katona C 1992 Psychiatric morbidity among continuing care geriatric inpatients. International Journal of Geriatric Psychiatry 7: 517–525

Sharpe M, Hawton K, Seagroatt V et al 1994 Depressive disorders in long-term survivors of stroke: associations with demographic and social factors, functional status, and brain lesion volume. British Journal of Psychiatry 164: 380–386

Sheikh J I, Yesavage J A 1986 Geriatric depression scale (GDS): recent evidence and development of a shorter version. Haworth Press, New York. Clinical Gerontologist 5(1/2): 165–173

Sholomskas A J, Chevron E S, Prusoff B A, Berry C 1983 Short-term interpersonal therapy (IPT) with the depressed elderly: case reports and discussion. American Journal of Psychotherapy 37(4): 552–566

Shulman K I 1989 The influence of age and ageing on manic disorder. International Journal of Geriatric Psychiatry 4: 63–65

Shulman K I , Tohen M 1994 Unipolar mania reconsidered: evidence from an elderly cohort. British Journal of Psychiatry 164: 547–549

Snowdon J 1991 A retrospective case-note study of bipolar disorder in old age. British Journal of Psychiatry 158: 485–490

Stone K 1989 Mania in the elderly. British Journal of Psychiatry 155: 220–224

Wade B 1993 The changing face of community care for older people: year 1, setting the scene. The Daphne Heald Research Unit, Royal College of Nursing, London

Weissman M M, Myers J K, Tischler G L et al 1985 Psychiatric disorders (DSM-III) and cognitive impairment among the elderly in a US urban community. Acta Pychiatrica Scandinavica 71: 366–379

Williams E I, Wallace P 1993 Health checks for people aged 75 and over. British Journal of General Practice Occasional Paper No. 59

Woods R T 1993 Psychosocial management of depression. International Review of Psychiatry 5: 427–436

Worden J W 1991 Grief counselling and grief therapy: a handbook for the mental health practitioner, 2nd edn. Routledge, London

World Health Organization 1992 The ICD-10 Classification of Mental and Behavioural Disorders: clinical descriptions and diagnostic guidelines. World Health Organization, Geneva

Yassa R, Nair V, Nastase C, Camille Y, Belzile L 1988 Prevalence of bipolar disorder in a psychogeriatric population. Journal of Affective Disorders 14: 197–201

Yesavage J A 1988 Geriatric Depression Scale. Psychopharmacology Bulletin 24(4): 709–710

Yesavage J A, Brink T L, Rose T L et al 1983 Development and validation of a geriatric depression screening scale: a preliminary report. Journal of Psychiatric Research 17(1): 37–49

RECOMMENDED READING

Gearing B, Johnson M, Heller T 1988 Mental health problems in old age. John Wiley, Chichester. *An important volume reflecting the complexities and challenges of this field and encouraging a positive multidimensional approach to care. Part of the Open University study pack of the same name.*

Gilbert P 1992 Depression: the evolution of powerlessness. Lawrence Earlbaum, Hove. *A comprehensive review of theories of the depressive disorders. It also offers a new perspective on depression derived from evolution theory and argues strongly for the adoption of the biopsychosocial model.*

Murphy E 1986 Affective disorders in the elderly. Churchill Livingstone, Edinburgh. *The classic text. Although now looking out of date in places, it is still a mine of information.*

Wattis J, Martin C 1994 Practical psychiatry of old age. Chapman and Hall, London. *A thoroughly up-to-date and practical reference book with case histories to illustrate clinical issues. The chapter on depression and mania is a comprehensive summary of current knowledge and treatment approaches.*

9

Suicide in later life

James Lindesay

INTRODUCTION

Just how important is suicide as a cause of death in the elderly population? It all depends on how you define the problem. In terms of rates, the very elderly are still the age group most likely to die by their own hand, but they are outnumbered by younger suicides, and suicide makes a much less significant contribution to total mortality in old age than it does in younger age groups (Fig. 9.1). Indeed, suicide in old age is regarded by public and professionals alike as somehow more understandable and 'rational' than in younger people, and this attitude probably explains the relative neglect and tolerance of elderly suicide as a public health

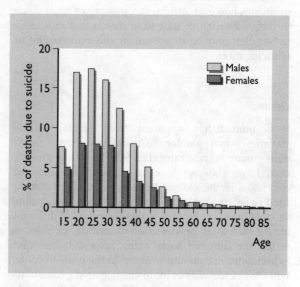

Figure 9.1 The contribution of suicide to total mortality at different ages.

problem compared to the concern expressed about rates in younger age groups. In his book, *The Savage God*, Alvarez (1971) refers to 'the extraordinary realism' of elderly suicides, 'who were willing to face and judge the unacceptable terms of the life they were living, without taking refuge in the delusions, self-pity and crotchety egoism of old age' (Alvarez 1971, p. 102). This is a view of late life that few elderly people will recognise or endorse (Thompson et al 1990). In fact, there is no reason to suppose that suicide in old age is any more or less rational than at other times of life; as the evidence discussed in this chapter makes clear, there is ample scope for prevention and the health professions have an important role to play in this respect.

EPIDEMIOLOGY

When considering the official suicide statistics it is important to bear in mind that they only record a proportion of the true rate. Suicide is a legal verdict and not a medical diagnosis, and is only recorded if there is clear evidence both of intent and self-inflicted injury. If there is any doubt, then the death is recorded either as an accident or else as an undetermined death. It is usual practice to combine suicides and undetermined deaths when estimating the true suicide rates but this will still be an underestimate, particularly in the elderly, when 'passive suicide' through self-neglect or non-compliance with medical treatment will be recorded as death by natural causes. Despite these problems, however, official statistics are of some value in the monitoring of long-term trends and indicating factors that may be important in either increasing or reducing rates.

Gender

It is immediately apparent from official suicide statistics that gender is an important factor determining suicide rates (Fig. 9.2). In all age groups, men have a higher rate of suicide, although the difference in the elderly is now less marked than it used to be, due principally to a greater secular decline in male rates (see below). Is this the result of different innate biological propensities to suicide, or does it reflect the different social roles, responsibilities and expectations of men and women? In the years to come, will the suicide rates of more emancipated generations of elderly women catch up with those of their male counterparts?

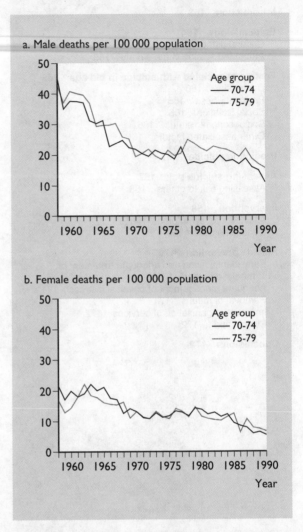

Figure 9.2   Recent trends in elderly suicide (England and Wales).

Suicide rates in the 20th century

In the early years of this century, suicide rates in the UK elderly were considerably higher than in younger age groups, particularly for men. Following a marked drop associated with the Second World War, elderly rates rose until the 1960s when they again declined, and since the mid-1970s they have remained relatively static, although there is some evidence of further decline in recent years in the older age groups (Fig. 9.2). The average annual death rate from suicide and undetermined deaths between 1986 and 1991 in men was 19 per 100 000 in the 65–74-year-olds and 29 per 100 000 in those aged 75 years and over. The equivalent rates for women over this period were about 11 per 100 000 for both age groups. In recent years, the most important trend has been the sharp increase in young male suicides (25–44 years), and the overall rates for men are now higher for the 25–54 year age group than in those aged 65–74 years. However, the highest rates still occur in the over-75-year-old male population. Suicide rates for women continue to rise steadily with age. The post-war decline in UK elderly suicide rates was probably the result of removing one of the most popular methods, namely the detoxification of the domestic gas supply in the 1960s. It appears that, having been deprived of this means, elderly people resorted less than the young to alternatives, with the result that that their overall rates fell. Other factors, such as improvements in the socioeconomic status of the elderly population, may also have contributed to this decline but there is unfortunately little evidence that improvements in medical and psychiatric treatment and care have made any impact on trends. The fact that removing a popular means of suicide may have a measurable impact on suicide rates has important implications for future prevention strategies (see below).

Common means of suicide

The commonest means of suicide in the UK elderly are currently overdose of prescribed and over the counter drugs and hanging, the latter being much more frequent in men than in women. In general, men favour violent methods of suicide more than women, and in countries where alternative violent means such as guns are more widely available, such as in the USA, these are also widely deployed in elderly suicides. In recent years, the rates of suicide by self-poisoning in the elderly have been declining, principally as a result of the reduction in the prescription and consumption of barbiturate tranquillisers. However, the decline in barbiturate-related deaths has been offset by an increase in the number of suicides involving benzodiazepines and non-opiate analgesics, specifically paracetamol and dextropropoxyphene preparations (Lindesay 1986). Another means-specific trend in recent years has been the increase in elderly male suicides using car exhaust fumes; this may be a result of the increasing numbers of elderly people who own cars and therefore have ready access to this means.

Cultural differences

The association between age and suicide is not a universal finding across all societies and cultures. In India, for example, suicides tend to decrease rather than increase with age (Bhatia et al 1987) and, in the UK, rates in elderly first generation immigrants originating from the Indian subcontinent also appear to be very low compared to the indigenous elderly population (Merrill & Owens 1986, Raleigh et al 1990). This may be because old people in these cultures are more respected and integrated into society, and it will be interesting to see if these attitudes and values survive in the younger, British-born generations of these communities. The evidence from India is not encouraging, since increasing urbanisation and fragmentation of the extended family are associated with increasing rates of depression and suicide in the elderly (Rao 1991). The important lesson to be drawn from these cross-cultural differences is that the increased suicide risk associated with age in developed societies such as ours is not innate and inevitable but is due in great part to the marginalisation of elderly people and the limited social roles that they are currently afforded.

To what extent can future trends be predicted from past and present data? It has been suggested that different birth cohorts have different suicide risks, and that high rates in early adulthood may be predictive of higher rates later in life. The evidence for such an early and enduring cohort effect is mixed; it does not appear to be a significant influence in those cohorts who are now elderly (Murphy et al 1986, Wetzel et al 1987), but there may be an increasing effect attributable to cohort membership in young cohorts (Woodbury et al 1988). If so, then the high rates of suicide in young males in recent years may persist to some extent into their old age.

Attempted suicide in the elderly

In contrast to completed suicide, elderly people are under-represented in those known to services who deliberately harm themselves. In the younger deliberate self-harm population there is rarely evidence of psychiatric disorder or serious suicidal intent, but the attempts of elderly people are more likely to represent serious bids that have failed, perhaps because they overestimated the lethal potential of an overdose, the commonest method employed by this group (Pierce 1987, Nowers & Irish 1988, Hawton & Fagg 1990). Elderly attempters therefore provide a valuable source of information about the factors associated with suicide in old age.

FACTORS ASSOCIATED WITH SUICIDE IN OLD AGE

Studies of completed and attempted suicide by elderly people have consistently demonstrated that a number of factors are powerfully associated with this behaviour. Chief among these are depression, physical illness and social isolation.

Depression

In Barraclough's classic study of completed suicides, 87% of his elderly sample were identified as depressed before death, and in most cases this depression was a first episode of a mild to moderate illness of relatively short duration (Barraclough 1971). Cattell (1988) found that 79% of his series of elderly suicides had depressive symptoms prior to death and that a positive psychiatric history was relatively common, with 43% known to have had depression in the past. Studies of elderly attempters have found similar high rates of depression; for example, in Pierce's prospective study 93% of the sample were depressed (Pierce 1987), and in that of Nowers (1993) the proportion was 61%, with the highest rates in younger females (65–74 years) and older males (over 75 years). Other psychiatric disorders, such as dementia and schizophrenia, are found less commonly in elderly people who commit or attempt suicide. Some studies have reported increased rates associated with the early and mild stages of dementia, perhaps because individuals have insight into the implications of the diagnosis (Sainsbury 1962, Draper 1994). Alcohol abuse is associated with suicide in old age, but less strongly than in younger age groups (Goodwin 1973, Cattell 1988); those who start abusing alcohol in old age may be at particular risk.

Physical illness

Completed elderly suicides have rates of post-mortem abnormalities considerably in excess of the general elderly population (Barraclough 1971, Cattell 1988), and elderly attempters report similar high rates of significant physical illness (Pierce 1987, Nowers 1993). Physical illness probably contributes to suicide in several ways: as a life event it is a significant cause of depression, either directly because of pain, disfigurement and disability, or indirectly through social isolation and loss of valued social roles. Certain physical disorders or their treatments may cause depression by direct action on the brain, for example cerebral tumours, carcinoma, endocrine disorders, and treatment with drugs such as steroids. Physical illness and depression may have a common antecedent cause, in particular loss events such as bereavement (Parkes et al 1969, Murphy 1982). Finally, physically ill individuals are likely to have greater access to the means of suicide in the form of prescribed medication and over the counter analgesics.

Social isolation

Barraclough (1971) found that for elderly people, living alone was the social variable that had the highest correlation with suicide. Similarly, in Cattell's sample of elderly suicides, nearly two-thirds were living alone and 16% had no contact at all with family or friends (Cattell 1988). At all ages, non-married (i.e. single, divorced and widowed) individuals have a higher rate of suicide than those who are married. In the elderly, widowhood is the commonest reason for not being married, with suicide most likely in the year following the bereavement (Sainsbury 1962, McMahon & Pugh 1965). Men appear to be at greater risk in this respect (Hawton & Fagg 1990). In a study of suicide at all ages, Vogel & Wolfersdorf (1989) pointed out that the breakdown of 'cardinal interpersonal relationships' such as death of relatives and family conflicts were important factors distinguishing elderly from younger suicides.

Socioeconomic status

Another social factor that has been implicated in elderly suicide, particularly in men, is the decline in socioeconomic status following retirement (Solomon 1981). Financial status is certainly an important variable influencing life satisfaction in old age, but the relationship between this and suicide is not simple, as some of the most disadvantaged elderly groups have the lowest suicide rates; for example, rates in elderly blacks in the USA are much lower than those of the whites (MacIntosh 1984). It is likely that it is the decline from pre-retirement levels rather than the absolute level in retirement that is important. Retirement is also an important social ritual marking the marginalisation of elderly people in our culture, and this aspect may also contribute to the increased suicide risk in old age.

Other associated factors

While factors such as depression, physical illness and social isolation are frequently associated with suicide in the elderly, it is nonetheless the case that the great majority of depressed, ill and isolated elderly people do not kill themselves, so what is it that provokes a vulnerable few into taking their own lives? Among those who are depressed, particular cognitions such as intense hopelessness and guilt may be more sensitive indicators of suicide risk than overall severity (Hill et al 1988, Weishaar & Beck 1992). Barraclough (1971) found that complaints of insomnia and hypochondriasis were common among those elderly patients who went on to kill themselves. Among severely depressed patients, those with an agitated, anxious form of the illness are more at risk of suicide than those who are retarded and who may not be able to formulate or initiate an attempt.

Physical illness

In the case of physical illness, it appears that chronic, painful and debilitating conditions are most directly associated with the decision to attempt suicide (Pierce 1987). Cancer carries a particular stigma, and it may be that this leads to increased risk of suicide over and above the illness and disability it causes, particularly in the period following the diagnosis or after a major recurrence.

Personality traits

Long-standing personality traits such as an incapacity for close relationships (Murphy 1982), a tendency to be helpless, hopeless and dependent (Ovenstone & Kreitman 1974, Sendbuehler 1977) and inability to tolerate change or loss of control (Wolff 1969, Ovenstone & Kreitman 1974, Hedlin 1982) may also be important in facilitating suicide in vulnerable individuals.

Biological factors

It is also possible that biological factors play a part. There is some evidence that suicidal acts are associated with reduced levels of 5-hydroxytryptamine (5-HT) in the cerebrospinal fluid (CSF) (Asberg et al 1976, van Praag 1982) and with a reduction in 5-HT2 binding sites in the frontal cortex (Arora & Meltzer 1989). Since there is a fall in 5-HT binding sites in the brain with age, this might render severely affected individuals more vulnerable to acting on suicidal thoughts; however, this interesting hypothesis is far from being proved (Rifai et al 1992). Metabolites of noradrenaline and dopamine have also been found to be reduced in the CSF of elderly depressed suicide attempters

compared to non-suicidal depressed elderly patients and normal controls (Jones et al 1990).

PREDICTING SUICIDE

Suicide is a rare event, even among those elderly people with a full house of the known demographic risk factors. Consequently, much energy and effort has been expended on attempts to identify particular clinical and biological features of at-risk patients that might provide sensitive and specific short-term indicators of suicidal behaviour; the results so far have been disappointing (Balon 1987), with measures of hopelessness perhaps offering the least bad performance in this respect (Beck et al 1990). Suicide is not the end-point of a deterministic biological process, but a behaviour that is highly dependent on circumstance and opportunity, and this is a good reason for believing that any attempt to identify potential suicides by screening populations at risk will always be doomed to failure. This is not to say that suicide is inherently unpredictable; as Pokorny (1983) has pointed out, clinical judgements are not based purely on statistical prediction, but involve detailed, personal knowledge of the individual and can be continuously revised as that knowledge increases. At the individual level, details of history, personal circumstances and behaviour are probably more useful in the short term as indicators of suicidal intent than the presence or absence of the general factors such as depression and physical illness that increase risk at the population level. For example, the particular circumstances known to have precipitated previous suicide attempts in an elderly patient will be useful in judging if and when they are at particular risk in the future. Similarly, anniversaries of important bereavements may be times of high risk for elderly people, as may the period around the individual's birthday (Barraclough & Shepherd 1976). Preoccupation with thoughts of suicide may be communicated indirectly by such activities as sudden changes in religious interest, putting affairs in order, making a will and giving possessions away (Osgood 1982), and those contemplating killing themselves may test the attitudes of those around them by raising the subject in an impersonal way. Direct threats of suicide by elderly people should always be taken seriously.

ASSESSING SUICIDE RISK

It may not be possible to predict with any accuracy who will commit suicide, but general and individual risk factors are of value in identifying patients in whom greater clinical vigilance and more rapid intervention are indicated. Assessment of suicide risk should always form part of the initial and on-going clinical evaluation of elderly depressed patients, and should cover all of the various social, clinical, cognitive and behavioural aspects discussed above (see also Box 9.1). When assessing an elderly patient who has attempted suicide, it is important to distinguish between the medical and psychiatric severity of the bid, as medically trivial overdoses may result from serious suicidal intent if the patient is unaware of the lethal potential of what they have taken. Patients should always be asked about any suicidal thoughts or plans they might have, and the extent to which they are preoccupied with these. Raising the issue will not put the idea into patients' heads, and a positive response to this enquiry is a very valuable indicator of risk. Close family and friends should also be asked about any direct or indirect expressions of suicidal intent that may have been made to them, as the patient may deny suicidal ideation when interviewed by a professional stranger. In patients with marked diurnal variation in mood, it is important to bear in mind that an assessment late in the day may underestimate the intensity of suicidal ideation when they are at their worst in the early hours of the morning. It is worth noting that most suicides occur at this time of day.

Box 9.1 Factors increasing suicide risk in elderly people

- **Older age**
- **Male gender**
- **Depression** Hopelessness
  Pathological guilt and
     self-blame
  Hypochondriasis
  Agitation
  Insomnia
  Weight loss
  No or inadequate treatment
- **Physical illness** Pain
  Chronic disability
- **Alcohol abuse**
- **Social isolation** Single, divorced, widowed
  Bereavement
  Living alone
- **Vulnerable personality** Hopeless/helpless
  Rigid
  Unable to sustain close
     relationships
- **Strong intent** Previous attempts
  Plans
  Threats
- **Recent contact with
  primary care services**

Assessing risk to others

A special consideration when assessing suicide risk is judging the extent to which others may be at risk. Suicide pacts and homicide followed by suicide are rare, but are particularly tragic when they do occur. There are certain circumstances in which this possibility needs to be considered in elderly patients. If the patient has depressive delusions of catastrophe, punishment or damnation involving others (usually the spouse), then suicide may be accompanied by their murder in order to save them from the imagined horrors to come. Another dangerous scenario in this respect can arise if the elderly carer of a demented or disabled spouse develops a terminal illness, becomes depressed, and believes their partner will be abandoned when they die. Suicide pacts may occur if the dominant member of a highly interdependent relationship becomes depressed and suicidal.

INTERVENTION

Whenever possible, depressed patients judged to be at acute risk of suicide should be admitted to hospital for treatment. Sometimes the intensity of the patient's hopelessness is such that they will refuse treatment, and will require formal admission to hospital (in the UK, under the appropriate section of the Mental Health Act, 1983). Compulsory admission is not an option for those rare cases in which the suicidal patient is not suffering from a mental disorder and alternative options will need to be negotiated, such as medical admission in order to improve pain control or home care under the close supervision of family and community health professionals. Hospital admission of suicidal patients is not of itself a guarantee of safety; in-patient suicides do occur, often in the first week of admission before treatment has had time to take effect and the patient is still a relatively unknown quantity. Supervision and observation should be continuous until such time as the critical factors underlying the acute risk of suicide are brought under control. Continuous observation is restrictive and undignified, and this can sometimes be difficult for nursing staff to come to terms with. However, in well-designed in-patient psychiatric units, it should be possible for staff to observe effectively more intimate activities such as toileting and bathing without being unduly obtrusive.

Alleviation of symptoms

Once admitted, it is important to alleviate the most distressing symptoms of the depressive illness as quickly as possible. Since severe anxiety and agitation are powerful provokers of suicidal behaviour, these should be treated immediately with an appropriate anxiolytic or sedative neuroleptic. Benzodiazepines carry the risk that they may disinhibit the patient and so increase the likelihood of patients acting on their suicidal impulses; conversely, neuroleptics may cause akathisia (mental and physical restlessness) and so increase still further the patient's agitation; the patient's individual response to the chosen sedative regime must be carefully monitored. Oral antidepressant treatment should be started at the same time, although this will take some 4–6 weeks to show an effect. Needless to say, the antidepressant chosen should be one that is safe in overdose (see below), since this is the medication that the patient will be discharged with, and perhaps continue to take indefinitely. In patients who are at extreme risk of death by suicide or self-neglect, or who are tormented by accusatory and punitive hallucinations and delusions, a course of electroconvulsive therapy (ECT) is indicated, in order to bring about a more rapid resolution of the depressive symptoms than may be possible with drugs alone. Old age is not a contraindication to ECT, which can be a life-saving procedure in severely depressed elderly patients.

Psychological treatments

Psychological treatments such as cognitive therapy, guided mourning and individual, group and family psychotherapy are also important in the management of the elderly suicidal patient. Cognitive therapy focuses on the content of the depressed patient's 'automatic' thoughts, particularly the hopeless/helpless cognitions, and helps them test these against reality. Guided mourning is a treatment strategy involving both cognitive and behavioural approaches which assists patients in dealing with abnormal or unarticulated grief following a bereavement. The dynamic psychotherapies have traditionally been thought to be less effective in elderly patients, and are rarely offered to this age group in the UK, where access to these forms of treatment is severely rationed in the National Health Service. In fact, an understanding of the psychodynamics of old age is very useful in the management of elderly depressed patients, and can be effectively deployed in a wide range of both brief and longer-term individual and group settings (Martindale 1995). Psychological and psychotherapeutic treatments in elderly suicidal patients are best used in combination with antidepressants and other physical treatments, once the patient has started to recover and can participate fully.

Continuing care

Once the period of acute suicide risk has passed, attention should turn to those factors such as physical disability and social isolation that are putting the patient at chronic risk. The opportunity should be taken while the patient is in hospital to optimise their physical condition, particularly with regard to eyesight, hearing, mobility, continence and freedom from pain. Discharge must be planned to ensure a seamless continuity of care between the hospital and community services; this is particularly important in the case of suicidal patients, since the immediate post-discharge period is known to be a time of increased risk of suicide, even in apparently 'recovered' patients. The key worker who will be responsible for monitoring their treatment and care at home should introduce themselves and establish a therapeutic relationship before the patient leaves hospital; the necessary practical support services such as home helps and meals on wheels should be arranged and ready to start as soon as the patient goes home; and every effort should be made to ensure that they are not returned to the same state of social isolation from which they came. The psychogeriatric day hospital is very valuable in this regard; a period of attendance here following discharge from hospital allows for further monitoring of recovery from depression, and for assessment of and planning for their particular social support needs. A few patients with chronic mental and physical problems may need to be supported by the day hospital indefinitely. When planning the long-term care of suicidal patients, it is important to ensure that antidepressant treatment is continued to prevent relapse and recurrence of the depression. Evidence is accumulating that elderly people need to be maintained on the dose of medication that got them well for at least 2 years and possibly indefinitely in order to obtain the maximum benefit. All patients who fail to comply with medication or who lose contact with services should be actively followed up and encouraged to persist with their treatment plan.

Evidence of the effectiveness of psychiatric interventions in elderly suicidal patients is limited, but some studies of elderly attempters assessed by specialist deliberate self-harm teams and/or admitted for psychiatric care have reported relatively low rates of repeated attempts at follow-up (Pierce 1987, Hawton & Fagg 1990), which suggests that appropriate treatment and support are important in reducing the long-term suicide risk in this particularly vulnerable group. Further research is needed on this important issue.

SUICIDE PREVENTION

The issue of suicide prevention is particularly topical in the UK, given the targets for mental health that have been set by the present government in its White Paper, *The Health of the Nation* (Department of Health 1992). Two of these refer specifically to suicide, and require an overall reduction in the suicide rate by at least 15% by the year 2000, and a reduction in the rate of suicide of severely mentally ill people by at least 33% over the same period. As performance indicators for mental health services, these are of limited value, given the problems inherent in accurate prediction of suicide risk and the overwhelming lack of evidence that any of the post-war advances in psychiatric treatment and care have had any direct impact on trends. However, it is incumbent upon health services to do what they can to minimise suicides among those under their care, and to ensure that their 'product' is as safe as it can be in this respect.

Early identification and adequate treatment of mental disorder

Given the importance of depression as a precursor and final common pathway to suicide, anything that contributes to improvements in its identification and treatment will reduce the population at risk. The role of primary care services is particularly important in this respect, given that many suicides present themselves to their general practitioners shortly before death (Barraclough 1971, Murphy 1975, Cattell 1988), and that a high proportion of all elderly people will be in contact with these services at least once a year. While accurate prediction is not possible, there is room for improvement in the early detection and effective treatment of elderly depressed patients in primary care. The diagnostic performance of GPs with regard to depression in the elderly is variable, and even if it is identified, many are insufficiently enthusiastic about treating it or else do so with inappropriate drugs at subtherapeutic doses for inadequate periods of time (Macdonald 1986). Studies of suicides and self-harm have found that only a minority of those who were depressed were receiving any treatment for this (Cattell 1988). Education has an important role to play here, both at the undergraduate and postgraduate

levels (Michel & Valach 1992), and training packages are being developed for use in general practice as part of the 'Defeat Depression' campaign being run in the UK by the Royal Colleges of Psychiatrists and General Practitioners. In a Swedish study, Rutz et al (1989) showed that following an intensive primary care postgraduate training programme on the diagnosis and management of depression, the suicide rate in the area served by these GPs dropped significantly; however, it should be noted that this study lacked a well-matched control group, and suicide rates were already falling before the introduction of this programme (Sheldon et al 1993).

Not all depressed elderly people come into contact with their GPs, and strategies also need to be developed for identifying and treating them. The mandatory annual health check that is now offered in the UK to all registered patients aged 75 years and over provides one important opportunity for detection, and some practices now include brief depression questionnaires such as the shorter 15-item Geriatric Depression Scale (GDS) (Yesavage & Brink 1983) in their screening packages. It remains to be seen just how efficient these screens are at detecting those with significant and treatable levels of depression. Another strategy is to train those who are frequently in contact with vulnerable elderly people, such as district nurses, home helps, residential care staff, chiropodists and voluntary workers, to be alert to the signs and symptoms of depression in those under their care.

Another group known to health services who would benefit from improved identification and treatment of depression are physically ill elderly in-patients in geriatric and medical wards. A significant minority are depressed (Shuckit et al 1980, Cooper 1987), but this often goes undetected by ward staff, who are understandably preoccupied with the physical aspects of management. The inclusion of a brief screen for depression, such as the GDS, in the routine assessment and monitoring of geriatric in-patients would help improve detection rates (Koenig et al 1988), as would greater collaboration between doctors and nurses in identifying psychiatric morbidity (Bowler et al 1994). Elderly patients who have attempted suicide are clearly a group at extremely high risk of repeat attempts, and all should receive specialist psychiatric assessment before being discharged from in-patient units or the Accident and Emergency (A & E) department (Leeds Consensus Conference 1996). Fortunately, it appears that only a few elderly attempters are discharged from A & E departments in the UK without receiving such an assessment (Owens et al 1991).

A significant proportion of elderly people in residential and nursing home care are depressed, much of which goes undetected and untreated (Ames 1990). They are also at increased risk of suicide for other reasons, such as physical illness and disability, loss of independence, loss of identity, and poor quality of life in bleak and unstimulating surroundings. In fact, rates of officially recorded suicides tend to be lower in the institutionalised elderly, perhaps because active attempts at suicide are limited by the restricted access that residents have to means and opportunity. They may be more likely to commit 'passive suicide' by turning their face to the wall and refusing nourishment and necessary treatment. Staff in these settings need to be more alert to the signs and symptoms of depression, and to be more aware of the impact that the process of care has on the lives of residents, for both good and ill.

Depression in old age is discussed in detail in Chapter 8.

Adequate management of physical distress

The proper management of physical illness also has a part to play in suicide prevention, since the associated pain and disability can drive some elderly people to becoming depressed and suicidal. Effective palliative care in terminal illness is particularly important in this respect; there is no longer any reason why anyone should suffer intolerable pain, and effective control of this would remove the justification and motivation for many of the so-called 'rational' suicides by the terminally ill. It is also important to identify and correct apparently minor disabilities, as these can have a quite disproportionate effect on the quality of life of vulnerable patients. For example, effective chiropody may make the difference between being mobile and having a social life, or being housebound and isolated.

Removal of means

The epidemiological evidence of substantial decline in suicide rates in the elderly following the removal of popular methods such as the toxic component of domestic gas and barbiturates suggests that this is a potentially powerful strategy for suicide prevention. The medical profession has an important role to play in this respect, since self-poisoning is the commonest means of suicide, and many of these deaths involve prescribed drugs. The elderly are considerable consumers of benzodiazepines as tranquillisers and hypnotics, but the benefit they derive from these is often limited, and a reduction in their use in favour of non-pharmacological alternatives such as relaxation training and advice on effective sleep hygiene would do much to remove an increasingly popular component of fatal suicidal self-poisonings.

Antidepressant drugs

Antidepressant drugs are less important as a cause of suicide in the elderly than in younger adults, but in view of the importance of depression as a precondition for suicide in old age, it is vital that its treatment should be safe as well as effective. One implication of improving the detection and treatment of depression in elderly patients is that greater numbers will have access to antidepressant drugs as a means of suicide, and this is another important reason for ensuring that they should be prescribed safely. The older tricyclic antidepressants such as dothiepin and amitriptyline are cheap and effective in adequate doses, and are still commonly prescribed to elderly depressed patients by general practitioners as a first line of treatment. However, they are dangerous when taken in overdose, and since they are often prescribed in sub-therapeutic doses on repeat prescriptions, the result is that many at-risk patients are being given ineffective doses of toxic medication which may eventually be hoarded and used in a suicide attempt. A new generation of antidepressants, such as the serotonin re-uptake inhibitors (SSRIs) and less toxic tricyclics and monoamine oxidase inhibitors such as lofepramine and moclobemide, is now available. They are as effective as the older drugs, are much safer in overdose, have fewer troublesome side-effects that reduce compliance, and there is much less potential for sub-therapeutic prescribing; in this author's opinion they should now be the first choice of treatment for depression at the primary care level. There is still a role for the older tricyclics in the treatment of depression in the elderly, but it is arguable that nowadays they should only be given under expert psychiatric supervision to those in whom the newer, safer drugs are ineffective. There is some evidence that GPs' prescribing practices are now changing in the desired direction (Grace 1994).

Analgesics

There is less scope for doctors to influence the availability of analgesics, since drugs such as paracetamol are available without prescription, and reduction of their suicide potential will require strategies such as packaging in sub-fatal quantities, the use of blister packs and the incorporation of antidotes and emetics in commercial preparations. However, it is important that doctors should be aware of the toxicity of prescribed analgesics such as dextropropoxyphene in overdose, and adjust their prescribing habits accordingly to ensure that patients at risk of suicide do not have the opportunity to accumulate fatal quantities of these drugs.

Improved organisation of services

The efficient detection, treatment and support of elderly patients at risk of suicide depends to a great extent upon an adequate health service infrastructure. Developed psychogeriatric services in the UK operate an advanced form of community psychiatry, providing a readily available, responsive, acceptable service that has close links with primary care, social services, voluntary agencies and the independent providers of residential and domiciliary care to elderly people. There is good case management, with community team workers retaining contact and responsibility for patients as they move through the various elements of the service, and ensuring that those at significant risk are not lost to follow-up.

While community-based services are central to the long-term care and support of elderly patients at risk of suicide, the role of other parts of the service should not be ignored. As community services develop, there is a tendency for in-patient units, especially those in old mental hospitals, to become isolated and under-resourced (Morgan 1992). It is important that the standards and resourcing of such units are maintained, and that their activities are fully integrated into the rest of the service. Likewise, day hospitals have an important role in providing long-term support to depressed elderly patients, and need to be adequately resourced as part of the spectrum of care available.

Clinical audit

Audit is the process by which clinical practice is observed, shortcomings identified and improvements made. All suicides that occur while patients are under the care of psychiatric services should be examined by those involved, not as a fault-finding exercise, but as a process for improving patient care. The multidisciplinary audit of suicides known to services is an important source of information, and is being encouraged in the UK at local and national levels. King and Barraclough (1990) have emphasised the importance of local clinical audit, and have described an audit of suicides in one district catchment area. At the national level, the Department of Health has established a Confidential Enquiry into homicides and suicides by mentally ill people. Suicides are identified at district level, and those health care professionals involved are sent a questionnaire for completion on a voluntary and confidential basis. Suicides not known to psychiatric services should be reviewed at the primary care level, and this is currently being undertaken by local Medical Audit Advisory Groups under the auspices of the Family Health Services Authorities (FHSAs).

CONCLUSIONS

Most of the suicidal behaviour of elderly people is motivated by mental and physical illness. It should never be dismissed or condoned as a rational response to circumstances without every effort being made to identify and treat these, and to address other problems such as social isolation that impair the quality of life in old age.

ACKNOWLEDGEMENT

I should like to thank Professor Richard Farmer for his permission to reproduce Figures 9.1 and 9.2.

REFERENCES

Alvarez A 1971 The savage god: a study of suicide. Penguin Books, London

Ames D 1990 Depression among elderly residents of local authority (Part III) residential homes in one London borough: its nature and the efficacy of intervention. British Journal of Psychiatry 156: 667–675

Arora R C, Meltzer H Y 1989 Serotoninergic measures in the brains of suicide victims: 5-HT2 binding sites in the frontal cortex of suicide victims and control subjects. American Journal of Psychiatry 146: 730–736

Åsberg M, Traskman C, Thoren P 1976 5-HIAA in the cerebrospinal fluid: a biochemical suicide predictor. Archives of General Psychiatry 33: 1193–1197

Balon R 1987 Suicide: can we predict it? Comprehensive Psychiatry 28: 236–241

Barraclough B M 1971 Suicide in the elderly. In: Kay D W K, Walk A (eds) Recent developments in psychogeriatrics. Headley Bros, Ashford

Barraclough B M, Shepherd D M 1976 Birthday blues: the association of birthday with self-inflicted death in the elderly. Acta Psychiatrica Scandinavica 54: 146–149

Beck A T, Brown G, Berchick R J et al 1990 Relationship between hopelessness and ultimate suicide: a replication with psychiatric out-patients. American Journal of Psychiatry 147: 190–195

Bhatia S C, Khan M H, Mediratta R P et al 1987 High risk suicide factors across cultures. International Journal of Social Psychiatry 33: 226–236

Bowler C, Boyle A, Branford M et al 1994 Detection of psychiatric disorders in elderly medical in-patients. Age and Ageing 23: 307–311

Cattell H R 1988 Elderly suicide in London: an analysis of Coroners' inquests. International Journal of Geriatric Psychiatry 3: 251–261

Cooper B 1987 Psychiatric disorders among elderly patients admitted to hospital medical wards. Journal of the Royal Society of Medicine 80: 13–16

Department of Health 1992 The health of the nation. HMSO, London

Draper B 1994 Suicidal behaviour in the elderly. International Journal of Geriatric Psychiatry 9: 655–661

Goodwin D 1973 Alcohol in suicide and homicide. Quarterly Journal of Alcohol 34: 144–156

Grace J 1994 Depression: your views. Geriatric Medicine 24: 44–48

Hawton K, Fagg J 1990 Deliberate self-poisoning and self-injury in older people. International Journal of Geriatric Psychiatry 5: 367–373

Hedlin H 1982 Suicide in America. Norton, New York

Hill R D, Gallagher D, Thompson L W, Ishida T 1988 Hopelessness as a measure of suicidal intent in the depressed elderly. Psychology and Aging 3: 230–232

Jones J S, Stanley B, Mann J J et al 1990 CSF 5-HIAA and HVA concentrations in elderly depressed patients who attempted suicide. American Journal of Psychiatry 147: 1225–1227

King E, Barraclough L B M 1990 Violent death and mental illness: a study of a single catchment area over eight years. British Journal of Psychiatry 156: 714–720

Koenig H G, Meador K G, Cohen H J et al 1988 Self-rated depression scales and screening for major depression in the older hospitalized patient with medical illness. Journal of the American Geriatrics Society 36: 699–706

Leeds Consensus Conference 1996 The general hospital management of adult deliberate self-harm: a consensus statement of minimum standards for service provision. (in press)

Lindesay J 1986 Trends in self-poisoning in the elderly: 1974–1983. International Journal of Geriatric Psychiatry 1: 37–43

Macdonald A 1986 Do general practitioners 'miss' depression in elderly patients? British Medical Journal 292: 1365–1367

MacIntosh J L 1984 Components of the decline in elderly suicide: suicide among the young-old and old-old by race and sex. Death Education 8: 113–124

McMahon B, Pugh T F 1965 Suicide in the widowed. American Journal of Epidemiology 81(23): 23–31

Martindale B 1995 Psychological treatments: (2) psychodynamic approaches. In: Lindesay J (ed) Neurotic

disorders in the elderly. Oxford University Press, Oxford (in press)

Mental Health Act 1983. HMSO, London

Merrill J, Owens J 1986 Ethnic differences in self-poisoning: a comparison with Asian and white groups. British Journal of Psychiatry 148: 708–712

Michel K, Valach L 1992 Suicide prevention: spreading the gospel to general practitioners. British Journal of Psychiatry 160: 757–760

Morgan H G 1992 Suicide prevention: hazards in the fast lane to community care. British Journal of Psychiatry 306: 1626–1627

Murphy G E 1975 The physician's responsibility for suicide. Annals of Internal Medicine 82: 301–309

Murphy E 1982 Social origins of depression in old age. British Journal of Psychiatry 141: 135–142

Murphy E, Lindesay J, Grundy E 1986 60 years of suicide in England and Wales: a cohort study. Archives of General Psychiatry 43: 969–976

Nowers M 1993 Deliberate self-harm in the elderly: a survey of one London borough. International Journal of Geriatric Psychiatry 8: 609–614

Nowers M, Irish M 1988 Trends in the reported rates of suicide by self-poisoning in the elderly. Journal of the Royal College of General Practitioners 38: 67–69

Osgood N J 1982 Suicide in the elderly: are we heeding the warnings? Postgraduate Medicine 72: 123–130

Ovenstone I, Kreitman N 1974 Two syndromes of suicide. British Journal of Psychiatry 124: 336–345

Owens D, Dennis M, Jones S et al 1991 Self-poisoning patients discharged from Accident and Emergency: risk factors and outcome. Journal of the Royal College of Physicians 25: 218–222

Parkes C M, Benjamin B, Fitzgerald R G 1969 Broken heart: a statistical study of increased mortality among widowers. British Medical Journal i: 740–743

Pierce D 1987 Deliberate self-harm in the elderly. International Journal of Geriatric Psychiatry 2: 105–110

Pokorny A D 1983 Prediction of suicide in psychiatric patients. Archives of General Psychiatry 40: 249–257

Raleigh V S, Bulusu L, Balarajan R 1990 Suicide among immigrants from the Indian subcontinent. British Journal of Psychiatry 156: 46–50

Rao A V 1991 Suicide in the elderly: a report from India. Crisis 12: 33–39

Rifai A H, Reynolds C F, Mann J J 1992 Biology of elderly suicide. Suicide and Life-Threatening Behaviour 22: 48–61

Rutz W, Walinder J, Eborhard G et al 1989 An education program on depressive disorders for general practitioners on Gotland: background and evaluation. Acta Psychiatrica Scandinavica 79: 19–26

Sainsbury P 1962 Suicide in later life. Gerontologica Clinica 4: 161–170

Sendbuehler J M 1977 Suicide and attempted suicide among the aged. Journal of the American Geriatrics Society 25: 245–248

Sheldon T A, Freemantle N, House A et al 1993 Examining the effectiveness of treatments for depression in general practice. Journal of Mental Health 2: 141–156

Shuckit M A, Miller P L, Berman J 1980 The three year course of psychiatric problems in a geriatric population. Journal of Clinical Psychiatry 41: 27–32

Solomon K 1981 The depressed patient: social antecedents of psychopathological changes in the elderly. Journal of the American Geriatrics Society 29: 14–18

Thompson P, Itzin C , Abendstern M 1990 I don't feel old: the experience of later life. Oxford University Press, Oxford

van Praag H M 1982 Depression, suicide and the metabolism of serotonin in the brain in affective disorders. Journal of Affective Disorders 4: 275–290

Vogel R, Wolfersdorf M 1989 Suicide and mental illness in the elderly. Psychopathology 22: 202–207

Weishaar M E, Beck A T 1992 Hopelessness and suicide. International Review of Psychiatry 4: 177–184

Wetzel R D, Reich T, Murphy G E et al 1987 The changing relationship between age and suicide rates: cohort effect, period effect or both? Psychiatric Developments 3: 179–218

Wolff K 1969 Depression and suicide in the geriatric patient. Journal of the American Geriatrics Society 17: 668–673

Woodbury M A, Manton K G, Blazer D 1988 Trends in US suicide mortality rates 1968 to 1982: race and sex differences in age period and cohort components. International Journal of Epidemiology 17: 356–362

Yesavage J A, Brink T L 1983 Development and validation of a geriatric depression screening scale: a preliminary report. Journal of Psychiatric Research 17: 37–49

RECOMMENDED READING

Jacoby R, Oppenheimer C (eds) 1991 Psychiatry in the elderly. Oxford University Press, Oxford. *This comprehensive and extensively-referenced textbook is an excellent starting point for those wishing to explore further any of the clinical issues raised in this chapter.*

Katona C 1994 Depression in old age. Wiley, Chichester. *This monograph provides a useful up-to-date review of what is currently known about depression in the elderly.*

Lester D, Tallmer M (eds) 1994 Now I lay me down: suicide in the elderly. The Charles Press, Philadelphia. *This is one of the few books devoted to this subject, and it contains much useful information, particularly on therapeutic interventions.*

Murphy E (ed) 1986 Affective disorders in the elderly. Churchill Livingstone, London. *Although somewhat out of date, this book is valuable background reading for those interested in depression and suicide in the elderly.*

Stillion J M, McDowell E E, May J H 1989 Suicide across the life span. Hemisphere Publishing Corporation, New York. *This is an introductory text for those in the 'helping professions', which contains a great deal of useful factual and illustrative information about suicide at all ages.*

10

Acute and sub-acute confusional states (delirium) in later life

E Jane Byrne

INTRODUCTION

'Confusion, this ambiguous and overworked, term ... should not be used as if it referred to a diagnosis.' (Lipowski 1992, p. 41).

This indictment of the use of the word 'confusion' may startle some readers as it is so commonly used in relation to mental state abnormality in older people. I agree with Lipowski (1990) for several reasons: first, every health or helping profession thinks they know what 'confusion' means but when you (or researchers) ask them, they each mean different things (Simpson 1984); secondly, there are well defined and well validated syndromes of global cognitive impairment in old age delirium (acute or sub-acute) and dementia (chronic) which have different morbidity and mortality (Rabins & Folstein 1982); thirdly, the ambiguity and lack of precision inherent in the word itself are often reflected in the thought processes of those who use it (without qualification). Lishman (1987, p. 4) defines 'confusion' as 'thinking with less than accustomed clarity'. So defined, 'confusion' is a feature of many syndromes of late life and may be related to the ageing process itself.

'Confusional state' therefore simply describes those syndromes in which 'confusion' – thinking with less than accustomed clarity – may be a feature. When one qualifies the term 'confusional state' with the word acute, it implies a confusional state with a sudden onset. Used in this way 'acute confusional state' has become synonymous with delirium, although there is no logical reason for this as consistent with the above would be the use of 'acute confusional state' to describe depression in old age.

Furthermore, the term 'acute confusional state' has a plethora of synonyms, including acute organic psychosis, acute brain failure, acute organic brain syndrome. This terminological confusion would be

---

Box 10.1 DSM-IV – diagnostic criteria for delirium (APA 1994)

A. Disturbance of consciousness (i.e. reduced clarity of awareness of the environment) with reduced ability to focus, sustain, or shift attention.

B. A change in cognition (such as memory deficit, disorientation, language disturbance) or the development of a perceptual disturbance that is not better accounted for by a pre-existing, established, or evolving dementia.

C. The disturbance develops over a short period of time (usually hours to days) and tends to fluctuate during the course of the day.

D. There is evidence from the history, physical examination, or laboratory findings that the disturbance is caused by the direct physiological consequences of a general medical condition.

Box 10.2 ICD-10 – diagnostic criteria for delirium (WHO 1991)

A. There is clouding of consciousness, i.e. reduced clarity of awareness of the environment, with reduced ability to focus, sustain or shift attention.

B. Disturbance of cognition is manifest by both:
(1) impairment of immediate recall and recent memory, with relatively intact remote memory
(2) disorientation in time, place or person.

C. At least one of the following psychomotor disturbances is present:
(1) rapid, unpredictable shifts from hypoactivity to hyperactivity
(2) increased reaction time
(3) increased or decreased flow of speech
(4) enhanced startle reaction.

D. There is disturbance of sleep or of the sleep-wake cycle, manifest by at least one of the following:
(1) insomnia, which in severe cases may involve total sleep loss, with or without daytime drowsiness or reversal of the sleep-wake cycle
(2) nocturnal worsening of symptoms
(3) disturbing dreams and nightmares, which may continue as hallucinations or illusions after awakening.

E. Symptoms have rapid onset and show fluctuations over the course of the day.

F. There is objective evidence from history, physical and neurological examination or laboratory tests of an underlying cerebral or systemic disease (other than psychoactive substance-related) that can be presumed to be responsible for the clinical manifestations in criteria A–D.

---

greatly eased if reference were made to current nosological systems (such as DSM-IV and ICD-10) where precise descriptions of mental state changes in different syndromes are given. This chapter will consider delirium as defined in DSM-IV (American Psychiatric Association 1994) and ICD-10 (World Health Organization 1991) in old people in detail (see Boxes 10.1 and 10. 2).

THE SIZE OF THE PROBLEM

Delirium is very common in old people, especially in those in hospital or residential care. Studies of old people living in the community are rare and show low prevalence (<1%, Folstein et al 1991). In hospital it has been estimated that a quarter of old people will suffer from a delirium at some point in their admission, the prevalence in several hospital studies ranging from 13–61% (Byrne 1994), the highest rates being seen in old people with hip fractures. Prevalence in residential homes is less well defined but is probably around 6% of residents at any one time.

That delirium is a serious condition is evidenced by the high mortality rate in delirious old people which, in recent careful studies, ranges from 15–40%. Delirium is also associated with significant morbidity, most studies showing that delirious old people have serious physical illness (often multiple) and have prolonged hospital stays compared to non-delirious old people (Francis et al 1990)

DIAGNOSIS

Despite the fact that delirium is a common and serious condition, it is quite frequently unrecognised. The reason for this is complex, partly due to ageism in health professions (and society) – old people being expected to be 'confused' – partly to the altered presentation of many syndromes in old people, such that delirium may be less florid than in younger patients, and partly due to lack of knowledge on the symptoms and progress of the syndrome. Rockwood et al (1994) have shown that a simple educational programme for junior doctors increases the recognition of delirium and, most importantly, improves the outcome for the patients.

Several rating scales for delirium now exist for use by various health professions, such as the scales of Trzepacz et al (1988), Johnson et al (1990), and Inouye et al (1990). One of the most important features of delirium is the changeability of the symptoms over time; this may explain why cross-sectionally administered cognitive screening tests are not highly sensitive for delirium. The rating scales above all require observations over time. A simple bed-side test of cognitive function, which may be repeatedly administered and graphically illustrates the changing cognitive abilities over time, is the clock-drawing test (Schulman et al 1986), which involves asking the person to draw a clock face within a pre-drawn circle; this test has been evaluated on busy medical wards (Huntzinger et al 1992). Diagnostic criteria most widely used are those of DSM III-R (now DSM-IV) and ICD-10 (see Boxes 10.1 and 10.2). A useful 'bedside' definition is that of Lipowski (1990, p. 490), that delirium is 'a transient organic mental syndrome of acute onset and featuring concurrent disturbance of consciousness, a global cognitive and attentional disorder, reduced or increased psychomotor activity and a disrupted sleep–wake cycle'.

SYMPTOMS AND COURSE

Acute onset in reference to delirium refers to hours or a few days. In most cases, before the onset of the full-blown syndrome there are warning symptoms (a prodrome), the features of which are listed in Box 10.3.

In people aged 65 years or more, the duration of delirium has recently been studied. Mean durations in such studies of hospital patients range between 19 and 21 days (Thomas et al 1988, Koponen & Reikkinen 1993). There is, however, a wide range of duration; some patients are delirious for up to 3 months.

The clinical features of delirium are shown in summary form in Box 10.4. Because of the changing nature of the syndrome these features are not always present in one person, at one time. The time when all the symptoms of delirium is most likely to be seen is during the night.

Box 10.3 Features of the prodrome of delirium (after Lipowski 1990)

Poor concentration
Difficulty in thinking
Feelings of restlessness and anxiety
Irritability
Hypersensitivity to light and sound
Drowsiness, insomnia
Vivid dreams or nightmares
General malaise
Tiredness or fatiguability
Occasional perceptual abnormalities

Box 10.4 Clinical features of delirium (derived from DSM-IV and ICD-10)

Acute onset – over hours or a few days
Fluctuation over time – within or a day, from day to night (often symptoms worse at night), from day to day
Reduced attention – inability to maintain, focus or shift attention to external stimuli
Disorganised thought – reduced comprehension, perplexity, rambling, irrelevant or incoherent speech
Altered perceptions – misinterpretations, illusions, perceptual distortions, hallucinations
Altered psychomotor activity – hypoactivity or hyperactivity, often shifting from one to another, increased reaction time
Altered sleep-wake cycle – insomnia, sleep-reversal, daytime drowsiness, disturbing dreams
Disturbance of emotion – anxiety, depression, euphoria, apathy, irritability, fear
Altered memory – reduced recall of recent events, reduced new learning, lesser impairment of recall for remote events
Impaired orientation – time, place, and rarely for person

Attention

Disordered attention has been given greater prominence in DSM systems over the years and now is required for diagnosis. Patients have difficulty in directing attention, for example they may appear to have difficulty concentrating on what one says to them and are easily distracted by extraneous stimuli. They have difficulty sustaining their attention and may seem to drift in and out of a conversation. They have difficulty in shifting their attention appropriately; one sometimes gets a correct answer to a question which is then repeated for subsequent questions (perseveration). One reason for the increased importance ascribed to disorders of attention in delirium may be the difficulty in defining or measuring change in consciousness level, which used to have pre-eminence. Altered consciousness is easy to adduce when one observes patients muttering to themselves, plucking at their clothes and showing an exaggerated startle response, but is less easy in patients who lie or sit quietly and are apathetically out of touch with their surroundings.

Activity

The speed of thought (psycho) and movement (motor) may be either increased or decreased in delirium. It is perhaps easy to see why in hospitals (not the most psychologically sophisticated environments) the overactive person is likely to be seen as disturbed or at least as non-conforming, and thus more likely to be noticed.

Sleep–wake cycle

Insomnia, sometimes with vivid dreams, is a feature of the prodrome and of the full syndrome. In severe cases there may be total reversal of the normal day-time alertness and night-time sleep. Dreaming is often intense and may be followed by day-time hallucinations or persistence of a dream-like quality to awareness. In experimental delirium (induced by anticholinergic agents) normal subjects showed altered sleep with reduction in REM sleep (rapid eye movement or dream sleep) (Ital & Fink 1966). Day-time drowsiness is frequently present.

Altered perceptions

Hallucinations (which may occur in any sensory modality) as a feature of organic mental states are so dramatically different to normal human experience that most observers (if aware of them) might conclude there is something wrong. Equally common in delirium are a group of perceptual experiences which are more closely related to 'real life'. For example at night, in poor light and when half-asleep, a normal person might, for a moment, see an article of clothing hanging over the chair as if it were a burglar crouched ready to spring. An instant later, when more awake, the correct interpretation is placed on the perception. Delirious people have great difficulty in re-interpreting perceptual distortions or misidentifications. When they are able to do so we say they have had an illusion; the experience had an 'as if' quality.

Altered emotion

Altered emotions are part of the prodrome and the full-blown syndrome of delirium. Anxiety, both psychic (a fearfulness which may be focused or generalised) and somatic (physical manifestations such as increased heart rate, sweating palms, dry mouth) is usual. Depression is also common, but less common is elation or euphoria. Characteristically these emotional states are rarely sustained throughout the whole course of the delirium. A delirious person may be weeping bitterly on one occasion and apathetic and unconcerned on another. When present, however, they may be very intense and have been associated with suicidal ideation or attempts.

PREDISPOSING OR RISK FACTORS

Increasing age is one of the most important predisposing factors for the development of delirium (Lipowski 1983, Erkinjuntti et al 1986). The underlying mechanism(s) are unknown but may include increased prevalence of degenerative brain disease, reduction in cholinergic transmitters in normal ageing, multiple disease states and impaired peripheral senses.

Alzheimer's disease and other causes of dementia predispose to delirium (Erkinjuntti et al 1986); as all causes of dementia are commoner in old people this is an important predisposing factor. Levkoff et al (1988) identified five risk factors associated with delirium in hospital patients: urinary tract infection, low serum albumin, raised white count, protein and urea (the latter three in the absence of preceding factors).

Whittaker (1989) suggests that delirium following surgery in old people is associated with the following risk factors: age, previous drug or alcohol abuse and prolonged operations. Also, premedications before surgery that include anticholinergic drugs that cross the blood–brain barrier, such as atrophine and hyoscine (Platzer 1988). Lipowski (1990) suggests that four factors may facilitate delirium in old people (increase the severity and possibly prolong its course): psychosocial stress, sleep deprivation, sensory underload or overload and immobilisation. Perhaps the most famous instances of these facilitating factors are the putative increased incidence of deliriums in patients undergoing eye surgery, and intensive-care 'syndrome' (Wilson 1972).

SUB-TYPES OF DELIRIUM

The early intensive studies by Engel & Romano (1959) suggested that delirium was of two types, the hypoalert-hypoactive type and the hyperalert-hyperactive type. Studies more recently confirm the presence of the two types in hospital populations but suggest they are not mutually exclusive, some patients shifting between the two states, whereas others have a more sustained course in one type or another (Liptzin et al 1992). Sub-acute confusional state is of less acute onset and less florid clinical picture, usually of the hypoalert-hypoactive type.

DIFFERENTIAL DIAGNOSIS

The main differential diagnosis of delirium is the dementia syndrome. There are a few causes of dementia which have an acute onset, including stroke and infection, but most causes of dementia have a gradual onset over months or years and marked impairment of attention or consciousness is not a feature of most dementias. The two syndromes may coexist and dementia is a predisposing factor for delirium.

Occasionally mood disorders may mimic delirium, especially hypomania and, more rarely, severe depression. Severe depression is, however, more likely to mimic dementia than delirium.

CAUSES OF DELIRIUM IN OLD PEOPLE

The reader is referred to the reviews cited in the recommended reading (Liston 1982, Beresin 1988, MacDonald et al 1989) for complete listings. Delirium may be caused by many different diseases and metabolic imbalances. The commonest causes in old people are cerebrovascular disease, carcinomatosis, drugs, infection, cardiovascular disease (especially heart failure), metabolic disorders (including disorders of fluid or electrolyte balance, renal failure) and anoxia (from whatever cause) (Royal College of Physicians 1981, Lipowski 1992). In old people the cause of delirium may be multifactorial. Francis et al (1990) found more than one cause for delirium in 44% of delirious old people in hospital. This is perhaps not surprising as old people in hospital are more likely than not to have more than one medical problem. This same study found that three factors predicted the emergence of being dependent in activities of everyday living: being cognitively impaired, being severely unwell and being admitted as an emergency. Of these factors, being cognitively impaired on admission requires further discussion.

Aggravation of pre-existing cognitive impairment

The abnormal brain is more sensitive to changes in its homeostatic milieu than the normal brain. Such changes may include sensory impairment or deprivation, metabolic abnormalities, difficulties with thermo regulation and environmental changes. Thus someone who has had a stroke, who is not demented, but who has some impaired cognition (e.g. dysphasia), is at increased risk of delirium when they develop pneumonia. Such a person is also at risk of an aggravation of their dysphasia or other cognitive difficulties which is often noted as an 'increase in confusion', but which is not delirium. This distinction is important to identify and to understand, so it can be managed appropriately, but does not necessarily increase mortality.

A list of such aggravating factors is given in Table 10.1.

It is important to note that the aggravation may take the form of a change in behaviour. Thus discomfort of constipation, for example, may be shown by the development of restless wandering. One should always be on the alert for dis-ease (discomfort) as well as disease!

INVESTIGATIONS

Most experts are agreed as to which investigations are the most useful or should be routine for delirium in old people (Beresin 1988, Lindesay et al 1990, Lipowski 1992). They are:

- full blood count
- erythrocyte sedimentation rate
- blood chemistry – electrolytes, calcium
- phosphate, liver function tests and glucose
- serology for syphilis
- electroencephalogram
- thyroid function tests
- urea and creatinine.

Other tests may be required in a selective fashion and are usually suggested by the results from the above or the previous medical history.

Table 10.1 Factors which may aggravate pre-existing cognitive impairment in old people (adapted from Byrne & Arie 1990)

Discomfort	Pain, wetness, constipation, corns
Environment	Excessive noise, extremes of temperature, change in the environment (e.g. a move, holiday)
Sensory impairment	Sight, hearing
Alcohol	Even small amounts
Physical illness	In any system, of any severity
Treatment	Drugs, especially cholinergic agents
Psychological factors	Anxiety, depression, psychotic experiences, anger, frustration, bereavement, insight into failing cognition

MANAGEMENT

The basic principle of management is to identify and treat the underlying cause whilst providing supportive measures (environmental, fluid, nutrition, comfort and safety). The environment is important in the management of the delirious patients but has received little research attention. It must be remembered that environmental measures relate to the core features of the syndrome. For example, delirious patients have problems with arousal and so the level of stimulation must be adjusted according to their level of arousal; highly aroused patients benefit from quiet environments, but not too quiet. The balance can be difficult to achieve but is possible as work on intensive care units has shown (Tesar & Stern 1986). Patients with delirium are often fearful and need reassurance. A good model is the way experienced handlers deal with frightened animals – they frequently repeat themselves and reassure in a firm audible voice.

Delirious patients, especially those who are hyperalert and hyperactive, can easily become dehydrated. Considerable ingenuity is sometimes required to ensure adequate hydration as over-aroused patients do not easily tolerate intravenous drips. Fluids may have to be given opportunistically, in periods of relative lucidity rather than adhering to standard ward regimes. Sometimes, presenting very small quantities (a medicine glass of about 10 ml) frequently is more successful than larger quantities less frequently. Nutritional requirements likewise require ingenuity in presentation. Liquid nutritional supplements are useful in this regard. B complex vitamins may need to be added to the fluid and nutritional regime. If sedation is required, haloperidol is the drug of choice (Lipowski 1990, Taylor & Lewis 1993). Some elderly delirious patients will respond to low doses (0.5 mg twice or three times in 24 hours); others require more. This author has never needed to give as high a dose as 5–10 mg in 24 hours although this is recommended by some. It is preferable to avoid hypnotics in delirious patients. Chlormethiazole is useful as an adjunct for severe sleep disruption.

Psychological interventions are infrequently described and little researched; there is some evidence they may be of benefit (Richeimer 1987). One of the most important is listening to the patient: in amongst their disjointed communications are nuggets of important information which may guide the intervention. If fear is expressed, reassurance and explanation, which may require frequent repetition, will often substantially reduce arousal or anxiety levels. The delirious patient in hospital shares the common anxieties of their non-delirious fellows, including fear of dependency as well as worries about their illness and its likely outcome, their family or their pets, who is caring for them, and past events (traumatic experiences, perceived misconduct, etc.).

Reorientation is also helpful but, as with most interventions, needs repetition, and often succeeds best at a personal level. Having one nurse who always introduces himself and, when appropriate, mentions the name of the hospital, is helpful to a delirious old person. Consistency of staff will also increase the likelihood of the identification of delirium in the first place.

Acknowledging the intensity of affect associated with psychiatric experiences such as hallucinations is more helpful to the old person than dismissing these experiences as unreal or a product of their imagination. If a delirious old person points to the insects crawling on the bed, ask how they feel and acknowledge these feelings.

Attention to the potential aggravating factors listed in Table 10.1 is always helpful. Changing the battery in the hearing aid can be a useful treatment for paranoid ideas. Restlessness may be reduced by the relief of pain or constipation.

Most of the interventions described above require time, which may be in short supply in busy wards. The lack of such an investment of time will, however, not only worsen the patient's state but inevitably require more staff time later in the course of the condition.

Delirium is a serious, common but often unrecognised syndrome in old people. Early recognition may influence morbidity and mortality.

REFERENCES

American Psychiatric Association 1994 DSM-IV. American Psychiatric Association, Washington DC

Beresin E V 1988 Delirium in the elderly. Journal of Geriatric Psychiatry and Neurology 1: 127–143

Byrne E J, Arie T 1990 Coping with dementia in the elderly. In: Lawson D H (ed) Current medicine 1. Churchill Livingstone, Edinburgh

Byrne E J 1994 Confusional states in older people. Edward Arnold, London

Engel G L, Romano J 1959 Delirium: a syndrome of cerebral insufficiency. Journal of Chronic Disease 9: 260–277

Erkinjuntti T, Wikstraun J, Polo J, Aetio L 1986 Dementia among medical in-patients evaluation of 2000 consecutive admissions. Archives of Internal Medicine 146: 1923–1926

Folstein M F, Bassett S S, Romanoski A J, Nestadt G 1991 The epidemiology of delirium in the community: the Eastern Baltimore mental health survey. International Psychogeriatrics 3: 169–176

Francis J, Martin D, Wishwan Kapoor W N 1990 A prospective study of delirium in hospitalised elderly. Journal of the American Medical Association 263: 1097–1101

Huntzinger J A, Rosse R B, Schwartz B L, Ross L A, Deutsch S I 1992 Clock drawing in the screening assessment of cognitive impairment in an ambulatory care setting: a preliminary report. General Hospital Psychiatry 14: 142–144

Inouye S K, Van Dyck C H, Alesi C A, Baltan S, Seigal A P, Horwitz R I 1990 Clarifying confusion: the confusion assessment method – a new method of the detection of delirium. Annal International Medicine 113: 941–948

Ital T, Fink M 1966 Anticholinergic drug-induced delirium: experimental modification, quantitative EEG and behavioural correlations. Journal of Nervous and Mental Diseases 143: 492–507

Johnson J C, Gottlieb G L, Sullivan E et al 1990 Using DSM-III criteria to diagnose delirium in the elderly general medical patients. Journal of Gerontology 45: 113–119

Koponen H J, Riekkinen P J 1993 A prospective study of delirium in elderly patients admitted to a psychiatric hospital. Journal of Neurology, Neurosurgery and Psychiatry 52: 980–985

Levkoff S E, Safron C, Cleary P D, Gallop J, Phillips R S 1988 Identification of factors associated with the diagnosis of delirium in elderly hospitalised patients. Journal of the American Geriatric Society 36: 1099–1104

Lindesay J, Macdonald A, Starke I 1990 The management of delirium. In: Lindesay J, MacDonald A, Starke I (eds) Delirium in the elderly. Oxford University Press, Oxford

Lipowski Z J 1990 Delirium: acute confusional states. Oxford University Press, New York

Lipowski Z J 1983 Transient cognitive disorders (delirium, acute confusional states) in the elderly. American Journal of Psychiatry 140: 1426–1436

Lipowski Z J 1992 Delirium and impaired consciousness In: Evans J G, Williams T F (eds) Oxford test book of geriatric medicine. Oxford University Press, Oxford

Liptzin B, Levkoff S E, Cleary P D et al 1992 Diagnostic criteria for delirium: an empirical study. American Journal of Psychiatry 148: 454–457

Lishman W A 1987 Organic psychiatry. Blackwell, Oxford

Platzer H 1988 A study into the causes of post-operative confusion in the elderly. Unpublished MSc Thesis, Kings College, London

Rabins P V, Folstein M F 1982 Delirium and dementia: diagnostic criteria and fatality rates. British Journal of Psychiatry 140: 149–153

Richeimer S H 1987 Psychological intervention in delirium. Postgrad Med. 81: 173–180

Rockwood K, Cosway S, Stolee P et al 1994 Increasing the recognition of delirium in elderly patients. Journal of the American Geriatric Society 42: 252–256

Royal College of Physicians 1981 Organic mental impairment in the elderly. Journal of the Royal College of Physicians 15: 141–167

Schulman K I, Shedletsky R, Silver I L 1986 The challenge of time: clock drawing and cognitive function in the elderly. International Journal of Geriatric Psychiatry 1: 135–140

Simpson C T 1984 Doctors and nurses use of the word confused. British Journal of Psychiatry 145: 441–443

Taylor D, Lewis S 1993 Delirium. Journal of Neurology, Neurosurgery and Psychiatry 56: 742–751

Tesar G E, Stern T A 1986 Evaluation and treatment of agitation in the intensive care unit. Journal of Intensive Care 1: 137–148

Thomas R I, Cameron D J, Fahs M C 1988 A prospective study of delirium and prolonged hospital stay. Archives of General Psychiatry 45: 937–940

Trzepacz P T, Baker R W, Greenhouse J 1988 A symptom rating scale for delirium. Psychiatry Research 23: 89–97

Whittaker J J 1989 Postoperative confusion in the elderly. International Journal of Geriatric Psychiatry 4: 321–326

Wilson L M 1972 Intensive care delirium. Arch. Intern. Med. 130: 225–226

World Health Organization 1991 ICD-10 Classification of mental and behavioural disorders. WHO, Churchill Livingstone, Edinburgh

RECOMMENDED READING

Lipowski Z J Delirium: acute confusional states. Oxford University Press, Oxford. *The most complete and authoritative work on delirium, covers the history of the concept, pathophysiology, causation, treatment and management.*

Byrne E J 1994 Confusional states in older people. Edward Arnold, London. *A paperback book written for the general reader, includes chapters on dementia as well as delirium.*

Lindesay J, MacDonald A, Starke I 1990 Delirium in the elderly. Oxford University Press, Oxford. *A book midway between the above in terms of complexity. Covers the same general ground as Lipowski, but in less detail.*

Liston E H 1982 Delirium in the aged. Psychiatric Clinics of North America 5: 49–66. *A good general review of delirium in old people.*

Beresin E V 1988 Delirium in the elderly. Journal of Geriatric Psychiatry and Neurology 1: 127–143. *Similar to the above.*

MacDonald A J D, Simpson A, Jenkins D 1989 Delirium in the elderly: a review and a suggestion for a research programme. International Journal of Psychiatry 4: 311–319. *A clinical appraisal of delirium in old people, challenges some long-held management strategies and suggests a programme of further research. Thought provoking.*

11

Dementia

Trevor Adams

The past 20 years have seen many developments in the ways in which dementia is conceived and understood and the introduction of many innovations in the care of dementing people and their families. Today we see continued interest in biological theories and explanations of dementia being complemented by models of dementia which emphasise the impact of psychosocial factors and those which highlight the effects of dementia on family carers. The first part of this chapter presents an overview of models of dementia and touches on the implications of these models for clinical practice. Readers are directed to relevant chapters in this volume for detailed discussion of brain changes in dementia and care practices. In the second part of the chapter we turn to discuss some practical issues in the family care of dementing people: assessment, helping families in crisis – including those prematurely grieving their loss and those in which there is high expressed emotion – and abuse of dementing people by caregivers.

HISTORICAL ORIGINS

First we consider the historical origins of the term 'dementia'. The concept of dementia is not fixed but has evolved and changed over time. 200 years ago, dementia was neither specifically defined in terms of cognitive deficit nor associated with a particular age group (Berrios 1987) and even now there is lack of agreement as to exactly what clinical features constitute 'dementia'. As we shall see later, there are differences of opinion over such issues as whether the term 'subcortical dementia' should be used and the importance of diffuse Lewy body disease as a type of dementia.

Berrios and Freeman (1991) trace the origin of dementia to the Latin works of Lucretius where it meant 'being out of one's mind', and note the *Oxford*

English Dictionary's earliest use in English as 1644. The term was apparently in common use in the early part of the 18th century since it was included in the 1726 edition of Blanchard's popular *Physical Dictionary* where dementia was considered to be equivalent to 'anoea' or 'extinction of the imagination or judgement'. Although at this time dementia was understood in broad terms, Berrios (1987) argues that throughout the 18th century the concept became more precisely defined. By the mid 19th century, the clinical boundaries of dementia marked it off clearly from other psychiatric phenomena. Important factors in this process were the development of knowledge about morbid anatomy, the reaffirmation in psychology of the importance of intellectual functions and the view that senility was an exaggerated form of ageing. Dementia was thus set within a cognitive paradigm which emphasised intellectual and memory impairment and was linked with the idea of social incompetence. It was believed that psychosocial incompetence resulted from intellectual failure and was related to degeneration theory – the belief that acquired social perversions (such as alcoholism) caused behavioural and physical stigmata which would be passed to later generations to form melancholia, mania and finally, dementia.

The concept of dementia was developed further by Alzheimer, who published a paper describing the case of a 51-year-old woman who presented with progressive cognitive impairment, hallucinations, delusions and marked psychosocial incompetence (Alzheimer 1907). On post-mortem her brain showed atrophy, arteriosclerotic changes, senile plaques and neurofibrillary tangles. The case was quickly taken up by Kraepelin as illustrating a new disease (Berrios 1990). The concept of dementia was further refined and arteriosclerotic dementia was distinguished from Alzheimer's original notion. These developments laid the foundation for understanding dementia up until the 1970s. At this time, new technology, including the electron microscope and computerised tomography, opened the way for research that gave credibility to the biomedical perspective of dementia. Kitwood (1987) argues that this research closed, temporarily at least, all discussion concerning the contribution of psychosocial factors in the causation of dementia. More particularly, it led to expansion of the concept of Alzheimer's disease to include both young and old people and the use of the term multi-infarct dementia to describe what had previously been called by the medical profession 'arteriosclerotic dementia'.

Alongside this dominant medical model there developed a subordinate, psychosocial model of dementia. Gilhooly (1984) describes various studies that clearly identify psychosocial factors which play a central role in the development of dementia. She cites Gruenthal (1927) and Rothschild (1937, 1942), who both claimed that brain damage alone could not account for the dementing process, Wilson (1955), who suggested that dementia might be viewed as a psychosomatic disease, and Williams et al (1942), who proposed a relationship between poor social lives and social skills and the development of dementia.

There has been a recent resurgence of interest in psychosocial models of dementia for a number of reasons. First, a powerful critique of what has become known as the 'biomedicalisation of dementia' has developed against a background of general suspicion against the activity of science and medicine in society. The critique has been carried out at various levels. At an empirical level, Kitwood (1993) argues that the assertion of the biomedical model, that there is a correspondence between brain damage and behaviour in people with dementia, is untenable. At a sociopolitical level, Fox (1989) has argued that the way in which Alzheimer's disease has been constructed in western society is related to the political manoeuvres between various agencies in their pursuit of much-sought-after research funding.

Secondly, western societies have moved from providing institutional care for people with dementia to the provision of care in the community. This has highlighted, and has perhaps created, the plight of informal caregivers – mainly family members – who are expected to provide a substantial part of the care required. As a result, health professionals have increasingly been called upon to develop new strategies aimed at helping informal caregivers maintain their dementing relatives at home.

Finally, there has been increasing multidisciplinary team work in the provision of care to people who are dementing. This has challenged medical provision for dementing people and has led to the application of new concepts and techniques regarding the nature and treatment of dementia. Clinical psychologists have been particularly active. They introduced psychological assessment and pioneered the development of psychological therapies for dementing people and their relatives. These approaches have now been taken on and developed by other professionals such as social workers and mental health nurses.

USES OF THE TERM DEMENTIA

A collective term

There are two ways in which the term dementia is

commonly used (Lishman 1987). The first is as a collective term and the second is as one of a variety of conditions with common features.

Dementia as a collective term suggests that dementia is one clinical entity. For example, The Royal College of Physicians defines dementia as:

> ... the acquired global impairment of higher cortical functions including memory, the capacity to solve the problems of day-to-day living, the performance of learned perceptuo-motor skills, the correct use of social skills and the control of emotional reactions, all aspects of language and communication and the control of emotional reactions, in the absence of gross clouding of consciousness. The condition is often progressive though not necessarily irreversible.
>
> (Royal College of Physicians 1982)

Clinical features

Within this wide definition the clinical features of dementia affect the following:

Memory. Memory of current events and learning of new information are adversely affected. As the disorder progresses, earlier memories are lost and concentration becomes poor. Memories of past events may appear as if they are in the present.

Orientation. Ability to recall the time and the place becomes difficult as eventually does the ability to identify other people. Some people tend to hide their memory deficits by confabulating. 'Reduplications' of place and person can occur when people think that they are in a different (although duplicated) place or that familiar persons are 'different' or even acting as impostors (Miller & Morris 1993).

Intellect. Increasing difficulty develops in understanding what is going on and what is being said, particularly if events are moving quickly. Thinking becomes slow and content is impoverished. There may be concrete thinking, reduced flexibility, and perseveration. Judgement becomes impaired.

Behaviour. Behaviour is often disorganised, inappropriate, distractable and restless. Antisocial behaviour such as shop-lifting and sexual disinhibition may also occur. Incontinence of urine and faeces develops in the later stages.

Mood. Changes of mood may occur, characterised by anxiety, depression, irritability. Severe agitation may also occur.

Neurological impairment. Neurological impairment may occur such as apraxia, agnosia and aphasia.

As dementia is a progressive condition, these clinical features should be seen as developing and changing over a period of time. This is important and relevant to the assessment of people who are dementing and their relatives.

One of a variety of conditions

The second understanding of dementia is as one of a variety of conditions: Alzheimer's disease, Pick's disease, diffuse Lewy body disease, vascular dementia and subcortical dementia.

Alzheimer's disease

There have been reports of a possible biochemical marker for the detection of Alzheimer's disease but this work needs to be replicated and made practicable for routine clinical practice (Ghanbari et al 1990). Thus, at present, it is not possible to give a definite diagnosis of Alzheimer's disease before death.

Neurophysiology and neurochemistry. In Alzheimer's disease there are four types of pathology (Mountjoy 1993). First, there is an excessive loss of neurones. Neuronal loss occurs in normal ageing but is more extensive in Alzheimer's disease. Secondly, there are large numbers of neuritic (senile) plaques. Plaques consist of altered axons and dendrites of neurones surrounding an extracelluar mass of thin filaments. Each plaque takes years and even decades to evolve. Thirdly, there is the development of neurofibrillary tangles which consist of dense bundles of abnormal fibres in the cytoplasm of neurones. These are paired helical structures composed of a protein called tau. Finally there is amyloid deposition which occurs in the cortex blood vessels and the core of the neuritic plaques.

Plaques and tangles are plentiful throughout the cortex and are particularly common in the temporal and parietal lobes, especially the hippocampus, amygdala, parahippocampus gyrus and basal nucleus of Meynert. These areas of the brain are known to play a central role in memory. The reader is referred to Chapter 3 for a more detailed discussion of physiological changes in Alzheimer's disease.

In Alzheimer's disease there is a gross depletion of acetylcholine and the enzymes involved in its metabolism, particularly in the hippocampus. Other neurotransmitters are also depleted, including noradrenaline, 5-hydroxytryptamine (5-HT), and to a lesser extent gamma-aminobutyric acid (GABA), glycine and somatostatin (Jagger & Lindesay 1993).

Risk factors associated with Alzheimer's disease. Risk factors linked with the incidence of Alzheimer's disease include:

Old age. Neurophysiological and community studies have found that advanced old age is associated with the development of dementia, and especially raised numbers of senile plaques (Hagnell et al 1983). This has led to the hypothesis that Alzheimer's disease is really accelerated or aggravated normal ageing. However, this is not supported by studies that show more cell loss in younger people with Alzheimer's disease than in older people (Wilcock & Jacoby 1991a).

Gender. The prevalence of Alzheimer's disease is higher in women because they are more likely to live longer than men.

Family history of Alzheimer's disease. Relatives of people with Alzheimer's disease have an increased likelihood of developing the disorder, particularly if the onset is early (Amaducci & Lippi 1994). A number of studies reveal an autosomal dominant gene in people with Alzheimer's disease, particularly for early onset disease, but most cases fail to demonstrate this pattern.

Down's syndrome. Since the early 1980s, interest has focused on establishing the genetic basis of Alzheimer's disease. It has been found that the gene sequence which codes beta-amyloid is located on chromosome 21. Early onset Alzheimer's disease is more common in families in which there is a history of Down's syndrome (Holland 1994) and the association between the two conditions is supported by the finding that people with Down's syndrome have beta-amyloid deposits (Heston et al 1981).

Aluminium. Interest has focused on raised aluminium levels in the brains of people with Alzheimer's disease and levels of aluminium in drinking water (Martyn et al 1989). However, the evidence to suggest that oral ingestion of aluminium can lead to Alzheimer's disease is very weak (Williams & Miller 1992), and the exact role of aluminium in Alzheimer's disease is unclear.

Smoking. Smoking is associated with the incidence of multi-infarct dementia but, interestingly, there is a reduced incidence of Alzheimer's disease in people who smoke (Graves et al 1991).

Head injury. A number of studies have investigated head traumas as a risk factor in Alzheimer's disease. Although the findings are not clearcut, the EURODEM Risk Factors Research Group report an association between head trauma and Alzheimer's disease in men and in cases without a previous history of dementia (Mortimer et al 1991).

Pick's disease

Pick's disease is a rare progressive disorder in which damage is localised in the frontal lobes of the brain with occasional temporal lobe damage. Family studies strongly suggest that there are genetic factors associated with its causation (Wilcock & Jacoby 1991b).

Women are nearly twice as likely to be affected by Pick's disease as men. Onset tends to be between 50 and 60 years and the progress of the illness is slower than Alzheimer's disease. Early clinical features usually involve lack of self-control rather than defective memory. Impairment of motivation may occur with episodes of tactlessness and gross insensitivity. Lack of restraint may lead to stealing or sexual misadventures. Facial expression becomes vacant and the person may indulge in foolish jokes. As the disorder develops, speech becomes noticeably perseverative with a marked reduction in vocabulary.

Diffuse Lewy body disease

Diffuse Lewy body disease, or a Lewy body variant of Alzheimer's disease (Hansen et al 1990), is a newly emerging diagnostic category characterised by the presence of senile plaques in the cortex of the brain but very few neurofibrillary tangles. In addition, Lewy bodies are present in the cortex and the brain stem nuclei. Some neurones are also lost (Tobiansky 1994b).

Increased recognition of diffuse Lewy body disease has altered the earlier beliefs that vascular dementia is the second most common form of dementia. It is now acknowledged that up to 20% of people diagnosed as having dementia in fact have diffuse Lewy body disease (Perry et al 1990).

The clinical features of the condition include:

- fluctuating cognitive impairment affecting both memory and higher cortical functions such as language, visuospatial ability, praxis and reasoning skills
- visual and auditory hallucinations with paranoid delusions and depression
- mild symptoms of Parkinson's disease are frequently present. The onset of the condition varies as does its progress.

Vascular dementia

Vascular dementia arises from a variety of cerebrovascular diseases in which there is a disturbance in the flow of blood to the brain. Until the mid 1970s, 'arteriosclerotic dementia' was often used to describe memory deterioration resulting from cerebral arterial pathology. The term implied that its cause was related to 'hardening of the arteries' but it has since been found that vascular dementia is related more to the occurrence of strokes both large and small.

Accordingly, 'multi-infarct dementia' is now more commonly used.

Vascular dementia may arise in the cerebral cortex or the subcortex. In the cortex it usually arises from a thrombus (a clot forming in a blood vessel leading to an occlusion), cerebral haemorrhage or emboli (detached clots). In cases of subcortical vascular dementia, ischaemia occurs in the white matter of the brain resulting in diffuse areas of demyelination (loss of the outer myelin sheath of neurones). There is also fibrotic thickening of small arterioles by fibrillary connective tissue, resulting in reduced blood flow in the terminal arterioles (Tobiansky 1994a).

The risk factors associated with vascular dementia are those normally associated with strokes, which include hypertension, cigarette smoking, cardiac arrhythmias and obesity.

The clinical features of vascular dementia vary according to the extent and location of damage (O'Brien 1994). Neurological deficits vary according to which cerebral hemisphere is affected. Left hemisphere deficits commonly include aphasia (loss of the power of speech or of understanding the written or spoken word), apraxia (inability to recognise common articles or perform correct movements because of a brain lesion), agraphia (loss of the power to express thought in writing) and acalculia (loss of the ability to do simple arithmetic), whereas right hemisphere injury often results in visuospatial deficits, amusia and dysprody in people whose dominant hemisphere is their left (right-handed people) (McKeith 1994).

Subcortical dementia

Subcortical dementias refer to conditions in which memory impairment occurs from pathology in the subcortex rather than the cortex of the brain. It should be noted though that the use of the term 'subcortical dementia' is not yet fully established by clinicians.

Millar & Morris (1993) suggest that conditions to which subcortical dementia is applied are not homogeneous enough to constitute one category and they may have less in common with each other than they do with Alzheimer's disease. However, the term subcortical is useful and is used in this chapter to identify a number of conditions in which dementia develops.

Subcortical dementia has been described mainly in cases of Parkinson's disease, Huntington's chorea, Wilson's disease, progressive supranuclear palsy and forms of multi-infarct dementia in which there are pathological changes in the subcortex. In addition, there are other conditions in which pathology is predominantly subcortical, such as progressive supranuclear palsy (Steele–Richardson–Olszewski syndrome), multiple sclerosis, Binswanger's disease, Creutzfeldt–Jakob disease and HIV dementia.

Overt dementia occurs in 30–40% of cases of Parkinson's disease and more subtle changes are present in a further 40% (Cummings 1988). In addition to features of dementia, people with Parkinson's disease display tremors, mask-like expression, shuffling gait and hyper-salivation, and about half have signs of depression (Absher & Cummings 1994).

Huntington's chorea is a genetic disease that usually affects people under 60 years old. Dementia is present in virtually all cases and its onset is gradual and insidious. Dementia is rarely conspicuous and eventually it becomes submerged within the other features of the condition such as poor attention, poor concentration, muteness and the characteristic swaying movements.

Wilson's disease is a rare inherited disorder affecting the liver and the central nervous system. It tends to develop in younger people but its onset may be as late as the 5th decade (Lishman 1987). Various psychiatric features may be apparent in cases of Wilson's disease, such as a change in personality and behavioural changes. Psychotic features are not uncommon. Dementia may occur during the course of the illness and progressive dementia often marks the terminal stages (Lishman 1987).

Progressive supranuclear palsy is characterised by initial vague mental slowing and behavioural problems which might be mistakenly diagnosed as Alzheimer's disease. However, other clinical features develop, such as supranuclear paralysis of external ocular movements, particularly in the vertical plane, dysarthria (a neuromuscular disorder affecting the actual articulation of words: linguistic ability remains unimpaired) pseudobulbar palsy, dystonic rigidity of the neck and trunk and dementia. In the latter stages, the eyes are fixed centrally and there is widespread rigidity of limbs. McKeith (1994) suggests that the condition is probably not rare and that many cases are diagnosed as Parkinson's disease.

Some people develop more than one of the degenerative dementias such as Alzheimer's disease and vascular dementia and are described as 'mixed cases'. Studies suggest that the prevalence of the pure Alzheimer's group ranges from 22–68%, the pure vascular dementia group from 9–59%, and the mixed Alzheimer and vascular group from 4–23% (O'Brien 1994).

DISTINGUISHING DEMENTIA FROM OTHER CONDITIONS

Acute confusional states, sometimes known as deliria, and depression can closely resemble dementia and accurate differential diagnosis is crucial. These conditions may occur at the same time as dementia and it is not uncommon for people with mild dementia to develop an acute confusional state. When treated appropriately, the acute confusional state disappears to leave the person with the residual dementia.

Mistaking dementia for depression is easy because both conditions share common features such as low mood, poor concentration and poor social skills. Sometimes depression so closely resembles dementia that it is termed 'pseudodementia' (Kiloh 1961). Post (1965) found that 16–18% of elderly depressed people 'exhibited a learning defect of the same kind as characteristic of elderly persons with diffuse brain damage'. The main difference is that pseudodementia is reversible whereas true dementia is not. Depression in old age is discussed in detail in Chapter 8.

Unlike dementia, acute confusional states develop very quickly. The majority of cases are reversible when the underlying physical cause is treated. However, some acute confusional states become chronic as in some traumatic syndromes or Wernicke's syndrome. The clinical features of acute confusional states arise from disruption of normal brain function and are surprisingly similar whatever their underlying cause. Confusional states are discussed in detail in Chapter 10.

PSYCHOSOCIAL MODELS OF DEMENTIA

As described in the previous section, various biological models (medical conditions) have been developed that attempt to explain the development of dementia. With Alzheimer's disease risk factors have been identified but causal explanations are yet to be established. More straightforward are biological explanations outlining the contribution of various risk factors to the vascular dementias; for example, smoking leads to impairment of the cerebral blood supply and in turn to cerebral infarction.

In spite of the power of biological theories of dementia they can provide only a partial explanation of the syndrome of dementia. Rothschild (1956) argues that 'the qualities of the living person and his life experiences are the most important factors in the origin of the mental breakdown', and that dementia is 'the end state in a long process which has its roots not just in certain impersonal tissue alterations but in psychological stresses and in special problems which affect the ageing population' (cited in Post 1965, p. 69). These early ideas resonate with more recently developed psychosocial models of dementia. Here we outline Miesen's and Kitwood's models and comment on their implications for clinical practice.

Miesen's attachment model of dementia

Miesen (1992) has developed a model of dementia based on Bowlby's attachment theory. Bowlby (1969) argued that people respond to situations as a consequence of pre-programmed patterns of behaviour becoming focused upon another individual. The effect of these 'attachment behaviours' solidify the relationship between two people, conventionally mother and child. Patterns of attachment behaviour vary according to age, sex and circumstances, and experiences with attachment figures earlier in life. For adults, attachment behaviours are seen most at times of distress and illness.

Within this framework, Miesen argues that attachment behaviours are displayed by people at varying levels of dementia. Alzheimer's disease clients with mild dementia, Miesen observes, are especially prone to touching when meeting family members unexpectedly. For clients with severe dementia, the sudden departure of family members triggers certain behaviours, especially turning towards them (while they are departing) and calling after them (when the family has departed). Miesen consequently links attachment behaviours with the level of cognitive functioning.

Miesen argues that the process of dementia can be understood as a 'strange situation' which gradually becomes more permanent. The more unsafe a situation appears the more attachment behaviours are evoked. As their bond with the outside world deteriorates dementing people will seek some kind of anchorage. However, since their memory is deteriorating the attachment bonds are not durable. Consequently, a vicious circle develops in which the person's need for security can never be fulfilled.

According to Miesen, the increasingly frequent feelings of being insecure in the early stages of dementia act as a 'retrieval cue' in which attachment behaviours are activated, especially turning towards, touching and calling after. Parent fixation, that is when dementing people continue to maintain that their parents are still living, does not occur at this early stage because the security provided by attachment figures is temporarily sufficient. If it does occur it can be explained as unreciprocated attachment behaviour. At a later stage the 'strange situation' remains constantly present and the experience of being unsafe becomes permanent. The care-requiring situations of the dementing person then act as a 'retrieval cue'. Parent fixation and touching are particularly evident at this later stage. Parent fixation has now become attachment behaviour which reciprocates the need for security from within the sufferers themselves. However, Miesen acknowledges that in the latter stage of Alzheimer's disease it is only possible to speculate upon the meaning of parent fixation and suggests that parent fixation then occurs when there is no other attachment figure around.

Miesen's work is potentially valuable to health care professionals working with dementing people although it needs development and research to replicate her findings. If parent fixation in early stage dementia indicates feelings of insecurity, then carers can seek to promote security, possibly through validation techniques (discussed in Ch. 21), which may raise self-esteem and show dementing persons that they are understood.

Kitwood's approach to dementia

Over the last few years, Kitwood and his colleagues at the Bradford Dementia Research Group, University of Bradford have developed a psychosocial model of dementia (Kitwood 1993) which is briefly described here and discussed in detail in Chapter 21.

Kitwood's starting point is the inadequacy of the dominant biological model of dementia which he describes as the 'standard paradigm' or the 'dominant discourse', and which he represents as follows:

X $\rightarrow$ neuropathic change $\rightarrow$ dementia
(Kitwood 1993, p. 139)

In this model X represents physical phenomena.

In the case of vascular dementia, the nature of X and the neuropathic change is fairly well understood whereas, with Alzheimer's disease, the identity of X is unknown in spite of many hypotheses and much controversy.

Kitwood points out that the model of dementia within the standard paradigm contradicts experimental findings such as the lack of correlation between:

- the degree of dementia and the measured extent of damage to the grey matter in the brain
- the rapid decline in the mental ability of people who are dementing when their life-style is changed

- the observation that people with dementia often stop deteriorating when their life-situation becomes stable and even undergo a degree of 'rementia' (Kitwood 1993).

Kitwood argues that the extent of a person's dementia does not simply depend on the extent of the brain lesion but upon a variety of factors including personality, biography, physical health, neurological impairment and social psychology (Kitwood 1993). In this context, biography refers to everything that has happened to a person in her life and also what is happening to that person moment by moment, as she attempts to be, to do, to relate, or to communicate and whether or not there is an enabling and helpful response from others.

Kitwood's perspective allows for the inclusion of a variety of factors in the presentation of dementia and these he develops in relation to aetiology, interpersonal psychology and implications for care. For example (Kitwood 1990a), he argues that the dementing process should be viewed as the outcome of a dialectical interplay between two tendencies: neurological impairment and a combination of personal psychology and social psychology. He puts forward various crucial life events which he has found in 'psychobiographical accounts' by relatives of dementing people that contribute to the precipitation of dementia (Kitwood 1993). These life events fall into the following categories:

- retirement, redundancy or major role loss
- bereavement
- rejection or disgrace
- stressful conflict
- geographical change
- accident
- assault or burglary
- major physical illness or operation.

In addition, Kitwood (1990a) developed the concept of 'malignant social psychology', in which particular processes and interactions experienced by dementing people are hypothesised to adversely affect their self-esteem and tend to diminish their personhood. These include treachery, disempowerment and infantalisation.

Kitwood also argues (Kitwood & Bredin 1992) that the standard interpersonal psychology paradigm represents dementia in terms of 'them' and 'us'; a clear division between we who are in the normal population and they who have dementia. This approach is taken by professional caregivers who do things to their patients, whether it be reality orientation or reminiscence therapy, and so locate the problem of dementia within the dementia sufferer rather than themselves. Adopting a 'them' and 'us' mentality places the caregiver in the comfortable, even smug, position of being absolved from any responsibility for the development of dementia. However, Kitwood argues that we (the carers) contribute to the problem of dementia, as well as the dementing people themselves. We and they are human beings with failings, limitations and suffering and consequently share the responsibility for the development of dementia in people. Moreover, Kitwood argues, the problem of dementia is in part due to the hypocrisy, competitiveness and pursuit of crass materialism in contemporary society. These are moral conditions which give rise to adverse life events which contribute to the development of dementia. They are as pathological as anything that exists in the person with dementia and constitute a largely unacknowledged 'pathology of normalcy'. Indeed, Kitwood goes so far as to suggest that 'they' are rather less of a problem than we are.

With regard to care, Kitwood argues that the central factor in caring for people who are dementing should be the preservation of personhood. This, he maintains, is not the same thing as cognitive ability but is a social phenomenon which is not 'at first, a property of an individual; rather, it is provided or guaranteed by the presence of others' (Kitwood & Bredin 1992, p. 275). Indeed, the preservation of personhood is linked by Kitwood and Bredin to the extent of intersubjectivity between the person with dementia and the caregiver; by dissolving the dichotomy between them and us in dementia care, personhood is preserved. The wellbeing developed by this means may be demonstrated by various factors such as the assertion of desire or the will and the initiation of social contact and humour. The outcome will be various global sentient states such as a sense of personal worth, agency, social confidence and hope.

Kitwood and Bredin's work is important for clinical practice for several reasons. First, whilst not forgetting the dementing person's family, Kitwood's model reinstates the dementing person as the most important consideration when planning and delivering services; this is a corrective to the family models of dementia discussed in the next section which emphasise family support sometimes to the exclusion of the dementing person. Second, Kitwood's model of dementia underpins his development of a quality care assessment procedure – 'dementia care mapping' – which seeks to take account of the dementing person's perspective. Third, the emphasis of the model upon

the self provides a theoretical basis for psychological interventions (such as validation therapy, discussed in Chapter 21) which aims to improve the dementing person's self-concept. Overall, Kitwood's ideas and care initiatives highlight the fact that those who are dementing are first and foremost people like ourselves, who deserve our respect.

FAMILY MODELS OF DEMENTIA

In addition to psychosocial models of the dementing process, models have developed that incorporate the experience of the family as well as that of the dementing person. Family models are of a different order to psychosocial models of dementia because they do not purport to explain dementia, but seek instead to address the effects of dementia on informal carers. In this section we focus on the family burden model of dementia.

Family burden and dementia

Grad & Sainsbury's (1965) early work on families giving care to their elderly relatives distinguished between the 'objective and subjective burden'. Objective burden consists of behavioural problems displayed by the elderly dementing person which the caregiver has to endure and the subjective burden is the emotional response of the caregiver. More recently, Gilleard (1984) has developed the idea of 'daily hassles' to refer to the day-to-day difficulties informal caregivers encounter and which may lead to the onset of psychiatric disorders in the caregiver.

In terms of objective burden, studies identify a range of problems encountered by informal caregivers of dementing people. Sanford (1975) found that the problems reported by caregivers included nocturnal wandering, faecal incontinence, an inability to wash and immobility.

In terms of subjective burden, the emotional effect of giving informal care to people who are dementing gives rise to a higher than average incidence of mental disorder in caregivers. Gilleard et al (1984) found that 68% of their sample of carers fitted the criteria constituting a 'case' for mental illness on the General Health Questionnaire (Goldberg 1978) and several studies (e.g. Coppel et al 1985) have found a high level of depression among informal caregivers of dementing people. However others, most notably Gilhooly (1986) and Eagles et al (1987), suggest that the mental health of caregivers is no worse than that of a community sample. One reason for this discrepancy is that some caregivers are better adjusted to their situation than others, particularly if they are looking after someone in the early stages of dementia (Miller & Morris 1993).

Discrepant findings do suggest, however, that the relationship between the objective and the subjective burden is not straightforward and this has given rise to the use of transactional models of stress (discussed later) to explain the experience of caregivers. Various studies have found that the level of the dementing person's impairment is not a good predictor of caregiver burden (Scott et al 1986, Zarit et al 1980), morale or mental health (Hirschfeld 1983), or caregiver wellbeing (George & Gwyther 1986). This suggests that there are mediating factors in the stressor–caregiver relationship. These include the following:

The nature of the relationship

Horowitz & Shindelman (1983) identify closeness and affection and Williamson & Schulz (1990) the closeness of the past relationship as important in determining the caregiver's experience of burden; and Hirschfeld (1981) regards mutuality as crucial in determining a family's ability to continue caring for a dementing person at home. Several studies have found that the greater the emotional distance between the caregiver and the dementing person the less the strain experienced by the caregiver (Gilhooly 1986). Conversely, positive feelings for the dementing person have been found to be positively correlated with the mental health of the caregiver. Morris et al (1988) found that higher levels of past marital intimacy correlated with low levels of strain and depression but that a decrease in intimacy was likely to be perceived as loss, and result in anticipatory grief.

Gender

Caregiving is often a more stressful experience for women than it is for men. Women caregivers are more likely to suffer depression and low morale because, though willing, they feel unable to give much practical help to their dementing relatives (Morris et al 1992, Horowitz 1985). However, men have been described as better able to manage the care of their dementing relative: to set limits assertively, to delegate and to take short cuts in housework (Colerick & George 1986). Also male caregivers are more willing to continue giving care beyond what would be considered to be a reasonable level of endurance (Mathew et al 1990).

Factors differentiating male from female caregivers have been identified as significant in influencing their approach: women more often feel obliged to give care than men and have more difficulty in coping with the dependency and demands of their dementing relative (Fitting et al 1986). This may explain why women are more likely to experience guilt than men when their dementing relative enters institutional care. Additional factors that make caregiving more stressful for women, particularly daughter caregivers, is that they are often expected to give care to other people too, such as their own children and spouse. When these expectations are combined with full- or part-time employment, the obligation to give care often results in emotional ill health (Gilleard et al 1984). These problems are exacerbated by the development of a model of community care that is dependent on family care which is, in reality, woman's care.

Coping strategies

Pearlin et al (1990) outline three types of coping strategies used by people giving care to dementing relatives. The first type focuses on managing the situation and involves strategies designed to minimise the burden upon the caregiver. Such behaviours include:

- asking the help of another relative
- successfully managing burdensome behaviours, such as nocturnal incontinence or aggressive behaviour
- strategically placing locks on doors to prevent the dementing relative from being exposed to the danger of leaving the house
- obtaining anticipatory legal assistance.

Another strategy is for caregivers to reorder their priorities so that these are more consistent with their dependant's behaviour. This may involve giving up full-time paid work or deciding not to do all the caregiving themselves.

The second type of coping strategy involves managing the meaning of the situation. Strategies include making positive comparisons with other people across time. For example, a caregiver might say, 'Well, it could have been worse – Mr Smith died when he was 40!'; or, 'He is no worse than at this time last year'; or, 'I will just go on one day at a time'. Alternatively, the caregiver may refer to something in the past that gives added meaning to their present situation; for example, 'When I got married to her I promised that it was for better or for worse' or, 'I know he would do the same for me'. Humour, for example a spouse laughing at the time when she lost her dementing partner on a shopping trip to later find him unharmed; or sometimes prayer may be used by caregivers to give new meaning to their situation. Pearlin et al (1990) found that caregivers sometimes prayed for a cure while others used prayer to generate inner strength. Another common way of coping is to convert their personal tragedy into some good by getting involved in support groups for caregivers. In this way some caregivers find that their tragedy has some purpose.

The third type of coping strategy employed by caregivers (Pearlin et al 1990) focuses on managing their distress. This involves a variety of activities including talking with others, pursuing a new hobby, relaxation exercises, watching television, smoking and sleeping. Although these strategies may give short-term relief they may also generate long-term problems, such as excessive drinking.

Support

Various studies indicate that increased social support enhances the mental health of caregivers (Gilhooly 1984); both formal support from people such as social workers and nurses, and informal support from family, friends and neighbours. However, as the illness progresses caregivers often find themselves increasingly isolated because the behaviour of their dementing relative stops family, friends and neighbours from visiting.

Morris et al (1989) examined the emotional, instrumental and financial help received by caregivers, and the web of social relationships that surround them. They found that caregivers who were well supported were less depressed and experienced less strain than those whose support was poor. Kielcolt-Glasser et al (1991) found that low levels of social support in caregivers, together with being distressed by dementia-related behaviours, correlated with changes in their immune function. Miller & Morris (1993) argue that it is the quality of support received by the caregiver that is important in maintaining the emotional stability of the caregiver, not the frequency of contact. Supporting informal carers at home is discussed in detail in Chapter 25.

MODELS OF CAREGIVING AND DEMENTIA

Various models of caregiving for a person with dementia have been developed. They are of three types: models based on an 'engineering' model of stress; models based on a transactional model of stress; and process models of caregiving.

Engineering models of caregiving

Early models of caregiving were underpinned by a model of psychological stress proposed by theorists such as Cannon (1932) whose work drew on an engineering model of stress, in which there is a direct relationship between the stress placed upon an object and its response. In the context of dementia, the influence of this engineering model of stress is evident in the work of Grad & Sainsbury (1965) who identified the relationship between objective stress-provoking behaviours of the dementing person (such as urinary and faecal incontinence, wandering and aggressive behaviour) and the subjective experience of the caregiver.

Engineering models of caregiving for clinical practice remove responsibility from individuals for the stress they experience. People are seen as simply responding to stressors rather than exercising control over their individual circumstances. Consequently, engineering models of caregiving are of limited value as a basis of interventions to help families cope.

Transactional models of caregiving

Transactional models of stress are more sophisticated than engineering models because they incorporate factors that mediate the relationship between the stress and its response. Typically, transactional models identify internal or external demands which result in perceived harm, threat or challenge. The demands are appraised by the individuals involved who act in accordance with their coping mechanisms within the context of their supportive network.

Transactional models of stress have been increasingly used to describe the experience of caregivers of dementing people (Schulz et al 1990). See, for example, Haley et al's (1987) model of stress and coping in caregiving which is described in Figure 11.1. In this model the stressors acting on the caregiver are mediated by their appraisal of the situation, the coping responses at their disposal and the available social support. These factors combine to determine the degree to which the caregiver is able to adapt to her situation.

Transactional models of caregiving are valuable in helping us understand the various factors that contribute to the caregiver's experience of stress. Thus interventions may be developed which address one or more aspects of the models: appraisal, coping responses and social support. However, for many caregivers the experience of dementia is perhaps more unified than transactional models suggest; separating

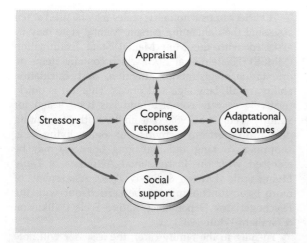

Figure 11.1 A model of stress and coping in caregiving (Haley, Levine, Brown and Bartolucci 1987).

out the elements of the experience is possible, but only to a limited degree. Further information on stress and coping, but of formal care workers, is provided in Chapter 26.

Process models of caregiving

The third type of model of family caregiving in dementia emphasises the process of giving care and so takes a longitudinal perspective on dementia in the family. Underlying process models are the concepts of 'career' and 'trajectory' in which illness is conceptualised as occurring over a period of time. This contrasts with other models of caregiving which portray the situation as 'a slice of time' (Goffman 1968, Corbin & Strauss 1991). A common feature of process models is that they have been developed using qualitative research methodologies such as grounded theory (Glaser & Strauss 1967).

One example of a process model is that of Willoughby & Keating (1991), which regards issues relating to taking on and relinquishing control as central to giving care to someone with dementia. The model contains five stages in the caregiving process. The first two stages, which relate to assuming control of caregiving, are 'emerging recognition' and 'taking control: making my own decisions'. The third and fourth, which relate to relinquishing control, are 'losing control: accepting decisions of others' and 'adjusting to the psychiatric institution'. The final stage, 'moving on', relates to retaking one's control of life outside caregiving.

Process models of caregiving in dementia have been developed through studies of very small samples and few models have been systematically validated. This raises questions about their generalisability and thus their value in guiding the development of interactions to support family carers.

INTERVENING WITH DEMENTING PEOPLE AND THEIR FAMILIES

We now move to discuss some practical issues in the family care of dementing people: assessment; helping families in crisis, those prematurely grieving their loss and those in which there is a high level of expressed emotion; and abuse of dementing people by caregivers. A valuable starting point for practice under all these circumstances is *Living Well in Old Age* (King's Fund 1986), which sets out principles concerning the provision of services to people with dementia and their informal caregivers. These principles are drawn upon in Box 11.1 to develop practice guidelines for health care professionals working with dementing people and their carers.

Aspects of assessment

Assessment of elderly people is discussed in Chapter 6. Here we emphasise those features which are particularly important with respect to dementing people and their carers.

Assessment provides the practitioner with an opportunity to start to build a supportive relationship with the dementing person and her family carer. As Kitwood's work reminds us, relationships which emphasise a division between 'us' (the professionals) and 'them' (the dementing person and caregiver) are counter-productive. Accordingly, assessment should be, as far as possible, a collaborative venture which encourages joint participation and responsibility for developing the caregiving package. In this way, the assessment is not disabling but rather increases clients' awareness of their strengths and abilities (Patterson & Whitehouse 1990).

A comprehensive assessment will include personal, family and social details; for example, the EPIC (Elderly People in the Community) project, based in Scotland, includes the client's housing, financial needs, accidents and emergencies, physical and mental health, help and support received, and ability to manage daily living (Myers & Crawford 1993). Reassessment at 6-monthly intervals keeps professional carers up to date with changing health and social circumstances.

Box 11.1   Practice guidelines based on the King Edward's Fund (1986) principles of dementia care

Principle 1
People with dementia have the same human value as anyone else, irrespective of their degree of disability or dependence. Recognising the status and worth of people with dementia.
People with dementia should:
- always be listened to
- not be physically, psychologically or socially abused – even if it is called 'teasing' by care staff (who like doing it)
- be spoken to kindly, as one would expect to address a senior and respected member of society.

Principle 2
People with dementia have the same varied human needs as anyone else. Responding to a full range of needs within the mainstream of society.
People with dementia:
- have got the right to the same sources of health care provision as anyone else
- have the right to a secure and safe environment
- should have a good diet that optimises their health
- have the right to expect relaxation and recreation.

Principle 3
People with dementia have the same rights as other citizens. Promoting the rights of people with dementia who use services.
People with dementia have the right to:
- express their views about the service
- be able to make choices
- independent advocacy
- expect first class care which aims to satisfy the interests of the demented person not that of the formal carer.

Principle 4
Every person with dementia is an individual. Creating individual centred care.
People with dementia have the right to:
- express their individuality
- satisfy their individual taste
- have their own clothes and belongings.

Principle 5
People with dementia have the right to forms of support which do not exploit family and friends. Safeguarding the quality of life of families and other caregivers.
People with dementia have got the right to expect that:
- the care they require will not place excessive strain upon the people they love and respect
- their informal caregivers receive the appropriate professional support
- their informal caregivers receive the information they require about dementia and services available and appropriate referral to agencies from GPs.

A variety of psychometric scales may be used when assessing the dementing person. Mental state may be assessed with the Mini Mental State Examination (MMSE) (Folstein et al 1975) which contains items on orientation, registration, attention, and calculation ability, recall, language and praxis. This test is quick, relatively easy to complete and has been tested for validity (Teng et al 1987). The ability of the dementing person to perform activities of daily living (e.g. shopping, cooking and managing finances) may be assessed with the Instrumental Activities of Daily Living Scale (Lawton & Brody 1969). Assessment of more basic functioning can be carried out with the Psychogeriatric Dependency Rating Scale (Wilkinson & Graham-White 1982).

Turning to the family carer, the assessor will note not only the experience of caregiving at the time but also the contribution of significant events in the lives of the dementing person and the caregiver which will have shaped their relationship. In complex cases it may be useful to construct a genogram, which is a means of graphically illustrating information such as names, dates of birth, health status, and place of residence of the client and family members, as well as the date and cause of death of deceased family members. The genogram has been found to be a valuable teaching tool for nurses in training to help them piece together aspects of the family's past to help to explain the present (Ritter et al 1996).

The assessor should be sensitive to cues that the caregiver may give regarding interfamilial relationships and will also clarify allocation of any tasks within the family and establish whether the caregiver has now to take on many additional and unfamiliar tasks (paying bills, shopping, cooking, cleaning, etc.). It is often worth interviewing more than one member of the family to gain a comprehensive picture of family life and to raise other family members' awareness of the problems experienced by the primary caregiver.

There are a number of scales for identifying the existence and level of problems experienced by caregivers. Commonly used measures include the Caregiver Strain Questionnaire (Robinson 1983) and the Burden Interview (Zarit et al 1980). However, Keady & Nolan (1994) advise health practitioners against over reliance on rating scales and instead urge them to pay attention to the family caregiver's expert knowledge of the caregiving relationship. As a response to standardised scales these authors have developed the carer-led assessment process (CLASP). This approach, which involves the caregiver holding the assessment documentation, emphasises the role of the health care professional as an information-giver and enabler, reinforces the role of the caregiver as expert and has led to the development of new professional roles.

A further area for assessment is the extent of the caregiver's knowledge, attitudes and beliefs about mental illness generally and dementia in particular, and the services that are available and received. What the caregiver believes to be the circumstances underlying the dementia can be important. Sometimes caregivers believe that they have caused the dementia. One caregiver we worked with thought that she was responsible for the dementia because she was holding the ladder when her partner fell off and hit his head. This belief caused the caregiver unremitting guilt as she saw her partner slowly become demented. Another caregiver thought that her husband's dementia might have been caused by his venereal disease contracted through an affair he had earlier in their marriage and this caused her to feel ambivalent in caring for him.

In sum, assessment is a dynamic and skilled activity which is essential to appropriate interventions and high quality care of dementing people and their family carers.

HELPING TROUBLED FAMILIES

Families in crisis

Health practitioners working with families looking after people who are dementing often have to intervene at times of crisis. Indeed, it is common to find that failure to diagnose the client early enough, followed by poor coordination of services and ineffective case management, has allowed a situation to build up until a crisis occurs and quick and effective specialist help is needed.

Caplan (1961) understands a crisis to occur when a person faces an obstacle to important life goals that cannot be overcome with customary methods of problem solving. Associated with the idea of a crisis is that of threat and associated intense and urgent emotions. One couple referred to me was at crisis point because of poor case management which led to their emotional needs being inadequately addressed. After a particularly difficult weekend, the wife hit her dementing husband on the head causing minor injury. This episode was the outward manifestation of a build up of emotional tension in the woman over the previous few months. The tension did not simply result from the behaviour of her husband but also from events that had occurred throughout a difficult and often confrontational and violent marriage. This illustrates the point made earlier that it is misleading

to assume that everything occurring between the caregiver and the sufferer results solely from the dementia itself; the illness must be seen against the backdrop of their life together.

Various studies have found that crisis intervention is a valuable approach with people who are dementing. Ratna (1982) found that 67% of 'crisis' referrals to a 24-hour, community-orientated psycho-geriatric service were people suffering dementia and that prompt intervention prevented hospitalisation and mobilised supportive community networks. Ratna's findings were recently supported by another community psychogeriatric team (Dole & Varian 1994).

Models of family crisis have been adapted as a theoretical basis for practitioners working with family caregivers to dementing people who are in a state of crisis (Adams 1990). As depicted in Figure 11.2, Parad and Resnick (1971) have described a crisis as consisting of three stages: a pre-crisis stage, a crisis stage and a post-crisis stage.

During the pre-crisis stage, people giving care to their dementing relatives maintain an equilibrium in which the stress they encounter is balanced by their coping mechanisms. In the crisis stage, the caregiver becomes aware of the possibility of threat. This threat is often in the form of a particular incident; for example, the person with dementia getting lost or leaving the gas on. From then on caregivers experience a downward spiral in which they become disorganised, anxious and tense. This continues until a 'rock bottom' point is attained at which things cannot get worse. From that point onwards the post-crisis stage begins, during which caregivers begin to resolve the situation by trial and error. For example, they may go to their GP who gives them a diagnosis, tells them about dementia and puts them in touch with supportive services such as a community mental health nurse or a social worker. Individual input from practitioners is often directed at helping caregivers to resolve the situation themselves by enabling them to take constructive action.

Recovery will continue until one of three positions is attained:

1. The state of equilibrium experienced by the caregiver before the crisis is regained.
2. The caregiver has been strengthened by the experience and is emotionally better able to deal with life than before.
3. The crisis has permanently damaged the caregiver's ability to function and cope.

The objectives of therapeutic intervention with a caregiver in a state of crisis are:

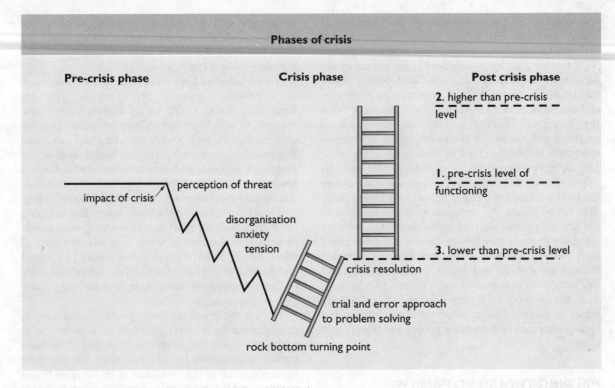

Figure 11.2 Phases of crisis. Source: Parad & Resnick (1971).

1. To help the caregiver reduce the feelings of anxiety, tension and loss of control that have resulted from the impact of the crisis.
2. To help the caregiver build an adequate support system, coping mechanisms and perception of the events that will reduce underlying feelings of vulnerability.

There are various techniques which practitioners may use to help carers in crisis. Cognitive restoration is a procedure designed to restore cognitive functioning by helping caregivers to understand why the crisis has happened and why their usual coping mechanisms failed. The practitioner can help clarify the relationship between events leading up to the crisis by encouraging the caregiver to make associations between events or by supplying an interpretation for the caregiver to consider. In one case a caregiver, who had slashed her wrist, spoke about her situation as hopeless and was helped to link her feelings with the endless burden of giving care.

Making suggestions and giving positive feedback on attempts by caregivers to resolve their problems is important, as is the support of mental defence mechanisms which result in adaptive responses.

Positive feedback will raise the self-esteem of carers, which will give them confidence to identify their problems and explore solutions in collaboration with the practitioner.

The case of Mr and Mrs Doyle (Box 11.2) describes intervening in a family which has reached a state of crisis following the slow decline of one dementing member. Mrs Doyle displays the emotional signs of being at rock bottom – crying, agitation and a sense of hopelessness. Crisis intervention in this case involved:

- raising Mrs Doyle's self-esteem by giving her a chance to tell her story
- cognitive restoration, achieved by helping Mrs Doyle piece together how she had arrived at the crisis point
- problem solving.

Families who are grieving

Various writers have understood the experience of some caregivers of relatives who are dementing in terms of loss and grief (Austrom & Gendrie 1990). This perspective draws on the work of Lindemann (1944)

Box 11.2 Crisis intervention in a family with dementia

Janet Doyle is a 'young' 54-year-old woman who is looking after her 68-year-old husband. Her husband has been demented for 3 years and has been receiving a mixture of private and health service day care so that Mrs Doyle can continue to have an independent life and go out to work. This has been very difficult for Mrs Doyle to manage as she can only use day care facilities that are on the way to work 12 miles away. Recently the private nursing home has suggested that Mrs Doyle should find another home as her husband is becoming too disturbed for the other residents in the home.

Mrs Doyle telephoned the community mental health nurse, Sally Jones, who had arranged the health service day care in a tearful and agitated state saying that she could not go on any more. Sally visited Mrs Doyle, who had taken the day off work, later that day. She found Mrs Doyle in an emotionally delicate state and near to the point of tears. Sally asked Mrs Doyle to tell her what had been happening and Sally listened to her account, asking for points of clarification when necessary. Asking Mrs Doyle about her problems and also listening to what she said helped Mrs Doyle raise her sense of self-worth in a situation in which she was feeling increasingly powerless.

Sally also tried to help Mrs Doyle restore an appropriate understanding of what had been happening. For example, when Mrs Doyle said, 'I do not know what I would do if I had to leave my job', Sally reflected back 'Do you think that perhaps you have tried too hard to keep the job going and look after your husband?' Also, Mrs Doyle talked about other recent stressful issues, including concern about a breast lump and the sudden death of her younger sister. Sally asked Mrs Doyle whether she thought that these things might be contributing to her present emotional state. Mrs Doyle said that she thought that was quite possible.

When Mrs Doyle had stopped crying, Sally suggested to her that she might like to suggest various things she could think of that might help her sort out the solution. Mrs Doyle initially had difficulty doing this. However, with a bit of encouragement from Sally, Mrs Doyle thought of a few ways in which she could sort out the situation.

Sally encouraged Mrs Doyle to look at the pros and cons of each of the suggested solutions. Eventually Mrs Doyle decided that she should think about leaving work and developing her circle of friends – which she had realised was the main reason why she was going to work – by joining night classes. When she was at night classes her daughter could stay with Mr Doyle, as she had done on many occasions. Sally reinforced the process by which Mrs Doyle had come to this decision by saying to Mrs Doyle that she had done well to think it out. Mrs Doyle seemed 'more steady' when Sally left her. Sally decided that she would call in a week to see how things were developing but said to Mrs Doyle that she could give her a ring if she wanted to see her earlier.

---

and, more recently, Parkes (1986) and Rando (1986), and is supported by the accounts that many caregivers give of their experience of finding out that their relative has dementia; for example, Pauline Taylor (1987) graphically describes her experience of caring for her dementing husband as a 'living bereavement'.

Grief may be understood as a psychological and physiological response to loss of a valued person, situation or object (Rando 1986). Grief that occurs before actual loss is described as anticipatory grief and is associated with situations in which the person is aware that the loss is imminent. Anticipatory grief is a separate experience from post-death grief.

Rando (1986) outlines three phases people go through when they are grieving:

1. Avoidance, characterised by initial shock, confusion and numbness on hearing news of actual or impending loss.
2. The confrontation phase, which involves feelings of anxiety, fear, guilt, loneliness and profound sadness about the loss. Physiological features may also develop, such as fatigue, anorexia, palpitations, dizziness and headaches.
3. Re-establishment, which involves successful adaptation to the loss and redirection of emotional energy into new people, things and ideas. The loss is not forgotten but is remembered and integrated into a new life.

That the relatives of people with dementia can have a grief reaction before their relative's death is well known (Barnes et al 1981). This pre-death experience of loss is followed by the experience of loss through bereavement when their dementing relative dies. Various studies have examined the experience of relatives of dementing people both before and after the death of their spouse. Collins et al (1993), in a longitudinal study of 350 people caring for a relative with Alzheimer's disease, identified six themes: loss of familiarity and intimacy, loss of hope, grief before death, expectancy of death, post-death relief, and post-death reflections.

Counselling people who are bereaved

Worden (1991) identifies various principles of counselling people who are bereaved which may be valuable when working with caregivers who are experiencing a pre-death experience of loss. These principles include:

Admit the loss. Counselling should be directed to helping caregivers actualise their loss. Accordingly, the practitioner may encourage caregivers to talk about what their dementing relative was like before they were ill. Talking about the qualities and attributes which their relatives have lost because of the dementia may help the caregivers adjust to the losses that have occurred.

Identify and ventilate feelings. Talking about the array of feelings such as anxiety, anger, guilt and helplessness that caregivers are experiencing may give some relief.

Exploration of what life is like without their dementing relative. The caregivers may be helped to explore the implications of losing their relative to dementia, possibly by considering problems consequent on the dementia and how they might be solved.

Discourage emotional withdrawal. Maintaining old and developing new friendships may be difficult because of the constraints that giving care places on caregivers. However, it is important for caregivers to maintain a supportive social network and resist emotional withdrawal.

Allow time for grief. Caregivers must be allowed time to grieve about what has happened to their dementing relative. Worden (1981) describes this process as 'grief work'.

Interpret normal behaviour. Following the loss of their relative to dementia, caregivers may have a sense that they are 'going mad' themselves. They need reassurance that what they are going through is a normal experience. Disturbing feelings may need interpretation and reflection to reassure them that their experiences are acceptable and to be expected.

Allow time for individual differences. Everybody reacts differently to losing someone to dementia and the reaction of some family members may cause difficulties for others. The practitioner may need to reassure the rest of the family that the way in which a particular family member is reacting is quite normal.

Provide continued support. Caregivers need continued contact with practitioners since strong feelings of loss may reoccur and be particularly acute at significant times, such as on birthdays and wedding anniversaries.

Examine mental defence mechanisms. Caregivers' mental defence mechanisms will be exaggerated during the period of loss. Some of these will be adaptive whilst others, such as excess alcohol consumption, will not. The practitioner may help

---

Box 11.3 Intervention in premature bereavement

Anne, aged 68, had cared for her husband with dementia for 4 years. She said, 'My sense of grief started the day that I got the diagnosis from the doctor. I used to go home and feel so upset about what had happened to my husband'. At other times, she said, when her husband was sleeping, she 'would fantasise and think that she could just wake her husband up and he would be like he used to be'.

Anne was visited by Sam the social worker, who took time to talk to Anne, get to know her and start to gain her confidence. He asked Anne questions about what her husband was like before he had become demented. Despite the fact that Anne eventually became tearful telling him about her husband, she was pleased to recall her husband in his earlier days.

Sam also encouraged Anne to tell him how she was coping at the moment. It was initially difficult for Anne to do this as she kept going off and back on to her husband. However, Sam was patient and kept listening to what she was saying.

Sometimes Anne asked Sam whether he thought she was going insane and whether she should be taken away to a mental hospital (not her husband). Sam explained to Anne that what she was going through was normal and was due to losing her husband to dementia. Anne was reassured by Sam's response. Sam visited Anne weekly for the next 6 weeks. The sessions took a similar format. Progress was slow but steady. The visits were changed to every 2 weeks and then every month until the social worker handed the case over to the day centre where Anne's husband had started going 2 days a week.

---

caregivers examine the impact of their mental coping mechanisms on their lives. A more detailed examination of bereavement and loss in old age is provided in Chapter 4.

The case of Anne who experienced premature bereavement when her husband was diagnosed with Alzheimer's disease is described in Box 11.3. In this example the social worker, Sam, applied bereavement counselling strategies to help Anne come to terms with her loss. Sam encouraged Anne to admit her loss – by talking about how she and her husband were prior to the onset of dementia and how things are now and encouraging her to identify and express her feelings and fears (e.g. that she was going insane), Sam interpreted Anne's present behaviour and feelings as normal in the circumstances.

Families with high levels of expressed emotion

The concept of expressed emotion (EE) arose from the work of Brown et al (1962) on people suffering from schizophrenia discharged from hospital into the community in the 1950s. The concept of EE concerns the behaviour displayed by relatives caring for dependants who have problem behaviours. A high EE family displays high levels of criticism and hostility towards their dependent relative and blames them for their behaviour whereas low EE families do not express criticism and hostility and accept the behaviour displayed by the dependent person. A number of studies have found that in high EE families there is a higher risk of relapse for the client than in low EE families.

The results of studies of EE in families with dementing members are equivocal. Orford et al (1987) found that many caregivers considered their dementing dependant's behaviour irritating and frustrating but they responded with compassion and understanding and failed to display high levels of EE. However, Bledin et al (1990), with a larger sample of 122 daughters caring for dementing relatives, found a positive relationship between high EE and emotional stress. In another study, Gilhooly and Whittick (1989) found that EE was positively associated with a number of caregiver and dependent characteristics including the sex of the caregiver, the caregiver's psychological wellbeing, contact with friends and the quality of the relationship between the caregiver and the dementing relative. These studies suggest the possible value of expressed emotion as a theoretical basis to underpin mental health interventions for people who are dementing and their relatives. Further empirical study of the application of the idea of expressed emotion in this field would be worthwhile.

Interventions to help reduce EE

There are a number of techniques which practitioners may use to help families reduce their EE. Asking questions that elicit the caregiver's perspective will help caregivers become aware of their feelings which may be giving rise to high levels of emotional expression. Sometimes the caregiver may not know the diagnosis or be unaware of the effects of dementia leading to misinterpretation of confused behaviour. Becoming angry is likely to elicit a negative response which exacerbates an already difficult situation.

An alliance between health care professional and caregiver is crucial to success in alleviating the stress of caring. The practitioner has professional knowledge and experience to contribute and the caregiver has personal knowledge of the dementing person plus first-hand experience of the difficulties encountered and will intuitively 'know what will work'.

It is important that the caregiver understands that the behaviour of dementing people can be a reaction to the manner of those around them. But the idea of responsibility or blame is simply not appropriate and needs to be set to rest. Focusing on problems that have arisen and the caregiver's responses to them can illuminate chains of behavioural events and ways in which emotionally charged family situations can be diffused.

Provision of information about dementia, possibly in the form of a booklet with contact telephone numbers and practical guidance on managing common problems, is often helpful. A particularly useful publication is Murphy's *Dementia and Mental Illness in Older People* which is comprehensive and clearly written. A follow-up visit provides an opportunity for the practitioner to clarify issues and answer questions.

The use of interventions in a family in which emotions are running high is illustrated in Box 11.4. The community occupational therapist, Joan, focused on the discord between Mr and Mrs Jackson and adopted strategies to decrease Mrs Jackson's displays of emotion towards her husband. These strategies were:

- information giving to help Mrs Jackson understand why her husband behaves as he does
- suggestion and diary writing to aid problem identification and solving, i.e. to help Mrs Jackson understand that she may be contributing to the situation and that she is able to alter it.

The abuse of dementing people by their caregivers

The term 'granny battering' was first used in the UK by Baker (1975). It is believed that about 5% of elderly people experience some degree of abuse, although the sensitivity of the issue on the part of both the abused and the abuser makes accurate assessment of its occurrence difficult. Abuse refers to a variety of ways in which caregivers can behave towards their dependent elderly relative and may include physical, psychological, or material abuse, and active or passive neglect (Wolf & Pillemer 1989).

Physical abuse includes physical harm, sexual molestation, medication misuse, unmet physical needs, physical restraint, and murder. Psychological abuse refers to inflicting mental anguish and may include subjecting the person with dementia to shame, blame, ridicule or rejection. Caregiver behaviours, such as insults or intimidation, which engender fear and agitation, are psychological abuse as is manipulation,

---

Box 11.4 High expressed emotion in the family

Mr Jackson has been demented for about 2 years and lives with his wife and their unmarried daughter. Although his daughter can deal with her father, Mrs Jackson has no time for her husband's confused behaviour. She gets angry with her husband when he cannot do things like getting himself dressed properly and when he drops food from his mouth while he is at the dining table. Mrs Jackson often ends up losing her temper and saying things like, 'Are you stupid or something!' Their daughter understands that whereas Mr Jackson could take his wife's outbursts when he was well, he now cannot; he always rises to the bait – shouting, swearing and banging on the table – and becomes upset.

The family was visited by Joan, a community occupational therapist. After listening to Mrs Jackson and her daughter describe the situation, and noting particularly the volatile relationship between Mr and Mrs Jackson, she decided to focus on the high levels of emotion expressed by Mrs Jackson in an attempt to reduce this.

Joan took time to get to know the family. The assessment took a few visits and Joan found out the perspectives of Mr Jackson, Mrs Jackson and their daughter. Joan gave Mrs Jackson a copy of a book on dementia and explained how her husband was not really responsible for all his actions. Joan also suggested to Mrs Jackson that Mr Jackson's behaviour might be in part a response to her efforts to deal with him and that she might like to think about how she could deal with her husband now that he was demented. Joan suggested that Mrs Jackson could start writing a diary on her husband's behaviour, noting those occasions when Mr Jackson was calm and other times when he was disturbed. Joan asked her to identify possible causes for each time her husband was difficult following something she had said to him. Mrs Jackson made a list of these situations and following discussion, with her daughter present, Mrs Jackson came to see that her husband had often become confused because of something she had said to him and the associated expression of high levels of emotion. Joan went through each 'difficult situation' in the diary, focusing on those situations that were cropping up repeatedly. Joan tried to get Mrs Jackson to think of alternative ways of dealing with each situation so that her husband might not become so distressed. On occasions, Joan got Mrs Jackson to role play various 'difficult' situations, which helped Mrs Jackson gain insight into how she might control her expressed emotion. The alliance Joan made with Mrs Jackson's daughter proved particularly helpful in getting Mrs Jackson to think about how she could deal with situations more appropriately. Joan visited the family on about 12 occasions over a period of 3 months and gradually Mrs Jackson got used to dealing with her husband without high levels of expressed emotion.

---

such as deliberately withholding or falsifying information in order to mislead. Material abuse refers to the illegal or improper exploitation and/or use of money or resources belonging to the dementing person. Role neglect occurs when there is neglect of or failure to perform the caregiving obligation and includes inadequate supervision or abandonment. Passive neglect occurs when there is a refusal or a failure to fulfil a care-taking obligation.

Various writers have attempted to identify the characteristics of elderly people who are abused. Glendenning (1993) cites Tomlin (1989), who suggests that the most likely victims are those with whom it is difficult to communicate and those with fluctuating difficulty. She comments that people with Parkinson's disease and dementia are the most commonly abused elderly people and states that 'American studies have shown the classic victim to be an elderly person over the age of seventy-five, female, roleless, functionally impaired, lonely, fearful and living at home with one child' (Tomlin 1989, p. 5).

Homer and Gilleard (1990) found that 45% of caregivers of elderly people openly admitted to some form of abuse. Their findings suggest that different types of abuse occur for different reasons and that physical abuse depends on the characteristics of the abuser rather than the abused. The most significant contributing factor was the consumption of alcohol by the caregiver. Other factors included poor pre-morbid relationship and previous abuse over many years. Few of the people in the study who were abused complained of abuse themselves.

Abuse in residential homes

Elderly abuse also occurs within residential homes and Horrocks (1988) lists various factors that contribute to this:

- sleeping areas being too large, unhomely and open, in which residents have few personal possessions
- sleeping areas being overcrowded with beds too close together
- poor or dilapidated carpets and furnishings
- a custodial atmosphere
- the excessive use of restraint (Tomlin 1989).

Cause and effect is difficult to disentangle here and more research is needed to identify the mechanisms through which the characteristics of residential homes contribute to abuse.

Assessment protocols

Davis (1993) describes two assessment protocols for identifying cases of elder abuse. The first, the Assessment Protocol for Elder Abuse, is a screening procedure and documents cases where there is suspicion of abuse or neglect. It is interesting to note that assessors are asked to use their powers of observation, instinct and 'gut feeling' when completing the assessment protocol.

The second assessment protocol is the Assessment Protocol for Carer Abuse which is designed to identify indications of possible stress and intensity. Assessment includes physical signs of abuse (e.g. bruising, abrasions, poor hygiene), cognitive and emotional functioning, interpersonal relationships and sexual abuse.

CONCLUSION

This chapter has looked at various approaches towards understanding dementia. The biomedical approach is valuable but we note increasing interest in psychosocial explanations of dementia, and models of dementia which incorporate the impact on families of living with a dementing member. These perspectives on dementia are sometimes presented as polar opposites but, in practice, they are not necessarily in conflict. All may be drawn on by clinicians to develop an in-depth understanding of the process of dementia, the dynamics of dementia within families and strategies for improving the quality of family life for dementing people and their family carers.

REFERENCES

Absher R, Cummings J 1994 Cognitive and non-cognitive aspects of dementia syndromes: an overview. In: Burns A, Levi R (eds) Dementia. Chapman and Hall, London

Adams T 1990 Crisis and the confused elderly. Nursing 4(6): 9–11

Alzheimer A 1907 Über eine eigenartige Erkrankung der Hirnrinde. Allgemeine Zeitschrift für Psychiatrie und Psychisch-Gerichtlich Medizine 64: 146–148

Amaducci L, Lippi A 1994 Risk factors. In: Burns A, Levy R (eds) Dementia. Chapman and Hall, London

Austrom M, Gendrie H 1990 Death of the personality: the grief responses of Alzheimer's family caregiver. American Journal of Alzheimer's Care and Related Disorders Research 5(2): 16–27

Baker A A 1975 Granny battering. Modern Geriatrics 8: 20–24

Barnes R F, Rashkind M A, Scott F R et al 1981 Problems with families caring for Alzheimer patients: the use of a support group. Journal of the American Geriatrics Society 14: 355–360

Berrios G E 1987 Dementia in the seventeenth and eighteenth centuries: a conceptual history. Psychological Medicine 17: 829–837

Berrios G E 1990 Alzheimer's disease: a conceptual history. International Journal of Geriatric Psychiatry 64: 355–365

Berrios G E, Freeman H 1991 Dementia before the twentieth century. In: Berrios G E, Freeman H (eds) Alzheimer and the dementias. Royal Society of Medicine Services Limited, London

Bledin K, MacCarthy L, Kuipers L et al 1990 Daughters of people with dementia: expressed emotion, strain and coping. British Journal of Psychiatry 157: 221–227

Bowlby J 1969 Attachment and loss, vols 1, 2, 3. Basic Books, New York

Brown G, Monck E M, Carstairs G, Wing J L 1962 The influence of family life on the course of schizophrenic illness. British Journal of Preventative and Social Medicine 16: 55–68

Cannon W B 1932 The wisdom of the body. Norton, New York

Caplan G 1961 An approach to community mental health. Tavistock, London

Colerick E J, George L K 1986 Predictors of institutionalisation among caregivers of patients with Alzheimer's disease. Journal of the American Geriatrics Society 7: 493–498

Collins C, Liken M, King S et al 1993 Loss and grief among family caregivers of relatives with dementia. Qualitative Health Research 2: 236–253

Coppel D B, Burton C, Becker J, Fiore J 1985 Relationships of cognition associated with coping reactions to depression in spousal caregivers of Alzheimer's disease patients. Cognitive Therapy and Research 9(3): 253–266

Corbin J, Strauss A 1991 A nursing model for chronic illness management based upon the trajectory framework. Image 5: 9–25

Cummings J L 1988 Intellectual impairment in Parkinson's disease. Clinical, pathologic and biochemical correlates. Journal of Geriatric Psychiatry and Neurology 1: 24–36

Davis M 1993 Recognising abuse: an assessment tool for nurses. In: Decalmer P, Lendenning F (eds) The treatment of elderly people. Sage, London

Dole H, Varian J 1994 Crisis intervention in psychogeriatrics: a round-the-clock commitment? International Journal of Geriatric Psychiatry 9: 65–72

Eagles J M, Beattie J, Blackwood G et al 1987 The mental health of elderly couples I: the effects of the cognitively impaired spouses. British Journal of Psychiatry 150: 293–298

Fitting M, Rabins P, Lucas M J, Eastham J 1986 Caregivers for demented patients: a comparison of husbands and wives. Gerontologist 26(3): 248–252

Folstein M F, Folstien S E, McHugh P R 1975 Mini-mental state: a practical method for grading the cognitive state of patients for the clinician. Journal of Psychiatric Research 12: 189–198

Fox P 1989 From senility to Alzheimer's disease: the rise of Alzheimer's disease movement. Milbank Quarterly 67: 58–103

George L K, Gwyther L P 1986 Caregiver well-being: a multi-dimensional examination of caregivers of demented adults. The Gerontologist 26: 253–259

Ghanbari H A, Miller B E, Haigler H J et al 1990 Biochemical assay of Alzheimer's disease-associated protein(s) in human brain tissue: a clinical study. Journal of the American Medical Association 263: 2907–2910

Gilhooly M L M 1984 The social dimensions of senile dementia. In: Hanley I, Hodge J (eds) Psychological approaches to the care of the elderly. Croom Helm, Beckenham

Gilhooly M L M 1986 The impact of care-giving on care-givers: factors associated with the psychological well-being of people supporting a dementing relative in the community. British Journal of Medical Psychology 59: 165–171

Gilhooly M L M, Whittick J E 1989 Expressed emotion in caregivers of the dementing elderly. British Journal of Medical Psychology 62: 265–272

Gilleard C 1984 Emotional stress amongst the supporters of the elderly mentally infirm. British Journal of Psychiatry 145: 172–177

Gilleard C J, Belford H, Gilleard E et al 1984 Emotional distress among the supporters of the elderly mentally infirm. British Journal of Psychiatry 145: 172–177

Glaser B G, Strauss A L 1967 The discovery of grounded theory: strategies for qualitative research. Aldine, Chicago

Glendenning F 1993 What is elder abuse and neglect? In: Decalmer F, Glendenning P (eds) The treatment of elderly people. Sage, London

Goffman E 1968 Asylums. Penguin, Harmondsworth

Goldberg D 1978 A manual for the General Health Questionnaire. NEFR-Nelson, Windsor

Grad J, Sainsbury P 1965 The effects that patients have on their families in a community care and a central psychiatric service: a two year follow-up. British Journal of Psychiatry 114: 265–278

Graves A, van Duijn C, Chandra V et al 1991 Alcohol and tobacco consumption as risk factors for Alzheimer's disease: a collaborative reanalysis of case-control studies. International Journal of Epidemiology 20(supplement 1): 548–557

Gruenthal E M 1927 Klinisch-anatomisch vergleichende Untersuchungen über den Greisen. Z. Ges. Neurol. Psychiatr. 111: 763. Cited in Gilhooly M L M 1984 The social dimensions of senile dementia. In: Hanley I, Hodge J (eds) Psychological approaches to the care of the elderly. Croom Helm, Beckenham

Hagnell O, Lanke J, Roreman B, Ohman R, Ojesjo L 1983 Current trends in the incidence of senile and multi-infarct dementia: a prospective study of a population followed over 25 years: the Lundy study. Archiv fur Psychiatrie und Nervenkrunkheiten 233(6): 423–438

Haley W, Levine E G, Brown S, Bartolucci A A 1987 Stress, appraisal, coping, social support as predictors of adaptional outcome amongst dementia caregivers. Psychology and Ageing 2(4): 323–330

Hansen L, Salmon D, Galasko D et al 1990 The Lewy Body variant of Alzheimer's disease: a clinical and pathological entity. Neurology 40: 1–8

Heston L L, Mastri A R, Anderson V, White J 1981 Dementia of the Alzheimer's type: clinical genetics, natural history and associated conditions. Archives of General Psychiatry 38: 1085–1090

Hirschfeld M 1983 Homecare versus institutionalisation: family caregiving and senile brain disease. International Journal of Nursing Studies 20: 23–32

Hirschfeld M J 1981 Families living and coping with the cognitively impaired. In: Copp A (ed) Recent advances in nursing, vol. 2: care of the aged. Churchill Livingstone, Edinburgh

Holland A J 1994 Down's syndrome and dementia of the Alzheimer type. In: Burns A, Levy R (eds) Dementia. Chapman and Hall Medical, London

Homer A C, Gilleard C 1990 Abuse of elderly people by their carers. British Medical Journal 301: 1359–1362

Horowitz A 1985 Sons and daughters as caregivers to older parents: difference in role performance and consequences. Gerontologist 25: 612–617

Horowitz A, Shindelman L W 1983 Reciprocity and affection: past influences to current caregiving. Journal of Gerontological Social Work 5: 5–20

Horrocks P 1988 Elderly people: abused and forgotten. Health Service Journal 22 September: 1085

Jagger C, Lindesay J 1993 The epidemiology of senile dementia. In: Burns A (ed) Ageing and dementia: a methodological approach. Arnold, London

Keady J, Nolan M 1994 The carer-led assessment process (CLASP): a framework for the assessment of need in dementia caregivers. Journal of Clinical Nursing 3: 103–108

Kielcolt-Glasser, Dura J K, Speicher C E et al 1991 Spousal caregivers of dementia victims: longitudinal changes in immunity and health. Psychosomatic Medicine 53: 345–362

Kiloh L C 1961 Pseudo-dementia. Acta Psychiatrica Scandinavica 37: 336–351

King Edward's Fund for London 1986 Living well in old age. King's Fund, London

Kitwood T 1987 Explaining senile dementia: the limits of neuropathological research. Free Associations 10: 117–140

Kitwood T 1990a The dialectics of dementia: with particular reference to Alzheimer's disease. Ageing and Society 10: 177–196

Kitwood T 1990b Understanding senile dementia: a psychobiographical approach. Free Associations 19: 60–76

Kitwood T 1993 Towards the reconstruction of an organic mental disorder. In: Radley A (ed) Worlds of disorder. Routlege, London

Kitwood T, Bredin K 1992 Towards a theory of dementia care: personhood and well-being. Ageing and Society 10: 269–287

Lawton M P, Brody E M 1969 Instrumental activities of daily living. Gerontologist 9: 179–186

Lindemann E 1944 Symptomatology and management of acute grief. American Journal of Psychiatry 101: 141

Lishman W A 1987 Organic psychiatry. Blackwell, Oxford

McKeith I 1994 The differential diagnosis of dementia. In: Burns A, Levy R (eds) Dementia. Churchill Livingstone, Edinburgh

Martyn C N, Barker D J P, Osmond C et al 1989 Geographical relation between Alzheimer's disease and aluminium in the drinking water. The Lancet 1: 59–62

Mathew L, Mattocks K, Slatt L M 1990 Exploring the roles of men: caring for demented relatives. Journal of Gerontological Nursing 10: 20–25

Miesen B 1992 Attachment theory and dementia. In: Jones G, Miesen B (eds) Care-giving in dementia. Routledge, London

Miller E, Morris R 1993 The psychology of dementia. Wiley, Chichester

Morris L W, Morris R G, Britton P G 1988 The relationship between marital intimacy, perceived strain, and depression in spouse carers of dementia sufferers. British Journal of Medical Psychology 62: 173–179

Morris L W, Morris R G, Britton P G 1989 Social support networks and formal support as factors influencing psychological adjustment of spouse caregivers of dementia sufferers. International Journal of Geriatric Psychiatry 4: 47–51

Morris R G, Woods R T, Davies K S, Morris L W 1992 Gender differences in carers of dementia sufferers. British Journal of Psychiatry 158 (Supplement 10): 69–74

Mortimer J A, van Duijn C, Chandra V et al 1991 Head injury as a risk factor for Alzheimer's disease: a collaborative re-analysis of case-control studies. International Journal of Epidemiology 20(Supplement 1): S28–S5

Mountjoy C Q 1993 Ageing and dementia: a nosological and neuropathological overview. In: Burns A (ed) Ageing and dementia: a methodological approach. Arnold, London

Murphy E Dementia and mental illness in older people. Macmillan, London

Myers K, Crawford J 1993 Assessment and care management of people with dementia and their carers. In: Chapman A, Marshall M (eds) Dementia: new skills for social workers. Jessica Kingsley, London

O'Brien M D 1994 Vascular dementia: definitions, epidemiology and clinical features. In: Burns A, Levy R (eds) Dementia. Churchill Livingstone, Edinburgh

Orford J, O'Reilly P, Goonatilleke A 1987 Expressed emotion and perceived family interaction in the key relatives of elderly patients with dementia. Psychological Medicine 17: 963–970

Oxford English Dictionary

Parad H J, Resnik H 1971 The practice of crisis intervention in emergency care. In: Resnik H J, Ruben H, Ruben D (eds) Emergency psychiatric care: the management of mental health crisis. Charles Press, Bowie, Md

Parkes C M 1986 Bereavement: studies of grief in adult life, 2nd edn. Penguin, Harmondsworth

Patterson M, Whitehouse P 1990 The diagnostic assessment of patients with dementia. In: Mace N (ed) Dementia care: patient, family and community. Johns Hopkins University Press, Baltimore

Pearlin L I, Turner H, Semple S 1990 Coping and the mediation of stress. In: Light E, Lebowitz B D (eds) Alzheimer's disease, treatment and stress: directions for research. Hemisphere Publishing, New York

Perry R H, Irving D, Blessed G et al 1990 Senile dementia of the Lewy Body type: a clinically and neuropathologically distinct form of dementia in the elderly. Journal of Neurological Science 95: 119–139

Post F 1965 The psychiatry of later life. Pergamon Press, Oxford

Rando T A 1986 Loss and anticipatory grief. Lexington Books, Lexington

Ratna L 1982 Crisis intervention in psychogeriatrics: a two year follow-up study. British Journal of Psychiatry 14: 296–301

Ritter S, Norman I J, Rentoul L, Bodley D E 1996 A model of clinical supervision for nurses undertaking short placements in mental health care settings. Journal of Clinical Nursing 5(3): 149–158

Robinson B 1983 Validation of a caregiver strain index. Journal of Gerontology 38: 344–348

Rothschild D 1937 Pathologic changes in senile psychoses and their psychobiologic significance. American Journal of Psychiatry 93: 757

Rothschild D 1942 Neuropathological changes in arteriosclerotic psychoses and their psychiatric significance. Archives of Neurobiological Psychiatry 48: 417

Rothschild 1956 (cited in Post 1965)

Royal College of Physicians 1982 Organic impairment in the elderly: implications for research, education and the provision of services. A Report of the Royal College of Physicians by the College Committee on Geriatrics, London

Sanford J R A 1975 Tolerance of debility in elderly dependents by supporters at home: its significance for hospital practice. British Medical Journal III: 471–475

Schulz R, Biegel D, Morycz R, Visintainer P 1990 Psychological paradigms for understanding caregiving. In: Light E, Lebowitz B D (eds) Alzheimer's disease, treatment and stress: directions for research. Hemisphere Publishing Corporation, New York

Scott J P, Roberto K, Hutton J T 1986 Families of Alzheimer's victims: family support to the care givers. Journal of the American Geriatrics Society 34: 348–354

Taylor P 1987 A living bereavement. Nursing Times 30: 27–30

Teng E L, Chui H C, Schneider L S, Metzer E 1987 Alzheimer's dementia: performance on the Mini-Mental State Examination. Journal of Consulting and Clinical Psychology 55: 96–100

Tobiansky R 1994a Understanding dementia II: vascular dementia. Journal of Dementia Care 1: 23–24

Tobiansky R 1994b Understanding dementia III: diffuse Lewy body disease. Journal of Dementia Care 1: 26–27

Tomlin S 1989 The abuse of elderly people: an unnecessary, and preventable problem. British Geriatric Society, London

Wilcock G, Jacoby R 1991a Dementias of old age: Alzheimer's disease. In: Jacoby R, Oppenheimer C Psychiatry in the elderly. Oxford University Press, Oxford

Wilcock G, Jacoby R 1991b Dementias of old age: dementia of the frontal lobe. In: Jacoby R, Oppenheimer C Psychiatry in the elderly. Oxford University Press, Oxford

Wilkinson I, Graham-White J 1982 Psychogeriatric Dependency Rating Scales (PGDRS): a method of assessment for use by nurses. British Journal of Psychiatry 137: 558–565

Williams L, Miller E 1992 The effects of prolonged high aluminium intake on cognitive functioning. Paper presented to the London Conference of the British Conference of the Psychological Society. As reported in Miller & Morris (1993)

Williams H W, Quesnel E, Fish V W et al 1942 Studies in senile and arteriosclerotic psychoses: relative significance of extrinsic factors in their development. American Journal of Psychiatry 98: 712–715

Williamson G M, Schulz R 1990 Relationship orientation, quality of prior relationship, and distress among caregivers of Alzheimer's patients. Psychology and Aging 5(4): 502–509

Willoughby J, Keating N 1991 Being in control: the process of caring for a relative with Alzheimer's disease. Qualitative Health Research 1(1): 27–50

Wilson D C 1955 The pathology of senility. American Journal of Psychiatry 111: 902–906

Wolf R S, Pillemer K A 1989 Helping elderly victims: the reality of elder abuse. Columbia University Press, New York

Worden J W 1991 Grief counselling and grief therapy: a handbook for the mental health practitioner, 2nd edn. Routledge, London

Zarit S, Reever K, Bach-Peterson J 1980 Relatives of the impaired elderly: correlates of feelings of burden. Gerontologist 20: 649–655

RECOMMENDED READING

Burns A (ed) 1993 Aging and dementia: a methodological approach. Edward Arnold, London. *This excellent book provides a clear account of developments in research relating to people with dementia and their relatives. Its focus is the development of research measures but it also covers the research findings.*

Burns A, Levy R 1994 Dementia. Chapman and Hall, London. *A comprehensive, state-of-the-art textbook which sets out a vast array of empirical research concerning dementia taken from the medical and social sciences. Some of the chapters, such as those on service provision and psychological approaches, are valuable for readers without a medical education.*

Chapman A, Marshall M (eds) 1993 Dementia: new skills for social workers. Jessica Kingsley Publishers, London. *This book is written for practitioners and describes various approaches that can be used to help people with dementia and their informal caregivers. It is written from a social work perspective but is relevant to other professions. The book includes practical accounts of strategies that may be used with people who are dementing and their informal caregivers. It explores new areas of working such as the use of systemic family intervention with elderly dementing people, the use of group work and empowerment approaches.*

Kitwood T, Bredin K 1992 Person to person, 2nd edn. Gale Centre Publications, Loughton. *A helpful little book designed to give practical guidance of caregivers to people with dementia. It puts into practice Kitwood and Bredin's theoretical approach to care.*

Opie A 1992 There's nobody there: the community care of confused older people. Oxford University Press, Auckland. *An interesting qualitative study that examines the practice of giving care to dementing people and implications for social policy. The study presents an account of the everyday lives of 28 family members giving care to people with dementia. The book, written from a feminist, postmodernist perspective, highlights the way in which responses to giving care cross gender boundaries.*

Miller E, Morris R 1993 The psychology of dementia. Wiley, Chichester. *An excellent book that explains the contribution of psychology to our understanding of dementia. Chapters cover memory and language of people with dementia, assessment and management and the provision of care to informal caregivers. It is valuable to both students and qualified practitioners.*

Wright L 1993 Alzheimer's disease and marriage. Sage, London. *A readable study that examines the effect of Alzheimer's disease upon people who are married. The study throws light upon day-to-day aspects of the marriage relationship such as household tasks, tension, companionship, affection and sexuality, and commitment. Guidelines for assessment and intervention are given.*

12

Substance misuse in the elderly

Declan M McLoughlin
Michael Farrell

INTRODUCTION

Drug and alcohol problems in the elderly are now more common than was previously acknowledged. The growth of drug dependence in the younger population is likely to persist into old age in a substantial minority of that population. It is also likely that substance-related problems will arise de novo in elderly populations and will become increasingly clinically relevant. The failure to recognise the extent of these problems and the virtual absence of research is generally accounted for by the relative size of the problem. However, the disparity in levels of epidemiological and research activity in the young compared to the elderly can only be accounted for by underlying social values which give priority to youth and an irrational assumption that such problems only arise in young people. Most of the research carried out to date has concentrated on the younger elderly (55–75 years) and little is known about the very old (over 80 years).

Ageing is a highly complex process dictated and modified by a wide variety of factors including social, economic, cultural, cellular and genetic ones (see Chs 1 and 3). Whilst it is a universal process, ageing is also a heterogeneous one with a large degree of inter-individual variation. Hence, as a group, the elderly can be said to have a lot in common but, as individuals, they are equally different. The elderly individual's response to a drug also needs to be similarly considered. Furthermore, the prevalence of dementia and of chronic illnesses (e.g. cardiac and respiratory disorders) is high in this population, compounding the response to drugs and further complicating the manifestations of drug-related problems.

This chapter describes how alcohol and drug-related problems present in the elderly, outlines the extent of the problem and provides guidelines for

---

Box 12.1 Definitions of commonly used terms

Substance. Any chemical, drug or medication that can be either prescribed or non-prescribed, licit or illicit. Most substances that are misused typically have psychoactive properties, i.e. they act on the central nervous system, particularly on the mind or psyche. Non-psychoactive medications can also be misused.

Use. Appropriate, socially-sanctioned consumption of a substance that does not lead to future harm, e.g. social drinking, taking prescribed medication as directed.

Misuse. Inappropriate use of a substance often contrary to instructions, e.g. under- and over-dosing or failure to take prescribed medications. The term has no implications for future harm.

Intoxication. A transient and reversible syndrome following the consumption of a psychoactive substance. The syndrome comprises maladaptive behavioural and psychological changes including altered level of consciousness, impaired cognition and changes in mood, judgement and perception sometimes associated with disinhibited and aggressive behaviour. The manifestation of intoxication usually depends upon the particular substance (e.g. drunkenness caused by alcohol) but may be unpredictable (e.g. agitation caused by antidepressant medication).

Abuse. In the DSM-IV (APA 1994) this is defined as a maladaptive pattern of substance use resulting in significant impairment or distress. This pattern is manifested by at least one of the following occurring in a 12-month period:
- failure to fulfil major occupational, educational or domestic roles on account of recurrent substance use

- recurrent use of the substance in dangerous situations, e.g. driving
- legal problems due to recurrent substance use, e.g. disorderly conduct, drunk driving
- use of the substance is continued with despite such use precipitating or worsening social and interpersonal problems, e.g. marital strife, domestic violence. This pattern of use occurs in the absence of evidence for substance dependence.

Tolerance. An increasingly greater amount of the substance is required to achieve the desired effect – usually intoxication – or the effect of the substance decreases with continued consumption of the same quantity; tolerance is decreased if intoxication begins to result with increasingly smaller amounts of the substance.

Craving. An intense subjective drive to use a particular substance.

Substance dependence. The ICD-10 (WHO 1992) and DSM-IV (APA 1994) criteria are shown in Table 12.1.

Substance withdrawal. A substance-specific syndrome occurring when use of the substance – previously consumed in large quantities over a prolonged period – is suddenly stopped or significantly reduced. The onset and course of the syndrome are time-limited and vary depending upon the nature of the substance used. The most serious and severe physical symptom is the development of convulsions. Psychological symptoms such as anxiety, mood and sleep disturbances are common. Withdrawal states include the 'shakes' and 'cold turkey' associated respectively with chronic heavy use of alcohol and opiates.

---

assessment and management. Definitions of the terms as used in this chapter are provided in Box 12.1. Early sections of the chapter provide an introduction to some of the general concepts of substance misuse with particular reference to the elderly. The remaining sections focus on the following specific substances: alcohol, sedative-hypnotics, prescription and over the counter medications, tobacco and illicit drugs.

RECOGNITION OF SUBSTANCE MISUSE IN THE ELDERLY

It is only recently that substance misuse for the elderly has come to be identified as a substantial public health concern. This is exemplified by the available evidence concerning alcohol use. A past history of heavy alcohol consumption at any stage in the life cycle is predictive of future social, physical and psychological problems (Colsher & Wallace 1990) and, even if heavy drinking is discontinued, is associated with at least a fivefold increase in the risk for late-life psychiatric disorder –

most notably depression and dementia (Saunders et al 1991). Countries with an upward trend in alcohol consumption coupled with an expanding elderly population will probably experience an increase in mental health problems in the elderly of the future.

Several theories have been advanced as to why substance misuse in the elderly has historically been under-recognised and to some extent been a subject of benign neglect. Signs and symptoms of substance misuse in the elderly often do not fit neatly into the textbook descriptions based on the young. The presentation may not be as obvious or as florid as that seen in younger adults. Atkinson (1990) has highlighted how substance misuse can mimic the symptoms of other medical and psychiatric conditions in the elderly, thereby obscuring the correct diagnosis. Moreover, substance misuse may precipitate new medical conditions or exacerbate already existing illnesses. In such instances the aetiological relevance of the substance misuse may not be considered and may even be ignored if detected. The social isolation experienced by many elderly people and the – sometimes inappropriate – taking-over of the elder's roles by well-meaning carers can militate against detection of substance-related problems. Even if these are recognised they have tended to be under-reported. Carers may be embarrassed by acknowledging the presence of substance misuse, may not consider it harmful or may inadvertently perpetuate such behaviour while not recognising it to be problematic and injurious to health. In fact, many carers may incorrectly condone substance misuse, notably alcohol abuse, believing it to be one the few pleasures left to a progressively incapacitated elderly relative or charge. Medical and social service personnel are also susceptible to the consequences of similar belief systems. Consequently, substance misuse problems often escape clinical detection, even in in-patients and, even when identified, patients may not be referred for specialist treatment (McInnes & Powell 1994).

Blazer & Pennybacker (1984) have identified research methodology shortcomings that account for some of the underestimation of alcohol-related problems in the elderly: heterogeneity of the populations between and within studies; lack of standardisation of diagnostic criteria and terminology used from study to study; and differences in data collection techniques employed across the studies they examined. Also, traditionally it was taught that conditions such as opioid and alcohol dependency were rare in the elderly. Much of previous clinical practice and thinking was influenced by earlier reports that these conditions were self-limiting due to abusers either dying young or recovering spontaneously in a 'maturing-out' process (Drew 1968, Winick 1962) and that the likelihood of a new substance-related problem developing after the age of 50 was negligible. It is not difficult to conceive how such thinking could lead to a low index of suspicion for substance misuse in the elderly and hence lower rates for investigation and detection. It is now recognised, and has been so for at least the past decade, that alcohol dependency, to use the best-studied example, can develop for the first time after the age of 60. In fact, late-onset alcoholism has been reported to account for approximately one-third of alcoholism in the elderly (Finney & Moos 1984, Atkinson 1990).

DIAGNOSIS AND ASSESSMENT OF SUBSTANCE MISUSE

Diagnostic criteria

The most commonly used diagnostic criteria for

substance dependence are the guidelines described in ICD-10 (WHO 1992) and the operationalised criteria of DSM-IV (APA 1994) which are detailed in Table 12.1. These contemporary criteria have reduced the previous emphasis on the physiological features of substance dependence and have incorporated both the psychological and social aspects of dependence into their diagnostic systems. The criteria for intoxication, abuse, dependency and withdrawal can be applied to practically all classes of substances as a framework for the development of a common biopsychosocial and behavioural model for these disorders (West & Gossop 1994). Some of the clinical features of a particular syndrome, such as dependence or withdrawal, are substance-specific. For example, some of the symptoms of the opioid withdrawal syndrome (e.g. pupillary dilation, piloerection and yawning) are not typically associated with withdrawal from alcohol.

Both the ICD-10 (WHO 1992) and DSM-IV (APA 1994) provide criteria for a wide range of disorders (dependence, abuse, intoxication, withdrawal as well as substance-induced conditions such as delirium, dementia, amnestic disorder, psychosis with delusions and/or hallucinations, affective disorder, anxiety and sleep disorders and sexual dysfunction) that, in part or in total, can be applied to a wide variety of substances including alcohol, opioids, cannabinoids, sedatives/ hypnotics, cocaine, other stimulants including amphetamines and caffeine, phenylcyclidine and ketamine, hallucinogens, nicotine, volatile solvents as well as polysubstance misuse. However, it is uncertain how applicable these diagnostic systems are to the elderly as they are based on research data mostly from younger adults. Although these diagnostic systems have not been validated in the elderly, they nonetheless serve as the most useful and practical guidelines available to establish, for both clinical and research purposes, the diagnoses of substance dependence and abuse. Reliable criteria specifically designed and validated for use in the elderly would be of major benefit to future research efforts and remain to be developed.

Psychosocial risk factors

The most commonly consumed substances by the elderly are alcohol, tobacco and prescribed sedative-hypnotics, especially benzodiazepines. In general, men tend to use the former while women use the latter, which are usually obtained by prescription. The psychosocial risk factors for late onset alcohol and other drug dependence is less than clear-cut.

Table 12.1 ICD-10 and DSM-IV diagnostic criteria for substance dependence.
For both diagnostic systems, at least three of the numbered criteria need to have occurred or been experienced within the same 12-month period

ICD-10	DSM-IV
1. Strong desire/compulsion to use the substance	1. Evidence of tolerance
2. Difficulty in controlling the onset, termination and level of use of the substance	2. Evidence of withdrawal (a) features of the substance-specific withdrawal syndrome or (b) the same or similar substance is used to relieve or prevent withdrawal symptoms
3. Evidence of withdrawal	3. The substance is used over a longer period or in larger amounts than was originally intended
4. Evidence of tolerance	4. Persistent desire or unsuccessful attempts to reduce or control the substance use
5. Progressive neglect of pleasures or activities; increasing amount of time devoted to obtaining, using and recovering from the effects of the substance	5. A great deal of time spent in obtaining, using and recovering from effects of the substance
6. Persistent substance use despite clear evidence and user awareness of harmful consequences	6. Important activities, e.g social, occupational or recreational, are given up or reduced due to substance use
Also required by ICD-10: (a) narrowing of personal repertoire of patterns of substance use, i.e. tendency to use the substance in the same way every day regardless of the circumstances and (b) a desire or subjective compulsion to use the substance is present	7. Continued substance use despite knowledge of substance-related persistent or recurrent physical or psychological problems

Atkinson et al (1992) have indicated that the relationship between life stressors and late life substance-related problems is complex. Old age can be a time of great upheaval in which the individual has to negotiate several novel life events – many of which are inevitable – such as retirement, loss of income, bereavements, gradual and occasionally sudden shifts in social and domestic roles and responsibilities, plus the curtailment on physical independence secondary to the effects of ageing. The relationship between substance consumption and stressors may be a reciprocal one in that individuals, due to intoxication, decreased risk awareness, physical and mental deterioration, etc., are more likely to encounter negative life events which, if not of initial aetiological import, may prove to be perpetuating factors. Ready availability of a substance can significantly influence the level of consumption and the risk of developing problems.

Some substances, such as alcohol and sedatives, may be incorrectly used as self-medication to relieve pain, insomnia and depression or anxiety, even though such use may obscure, perpetuate and aggravate the clinical picture. Such use is often inadvertently supported by well-intentioned relatives and condoned by health care workers as some comfort, albeit temporary, may well be derived from ingestion of these substances. Unfortunately such beliefs can lead to collusion with self-damaging behaviour and prevent or delay adequate identification, assessment and management of the true underlying difficulties.

Biological risk factors

There are age-related pharmacokinetic changes in the body's ability to process and to excrete alcohol and other drugs. In the elderly there is altered absorption of drugs from the gastrointestinal system, distribution of ingested drugs due to altered protein binding, decreased muscle mass and a decrease in the ratio of body water to fat. Metabolism and excretion are affected as a result of reduced hepatic blood flow and liver enzyme efficiency, as well as decreased clearance through the kidneys. The consequence of these pharmacokinetic changes is that smaller amounts of a substance, such as alcohol, can be intoxicating or toxic in the elderly (Atkinson 1990). Concomitant with this are alterations in the body's response with age to a given substance. For example, the same blood level of alcohol will have a greater effect on an elderly person than on a younger one.

There are also different levels of susceptibility between various organ systems in the elderly to the effects of alcohol, the central nervous system being the most vulnerable (Vogel-Sprott & Barrett 1984). The net result of these biological changes is that elderly people are more sensitive to and less tolerant of the effects of all types of drugs. The elderly consumer may not appreciate that a level of consumption previously deemed safe may no longer be so. Furthermore, this increased sensitivity is compounded by other age-related biological factors including an increased prevalence of cognitive impairment and medical disorders, coupled with a greater likelihood of inappropriate drug–drug interactions with medications prescribed for these conditions.

Assessment

The reason for referral may be only indirectly related to substance misuse or substance misuse may be an important, but as yet unidentified or unacknowledged aetiological factor. Ideally, patients should be accompanied by a reliable informant, preferably somebody they live with or who has known them for several years. Often patients are unwilling to provide full details about drug and alcohol consumption and may not be able adequately to describe their difficulties if there is cognitive impairment. A source of corroborating and collateral information is invaluable in such instances. Furthermore, if the informant is a spouse or other close and involved relative it provides them with an opportunity to become involved from the beginning in treatment and management decisions.

The main aim of the assessment is to outline a full drinking and drug using career and current pattern of consumption, the degree of dependence and the extent of substance-related problems. It is generally helpful to record a history without initially assuming the degree of problems associated with particular behaviour such as alcohol or drug consumption. Often the most neutral point of entry is the elucidation of the lifetime drinking career. Such an approach can provide a wealth of information on the drinking career and possible problems related to drinking. Similar information on the drug use career is helpful in contextualising current problems. It can also be done in a manner that does not appear to stand in judgement of current behaviour.

The first meeting with the patient is important not only for gathering information but also, perhaps more crucially, to obtain the patient's trust and create the foundations for a solid therapeutic relationship. Some patients will be ambivalent about their need for treatment and may feel that they have been coerced into attendance. For some it will be a potentially embarrassing and humiliating occasion, while others may demonstrate marked denial and refuse to engage in the assessment. Therefore, sensitivity is required and the patient's feelings and wishes must be respected. At the same time, the interviewer, if appropriate, should indicate concern over the issue of alcohol or drug consumption and not allow the topic to be glossed over.

Enquiries about substance use and misuse should be routine practice when interviewing an elderly patient, their relatives and other informants. Histories of alcohol use taken from elderly people on admission to hospital are frequently inadequate, interviewers omitting to obtain information about the amounts consumed (Naik & Jones 1994). Also, health care workers often have a fear that they may offend the sensibilities of others, especially their elders, and do not wish to precipitate an awkward situation. However, because substance misuse may not be considered a problem or may even be encouraged by carers, unless direct questions are asked, vital information may not be acquired and the diagnosis may be missed.

The majority of patients, both young and old, have no objections to being asked about their consumption of alcohol, tobacco and use of illicit drugs when this is done in a suitably tactful manner. Inordinately hostile or indignant responses should raise one's suspicions that a delicate matter has been broached. At the same time, it is important not to alienate the patient by a 'third degree' interview style. If the patient is adamant in refusing to discuss issues of substance use and abuse this information can usually be sought at another time or from another source. In the long term it is important to gain the patient's trust and concentrate on developing a therapeutic alliance that will facilitate future care.

To date, no single screening instrument has been devised that has been validated for general substance misuse in the elderly. The CAGE (Ewing 1984) is a popular brief screening tool for alcohol abuse. It consists of four simple questions:

1. Have you ever felt you should **C**ut down on your drinking?
2. Have people **A**nnoyed you by criticising your drinking?

3. Have you ever felt bad or **G**uilty about your drinking?
4. Have you ever had a drink first thing in the morning to steady your nerves or get rid of a hangover (**E**ye-opener)?

The CAGE has been evaluated in an elderly medical out-patient setting (Buchsbaum et al 1992), giving a sensitivity and specificity of 86% and 78%, respectively, when one positive response was elicited.[1] With two positive responses, sensitivity fell to 70% but specificity rose to 91%. One needs to bear in mind, however, that the prevalence of alcohol-related problems in a medical out-patient setting is relatively high. Thus, caution is required if the CAGE is to be used in the community where it has not yet been adequately validated for elderly populations.

The Michigan Alcohol Screening Test (MAST) (Selzer 1971) is longer and more complex than the CAGE and like the CAGE is derived from studies on young alcohol abusers. A geriatric version, the MAST-G, has been created and validated by one group, demonstrating a greater sensitivity and specificity than either the MAST or CAGE screening questionnaires in an elderly study population (Beresford et al 1990, Blow et al 1992).

Standard clinical interviews, supplemented by informant accounts, along with examination of mental state and cognitive function, continue to be the best method of assessment. A comprehensive history of the substance misuse is required; i.e. duration of use, quantity used, pattern of consumption and details of any resultant physical, social, psychological and legal complications. A useful direct question to ask the patient is what benefit is derived from the alcohol or drug use. A major part of treatment will be to change the balance that exists for the patient between the advantages and disadvantages of substance consumption. Evidence should be sought of changing tolerance, withdrawal phenomena or other symptoms, detailed in Table 12.1, that might indicate dependence.

---

[1] The 'sensitivity' of a test or an investigation provides a measure of how well it detects what is being sought. 'Specificity' is an index of how effective the test is at excluding what is not being sought. In the text example, when one positive response is obtained, the CAGE questionnaire will detect 86% of the cases of problem drinking but will miss 14% of such cases; the same response will also allow exclusion of 76% of the non-problem drinkers but will incorrectly identify 24% of these as problem drinkers. As the number of positive responses rises to two the screening tool becomes less sensitive (70%) but more specific (91%) in detecting problem drinking.

Details of personal history, relevant significant relationships and current social situation are necessary to provide a complete and rounded picture of the patient and to define the social context of the substance misuse and the extent of available social supports. Additional information is required about past medical and psychiatric history including current medications, as well as family history for substance misuse and psychiatric disorders. Pre-morbid personality can be confirmed and expanded upon by informants.

Mental state examination should be thorough and should include detailed questioning on mood state, suicidal thoughts and action and cognitive functioning.

Routine physical examination is also essential. Elderly patients need to be screened for common medical conditions which can be exacerbated by substance misuse, especially alcohol abuse. On examination, it is important to search for and document signs of substance misuse such as personal neglect of hygiene, malnutrition, needle marks, signs of head injury and bodily bruising from recurrent falls whilst intoxicated, features of liver failure and evidence of peripheral neuropathy.

Baseline and screening laboratory investigations are also necessary in the elderly. These should include a full blood count, vitamin B_{12} and folate levels, urea and electrolyte estimation, liver function tests, glucose level and thyroid function tests. Baseline electrocardiogram and chest X-ray, which may indicate a history of multiple rib fractures, should be obtained. If deemed necessary, a urine sample can be used for drug screening. Other investigations (e.g. serum amylase levels, endoscopy, neuroradiology, electroencephalogram, etc.) will be dictated by the history and findings on mental state and physical examination. A home visit by members of the multidisciplinary team provides a unique opportunity to examine the patient's living conditions and assess ability to perform activities of daily living in an ecologically valid way. Note can be made of how well the home is being maintained, the level of hygiene, the patient's awareness of danger in the home and the extent to which cognitive impairment, if present, is interfering with the ability of the patient to care for herself. Whilst in the home, the opportunity should be taken, with the patient's consent, to inspect the premises. One occasionally finds empty bottles stashed in unlikely places and toilet cabinets overflowing with a bewildering range of medications. If possible, substances with a potential for misuse should be removed. During the course of follow-up, visits can be made to the home on a regular basis by either a district nurse or a community psychiatric nurse to oversee progress.

MANAGEMENT ISSUES IN SUBSTANCE MISUSE

Management decisions are usually made by the multidisciplinary team comprising medical, nursing, clinical psychology, occupational therapy, social worker and community-based staff, including outreach workers, community psychiatric nurses and district nurses. Other agencies may also be involved such as home helps, 'meals on wheels', day centre staff and local voluntary organisations. Three major aspects of the management of substance misuse by the elderly have been identified by Atkinson et al (1992):

- reduce the inappropriate consumption of the substance(s)
- identify and treat any coexisting problems
- organise suitable social interventions.

In mild cases, when consumption is not high and of short duration, the risk of dangerous withdrawal symptoms is low. If the patient is well-supported and cooperative, consumption can be gradually reduced as an out-patient or a day patient. If the opposite is the case and withdrawal is considered to be potentially hazardous, it is best to admit the patient to hospital before attempting to reduce the intake of the substance. Hospital admission will enable close medical supervision of the patient during withdrawal and also provide an opportunity for close observation and detailed assessment.

Admission to a day hospital or as an in-patient will also allow for more ready identification of any comorbid conditions that might be amenable to treatment; for example, depression, delirium, anxiety, cognitive impairment, insomnia, chronic pain and other medical problems. While the patient is withdrawing from the substance and remains off it, it should be possible to determine whether these conditions are primary or secondary to the substance misuse and to what extent they are contributing to and are worsened by it. Persisting depression or other symptoms should be appropriately treated.

The patient's social situation and level of support in the community also needs to be ascertained with particular reference to alcohol and drug free social support. If it proves impossible to support and care for the patient safely in the community, admission to hospital will need to be considered. There are no strict rules and each patient's care programme will need to be tailored to her needs. The social worker in the multidisciplinary team will be able to provide invaluable advice and help with housing, legal and financial matters. Many elderly people are often unaware of their entitlements and what benefits are due to them. Simple practical advice and help can be instrumental in improving the patient's social welfare. Other social interventions can range from the simple to the complicated, for example, from organising attendance at a local day centre or coordinating home help, to arranging long-term placement in a local authority accommodation or a nursing home.

ALCOHOL ABUSE AND DEPENDENCE

Epidemiology

Alcohol is the substance that has been best studied in the elderly. In a Liverpool community-based study, 46% of males and 14% of females aged 65–69 drank alcohol at least once per week; these figures fell to 25% of males and 8% of females in the over-80 age group (Saunders et al 1989). Another method of gauging alcohol use is to examine levels of abstinence within a community. Of 624 respondents in an earlier US survey 35% of the males and 56% of the females were considered to be abstainers as they had less than one drink per year (Cahalan & Cisin 1968).

The results of several useful studies from different sites with varied methodologies are available but all have methodological limitations of self-report and recall in the elderly. In the above Liverpool study (Saunders et al 1989) approximately 20% of the regular drinkers were consuming more than the recommended weekly maximum intake of 21 units for men and 14 units for women (one unit is the equivalent of 8 g of alcohol or the alcoholic content of a half pint of regular beer, a glass of wine or a measure of spirits). The overall point prevalence for alcohol-related problems in the over 65 age group was 0.9% (1.5% in males, 0.6% in females).

A small community study from Newcastle reported that 13% of respondents, aged over 60, drank sufficiently to put themselves at risk for developing hepatic damage (Bridgewater et al 1987). Using data from three of the US Epidemiologic Catchment Area sites, consisting of 4600 respondents 60 years and older, Robins (1986) has reported that approximately 3% of males and 1% of females over 65 met DSM-III-R criteria for either alcohol abuse or dependency. In Cahalin & Cisin's (1968) study 20% of the male and 2% of the female non-abstainers were deemed to be heavy drinkers. The prevalence figures are higher in general medical and psychiatric patient populations whether they be in-patients or out-patients. Alcoholism was a feature in 9% of elderly patients seen on home visits in Liverpool (Malcolm 1984) and in 10% of a similar population in Seattle, USA (Reifler et al 1982). In the total population of alcoholics 10% have been reported to be over 60 years old (Schuckit 1977).

Late-onset alcohol misuse

Late-onset alcohol abuse and dependency have conventionally been considered to be rare. This view has changed in the past 2 decades. However, there is some confusion in the literature surrounding the definition of 'late-onset'. One group of researchers has used 25 (Irwin et al 1990) as a cut-off age whilst another has used 40 (Atkinson et al 1985). Irrespective of what cut-off point was used, compared to the late-onset group, the early-onset alcoholics had more psychopathology, more complicated alcohol-induced social, marital and health problems, plus a greater family history of alcoholism, alcohol- and non-alcohol-related violence, and illicit substance use, thereby reflecting a more severe course.

Studies employing a cut-off age of 60 have supported the above findings in the early-onset subjects and generally agree that alcohol-related problems of late-onset tend to be more limited and less severe, with less evidence of a family history for substance misuse (Atkinson et al 1990, Schonfeld & Dupree 1991). Moreover, nearly 30% of the sample in the Atkinson et al (1990) study reported an age of onset after 60, while for nearly 50% the age of onset was after 45.

The reasons for late-onset alcohol misuse are not clear. Nevertheless, the fact that alcohol abuse can begin for the first time in late life and that this group has significant differences from the earlier onset group, implies the existence of predisposing factors which either persist into late life or arise de novo. To date, no single risk factor has been identified. Contrary to popular conceptions, psychiatric comorbidity has been shown to be lower in late-onset than in early-onset groups (Schonfeld & Dupree 1991, Atkinson 1994). Thus, although late-onset alcohol abuse can be secondary to other psychiatric disorders, this is not necessarily always so and, in fact, it accounts for only a minority of cases.

Later onset may be more common in higher socioeconomic groups (Atkinson 1984) and the proportion of women has been reported to be higher than in early-onset groups (39% versus 22%, Moos et al 1991). An age-related increase in sensitivity to alcohol, use of alcohol as self-medication, and increased free time coupled with readily available money may all be risk factors, but not yet adequately studied, in some late-onset cases (Atkinson 1994).

Age-determined stressors have been adduced as causes for late-onset alcohol misuse but the evidence for this is conflicting and can be difficult to interpret. In putative stress-related conditions, such as late-onset alcoholism, it can be a difficult task to distinguish between stressors that are a consequence of the problem or that may be of aetiological significance. Furthermore, some age-related stressors, e.g. physical disability and poverty, will limit access to alcohol and reduce consumption and may provoke spontaneous recovery.

Finney & Moos (1984) have proposed a model for late-life problem drinking that incorporates exposure to stressors, acute and chronic, as well as coping skills. Employing a systems perspective, there are several factors that need to be considered in the elderly person's vulnerability to alcohol abuse, its precipitation and perpetuation:

- personal characteristics, e.g.: marital status, cognitive impairment, physical debility
- negative life events, notably loss events such as bereavements, retirement, relocation
- chronic stressors e.g.: lack of money, interpersonal discord
- social resources, particularly family support
- personal coping skills and help-seeking behaviour which may be ineffective.

These factors can all interact and, of course, there is a reciprocal relationship between them and alcohol use disorders. Although late-onset problem drinkers report more recent acute negative life events and more chronic stressors than age-matched controls (Brennan & Moos 1990, Wells-Parker et al 1983), there does not appear to be an association between the onset of late-life alcohol misuse and age-related loss events (Brennan & Moos 1991).

The prevalence of alcohol abuse, as well as of other substances, is lower in the elderly than in the young. There are several reasons for this. Substance-related increased mortality means that many do not survive into old age. Spontaneous remission or assisted remission will have peaked and reached a plateau in the longer term population. Fewer people start to abuse alcohol and other substances for the first time in old age. Life stressors, such as reduced income, and the symptoms of end-organ damage may provide an incentive to reduce consumption, if not stop it altogether. Furthermore, the long term sequelae of substance misuse may have rendered elderly subjects so incapacitated that they are no longer capable of obtaining the relevant substances (Crome 1991). Some of these elderly people will end their days in nursing homes and similar institutions where alcohol will not be readily available and its consumption may not be tolerated. This may cause problems for individuals who persist in drinking or other drug use.

Cohort effect and implications for future alcohol abuse

There is some evidence to predict that alcohol abuse by the elderly is going to increase in the future. The prevalence rates for tomorrow's elderly population are influenced by the rates of alcohol consumption and misuse by today's young adults which rose steadily in the UK between the 1950s and the 1980s but have levelled off since. This is referred to as a 'cohort effect'. The major social and economic changes that have occurred since the 1950s – e.g. changing expectations of the roles of women in western countries, increasing numbers of females in the workforce – have had an even greater impact on the pattern of consumption of alcohol, as well as other substances, by women (Szwabo 1993). For example, while the average weekly alcohol intake for young men aged 18–24 in the UK fell during the 1980s from 26 to 21 units, it rose from 4.5 to 6 units in young women (Goddard & Ikin 1988). As the number of economically independent working women increases, it is possible that this trend will continue.

Patterns of alcohol consumption

It now appears that alcohol consumption remains relatively stable throughout life and does not fall as dramatically with age as was previously thought. On following up more than 1800 men in the USA aged 28–87 over nearly 1 decade, as part of the Veterans Administration's normative study of ageing, Glynn et al (1985) found that, although older cohorts consumed less alcohol, there was little change in mean alcohol consumption for all age cohorts over the study period. Therefore, it is possible that the pattern of alcohol consumption established as a young adult tends not to change dramatically in later life. These findings suggest that the extent of alcohol use seen in today's cohort of young adults will continue as the current cohort grows into old age. If this proves to be the case it will translate into increased alcohol-related health care problems and needs for future elderly generations.

Period effect

An historical factor can also shape the use of alcohol and is known as a 'period effect'. For example, there is a decrease in the use of alcohol by elderly Americans who were young adults during the famous Prohibition period (1920–1933) when, for over a decade, it was illegal to buy or sell beverage alcohol in the USA. Another example, this time due to technological advances, was the introduction of barbiturates and benzodiazepines in the 1960s and 1970s. When studying alcohol and other substance misuse in the elderly, it is important to distinguish between both cohort and period effects and specific ageing effects. As indicated above, this already has implications for the planning and development of future health care resources for the elderly.

Clinical features

Alcohol misuse in the elderly leads to increased mortality and is associated with death from suicide, cirrhosis, accidents, cardiovascular disease and cancer. It is likely that data garnered from death certificates underestimate the number of deaths attributable directly and indirectly to alcohol as the clinical manifestations of alcohol misuse in the elderly are protean and often non-specific. Owing to age-determined biological factors, the elderly are at greater risk than their younger counterparts from the adverse effects of substance misuse. Rather than simply presenting with a history of signs and symptoms of dependency, alcohol misuse by an elderly person needs to be considered in cases of recurrent falls, deterioration in self-care and hygiene, memory problems, etc. Indeed, alcohol can have wide-ranging effects on every major organ system in the body.

Physical complications of alcohol abuse

The medical complications of alcohol abuse are itemised in Box 12.2. These complications are occasionally advanced and irreversible by the time of discovery, due to the low level of suspicion there is for alcohol abuse in the elderly. As a rule, alcohol abuse should be considered for any disorder in an elderly patient, particularly if recurrent, for which no obvious cause can be found. The same principle applies to other substances of abuse in the elderly, notably sedative-hypnotic drugs.

Psychiatric consequences of alcohol abuse

The psychiatric consequences of alcohol abuse and dependency merit further consideration as the ageing central nervous system is particularly vulnerable to the

---

Box 12.2   Physical complications of alcohol abuse

- Gastrointestinal system
  - gastritis and gastric ulcers
  - Mallory–Weiss syndrome
  - acute and chronic pancreatitis
  - fatty liver
  - alcoholic hepatitis
  - cirrhosis
  - oesophageal varices
  - increased risk of oropharyngeal and oesophageal carcinoma
  - diarrhoea
  - malabsorption
  - incontinence
- Cardiovascular system
  - hypertension
  - arrhythmias
  - cardiomyopathy
- Haematology
  - impaired haemopoiesis secondary to direct toxic effect on bone marrow
  - vitamin deficiencies
- Metabolic
  - malnutrition
  - vitamin deficiencies (especially thiamine)
  - obesity
  - hypoglycaemia
  - hyperlipidaemia
  - hyperuricaemia
  - pseudo Cushing's syndrome
  - haemochromatosis
  - hyponatraemia ('beer drinker's potomania')
- Genitourinary system
  - sexual dysfunction
- Respiratory system
  - chemical pneumonia following aspiration of vomitus
- Nervous system
  - neuropsychiatric complications (see text)
  - peripheral neuropathy
  - 'Saturday night palsies' due to nerve compression
  - myopathy
  - cerebellar degeneration
  - central pontine myelinosis (secondary to hyponatraemia)
  - retrobulbar neuropathy
  - hepatic encephalopathy
  - Marchiafava–Bignami syndrome (demyelination of the corpus callosum)
- Miscellaneous
  - falls, head injury, burns, road traffic accidents
  - hypothermia
  - increased risk for tuberculosis

---

neurotoxic effects of alcohol. Mood disturbance, especially depression, coexists with alcohol dependency in approximately 50% of elderly cases

(Atkinson 1990). However, in the majority of these cases affective symptoms resolve spontaneously within 1 month of abstinence. In elderly patients hospitalised for the management of alcohol dependence, around 10% have been found to have major depression (Finlayson et al 1988). Self-medicating with alcohol as a hypnotic or analgesic or by a depressed or anxious patient needs also to be considered and investigated.

The approach employed by most doctors is, in the absence of sufficient symptoms to meet the diagnostic criteria for a major depressive illness, to inform the patient with lowered mood that this is most likely to be secondary to the effects of alcohol and that mood will improve and remain so as long as the patient perseveres with sobriety. This can provide a useful therapeutic lever and concretely demonstrate to the patient at least one of the advantages of abstaining. Mania is quite rare as a manifestation of alcohol misuse but, as with younger patients, increased alcohol consumption can be a feature of a manic episode. Apparent manic symptoms may occasionally feature prominently in the symptomatology of a withdrawal syndrome (Beresford 1993).

Withdrawal from alcohol

Withdrawal from alcohol in the elderly has a reputation for being difficult to manage (Liskow et al 1989, Brower et al 1994). The outcome can be a mild uncomplicated withdrawal syndrome, or a hallucinosis (occurring in clear consciousness) or sometimes, in more severe instances, seizures which can happen up to 2 weeks following withdrawal. However, the most serious complication, associated with a high mortality rate, is the development of delirium tremens, usually in an individual with a long history of heavy consumption. The patient typically presents with a short history of clouding of consciousness, disorientation, perceptual disturbances and is usually extremely agitated. This is associated with marked tremulousness and autonomic hyperactivity. The condition may arise following hospital admission of a previously unsuspected alcoholic for reasons not directly related to alcohol such as a chest infection or other intercurrent illness. The sudden cessation of alcohol intake precipitates this severe form of withdrawal and can result in death. This is a medical emergency and admission to a general hospital is imperative in order to appropriately sedate the patient, restore any electrolyte and fluid imbalances, treat associated metabolic disturbances, identify and manage any associated complications and monitor the patient's cardiovascular and respiratory status.

Causes of cognitive impairment

Cognitive impairment is an important feature of alcohol misuse in the elderly and its presence raises the issue of the differential diagnosis of the cause. It continues to be a contentious issue whether or not alcohol itself can cause a dementia syndrome as specific brain post-mortem findings have not yet been identified (Lishman 1990). Nonetheless, there is some evidence to show that alcohol does have a neurotoxic effect upon the brain causing possible neuronal loss with cortical shrinkage and ventricular dilatation which can be demonstrated by computerised tomography (CT) scan (Ron et al 1977). Interestingly, in some of this study group who succeeded, to some extent, in remaining abstinent during the 6–36-month follow-up period there was regression of the shrinkage (Ron et al 1982) suggesting the possibility of some reversal of alcohol-induced brain damage with abstinence. This neurotoxicity, when coupled with a deficiency in the vitamin thiamine, results acutely in Wernicke's encephalopathy which may progress to Korsakoff's syndrome. The pathological basis for these conditions is known to be the same and the two conditions are now usually considered to represent either end of a spectrum of reversibility and severity. The classical acute presentation, with the triad of confusion, ophthalmoplegia and ataxia, is responsive to treatment with thiamine whereas the chronic presentation of a persisting severe defect in short-term memory is, for the majority of sufferers, unresponsive to vitamin replacement therapy. The term Wernicke–Korsakoff syndrome is now used to describe the condition in its entirety.

Several other causes of cognitive impairment need to be entertained. Frequent episodes of intoxication compounded by increased sensitivity to alcohol place the elderly person at greater risk for falls and head injury. Such events may not even be remembered but can present later with a subdural haematoma which will manifest itself as slowly progressing cognitive impairment similar to a dementing syndrome. Neuroimaging of the brain is required to confirm the diagnosis and surgical intervention is necessary to remove the expanding clot. Cognitive impairment and delirium are features of many of the metabolic disturbances and other medical complications that can be attributed to alcohol, e.g. liver failure, atrial fibrillation, etc. Medical treatment should be directed towards the underlying problem.

Many elderly persons use other drugs – either appropriately or inappropriately – that can interact with alcohol, their effect being enhanced or diminished. As a rule polypharmacy should be avoided in the elderly and patients should be warned that certain prescribed medications are not compatible with alcohol use. Caution, therefore, is required when prescribing medications to both known and suspected heavy alcohol consumers.

Dementia is not uncommon in the elderly. 5–10% of the population over 65 are dementing, Alzheimer's disease being the most common cause (Jorm et al 1987). Because of established cognitive impairment, impaired risk awareness and sometimes disinhibited behaviour, this group is at increased risk for alcohol misuse and is particularly sensitive to the effects of alcohol and any other psychotropic substances which will exacerbate any existing cognitive impairment. Following withdrawal it will become apparent that there are residual cognitive deficits which, despite abstinence on follow-up, are progressing. Issues of future management and care will need to be reconsidered in such instances.

Social consequences of alcohol misuse

The social consequences of alcohol misuse are manifold. Society's expectations of the elderly are different from those of the young. Many elderly persons are no longer working or no longer have any major domestic commitments. Therefore, evidence of social decline and dysfunction will need to be sought in age-appropriate aspects of the person's life (e.g. contact with family and friends, ability to pursue hobbies and interests, level of self-care, etc.). Chronic alcohol misuse impairs social skills and functioning. Many elderly alcoholics will be divorced and estranged from their families and will have cut themselves off from normal social contacts. The legacy of their misuse will have detrimental effects upon their spouses and children extending even into the latter's adulthood. The ensuing social isolation perpetuates misuse as the few remaining social activities become increasingly centred around obtaining and consuming alcohol.

As with their younger counterparts, misuse of alcohol by the elderly leads to an increased risk of road traffic accidents and other driving offences that can mean loss of a driving licence. Such a loss will have a great impact upon the autonomy of an elderly person. There is little data available about violence and criminal behaviour in elderly alcoholics. Most likely, these are less frequent and troublesome than in younger alcoholics. However, one study found that alcohol use at the time of the offence was a feature in 20% of elderly offenders, a greater percentage than in the younger offenders in the study (Taylor & Parrott 1988).

Social disruption can be severe with elderly alcoholics becoming destitute, incapable of availing themselves of social service facilities and ultimately winding up homeless and roofless. Another, albeit unusual, extreme social end-point of alcohol misuse is 'Diogenes syndrome', or 'senile squalor', which is characterised by a severe decline in social standards and behaviour in a previously stable elderly person (MacMillan & Shaw 1965, Clark et al 1975). This results in gross self-neglect and squalor to which these individuals are remarkably oblivious – often to the dismay of their neighbours. Approximately 50% of these persons are found to be dementing or, less commonly, to be suffering from schizophrenia or alcohol dependency whereas, intriguingly, there is no evidence of a psychiatric disorder or of cognitive decline in the other half.

Treatment, course and prognosis

Treatment

The overall treatment approach is broadly similar to that for young adults (Beresford 1993) and the general principles described below can be applied to all types of substance misuse by the elderly. Once the assessment has been completed and the diagnosis made, every attempt should be made to foster a therapeutic alliance with the patient and relevant family members and friends, and engage them all in a treatment programme modified to meet the needs of the patient. Appropriate goals should be set based on the assessment of readiness to change. Initially the treatment plan may involve promoting an attitude of change and motivating the patient to set appropriate targets for their own behaviour change. Depending on the degree of the problem this may involve a reduction in amount consumed or may involve a goal of abstinence. For assessment and diagnostic purposes an initial goal of abstinence is more desirable if jointly agreed. If there is evidence of dependence the patient should be encouraged to abstain from alcohol.

If necessary, withdrawal symptoms can be ameliorated by using chlordiazepoxide prescribed on a reducing-dose schedule over a 5–7-day period. Vitamin supplements are usually co-administered. Clinicians need to be wary of co-dependence on benzodiazepines which may only become apparent following discontinuation of the chlordiazepoxide. Most elderly persons, if motivated, can be detoxified as out-patients, but admission to hospital may be warranted when this is repeatedly unsuccessful and also for severe cases to monitor withdrawal and initiate treatment of any other complications of alcohol abuse.

Whilst detoxification is underway the patient's rehabilitation and future care needs to be planned. Both patients and their families should be educated about the harmful effects of alcohol and substance abuse. Family therapy may be of use if family members live nearby and have been affected by, or have been facilitating the patient's drinking. Age-specific therapy appears to be associated with a better attendance for out-patient groups as well as a better short-term outcome for in-patient groups (Kofoed et al 1987, Kashner et al 1992). Alcoholics Anonymous can be a suitable alternative. In general, a gently supportive, encouraging, non-confrontational approach, yet one that does not avoid the issues, is the best therapeutic attitude to adopt (Atkinson et al 1993).

Because of its sedative properties and the risk of delirium and psychosis, the aversive agent disulfiram (Antabuse) is used infrequently for prophylactic purposes in the elderly. It is not sufficient to simply stop the intake of alcohol. Meaningful and constructive social activities are necessary to replace inappropriate alcohol-related behaviours and improve the patient's social network and support system, and enhance their self-esteem. Attendance at a local day centre or day hospital can provide a structured social outlet with a range of activities and opportunities for contact with the patient's peer group in a non-threatening environment. Follow-up home visits by a member of the multidisciplinary team will also be essential and will provide a realistic assessment of progress.

Course and prognosis

Treatment studies to date indicate that elderly people with alcohol-related problems do as well as, if not better than, young adults in treatment programmes. Although the course of late-onset alcohol use disorders can be fluctuating and the problem is milder than in early-onset cases and there is less comorbid psychiatric pathology, it is not yet clear whether the long-term outcome following treatment is better. Moos et al (1991), in a community survey of problem drinkers, found that the late-onset ones were the more likely to remit within a 1-year period. In particular, they reported that the late-onset group seemed to be more responsive to physical health problems and to external social pressures, e.g. from a spouse or a friend, to discontinue.

Mortality

Alcohol and other substance abuse in the elderly is

associated with higher mortality rates than that of the general population. On following up over 21 000 elderly (aged 55 and over) substance abuse patients over a 4-year period, Moos et al (1994) found that 24% of the cohort had died – a rate that was 2.64 times that expected. Alcohol-related psychosis and organic brain disorders, older age, and being single were some of the identified predictors of early death.

HYPNOTIC AND SEDATIVE MISUSE

Benzodiazepines

Benzodiazepines now account for the majority of this group of substances used by the elderly. They are used more frequently as hypnotics rather than sedatives. Barbiturates are no longer routinely prescribed and the prescription rate for benzodiazepines has been falling since the early 1980s. Nonetheless, there are probably still too many elderly people, women more so than men, being unnecessarily prescribed these drugs. Nearly 12% of the elderly population in a community survey from Liverpool were taking benzodiazepines, 60% of this group receiving the prescription for more than 1 year (Sullivan et al 1988). The latter finding is important as long-term users are more at risk of developing dependence. Elderly residents in nursing homes and similar institutions are liable to be regularly prescribed benzodiazepines, especially if they have been admitted from a hospital (Gilleard et al 1984). Other risk factors for benzodiazepine dependence include chronic pain, previous history of sedative abuse, current alcohol abuse, chronic insomnia and chronic depression (especially if unrecognised or misdiagnosed as anxiety). Benzodiazepines may well provide some immediate relief for some of these problems but, in the long term, tolerance develops and their use only obscures and complicates the underlying illnesses.

Whilst tolerance to their anxiolytic effects is small, tolerance to the hypnotic effects develops within a few weeks of regular use. Hence, benzodiazepines are not indicated for individuals with chronic sleep disorders. Besides, sleep disturbances in the elderly should be adequately investigated before any medication whatsoever is prescribed – insomnia could be a feature of depression, caused by pain, or be secondary to cardiovascular and respiratory disease.

Initially considered to be safe, benzodiazepines are now recognised as having a range of side-effects and complications that can result from prolonged use and sometimes even from brief use. The pharmacological properties of benzodiazepines dictate their potential for dependence and their toxicity. In general, short-acting benzodiazepines (e.g. lorazepam, triazolam) have a more rapid onset of action as well as a greater potency per milligram of the drug, whilst the medium- and long-acting benzodiazepines (e.g. diazepam, nitrazepam, flurazepam) take longer to exert their effects. The latter are less potent but have prolonged half-lives and lengthy durations of activity, sometimes lasting days. Consequently, the cumulative effect of daily consumption can lead to toxicity on what seems to be a standard dose. This can readily occur in the elderly whose drug metabolism is slower and less efficient than that of younger adults. Hence, the elderly are more susceptible to the side-effects of benzodiazepines.

Dependence usually occurs in the context of prolonged use, leading to tolerance and sometimes, but not necessarily, to escalation of dose (Higgitt 1988). The patient, typically with a substantial degree of persistence, may solicit benzodiazepines from several different doctors and from relatives and friends. Alternatively, the patient may inadvertently be being prescribed them by both the general practitioner and the hospital doctor. This most commonly occurs if there is poor communication between the patient's various doctors and also when the patient passively accepts the doctors' treatment plans.

Clinical manifestations of withdrawal

Attempts to suddenly reduce intake or stop use causes withdrawal symptoms in approximately half of users, lasting in most instances less than 4 weeks and rarely several months. The clinical manifestations of withdrawal are typically novel for the patient and can be quite diverse, ranging from tinnitus, headaches, restlessness, irritability and tremor to delirium, psychosis and occasionally seizures. Sometimes low-dose dependency – with doses as low as the equivalent of 6–10 mg of diazepam per day (Ashton 1987) – is uncovered when patients' supplies have been abruptly cut off.

'Rebound' phenomena can also occur following discontinuation. These are the same symptoms, usually anxiety, that initiated prescription of the drug. They appear rapidly after discontinuation but are less severe than the original symptoms and disappear within a few days. 'Reoccurrence' symptoms are the original symptoms – with their original intensity and severity – which appear after stopping the drug but which persist rather than fade away. Essentially, benzodiazepine use was only masking the symptoms rather than treating them.

Toxicity

Benzodiazepines can cause both acute and chronic toxicity. The potent ultra-short-acting agents are more associated with acute side-effects: sedation, cerebellar ataxia, memory 'blackouts'. Chronic ingestion may cause persistent ataxia associated with falls and an increased risk of fractured femur, sedation, incontinence, lowered mood and memory impairment which, if associated with other benzodiazepine-induced cognitive impairments, may be mistaken for a dementia syndrome. Memory impairment has been demonstrated to improve in nursing home residents when benzodiazepines have been discontinued (Salzman et al 1992). They can also cause respiratory depression and exacerbate underlying depression and dementing conditions. Effects and side-effects of hypnotics and sedatives are discussed further in Chapter 23.

Management of benzodiazepine dependence

Initial management of benzodiazepine dependence is similar to that described for alcohol dependence. Once the condition has been recognised and the patient is willing to discontinue the drug, the dose should be gradually reduced at a rate that is tailored to the patient in order to avoid withdrawal symptoms. The dose may need to be tapered over several months. During this time the patient should be reviewed on a regular basis and provided with encouragement and support. Hospitalisation may be indicated if use has been heavy (i.e. beyond therapeutic limits), severe withdrawal symptoms are already evident, there is polysubstance abuse, or if the patient lives alone without any community support. Group therapy can provide a suitable source of emotional support. Patients must be informed that sudden cessation of use may result in a severe withdrawal syndrome. Reoccurrence of symptoms requires investigation and specific management rather than reinstatement of benzodiazepines which will serve only to suppress rather than treat symptoms.

As public awareness of the risks of benzodiazepine use increases and the indications for their use decreases it is likely that prescription rates in the elderly will continue to decline. In the meantime, audit should contribute to improved prescribing practice. Limiting repeat prescriptions would also reduce the numbers of patients inappropriately receiving benzodiazepines on a long-term basis, thereby reducing the risk of future dependency.

MISUSE OF PRESCRIBED AND OVER THE COUNTER MEDICATIONS

The elderly account for the largest user group of both prescribed and non-prescribed medications (Abrams & Alexopoulos 1988). Apart from psychotropic drugs, many elderly are also taking medications for chronic medical conditions. As discussed in Chapter 23, it is not unusual to come across elderly patients who are being prescribed a bewildering array of medications, often with no clinical indication for use. Such polypharmacy greatly increases the chances of adverse drug interactions, especially if the patient is also taking over the counter medications of which the prescribing doctor has no knowledge. Elderly patients may inadvertently, and occasionally deliberately, underdose or over-dose their prescribed medications leading to therapeutic failure or toxicity.

Use of over the counter (OTC) medications increases with age and is possibly related to limited access to medical care and poverty. In one US study, up to two-thirds of individuals aged over 60 were taking at least one OTC medication on a daily basis (Abrams & Alexopoulos 1988). The harmful effects of such self-medication can be easily underestimated. For example, inappropriate use of laxatives and purgatives can result in severe life-threatening electrolyte abnormalities and excessive use of nonsteroidal analgesics can cause renal damage. Many OTC tonics, cough mixtures and cold remedies contain alcohol or the stimulant caffeine. Some have antihistamine and anticholinergic properties which can predispose them to being used for psychoactive effect and which can also result in toxicity. As many elderly people do not consider OTC preparations to be medications, it is essential in the assessment interview to enquire specifically about them and to consider the possibility of polysubstance abuse. Abuse of one substance increases the likelihood of abuse of other substances.

Nicotine

The most widely used OTC drug is, of course, nicotine in cigarette form. Approximately 15% of the over 65 population are smokers. Although not usually directly associated with psychological morbidity, psychological interventions may be useful in encouraging individuals to give up what is, for many, a dangerous addiction and predisposes elderly people to increased rates of upper respiratory tract and chest infections.

ILLICIT DRUG USE IN THE ELDERLY

Little is known about illegal drug use by the elderly. However, as this problem is becoming more common in younger cohorts it is likely that its prevalence in the elderly will rise in the future. Opioid addiction is mainly confined to survivors who started early in life and who have been able to maintain their habit into old age (Schuckit 1977) and is often associated with a previous criminal lifestyle. The attractions and few benefits to be derived from participating in and belonging to an illicit drug culture probably have little appeal for the opioid-naïve elderly person.

Abuse of psychostimulants is exceptional in the elderly but the occasional patient presents who has been in receipt of amphetamines for over 4 decades and problems arise when their elderly general practitioner dies. Such interruption of supply can result in fraudulent and deceptive behaviour in order to obtain their drug. Humane and sympathetic management is required but attempts should be made to fully exploit these opportunities for change.

Although benzodiazepine use is relatively common in the elderly it is uncommon for patterns of binge use and supratherapeutic or high dose use to occur. Opiate dependence related to analgesic medication occurs with some frequency. Appropriate pain-management strategies should be adopted and if pain control is achieved then opiates can be withdrawn but may result in a withdrawal syndrome. Parenteral analgesia should be instituted only for short-term acute pain control and any elderly patients presenting who have been inappropriately prescribed injectable pethidine or morphine should initially be switched to oral longer-acting opiates before detoxification. In situations where pain control cannot be achieved then it is appropriate to use opiates to achieve adequate control and this can be done with oral opiate medication.

The advent of HIV and AIDS has highlighted the risks of injecting drug use but has also brought to the fore the problem of HIV encephalopathy and dementia. This new young cognitively-impaired population with major illicit drug problems present a major challenge to hospital and community services. This type of clinical problem presents a vignette of the problems associated with unstable chaotic drug use and severe cognitive impairment and should galvanise us to ensure early effective community interventions to minimise alcohol and drug-related harm.

CONCLUSION

This chapter has provided considerable clinical detail on the approaches to alcohol and other drug-related problems in the elderly. Increasing diagnostic precision is likely to demonstrate the importance of substance misuse in elderly health care. The application of brief therapeutic interventions directed at modifying substance consumption behaviour could potentially deliver a substantial degree of health and social gain to the elderly population. For this reason, an increased index of suspicion and readiness to detect and intervene with alcohol and other drug-related problems at the generic and primary care level as well as at a specialist level will be a positive development in the delivery of health and social care to the elderly. The lack of attention to substance-related problems in elderly people has become one of the most glaring examples of ageism and requires direct attention by organisations representing their needs. We have little doubt that in a decade we will look back in puzzlement at the profundity of our blind spot to this pressing, overt and manageable clinical problem.

REFERENCES

Abrams R C, Alexopoulos G S 1988 Substance abuse in the elderly: over the counter and illegal drugs. Hosp Comm Psychiatry 39: 822–829

American Psychiatric Association 1994 Diagnostic and statistical manual of mental disorders, 4th edn. APA, Washington DC

Ashton H 1987 Benzodiazepine withdrawal: outcome in 50 patients. Br J Addict 82: 665–671

Atkinson R M 1984 Substance use and abuse in late life. In: Atkinson R M (ed) Alcohol and drug abuse in old age. American Psychiatric Press, Washington DC

Atkinson R M 1990 Aging and alcohol use disorders: diagnostic issues in the elderly. Int Psychogeria 2: 55–72

Atkinson R M 1994 Late onset problem drinking in older adults. Int J Geriatr Psychiatry 9: 321–326

Atkinson R M, Turner J A, Kofoed L L, Tolson R L 1985 Early versus late onset alcoholism in older persons: preliminary findings. Alcoholism: Clin Exp Research 9: 513–515

Atkinson R M, Tolson R L, Turner J A 1990 Late versus early onset problem drinking in older men. Alcoholism: Clin Exp Research 14: 574–579

Atkinson R M, Ganzini L, Bernstein M J 1992 Alcohol and substance-use disorders in the elderly. In: Birren J E, Sloan R B, Cohen G D (eds) Handbook of mental health and ageing. Academic Press, San Diego

Atkinson R M, Tolson R L, Turner J A 1993 Factors affecting outpatient treatment compliance of older male problem drinkers. J Stud Alcohol 54: 102–106

Beresford T P 1993 Alcoholism in the elderly. Int Rev Psychiatry 5: 477–483

Beresford T P, Blow F C, Hill E, Singer K, Lucey M R 1990 Comparison of CAGE questionnaire and computer-assisted laboratory profiles in screening for covert alcoholism. The Lancet 336: 482–485

Blazer D G, Pennybacker M R 1984 Epidemiology of alcoholism in the elderly. In: Hartford J T, Samorajski T (eds) Alcoholism in the elderly. Raven Press, New York

Blow F C, Brower K J, Schulenberg J E, Demo-Dananberg L M, Young L M, Beresford T P 1992 The Michigan Alcoholism Screening Test–Geriatric version (MAST-G): a new elderly-specific screening instrument. Alcohol Clin Exp Res 16: 372

Brennan P L, Moos R H 1990 Life stressors, social resources, and late-life problem drinking. Psychol Aging 5: 491–501

Brennan P L, Moos R H 1991 Functioning, life context, and help-seeking among late-onset problem drinkers: comparisons with non problem and early-onset problem drinkers. Br J Addiction 86: 1139–1150

Bridgewater R, Lee S, James O F W, Potter J F 1987 Alcohol consumption and dependence in elderly patients in an urban community. BMJ 295: 884–885

Brower K J, Mudd S, Blow F C, Young J P, Hill E M 1994 Severity and treatment of alcohol withdrawal in elderly versus younger patients. Alcohol Clin Exp Res 18: 196–201

Buchsbaum D G, Buchanan R G, Welsh J, Centor R M, Schnoll S H 1992 Screening for drinking disorders in the elderly using the CAGE questionnaire. JAGS 40: 662–665

Cahalan D, Cisin I H 1968 American drinking practices: a summary of findings from a national probability sample, I: extent of drinking by population subgroups. Quart J Stud Alcohol 29: 130–151

Clark A N G, Manikar G D, Gray I 1975 Diogenes syndrome: a clinical study of gross self-neglect in old age. The Lancet i: 366–368

Colsher P L, Wallace R B 1990 Elderly men with histories of heavy drinking: correlates and consequences. J Stud Alc 51: 528–535

Crome P 1991 What about the elderly? In: Belle-Glass I (ed) The international handbook of addiction behaviour. Routledge, London

Drew L R H 1968 Alcoholism as a self-limiting disease. Quart J Stud Alc 29: 956–967

Ewing J A 1984 Detecting alcoholism: the CAGE questionnaire. JAMA 252: 1905–1907

Finlayson R E, Hurt R D, Davis L J, Morse R M 1988 Alcoholism in elderly persons: a study of the psychiatric and psychosocial features of 216 inpatients. Mayo Clin Proc 63: 761–768

Finney J W, Moos R H 1984 Life stressors and problem drinking among older adults. In: Galanter M (ed) Recent developments in alcoholism. Plenum Press, New York

Gilleard C, Smits C, Morgan K 1984 Changes in hypnotic usage in residential homes for the elderly: a longitudinal survey. Arch Gerontol Geriatr 3: 223–228

Glynn R J, Bouchard G R, LoCastro J S, Laird N M 1985 Aging and generational effects on drinking behaviours in men: results from the Normative Aging Study. Am J Pub Health 75: 1413–1419

Higgitt A C 1988 Indications for benzodiazepine prescriptions in the elderly. Int J Geriatr Psychiatry 3: 239–243

Goddard E, Ikin C 1988 Drinking in England and Wales in 1987. HMSO/OPCS, London

Irwin M, Schuckit M, Smith T L 1990 Clinical importance of age at onset in type 1 and type 2 primary alcoholics. Arch Gen Psychiatry 47: 320–324

Jorm A F, Korten A E, Henderson A S 1987 The prevalence of dementia; a quantitative integration of the literature. Acta Psychiatr Scand 76: 465–479

Kashner T M, Rodell D E, Ogden S R, Guggenheim F G, Karson C N 1992 Outcomes and costs of two VA inpatient treatment programs for older alcoholic patients. Hosp Commun Psychiatry 43: 985–989

Kofoed L L, Tolson R L, Atkinson R M, Toth R F, Turner J A 1987 Treatment compliance of older alcoholics: an elder-specific approach is superior to 'mainstreaming'. J Stud Alcohol 48: 47–51

Lishman W A 1990 Alcohol and the brain. Br J Psychiatry 156: 635–644

Liskow B I, Rinck C, Campbell J, DeSouza C 1989 Alcohol withdrawal in the elderly. J Stud Alcohol 50: 414–421

MacMillan D, Shaw P 1965 Senile breakdown in standards of personal and environmental cleanliness. BMJ ii: 1032–1037

Malcolm M T 1984 Alcoholism and drug use in the elderly visited at home. Int J Addiction 19: 411–418

McInnes E, Powell J 1994 Drug and alcohol referrals: are elderly substance abuse diagnoses and referrals being missed? BMJ 308: 444–446

Moos R H, Brennan P L, Moos B S 1991 Short term processes of remission and nonremission among late-life problem drinkers. Alcoholism: Clin Exp Res 15: 948–955

Moos R H, Brennan P L, Mertens J R 1994 Mortality rates and predictors of mortality among late-middle-aged and older substance abuse patients. Alcoholism: Clin Exp Res 18: 187–195

Naik P C, Jones R G 1994 Alcohol histories taken from elderly people on admission. BMJ 308: 248

Reifler B V, Kethley A, O'Neill P, Hanley R, Lewis S, Stenchever D 1982 Five-year experience of a community outreach program for the elderly. Am J Psychiatry 139: 220–223

Robins L N 1986 Introduction to the ECA project as a source of epidemiological data on alcohol problems. In: Maddox G, Robins L N, Rosenberg N (eds) Nature and extent of alcohol problems in the elderly. Springer, New York

Ron M A, Acker W, Lishman W A 1977 Morphological abnormalities in the brains of chronic alcoholics: a clinical, psychological and computerised axial tomography study. Acta Psychiatrica Scandinavica 62(suppl 286): 41–46

Ron M A, Acker W, Shaw G K, Lishman W A 1982 Computerised tomography of the brain in chronic alcoholism: a survey and follow-up study. Brain 105: 497–514

Salzman C, Fisher J, Nobel K, Glassman R, Wolfson A, Kelley M 1992 Cognitive impairment following benzodiazepine discontinuation in elderly nursing home residents. Int J Geriatr Psychiatry 7: 89–93

Saunders P A, Copeland J R M, Dewey M E et al 1989 Alcohol use and abuse in the elderly: findings from the Liverpool longitudinal study of continuing health in the community. Int J Geriatr Psychiatry 4: 103–108

Saunders P A, Copeland J R M, Dewey M E et al 1991 Heavy drinking as a risk factor for depression and dementia in elderly men: findings from the Liverpool longitudinal community study. Br J Psychiatry 159: 213–216

Schonfeld L, Dupree L W 1991 Antecedents of drinking for early- and late-onset elderly alcohol abusers. J Stud Alcohol 52: 587–592

Schuckit M A 1977 Geriatric alcoholism and drug abuse. Gerontologist 17: 168–174

Selzer M L 1971 The Michigan Alcoholism Screening Test: the quest for a new diagnostic instrument. Am J Psychiatry 127: 1653–1658

Sullivan C F, Copeland J R M, Dewey M E et al 1988 Benzodiazepine usage among the elderly: findings of the Liverpool community survey. Int J Geriatr Psychiatry 3: 289–292

Szwabo P A 1993 Substance abuse in older women. Clin Geriatr Med 9: 197–208

Taylor P J, Parrott J M 1988 Elderly offenders. Br J Psychiatry 152: 340–346

Vogel-Sprott M, Barrett P 1984 Age, drinking habits and the effects of alcohol. J Stud Alcohol 45: 517–521

Wells-Parker E, Miles S, Spencer B 1983 Stress experiences and drinking histories of elderly drunken-driving offenders. J Stud Alcohol 44: 429–437

West R, Glossop M 1994 Commonalities in substance dependence. Addiction 89: 1355–1356

Winick C 1962 Maturing out of narcotic addiction. United Nations bulletin on narcotics 14: 1–7

World Health Organization 1992 The ICD-10 classification of mental and behavioural disorders. WHO, Geneva

RECOMMENDED READING

Abrams R C, Alexopoulos G S 1988 Substance abuse in the elderly: over the counter and illegal drugs. Hosp Comm Psychiatry 39: 822–829. *There is a tendency to forget about OTC medications. Their use by the elderly is widespread, unsupervised and often neglected by clinicians. This is one of the few papers to address this issue and examine the extent of OTC medication use in the elderly.*

Beresford T P 1993 Alcoholism in the elderly. Int Rev Psychiatry 5: 477–483. *The MAST-G is appended to this concise review.*

Glynn R J, Bouchard G R, LoCastro J S, Laird N M 1985 Aging and generational effects on drinking behaviours in men: results from the Normative Aging Study. Am J Pub Health 75: 1413–1419. *This important large study has led to a reappraisal of how patterns of alcohol consumption change with ageing. The finding that individual alcohol consumption does not alter dramatically with age was contrary to traditional assumptions.*

Lishman W A 1990 Alcohol and the brain. Br J Psychiatry 156: 635–644. *This is an informative account of the neuropsychiatric complications of alcohol abuse.*

Naik P C, Jones R G 1994 Alcohol histories taken from elderly people on admission. BMJ 308: 248. *A study need not be long and complex to be provocative. This recent succinct report once again highlighted that elder alcohol misuse continues to be under-recognised, even in a hospital setting.*

Saunders P A, Copeland J R M, Dewey M E et al 1989 Alcohol use and abuse in the elderly: findings from the Liverpool longitudinal study of continuing health in the community. Int J Geriatr Psychiatry 4: 103–108. *Given the increasing awareness of alcohol misuse in the elderly population and the implications that this is likely to have for informed planning of future health services it is surprising that there is so little epidemiological data available. This is the most useful and methodologically sound of the few available UK studies of alcohol misuse in the elderly.*

13

Schizophrenia in later life

Michael Morley
William Sellwood

INTRODUCTION

'Schizophrenia is a common condition. It attacks one person in every one hundred in all types of society and culture the whole world over. Yet it remains shrouded in secrecy, ignorance and fear.' (Howe 1991, Introduction).

Schizophrenia is one of the most significant illnesses any individual can have. Sufferers may be left permanently damaged and in need of some continuing support throughout their lives. In spite of this, it is a little understood disorder for which relatively little clinical input is provided other than brief follow-up interviews and regular prophylactic medication (Woof et al 1988, Patmore & Weaver 1990). As many as 30% of homeless people may have a diagnosis of schizophrenia (Fischer & Breakley 1986). In comparison to depression and dementia there are relatively few older people suffering from schizophrenia. Nevertheless, Arie & Jolley (1982) noted that 'some 50% of all mental illness beds in England are now occupied by people over 65 years, and the elderly account for between 20 and 40% of psychiatric admissions' (p. 225). Within the long-stay, or 'graduate' group the commonest diagnosis is schizophrenia, and it is this group that have been the focus for resettlement, when this is feasible (Campbell 1992). Although the onset of schizophrenia tends to occur mainly in adolescence or early adulthood, it is recognised that a 'variant' of this disorder also occurs later in life (Kay & Roth 1961).

Broadly speaking, schizophrenia in old age occurs in two population groups: those individuals first diagnosed in early adulthood who have grown old; and those who are first diagnosed later in life. The bulk of this chapter is devoted to the former group as they are more numerous. Late paraphrenia or late-onset schizophrenia is generally recognised as being fairly rare (Naguib & Levy 1992).

Schizophrenia has, from its earliest conceptual origin, been a controversial diagnosis (Kendell 1988). Considerable effort has been expended in clarifying and establishing diagnostic guidelines, yet perhaps more than ever the validity of this diagnosis is under question (Bentall 1990a).

Recent research on outcome for individuals with the diagnosis of schizophrenia indicates that the pessimism once associated with the diagnosis is inaccurate (Ciompi 1986). Moreover, the needs of this population, whether they are catered for in hospital or in the community, are going to increase with the increase in the over 65 age group. In spite of this, there has been a relative paucity of research to establish these needs, particularly for people who have survived into old age. Little work has been carried out on the management of the disorder in late life except with regard to pharmacological treatments.

The aim of this chapter is to summarise current knowledge concerning the nature of schizophrenia in the elderly, including methods of treatment and the provision of services. The first section deals with the relationship between ageing and schizophrenia. There follows a summary of what is known about the nature of the illness, including diagnostic criteria, a historical description and possible aetiological and mediating factors. Biological and pharmacological treatment approaches are then described. Although many of the approaches used have not specifically been studied in the elderly there is little or no reason to suppose that they are not applicable to elderly patients and where there are likely to be differences these are described. From the psychological viewpoint, treatment of late paraphrenia has yet to be studied in depth.

AGEING AND SCHIZOPHRENIA

Although the onset of the frank symptoms of schizophrenia often occurs in adolescence or the early 20s, the full impact of the illness will gradually unfold over a lifetime. Not infrequently, the story begins before the diagnosis is made, a history of behavioural difficulties in childhood has been noted as a predictor of poor outcome for adults with the disorder (WHO 1979). Most of us expect to progress through certain landmarks in life which help to define ourselves as individuals. Such development or progression may be severely limited or even absent if schizophrenia becomes chronic. Many people who suffer from schizophrenia are fortunate and settle down, finding a routine, a way of coping with the disorder, and a way of living in the community. However, if the disorder becomes chronic it tends to alter the person's lifestyle

---

Box 13.1 The case of Michael Harrison: a person with a long history of schizophrenia and many years spent in institutional care

Mr Harrison was born in an inner city district in Manchester in the early 1920s. During adolescence he was involved in petty crime. He was extrovert and had a number of friends and a wide social circle. During the Second World War he was drafted into the navy, where he served as able seaman. In 1943, his ship was sunk in battle; it was immediately after this that his mental illness became apparent. He was discharged from the navy on a pension with the diagnosis of dementia praecox. For the first 2 years of his stay in hospital he gained a reputation for aggressive behaviour presenting as a severe management problem. After this he was noted to be a passive, quiescent patient who said little. He stayed in the hospital continuously for the next 48 years. Throughout this time the most detailed accounts in his psychiatric notes concerned regular dental checkups during the 1970s. In 1991 he was discharged for the first time to the mental health services in his district of origin. He was admitted to the Care Hostel ward where it was noted that he seemed indifferent to this radical change to his lifestyle. The only significant relationship maintained during his illness career was with his sister who visited him every 2 weeks.

---

profoundly which, over successive periods of hospitalisation and recovery, leaves the sufferer continually out of step with the demands of society and family life. Instead of securing employment and forming supportive relationships, the person with schizophrenia may have to adapt to the loss of a university place, or encounter the reluctance of employers to offer him a job. Over the course of their lives they may find difficulties with interpersonal relations, face a quality of life far removed from their expectation and may even be homeless. Such losses create additional burdens for the individual and family particularly as the sufferer may be 'isolated' by virtue of the disorder (Howe 1991). Some individuals who are unable to find support within the community have entered and remained in large mental hospitals for most of their lives; this is illustrated by the case of Michael Harrison, discussed in Box 13.1.

WHAT IS SCHIZOPHRENIA?

A psychosis is a severe mental disorder in which the ability to judge and interpret reality is seriously impaired. In addition to this disruption, there are often marked changes in a person's emotional and thinking processes. Schizophrenia is a psychotic disorder. The two most common psychotic disorders are schizophrenia and manic depressive illness (also known as bipolar affective disorder) which is discussed in Chapter 8. For psychiatrists, the differential diagnosis between the two disorders is not often easy (Kendell 1988). Both manic depressive illness and schizophrenia are most likely to begin in late adolescence or in early adult life.

At present it is widely agreed that there are two main aspects to symptomatology. First are the 'positive' symptoms, consisting of delusions, which are culturally exceptional beliefs, held with great conviction, in spite of evidence to the contrary, and auditory hallucinations when the sufferer has the experience of hearing voices which do not exist. There are a number of themes commonly seen in delusions. Delusions of persecution involve ideas that some agency (e.g. the devil, the CIA or the next door neighbours) is doing something harmful to the patient. A further category of delusions involves the idea that thoughts or movements or other aspects of behaviour are being controlled externally. For example, 'thought insertion' is the experience that thoughts are being placed in one's head and 'thought broadcast' is the experience involving the realisation that other people can read one's thoughts. Individuals with schizophrenia can also experience 'grandiose delusions', whereby they believe that they have special powers or some purpose in life. It is, for example, not uncommon to come across patients who believe that they are a religious leader (Jesus Christ) or that they are responsible for items which appear in the news.

The commonest forms of hallucination are auditory-verbal in nature. Classically, people with schizophrenia hear one or more voices talking about them in the third person. However, this varies and many sufferers hear voices in the second person and may even 'hear' themselves thinking. They may also experience hallucinations in the other perceptual modalities.

'Thought disorder' is also usually included in the positive symptom category but can be classified separately (Liddle 1987). This involves a disorder in language production whereby the patient's speech is characterised by phrases and sentences which seem unconnected with each other. Sometimes the sufferer produces apparently meaningless words (neologisms) or uses words to represent things not usually associated with them.

The second category of symptom are 'negative' symptoms. Generally, negative symptoms involve behavioural deficits and include: apathy, anhedonia (loss of enjoyment/pleasure), flatness of affect, motor retardation, lethargy, lack of spontaneity, impoverished speech (quantity and content) and poor self care. People suffering from schizophrenia with marked negative symptoms may be difficult to communicate with. This is because the person responds minimally in conversation (poverty of speech), often providing only one word answers to questions and saying little spontaneously. In fact, there are examples of patients who are almost mute. In some cases there is little to indicate what emotion the patient is experiencing (flatness of affect) or the emotion being expressed is incongruous so that patients may seem to be amused by distressing events, or at least, not 'on the same wavelength' as the person they are conversing with.

In many cases sufferers complain of lethargy and find it difficult to initiate actions. This leads to self neglect which, in rare cases, can be so extreme that without continuing support and supervision they will not feed themselves or be concerned with cleanliness or hygiene.

Schizophrenia has a highly variable course, outcome and presentation. Some sufferers experience one or two episodes of psychosis with little or no long-term negative consequences. Other patients have many severe relapses throughout their life with impairment of social functioning between episodes and others still remain chronically affected by positive and negative symptoms throughout their adult lives. Shepherd et al (1987) found that only one-third of patients return to premorbid levels of functioning over the 5 years after their initial diagnosis.

As described above, a significant proportion of those initially diagnosed as suffering from schizophrenia continue to exhibit symptoms for the whole of their adult lives. In general, the onset is early in adulthood and, in men, onset is most frequently seen in those in their late teens and early 20s. By the time patients are elderly they have had a lifelong career of patienthood.

An historical perspective

The German psychiatrist Emil Kraepelin (1896, cited in Kendell 1988) proposed a classification of insanity with two major categories: manic depressive insanity and dementia praecox. Kraepelin viewed dementia praecox as a deteriorating condition (dementia) and its onset was early in life (precocious or praecox). He assumed that it was a disease entity with its own characteristic symptoms, aetiology and diagnosis. Kraepelin's view that the condition inevitably leads to deterioration is now known to be incorrect (Cutting 1986, Ciompi

1986). In a subsequent modification of this classification, Kraepelin added a new diagnostic entity under the heading dementia praecox, paraphrenia. He used this diagnosis to describe patients who developed a form of chronic mental illness with persecutory or grandiose delusions. Follow-up studies indicated that some of the patients diagnosed as having paraphrenia had symptoms similar to those of dementia praecox. The diagnosis of paraphrenia was thus largely abandoned, only to be 'revived' some years later by Roth and his co-workers in Newcastle (see section Does schizophrenia occur in elderly people?) and called late paraphrenia (Kay & Roth 1961).

Eugen Bleuler (1911) introduced the term schizophrenia to cover a group of illnesses which he considered could arise at any stage in life and that were characterised primarily by psychological disturbance. The identifying characteristic of the illness was not poor outcome but a characteristic psychological disturbance. Bleuler used the term schizophrenia, meaning 'split mind', because he thought that the illness was due to 'a loosening of associations' between different psychological processes. Essentially he viewed this loosening as disrupting both thought and speech, with consequent disruption of emotional, volitional and intellectual processes. The diagnosis of schizophrenia was based on the presence of one or more of the 'Four As' (blunting or incongruity of affect, loosening of associations or thought disorder, ambivalence and autism). The more prominent aspect of acute phases of the illness, the positive symptoms (hallucinations and delusions), were viewed as phenomena of lesser importance. In the decades up to the 1950s, Bleuler's term schizophrenia with his diagnostic criteria became predominant in classifying the disorder in the USA. Kendell (1988) has noted two fundamental problems with Bleuler's criteria: they are difficult to define and may well occur in normal people in times of stress.

Schneider (1959) emphasised the importance of specific symptoms that he believed to be characteristic of schizophrenia, and which he called first-rank symptoms. They include:

- Passivity experiences, that is believing and feeling that thoughts are being put into or taken out of one's head.
- Believing and feeling that one's body is being moved by an outside force; feeling shocks or other unpleasant sensations coming from outside the body.
- Auditory hallucinations which come from outside the head, consist of a group of voices that talk to

one another, and that discuss the person in the third person; thought broadcasting and reception, that is believing that one is able to send or receive thoughts through the air.

- Delusional perceptions, the sudden development of a delusional system from an actual perception; for example, seeing any object that exists and immediately developing a delusional system or interpretation.

No theoretical assumptions were made about these symptoms; rather they were viewed simply as valid indices for a diagnosis of schizophrenia. Schneider made the point that these symptoms could occur in other disorders but they were predominant in schizophrenia. Therefore, he drew a distinction between these and other 'second-rank symptoms'. The latter, emotional blunting, delusions and hallucinations, could occur in other illnesses, such as depression. Although Schneider's first-rank symptoms were able to be identified and reliably rated it has become clear that they have little significance for long-term prognosis.

In the 1970s the confusion surrounding the diagnosis of schizophrenia reached a turning point. Cooper et al (1972) showed that although patients in London and New York mental hospitals were admitted with similar symptoms, the diagnosis of schizophrenia was nearly twice as high in New York as London. Psychiatrists in the USA were four times more likely to diagnose psychotic depression and ten times less likely to label a psychotic patient as suffering from mania. In addition, the International Pilot Study of Schizophrenia (WHO 1973) found that psychiatrists in Washington had a different concept of schizophrenia compared with psychiatrists from seven other countries, drawn from Europe, Asia and Africa.

In the past 20 years, several operational definitions of schizophrenia have been proposed, mainly by clinical researchers and epidemiologists working in the USA. The principal aims behind these varying definitions have been to improve the reliability of diagnosis, and better predict the response to treatment and long-term prognosis. In 1980, with the publication of the American Psychiatric Association's Diagnostic and Statistical Manual (DSM-III), psychiatry in the USA moved from a very broad concept of schizophrenia to a much narrower one. In the revised third edition (see DSM-III-R; APA 1987) schizophrenia is conceptualised as a mental disorder with a tendency toward chronicity which impairs functioning. It is characterised by psychotic symptoms involving disturbances of thinking, feeling and behaviour.

Schizophrenia cannot be diagnosed unless someone has been continuously disturbed for a period lasting not less than 6 months. Therefore, brief schizophrenia-like episodes lasting less than 6 months are not defined as schizophrenia. Also, if a person does not show a clear deterioration in functioning then he is not suffering from schizophrenia. Those individuals who appear to be suffering from schizophrenia but fail to meet the other criteria may be diagnosed as suffering from brief reactive psychosis, schizophreniform disorder or atypical psychosis.

Outcome of schizophrenia

It is hard to imagine a more alien experience than a schizophrenic disorder. It is perhaps, with the exception of a dementing illness, potentially more disruptive of a person's life than any other psychiatric disorder. Kraepelin regarded recovery from the disorder as unlikely, and used this as a defining characteristic of dementia praecox. This pessimistic outlook was shared by most psychiatrists, the most significant development in terms of altering the expression of the illness generally being ascribed to neuroleptic drugs. However, there have also been attempts to treat the illness in a different manner by psychologists and psychiatrists influenced by behaviourism and social learning (discussed later).

There have been many studies of outcome, both in terms of long-term evolution of the disorder and its response to drug treatment. Until the mid 1980s there was little authoritative opinion to challenge the accepted wisdom of inevitable decline. Ciompi (1986) in a long-term follow-up study, re-examined 289 survivors from an original cohort of 1642 cases with an initial diagnosis of schizophrenia. The follow-up examination included a semi-structured interview. The outcome of the disorder was assessed across these dimensions: evaluation of psychotic symptoms, development of psycho-organic or other deteriorating disorders, the nature of the social adjustment, and global overall evolution. The average age of this group was 75.2 years for men and 75.8 years for women. Ciompi found that 20.1% had been completely free of any residual symptoms for at least 5 years and 42.6% were markedly improved. His broad conclusion was that in about half to two-thirds of the cases the long-term evolution of the disorder was relatively favourable. He reduced what he thought were 30 different types of long-term outcome to eight main evolutionary types; the most frequent of which were the undulating (25%) or continuous (24%) courses. In

those cases with the most enduring form of schizophrenia, he noted that over 50% had striking negative or amotivational symptoms.

Cutting (1986) reviewed 10 studies that examined the outcome of schizophrenia with those factors thought to affect prognosis. Following a first admission, one-quarter of patients recovered completely, one-quarter had some residual chronic impairment requiring further admissions or community support, and about one-half did well. Cutting noted that, at any one point in time, about 15% of discharged patients are suffering from delusions or hallucinations and up to 30% may display negative symptoms. Up to 70% may also have symptoms of depression.

Throughout the literature on schizophrenia, a large number of factors have been reported to affect outcome. These include personality factors, recent life experiences, cerebral dysfunction, family history or family environment, and the form of the illness. Ciompi (1986) makes the point that, although the onset and initial symptomatology may be important predictors, the way sufferers cope with various aspects of the disorder might have a greater significance on outcome. The International Pilot Study of Schizophrenia (WHO 1979) ranked 47 potential predictors of outcome according to their ability to account for the variance between individuals and grouped them into three categories: sociodemographic, past history and current episode. The most powerful overall predictors of poor outcome were:

- social isolation
- long duration of the episode
- a history of past psychiatric treatment
- a history of behavioural symptoms in childhood.

Only 37% of the variance was accounted for by the 47 potential predictors, with each category accounting for roughly the same amount of variance. Of particular note was the finding that the form of the current illness was an unreliable predictor of outcome and that the outcome was very different between various countries. The disorder seemed to have a better outcome in less developed countries (e.g. Nigeria) than in the more developed countries (e.g. Denmark).

The explanation for this and similar findings may be that in less industrialised societies the opportunities to engage in useful and socially meaningful activities, such as work, are greater. A further possibility is that families in the third world may provide more extended support for patients. In the UK, families from the Indian subcontinent fare better than other ethnic groups (including native British) and this also seems to be related to differences in family structure and social role (Birchwood et al 1992).

A recent analysis of 111 studies examined both recovery from the illness and its social consequences (Warner 1994). Social recovery was viewed in terms of the degree of independent living attained by patients. Recovery rates were found to be the same now as they were nearly 100 years ago. During times of economic recession, Warner noted, the level of recovery was reduced. He also pointed out that the proportion of patients remaining in hospital has been declining throughout this century, the bulk of this decline occurring before the widespread use of neuroleptic drugs.

DOES SCHIZOPHRENIA OCCUR IN ELDERLY PEOPLE?

The diagnosis of any form of mental illness within older adults is not always straightforward, due to the often complex interaction between organic and functional symptoms (see section on differential diagnosis). Comparisons between different studies is sometimes not easy because terms such as paranoia and paranoid may be used in different ways: sometimes to describe the illness, sometimes to describe the delusions, and at other times to describe personality (Campbell 1992).

Kay & Roth (1961) chose the term late paraphrenia to describe a group of patients that they thought resembled Kraepelin's original cases of paraphrenia. They described a specific group of older adults who exhibited a systematic set of hallucinations and delusions. Like Kraepelin, they viewed these patients as having a well preserved personality and affective response, and, in the majority of the cases, the illness started after the age of 60 years. Kay and Roth further refined the concept of late paraphrenia by noting that signs of organic dementia or confusion were absent, and that the delusions and hallucinations were not attributable to a mood disorder. Holden (1987), using the Camberwell and Maudsley Hospital case registers, estimated the annual incidence of paraphrenia to be 17–26 per 100 000 of the population. He concluded that only a proportion of his patients satisfied diagnostic criteria for schizophrenia and that paraphrenia was not homogeneous.

Over the last 30 years, several studies have used different definitions of schizophrenia, late paraphrenia or paranoid symptoms beginning in late life. For example, schizophrenia after age of 45, 'late-onset', could not be diagnosed using DSM-III (APA 1980).

Therefore many patients who could have been diagnosed as suffering from late-onset schizophrenia were instead diagnosed as suffering from atypical psychosis or paranoid disorder. In DSM-III-R (APA 1987) the 45-year cut-off had been abandoned and a diagnosis of late-onset schizophrenia can now be made; the category paranoid disorder has been replaced by delusional disorder. The diagnoses late-onset schizophrenia and late paraphrenia are often seen as interchangeable, without evidence to support this. The diagnosis of paraphrenia has been excluded from the World Health Organization's International Classification of Diseases, Tenth Edition (ICD-10; WHO 1992) on the basis that schizophrenia in older adults resembles the early-onset disorder (cf. Hassett et al 1992). ICD-10 therefore assigns the diagnosis 'paranoid schizophrenia' or 'delusional disorder' in such cases. This conclusion has been challenged on the basis that there is, in fact, sufficient evidence of different underlying aetiological processes to keep the diagnosis of paraphrenia separate (Quintal et al 1991, Almeida et al 1992).

Generally speaking, the number of women suffering from late-onset schizophrenia or late paraphrenia outnumber men. This female preponderance remains after statistical adjustment for the higher life expectancy of women (Pearlson et al 1989, Howard et al 1993). There are some reports of a low marriage rate in late paraphrenia of both sexes, and those late paraphrenics that do marry have low fertility rates (Kay & Roth 1961, Herbert & Jackson 1967). In addition, people who develop late-onset schizophrenia appear to be more socially isolated, which may be a consequence of being unmarried or not having children. It is difficult to discern whether the finding of more premorbid social isolation is itself a risk factor for the onset of schizophrenia in late life or whether it is a secondary effect of the unusual premorbid personalities often described.

Differential diagnosis

Generally speaking, when an older adult presents with psychotic symptoms, organic pathology must be ruled out. Many neurological disorders can be associated with the development of secondary psychotic symptoms. A careful neurological and psychiatric examination followed by routine medical tests (e.g. haematology, serum B12, folate, thyroid function and syphilis serology) are usually part of the assessment. Modern imaging methods (e.g. computerised axial tomography, magnetic resonance imaging) may also help identify structural or vascular abnormalities that coexist with a psychotic illness in an older adult. In addition, neurological assessment may aid in the process of differential diagnosis. Although the diagnosis of late paraphrenia is thought to be straightforward for the experienced clinician (Naguib & Levy 1992), several authors note problems of distinguishing between late paraphrenia, advanced deterioration of schizophrenia and dementing illness, especially if a person is presenting at hospital for the first time (Charlesworth et al 1993).

Depression is the commonest psychiatric disorder and should always be considered. It is common for patients who are psychotically depressed to describe nihilistic delusions when, for example, they may believe that they have no stomach. Delusions of poverty and guilt are also common. Differential diagnosis with respect to depression is facilitated by a thorough history, taking into account the patient's premorbid personality, family and past psychiatric history.

16% of patients with dementia experience delusions over a 12-month period (Burns et al 1990), delusions of theft and suspicion being the most common type. Burns et al also found that 13% of their sample reported visual hallucinations and 10% reported auditory hallucinations. As the dementing illness progresses these psychotic phenomena tend to recede. Naguib & Levy (1992) note that, due to the underlying cognitive impairment, the delusions are fragmented and much less elaborate and systematised than those encountered in late paraphrenia.

Delusional disorder also needs to be considered. This is distinguished from schizophrenia by the absence of hallucinations, thought disorder and negative symptoms. The delusions usually have a persecutory or grandiose content, without features such as thought broadcasting, thought insertion or delusions of control (APA 1987). Less commonly, delusions may have a jealous content or be erotomanic (where it is believed that one is loved by another).

Causes and influences on schizophrenia

There are few solid facts concerning the aetiology of schizophrenia. It is assumed to result from some unidentified disorder(s) of brain function because there is an association with general cognitive deficits (see below), changes in brain structure, increased risk amongst first degree relatives and the symptoms may be explicable in terms of neuropsychological deficits (Frith 1992). However, it is clear that psychosocial factors are related to course and outcome (Vaughn & Leff 1976) and so any model of schizophrenia should account for the interaction of physiological and psychological factors in order to be complete. Such models are the stress vulnerability models (Clements & Turpin 1992) the best known of which was developed by Zubin & Spring (1977). Their model is based on the assumption that schizophrenia is episodic in nature and that episodes are the result of a variety of possible stressors in people who are predisposed to the illness. This predisposition is held to be the result of both genetic and environmental factors, such as birth trauma and learning experiences. Much research has been directed at identifying markers of such predisposing factors. There is evidence that there may be biochemical, genetic, anatomical, psychophysiological and cognitive markers, although this evidence is not conclusive (Clements & Turpin 1992).

According to stress vulnerability models, relapses result from stress reaching a certain threshold, specific to the individual and dependent on their level of vulnerability. Patients who have fewest relapses are thought to be those experiencing the lowest levels of stress and the least vulnerable. This idea has been incorporated into psychological treatment approaches such as family interventions (Tarrier et al 1988, Falloon et al 1985), cognitive behavioural therapy (Kingdon & Turkington 1994), and early interventions (Birchwood et al 1992a). These psychological approaches have a certain face validity which patients' relatives and keyworkers understand readily.

BRAIN FUNCTION IN SCHIZOPHRENIA

There are two main psychological aspects of brain function which have been considered in schizophrenic patients: first, aspects of function which seem to underlie the core symptoms of this illness, and second, cognitive deficits which occur commonly but are not central to the diagnosis (Frith 1992). In this section a brief description of brain function in schizophrenia is preceded by clarification of some terminology.

Cognition refers to mental activities such as remembering, thinking and linguistic function and involves both conscious and nonconscious processing of information within the brain. Neuropsychology refers to the study of cognitive function and may involve investigations of abnormal cognitive function resulting from 'insults' to the brain. Inferences are then made about what aspects of cognition are required for normal function to take place.

Neuropsychological models

In developing models of neuropsychological function in schizophrenia, most work has focused on positive symptoms. It is widely accepted that hallucinations result from the misattribution of internal mental events as being alien (Haddock et al 1994) and there is some debate as to why this occurs. Hoffman (1986) suggests that patients suffering from auditory hallucinations have a discourse planning disorder with the consequence that subvocalisations (auditory-verbal information which is held in the mind but not spoken) are experienced unintentionally.

Bentall (1990b) argued that the deficit in monitoring inner speech is likely to be influenced by patients' beliefs and expectations about what kind of events are likely to occur. He also posited that reinforcement processes (particularly anxiety reduction) may facilitate the misclassification of inner speech which has an unpleasant content. David (1994) accounts for positive symptoms in terms of a cognitive neuropsychological model of language function. In this model there are several stages required in the process of thoughts being turned into speech and comprehension of incoming auditory-verbal information.

Frith (1992) accounts for a variety of positive and negative symptoms in his model. Certain positive symptoms (hallucinations, delusions of control, thought broadcast and thought insertion) are said to result from a deficit in a monitoring system responsible for identifying mental events which occur as the result of intention. In this model, inner speech and its content are normal. What is abnormal is that the patient fails to recognise that the content of inner speech is self-initiated which in turn leads inner speech to be perceived as alien. This kind of deficit is also said to lead to certain delusions (see below).

Few researchers have attempted to explain delusions in terms of possible cognitive abnormalities specifically underlying them. It can be argued that delusions reflect normal ideas about other abnormal experiences associated with mental illness (Mahr 1974). However, the little research carried out in this area suggests that this is not the case. It has been found that patients in this group are more willing to make decisions in the absence of adequate information than control subjects (Garety & Hemsley 1987). This suggests that deluded patients are impaired in their ability to make probabilistic judgements. Kaney & Bentall (1989) demonstrated that patients with persecutory delusions exhibit more global and stable attributions than normals and that, when these events are negative, they are more likely to be externally

attributed. When events are positive they are internally attributed. In addition, deluded patients are more likely to attribute other peoples' negative actions to those persons' general disposition rather than the specific context of the behaviour involved (Bentall et al 1991) and also have a selective bias for threat-related stimuli (Kaney & Bentall 1989).

Frith's (1992) model, mentioned above, includes an account of some forms of delusion. Delusions of control, for example, are surmised to result from patients not being able to recognise that their actions are self-initiated because of a fault in the mechanism which provides feedback on whether behaviours are willed or not.

Neuropsychological deficits

There is a variety of evidence to suggest that patients with schizophrenia are liable to some impairment in cognitive function. However, some patients exhibit little or no impairment whilst others show marked deficits. A further problem is that the variety of impairments in function makes it difficult to draw generally applicable conclusions about a typical profile of dysfunction in this disorder. For example, Frith (1992) has pointed out that many patients who suffer from schizophrenia have a general deficit in intellectual function compared with premorbid levels, and others will have attentional or memory problems. There are several neuropsychological deficits which are common enough in elderly patients with schizophrenia to need consideration when working with this patient group on a day-to-day basis.

If large groups of institutionalised patients are tested, a decline in performance on intelligence tests is found in the first 5 years after admission (Nelson et al 1990, Dunkley & Rogers 1994). This decline appears progressive, even though, as has been argued, the process of institutionalisation may lead to these deficits (see section on institutionalisation).

Many patients diagnosed as suffering from schizophrenia are impulsive, or apparently apathetic showing little evidence of being able successfully to organise their own behaviour. These behavioural abnormalities are also seen in patients with frontal lobe lesions. Schizophrenic patients also perform poorly on neuropsychological tests sensitive to frontal lobe dysfunction (see Pantelis & Nelson 1994). Liddle (1987) has gone so far as to suggest that specific areas of the frontal lobes are involved with specific clusters of symptoms (positive, negative and cognitive disorganisation – see above). Pantelis and Nelson, however, suggest that it is the neural pathways that connect the frontal cortex with certain subcortical structures which are compromised. This would account not only for poor performance on frontal lobe tests (patients with lesions to these connecting pathways also seem to exhibit 'frontal' behaviour) but also the occurrence of movement disorders and poor performance on tests which are sensitive to disruption of subcortical function.

Mnemonic function is also impaired in many patients who have been diagnosed as being schizophrenic. For example, McKenna et al (1990) found that performance on memory tests was worse than that predicted by level of intellectual functioning in a large group of schizophrenic patients.

A common neuropsychological problem relates to social perception. Frith's recent review summarises these deficits (Frith 1994). Schizophrenic patients show difficulty in making attributions about others' emotional states and this phenomenon is related to flattening of affect. This latter symptom has been attributed to patients' difficulties in identifying their own emotions; however, recent evidence suggests that many of these patients do understand their own emotions (Kring et al 1993). In addition, patients with thought disorder seem not to realise that the listener is unaware of what the patient is referring to when producing each phrase in a conversation. That is, patients assume that the listener has the same knowledge viewed from the same perspective as themselves. In addition to this handicap, a large number of patients have difficulties in identifying emotions expressed by others (Cramer et al 1989) and may also have problems in recognising faces (Archer et al 1992).

The importance of research into the neuropsychological deficits seen in schizophrenia for the clinician lies in understanding that some of the difficulties in working with this group are a direct result of them. Two examples could be, first, when a patient takes many weeks to learn what appears to be a simple task, or second, becomes aggressive as a result of misperceiving a member of staff to be threatening. Conceptual disorganisation is a common feature seen in people with schizophrenia and this, combined with a general impairment of cognitive function, including memory, will lead to slow learning. In addition, antipsychotic medication leads to impaired concentration, which may exacerbate difficulties in learning. In the second example, the inability to interpret facial expressions (relating to empathy and reassurance), in combination with delusional beliefs, may make the patient angry. In this example frontal lobe dysfunction might also be implicated as this can lead to disinhibition so that the patient feels little compunction

at apparently appearing to be abusive. Another important aspect of this type of research is that it may lead to specific interventions which account for the deficits involved (e.g. Brenner et al 1992) (see section on treatment below). Finally, assessing certain aspects of neuropsychological or cognitive function may be useful in predicting the level of supervision patients need in the long term and be useful in predicting rehabilitation outcome (Wykes & Dunn 1992). For example, Wykes (1994) found that impaired performance on complex reaction time tasks was associated with poor rehabilitation outcome. She concluded that: 'The group of patients who exhibit high levels of impairment could now be selected for special attention in order to develop innovative rehabilitation methods (cognitive rehabilitation) ... It could help patients take advantage of community provision, and if these impairments are found to be vulnerability factors, their remediation might also help to prevent further exacerbations of symptoms' (p. 491).

INSTITUTIONALISATION

Institutionalisation is a concept that can be applied to many aspects of society and to everyday social events that affect us all (see Ch. 27 for further discussion). Wing & Brown (1970) observed that several well-known authors, such as George Orwell, have illustrated the changes in attitude and behaviour that may occur when someone is placed in an environment which requires adherence to an arbitrary and depersonalising routine. Although much has been written about the syndrome of 'institutionalism' there has been little scientific scrutiny of such a process. It is somewhat unfortunate that, in addition to the paucity of research on institutions, most of what has been written is exclusively negative with very little reference to any positive aspects. In the first part of this century the profound pessimism with regard to the outcome of schizophrenia no doubt contributed to the lack of any real therapeutic culture within the mental hospital. The original function of the large asylums was to provide protection from the ordinary stresses of everyday life. Underpinning this approach was the assumption of a scientific basis for this 'moral' treatment. Whatever the rationale and intentions of such an approach, it is apparent from several accounts that the large hospitals became dismal places to spend one's life (Abrahamson 1993). Descriptions of wards as 'backward' have been elaborated upon by those attempting to resettle patients outside the hospital. Descriptions of inadequate case notes lacking detail with regard to the course and progression of the illness serve to highlight the absence of adequate medical and psychiatric follow-up (Abrahamson 1993). During the 1950s and 1960s, the political and social climate for reform was reinforced by the idea that exposure to mental hospitals for a substantial period could in itself lead to 'an illness' (cf. institutionalism).

In 1957, Greenblatt et al published *The Patient and the Mental Hospital,* which contained 38 separate papers examining such issues as custodial attitudes among staff, the depersonalising effects of hospital routine and the administrative process of entering a large mental hospital. Barton (1959) adopted the term institutional neurosis to refer to the clinical effects of poor hospital care which includes low self-esteem, withdrawal of interest, and inability to plan for the future. Barton hypothesised that certain features of the institution lead to a 'disease' that is independent of the original illness on admission, that increases with the duration of stay in the hospital, but that could be 'treated'. Some of the factors that Barton thought might be important in the development of institutional neurosis were: loss of contact with the outside world, enforced idleness, authoritarian staff attitudes, loss of personal friends and possessions, drug treatment and poor ward atmosphere.

Although he never specifically referred to schizophrenia, he believed that much of the 'end-state' thought to be characteristic of the disease was in fact the product of social and environmental factors. Another way of construing his basic argument would be that entirely normal people could resemble those with schizophrenia if they spent long enough in a mental hospital. This hypothesis would not gain much favour today. However, at the time it not only questioned the therapeutic value of the institution, but also raised serious doubts about the validity of the diagnosis of schizophrenia. At this time Kraepelin's idea of poor outcome as being a defining aspect of schizophrenia was still widely accepted in the UK and the rest of Europe.

Broadly speaking, elderly people who are suffering from schizophrenia are resident in institutions as a result of two different events:

• Individuals may have entered a large hospital setting suffering from schizophrenia when younger, and following repeated episodes eventually become long-stay patients.
• Older adults with early-onset (or late-onset) schizophrenia enter institutional care in the community. When the person moves from one location to another in the community this is viewed as a specific kind of relocation (cf. Tobin 1989). Resettlement

usually refers to a move from a large hospital setting to a community setting.

The complex organisation of mental hospitals with social, environmental and illness variables makes the scientific study of institutional life difficult. In spite of this, there have been a few studies which have attempted to examine whether the disabilities evident in sufferers of schizophrenia are related to the illness or social and environmental factors. Wing & Brown (1970) conceptualised three possible types of disability from which to examine this question. Those individuals who have had schizophrenia for many years may have:

• disabilities, in a relative sense, that were present before the onset of the illness and hospitalisation
• primary disabilities which are part of the illness, e.g. negative symptoms
• secondary disabilities which are not part of the illness, but have arisen solely because the person is ill (e.g. their attitude to discharge).

All the research has focused on the two latter categories.

Wing & Brown (1970) studied three hospitals that were selected because they seemed to differ markedly in social conditions and administrative policies. Samples of patients suffering from schizophrenia were drawn randomly from each hospital and followed longitudinally. Wing and Brown concluded that 'environmental poverty' was highly correlated with a clinical poverty syndrome. Thus patients in the 'richest' social environments displayed fewer negative symptoms (social withdrawal, flatness of affect and poverty of speech). The improvement in the social environment resulted in a significant proportion of patients being less disabled by these negative symptoms. These 'gains' were actually removed when, over the course of 8 years, there was a deterioration in the environment of two of the hospitals. At the time, these results were mistakenly viewed as evidence that the negative symptoms of schizophrenia are a consequence of institutional life. However, as Wing (1992) has pointed out, their main hypotheses regarding 'institutionalism' were related to secondary disabilities. Specifically, they hypothesised that attitudes held towards discharge would depend on the poverty of the social environment. In addition, they postulated that the length of stay would be related to level of disability. Thus they described a 'gradual adoption of an attitude of indifference to leaving' as illustrated by the case of Mr Harrison (Box 13.1). Curson et al (1992), in a cross-sectional re-examination of the original study, failed to confirm Wing and Brown's findings that the number of years spent in a large mental hospital was related to institutionalism, whether this was defined as a reluctance to leave, social withdrawal or negative symptoms. However, this study has been criticised because there appeared to be too little variation in the environment to adequately test Wing and Brown's original hypotheses (Abrahamson 1993).

Wing and Brown also found a strong relationship between inactivity and negative symptoms. Improving the social environment led to an improvement in negative symptoms and the longer patients remained in hospital, the less likely they were to want to leave. However, improving the environment in these hospitals did not remove negative symptoms entirely, suggesting that these are a core feature of chronic schizophrenia, rather than purely due to the effects of institutionalisation. In support of this idea, Johnstone et al (1985) found that schizophrenic patients discharged from hospital had similar levels of negative symptoms to those remaining in hospital, although they were less cognitively impaired. Manic depressive patients who had been in hospital for the same length of time as the schizophrenic in-patients had a significantly lower level of both positive and negative symptoms but similar levels of cognitive impairment. Conclusions from this study must be tempered to some degree because the age of admission for the schizophrenic group was significantly younger than for the manic depressive group. It is possible that admission at a younger age has a different impact on functioning than being admitted later in life. In addition, the authors assumed that not living in a large mental hospital inferred an optimally stimulating environment for discharged patients. Many of the out-patients studied may have been socially inactive, and thus living in a situation akin to that found in a large mental hospital.

RESETTLEMENT, COMMUNITY CARE AND CASE MANAGEMENT

It might be assumed that the relevance of the research on institutionalism may be declining as the large Victorian mental hospitals are being closed. However, a significant proportion of psychiatric patients, particularly elderly people, remain in large institutions and conditions for many of these patients have changed little. For example, Ford et al (1987) described conditions for patients over the age of 65 years as 'scandalous'. Only 27 out of 206 patients in this age group in the hospital they studied ever went out. This was largely attributed to lack of friendships, loss of contact with family and low staffing levels. Although the population in the hospital studied fell by approximately 50% between 1960 and 1985, the number of male patients aged over 65 years had declined little.

There are further risks for the occurrence of institutionalisation in modern times. The length of stay in district general hospital acute wards can be longer than planned, especially if there is little community provision or where such provision does not include enough supervision and care. For example, Salit and Marcos (1991) examined the factors leading to marked increases in the length of stay in general hospitals in New York City. They attributed the changes in admission patterns to changes in funding arrangements whereby health care reimbursement covers low cost long-term mental health care only. In addition, there has been a huge reduction in beds available in long-term care psychiatric institutions and a shortage of community care programmes. In the UK similar problems have occurred in district general hospitals where there has been a build-up of patients who are referred to as the 'new' long-stay. These patients require up to 24-hour nursing care and represent the most psychiatrically disabled of patients (Mann & Cree 1976). Although there have been strategies developed recently aimed at providing services for this group, many are likely to remain in hospital and so be at the risk of institutionalism. Elderly people residing in nursing homes, hostels, hostel wards and staffed group homes may be particularly at risk.

A small scale residential service does not necessarily avoid institutionalisation. Individuals with schizophrenia may spend little time engaged in structured activity or in contact with people away from the institution concerned. It is all too easy for small residential settings to become isolated from the community, even when the physical location is on an urban street.

Box 13.2 illustrates that the routine followed by elderly patients living in a community home may offer few advantages over life in hospital. In this example it is clear that without the integration of these two patients' residential care with that provided by the hospital and social services, they would lead lives very similar to some of those in long-stay wards in the large Victorian mental hospitals. Moving them away from the large institution did not lead them to have friends and increased contact with relatives. In spite of the efforts of the untrained staff who see to the day-to-day

Box 13.2   Institutionalism in a small group home

37 Wavertree Avenue is a small privately run group home on the edge of a large city centre. There are three male residents, one attends a local social services day centre most days of the week, and another attends the local psychiatric day hospital every weekday. Mr Andrews is visited by his sister and brother-in-law once per fortnight. He spends the greater proportion of his time each day searching for 'dimps' in the local shopping centre, picking them up from the pavement and searching litter bins. The rest of his time is spent watching television. Mr Newman spends his time at the group home smoking and drinking tea. At around 4 p.m. each day he exhausts his daily tobacco supply; he then invariably goes to bed until 11 p.m. when he goes to the local pubs at closing time in order to beg for tobacco and cigarettes. He usually returns at 1.30 a.m. The residents of the group home are not allowed access to food supplies except when the meals are prepared by members of staff. The only household activity residents are allowed to participate in is vacuum cleaning.

cooking and cleaning, there is little opportunity for stimulating activity.

The length of time people spend in hospital has been declining since the mid 1940s due to changes in outlook and therapeutic approaches within institutions as well as the development of community care policies. Ford et al (1987) found that between 1960 and 1985, the rate of decline of in-patient numbers appeared to be slowing but that nearly one-third of the population of the hospital had been resident since 1960. McGreadie et al's (1985) survey of new long-stay patients across 14 hospitals in Scotland found that only 20% of these patients had been discharged at follow-up 2 years later. Unless appropriate alternatives to psychiatric hospitalisation can be found, the new long-stay patients are going to become old long-stay patients.

Perkins et al (1989) have argued that residential and nursing accommodation for older people suffering from mental illness offers limited choice and flexibility. Although classed as 'homes for elderly people', many residents in this type of accommodation have disabilities very different to those with schizophrenia. Although it is known that such accommodation usually has a large number of confused people there have, in fact, been few studies that have examined the prevalence of mental disorder in nursing homes (Burns et al 1988). Moreover, a consumer survey of 100 residential homes showed that 65% had more than

40 residents and 20% more than 50 (Willcocks et al 1986). These types of care setting for older people have been noted for low levels of activity and social interaction, and consequent susceptibility to the development of passivity and dependence (Woods & Britton 1985). Clearly, attempting to abolish hospital institutionalism does not solve the problems of schizophrenia, and institutionalism in hospitals may be no different from institutionalism that develops in other care settings. A consensus view appears to favour smaller private accommodation for resettlement purposes where residents have greater choice about their lifestyle and privacy. If both staff and residents are intensively prepared before any move, then it has been found that patients' functioning improves (Morris et al 1988). Scores on behavioural rating scales improve due to less staff input in everyday activities such as bathing, dressing and going out.

Community care and case management

Community care embodies many assumptions, not least of which are the beliefs that the community is caring and therapeutic (cf. Hawks 1975). In the UK, the run-down of the large mental hospitals began in the 1960s under the then Minister of Health, Enoch Powell. Support for community care came from several sources. Critiques of psychiatric institutions highlighted the problems of separating illness symptoms and treatment and institutional effects (Barton 1959, Goffman 1961). At a societal level, considerable disquiet resulted from the occasional media reports of the poor conditions under which many patients were kept in the large mental hospitals. One of the most significant determinants at the time was the availability of the recently developed antipsychotic drugs with which it was thought the disorder might be satisfactorily managed in the community. Consequently, from 1960 to 1985 the number of in-patients fell from 128 000 to 64 000 (General Register Office 1964, DHSS 1986).

The implementation of this policy has been referred to as deinstitutionalisation. This policy can only be successful if the health care services are able to reduce the number of people who require long-term nursing care. In addition, mental health services have to find ways of preventing or managing acute exacerbation of mental illness. Within the elderly group several questions remain over the assumptions inherent in community care. Levene et al (1985) conducted a 1-day survey of 1087 people resident in two large mental hospitals. Over 50% of their sample was over 65 years old and over two-thirds of those had a primary diagnosis of dementia. Although this figure would appear to be unusually high for dementia (cf. Jorm et al 1987), it serves to highlight how little we know about the prevalence of other psychiatric syndromes within 'long-stay' patients. In addition, Levene et al found that three-quarters of all residents over 65 years had substantial social withdrawal, and two-thirds were not fully continent. They concluded that a large proportion of those studied could not be managed outside a residential setting.

Recent years have seen marked changes in care policy in the UK (DOH 1987, 1989a, 1989b) regarding the structure and function of health care. A greater degree of professional accountability and tighter financial control is expected, and the needs of any population should be made explicit in relation to current priorities. The aim is that health-related services in a hospital and community setting reflect the needs of the population they serve. Although there is information available on the epidemiology of mental disorders in elderly people, there is very little detailed information on both the need for long-term health and social care. Furthermore, it is not clear exactly how health and social care should be defined with reference to this patient group. Murphy (1992) has defined health care as: 'the specific diagnostic, investigatory and treatment interventions designed to reduce or eliminate symptoms and signs of mental disorder or to rehabilitate an individual to maximum social and occupational function' (p. 123).

She defines social care as the provision of assistance to individuals which allows them to sustain activities of daily life which are common to all humanity; assistance with provision of adequate income, shelter, food and clothing. A generally agreed way of providing such care is through multidisciplinary working in order that the sheer diversity of needs can be met. Case management is a way of delivering care to meet individual need through placing the responsibility for assessment and service coordination with one individual worker or team (Onyett 1992). The principal tasks of case management are:

- assessment
- planning
- implementation
- monitoring
- review.

The target of effective case management of patients suffering from schizophrenia is to:

- improve health and social functioning
- reduce mortality from suicide and physical illness.

Such a goal depends upon the development of adequate and appropriate community care services. Challis and Davis (1986) compared two groups of elderly people; one received standard provision and the other a community care approach coordinated and managed by a social worker. Most of the people included in the study lived in their own homes and were described as being 'on the margins of institutional care'. The latter approach led to fewer admissions to institutional care and was more cost effective. However, the small percentage of clients with a functional psychotic illness posed substantial management problems. A disproportionate amount of time was spent in liaison with other agencies in order to ensure that care provided was beneficial. In summary, adequate case management may lead to reduced relapse and readmission rates, but only if it allows the optimal use of a variety of treatment strategies which have been demonstrated to be effective.

TREATMENT
Neuroleptic medication

The predominant treatment for schizophrenia is neuroleptic medication. Neuroleptic drugs are major tranquillisers which have their therapeutic effect by blocking dopamine receptors in the brain. The efficacy of these drugs is closely related to their affinity for D2 dopamine receptors. The more of the drug that binds with these receptors, the smaller the dose that is needed to have a therapeutic impact. Neuroleptics first came to be used during the 1950s and had a marked impact on the management of schizophrenia. They are effective in the management of positive symptoms but their influence on negative symptoms is less certain (see below). Not only does this medication lead to a reduction in symptoms during acute episodes, but if administered during such episodes, outcome is markedly improved over the subsequent 3–5 years (Davis & Andriukaitis 1986). Between 8% and 16% of patients relapse per month if not taking medication (Davis & Andriukaitis 1986) and, over a 9-month period, 50% of patients relapse when not regularly taking their medication, compared with 14% of those who do (Vaughn & Leff 1976). Davis and Andriukaitis conclude that the rate of relapse is dramatically reduced in patients who receive long-term neuroleptic medication. Clear benefits for patients with late paraphrenia are also obtained when treated with neuroleptic medication (Howard & Levy 1992).

Prophylactic neuroleptic medication is often administered in depot form (this is by injection which lasts for a number of weeks) rather than orally. This is thought to improve compliance (Johnson & Freeman 1973) although there is little evidence to suggest that schizophrenics are less compliant than any other patient group (Young et al 1986). The treatment of early-onset schizophrenia in late life and late-onset schizophrenia is also mainly based upon neuroleptic medication although the doses used may be smaller (Gierl et al 1986) particularly in patients who have a late onset (Tran-Johnson et al 1992).

Problems and side-effects associated with the use of neuroleptics

There are a number of significant problems associated with the use of neuroleptics. Foremost amongst these are a number of common severe side-effects of which there are two main groups:

1. The first of these is extrapyramidal symptoms, which include acute dystonia, in which involuntary muscle contractions, particularly of the head and neck, occur. Patients can suffer also from lockjaw (trismus) and oculogyric crisis, in which the eyes are rotated upwards. A further extrapyramidal symptom is akathisia. Patients with this symptom exhibit marked restlessness, particularly of their legs, and they sometimes pace for hours at a time. The final extrapyramidal symptom is tardive dyskinesia. This occurs after chronic neuroleptic use (longer than 6 months) and involves involuntary movements of the tongue, lips and jaw. Tardive dyskinesia worsens if the medication is reduced.
2. The second group of common side-effects of neuroleptic drugs is parkinsonian symptoms. Patients are rigid, have slow movements and a tremor. The slowness induced by neuroleptic medication is sometimes mistaken for a negative symptom of the illness.

Both extrapyramidal and parkinsonian side-effects are pharmacologically treatable to some degree, however dose reduction is generally required (Schwartz & Brotman 1992).

Perhaps the most dramatic side-effect is neuroleptic malignant syndrome, which occurs 24–72 hours after administration in 2% of patients receiving neuroleptic medication. Patients suffer from pyrexia, unstable blood pressure and marked rigidity. 10–25% of patients with these symptoms die (Schwartz & Brotman 1992, Bristow & Hirsch 1993). The list of other neuroleptic side-effects is too long for a detailed

description in this chapter but nevertheless they have important consequences for the patient. Examples include impotence, anorgasmia (in women), confusion, dry mouth, weight gain, photosensitivity, constipation and amenorrhoea. Clinically these are often not assessed, sometimes leaving the patients to suffer unnecessarily.

It is widely accepted that the negative consequences of medication are more severe in elderly patients (Walker & Wynne 1994). Tardive dyskinesia is more frequent in older patients and this may be associated with the cumulative dosage they have received and organic brain disease (Bristow & Hirsch 1993). Jeste & Wyatt (1986) provide guidelines for the prescription of neuroleptic medication in the elderly, which are aimed at reducing the risk of tardive dyskinesia. They suggest that the smallest effective doses are used, that the use of anticholinergic medication is avoided, that patients and their relatives are fully informed of the risk of tardive dyskinesia, that patients are regularly reviewed, and that neuroleptic medication should be discontinued at the first signs of tardive dyskinesia. It has been suggested that treating patients suffering from severe side-effects with atypical neuroleptics such as remoxipride and clozapine which have different side-effect profiles may be a useful strategy (Lindström 1994). However, it should be noted that the side-effects of these alternative drugs can also be severe and require careful monitoring. In the USA there is a legal requirement in some states for patients to sign an informed consent form before receiving neuroleptic medication. In addition, patients who are held against their will (because of the risk of harming themselves or others) are permitted the right to appeal against the use of neuroleptic medication. The opportunity to appeal against treatment decisions is important, even when those decisions can be enforced under the law, because only the person treated with medication can relate the impact of side-effects. However, in many cases this must allow for some process of advocacy, so that patients who, because of their illness, find it difficult to express arguments coherently or lack insight, can have their interests fully represented.

Psychological treatments

Psychodynamic approaches to the management of schizophrenia have been investigated empirically only once (Gunderson et al 1984). It is often stated that such approaches may be harmful to patients. Gunderson et al found neither positive nor negative effects of the two psychodynamic treatments that they used.

The first psychological approaches to be used

successfully in the management of schizophrenia were behavioural techniques developed during the 1960s, and the main examples of these are discussed below.

Token economies

Token economies have largely been applied to in-patients and are based on the principles of operant conditioning. Patients are encouraged to carry out specified behaviours by giving them tokens which can be exchanged for items that each patient desires. Token economies were found to be effective in improving self-care skills, reducing apathy and aggression and generally improving social interaction (e.g. Paul & Lentz 1977).

There are a number of problems in applying token economies. First, removal of the economy can lead to return to baseline levels of behaviour, although there are some studies in which patients were able to maintain levels of behaviour above baseline levels (Hall 1983). The second problem is that they have largely been applied to in-patients, with only four known studies of their application in the community up until 1991 (Corrigan 1991). This is because they are much more difficult to apply in the community than in in-patient settings where competing reinforcers are less available, patients have less income and family members can interfere less.

A third problem is that the awarding of tokens can be seen as a demeaning process or rather childish. It is, however, possible to make the token economy run on an age-appropriate basis involving mutual respect on the part of patients and staff. In addition, it has been suggested that, for many patients, the administration of token reinforcement may be less important than resultant changes in staff behaviour. For example, staff should adopt a positive encouraging tone combined with the expectation of positive changes on the part of the patient (Hall & Baker 1986).

Social skills training

Wixted et al (1988) argue that social skills training is especially important for patients who predominantly suffer from negative symptoms. The rationale for its use is that negative symptoms interfere with the acquisition of social skills which normally occurs in early adulthood.

As well as improving specific aspects of interpersonal behaviour, this approach aims to help patients to develop social networks and to cope effectively with day-to-day stress. Overall, patients undergoing social skills training should improve their ability to solve everyday problems, develop mutually rewarding relationships and obtain relevant help and work (Anthony & Liberman 1986).

Interventions usually consist of instruction, modelling, and role playing and are often carried out on a group basis. Generalisation is facilitated by use of in vivo training and homework assignments. The content of social skills programmes varies greatly between centres and may focus on problem-solving skills, assertiveness, or specific interpersonal skills such as maintaining appropriate eye contact and using open questions. Social skills training is effective in that patients learn the skills taught; however, there is little evidence that these skills generalise to situations away from the training environment (Halford & Hayes 1991). Outcome studies have not focused specifically on those patients with negative symptoms. However, in general, outcome is thought to be positive (Bellack & Mueser 1993).

There have been no research studies directed at the use of social skills training in elderly patients. There is no reason to suppose that this approach would not be useful in this patient group; however, the slant of training may have to differ to account for differences between old and young groups. For example, training patients how to ask a member of the opposite sex for a date may be less relevant, but being able to identify and report physical health problems may be particularly pertinent for older patients.

Cognitive rehabilitation

As can be seen from the section on neuropsychological deficits above, schizophrenic patients exhibit a wide range of cognitive deficits. These interfere with learning, problem solving and attentional skills. There have been attempts to address these deficits in patients' rehabilitation programmes and design treatment strategies to overcome them (e.g. Green 1993, Erickson 1988).

Integrated psychological therapy (Brenner et al 1992) is such an approach. Patients undergo a programme of training which at first involves the acquisition of basic cognitive skills. Then patients are trained to use more complex social skills which are assumed to be dependent on the more basic skills learned earlier. Brenner et al found that patients learn the specific skills in which they are trained; however, they do not generalise to 'real life' and the skills learned are not particularly relevant to their lives. For example, it is difficult to see how learning to successfully complete a card sorting task will really lead to improved quality of life.

Family interventions aimed at reducing expressed emotion (EE)

During the 1970s, it was observed that certain patterns of interaction between family members of schizophrenic patients were related to increased relapse rates. These studies have been summarised by Vaughn and Leff (1985) and were based on a specific measure of family interaction, the Camberwell Family Interview (CFI). Certain variables measured on the CFI, when combined, constitute the expressed emotion construct. The most important elements of expressed emotion in predicting the course of schizophrenia are 'criticism', 'hostility' and 'emotional overinvolvement' (EOI). In this context 'criticism' relates to the expression of dissatisfaction of the patient in a critical tone of voice. 'Hostility' involves negative statements about the person as a whole, for example, concerning their personality or other general characteristics. EOI involves exaggerated emotional responses, where the relative may be over-anxious about the patient. Emotionally over-involved relatives tend to sacrifice their own welfare on behalf of the patient and ensure that negative experiences for the patient are avoided at all costs. As a result, patients lead restricted lifestyles in which they are not responsible for their own care.

There have been a number of family intervention studies aimed at reducing EE and thus relapse rates. Of the seven studies published up to 1991, five led to reduced relapse rates (Barrowclough & Tarrier 1992). Of the two studies in which there was no advantage for the family intervention one used a psychodynamic approach (Kottgen et al 1984) and the other treated family members without the involvement of the patient (Vaughan et al 1992). The effectiveness of the family interventions in reducing relapse rates is marked. 2 years after the interventions, relapse rates were reduced by at least 50% and in one study there remained a significant difference in outcome 8 years after the intervention (Tarrier et al 1994).

Each of the studies in which a family intervention was successful adopted a different approach to reducing EE but they shared certain aspects. First, all the studies included education regarding the illness and treatment. However, it is important to note that educating patients' relatives does not lead to a reduction in relapse rates (Tarrier et al 1988, Smith & Birchwood 1987) but can lead to a reduction in burden for relatives (Smith & Birchwood 1987). It is probably an important aspect of therapy, not just because information is provided, but because it acts as an aid in establishing a therapeutic relationship with families and allows them to ask relevant questions, often for the first time. Those intervention studies that were successful focused on interactions between family members with the goal of developing adaptive problem-solving skills. The results from studies where the interventions were delivered over a relatively long time period showed the best outcome. The interventions also tend to emphasise stress management for relatives as well as patients, combined with the assumption that the patient should lead as independent a lifestyle as is possible.

It should be noted that the positive outcome of these studies was not solely evaluated in terms of relapse rates. Social functioning has also been observed to improve as a result of these interventions (Barrowclough & Tarrier 1990) as well as burden and stress experienced by relatives (Falloon et al 1985). Family interventions can also lead to a reduction in service costs (Tarrier et al 1991, Cardin et al 1986).

Family interventions aimed at elderly patients obviously involve spouses and offspring more than parents and siblings. This, and the fact that maladaptive behavioural patterns may have become ingrained over decades, may lead to some differences in the intervention. There may need to be greater emphasis on practical support for the patient and spouse in order, for example, to account for physical health needs, finance and transportation (also see Box 13.3 below).

Cognitive behavioural treatment of positive symptoms

Initially, attempts to manage positive symptoms psychologically were reported on a case-by-case basis. Slade and Bentall (1988) summarise these studies and conclude that, as far as hallucinations go, three basic tactics had been useful:

- distraction
- focusing on the symptom
- reduction of arousal.

There have been fewer attempts to reduce delusions by psychological means. More recently, trials have been carried out to examine the effectiveness of a variety of interventions, only some of which are described below.

Bentall and his colleagues (Bentall et al 1994, Haddock et al 1995) have developed a novel treatment approach to the management of auditory hallucinations. Patients are asked to focus progressively on the characteristics of the voices heard. Initially the patient focuses on physical characteristics such as volume and gender gradually building up to concentrate on the content and underlying meaning of what the voices say. This is thought to have two effects. First, the process of focusing, in combination with feedback from the therapist, helps patients to identify their hallucinations as the product of their own mind and second, to become desensitised to the occurrence of voices and thus feel less anxious about them. In a preliminary trial this approach was as effective as training patients to distract themselves from hallucinations but led to an increase in self-esteem. Both interventions were successful compared with a control group (Haddock et al 1995).

Tarrier has taken a different approach to the management of positive symptoms. This is based on the observation that many patients who experience unremitting positive symptoms develop their own coping strategies to deal with them. In the coping strategy enhancement approach, patients are trained to use the strategies they have developed for themselves and apply them systematically. Alternatively, patients are taught to use strategies which have been developed by the therapist with the patient, aimed at countering the effects of contingencies influencing the occurrence of their psychotic symptoms. The patients are encouraged to practice coping strategies in vivo, if necessary deliberately generating the symptom of concern in order to practise the relevant strategy. The approach is based on a careful cognitive behavioural analysis and the coping strategies are developed with each patient on an 'if it works use it' basis. This means that the treatment can be very different for different patients.

Tarrier et al (1993) compared coping strategy enhancement with problem solving in a recent outcome trial. They found that the two psychological approaches were both successful in reducing psychotic symptoms compared with a control group.

Kingdon and Turkington (1994) have developed a more general cognitive behavioural approach to the management of schizophrenia. They aim to treat all aspects of the illness which cause distress for the patients. Patients are engaged in therapy by using education with a normalising rationale. Important events associated with the onset are also discussed fully with the patient and cognitive techniques applied as necessary with the aim of modifying maladaptive beliefs and automatic thoughts. They also target anxiety and depression, which often occur in schizophrenia. After this stage the psychotic symptoms themselves are treated. Hallucinations are explained to the patient as being something that many people can experience as a result of severe stress or sleep deprivation. Reality testing and inductive reasoning are used to test out possible explanations for the hallucinations. In dealing with entrenched psychotic symptoms, Kingdon and Turkington suggest that it is important to explore the patients' emotional invest-ment in the symptom of concern. When questioning the patient it is important not to challenge delusions or other strongly held beliefs directly but to attempt to draw out the patients' ideas. They also advocate using coping strategies that patients have developed for themselves. These are encouraged in a general sense rather than being systematically assessed and enhanced as in the approach taken by Tarrier and his colleagues. Negative symptoms are treated using long-term plans (5–10 years). Short-term achievable targets which act as steps towards achieving the long-term goals and which the patient can readily attain are also used. Kingdon and Turkington also suggest that activity schedules, often used in the treatment of depression, where possible combined with allowing the patient to decide on activities, are an effective means of reducing the impact of negative symptoms.

The approaches described above relate to symptoms which are present in spite of medication. Another psychological approach is to train patients and their relatives how to identify that a relapse may be imminent and to take appropriate avoiding action (Birchwood et al 1992b). A number of investigators have identified certain symptoms which occur in many patients who subsequently relapse (Hirsch & Jolley 1989). For example, approximately two-thirds of patients suffer anxiety and/or depression in the weeks before the onset of a full schizophrenic relapse. Each patient can also experience idiosyncratic symptoms which also consistently antedate relapses. The approach is particularly applicable to those patients who are in regular contact with carers or have good insight. In addition, patients who are on low doses of medication or who are often non-compliant are suitable. Each patient's 'relapse signature' is obtained by interviewing the carer and patient and then fed back to them in summarised form. They are then taught how to monitor the relevant symptoms on a regular basis and a specific plan of action is developed for each patient. This normally involves an increase in medication and an increase of contact with services. In some cases, perhaps where the prodrome has resulted from some stressor, the patient can receive help with appropriate coping.

Cognitive-behavioural interventions for the management of positive symptoms are a recent development and have yet to be fully evaluated. The results to date are promising and eventually this approach may be seen as a major aspect in the management of schizophrenia. However, the research success of family interventions has not yet led to their use as an everyday aspect of care for schizophrenic patients. This may also be a problem in the implementation of psychological treatments of positive symptoms in this patient group.

A further problem lies in applying these approaches to the elderly subset of patients. There are few, if any, theoretical reasons why these approaches should not be used with this group; however, there is little, if any, research on this matter. Some of the potential problems are highlighted in the case of Mr Davidson, described in Box 13.3.

In this case, the intervention initially thought to be most useful did not work. Several practical conside-

---

Box 13.3 Psychological approaches to schizophrenia in old age

Martin Davidson is a 67-year-old man who lives with his wife on a council estate near to the local hospital. He was first diagnosed as suffering from schizophrenia in the mid 1950s at the time he finished national service. Over the last 40 or so years he has been admitted to hospital for between 2–8 weeks on 10–15 occasions. His admissions have generally been short and symptoms marked by delusions that his wife has extra-marital affairs, that he is sexually inadequate and that neighbours believe that he has sexually abused children. In between relapses, his symptom profile is characterised by severe anergia (lethargy) and inactivity. He also spends most of his time smoking between 80 and 100 cigarettes per day, or borrowing money from neighbours to buy more cigarettes. At the time of referral he had a severe chest infection.

Mrs Davidson has coped with her husband's illness since it was first diagnosed by taking all responsibility for household tasks and income generation (he never gained employment after discharge from the army). Over the years she found that 'nagging' and criticism were effective methods of controlling his behaviour, and in sessions with the therapist openly insulted her husband. Soon after family therapy aimed at reducing expressed emotion was commenced Mr Davidson's physical condition deteriorated and he became increasingly restless, irritable and socially avoidant. His self-care also deteriorated. During a particularly severe family argument Mrs Davidson attacked her husband with a knife, but her arthritis prevented her from harming him.

At this point Mr Davidson deteriorated still further and was admitted to hospital 4 weeks later. His main problem at this time being delusions as described above, plus feelings of hopelessness, low self-esteem and other symptoms consistent with a co-existent depressive illness. It was clear that the family therapy was not succeeding, largely because Mrs Davidson found it difficult to either follow the advice given concerning her stress management (developing a social life, relaxation, etc.) or implement assertive, constructive responses to her husband's difficult behaviours. It had also been suggested that Mr and Mrs Davidson reduce the amount of babysitting they carried out for her son and daughter-in-law. There were 4 grandchildren which Mr and Mrs Davidson looked after for at least part of every day of the week. The couple felt unable to refuse to see their grandchildren.

From the time of Mr Davidson's admission, plans were made for his discharge. It was clear that, in the short-

term, Mrs Davidson would not be likely to reduce her hostility and critical comments. It was therefore decided to provide Mr Davidson with a weekly activity schedule which reduced his contact and dependence on his wife whilst being engaged in activities he found rewarding and constructive. It had also been noted that, while on the ward and engaged in activity, including general conversations with others, he smoked less. In light of his physical health problems this was held to be important. The following plan was implemented on discharge:

1. Mr Davidson will attend the industrial therapy unit each weekday (he had previously enjoyed this and appreciated the small amount of extra money he was able to earn). Mr Davidson will meet the clinical psychologist in the industrial therapy unit for a short weekly session. This will allow Mr Davidson to discuss ongoing problems and the psychologist to check that he feels comfortable in the unit's environment.
2. Mr Davidson will be picked up by taxi at the hospital's expense for the journey to and from the industrial therapy unit – this worked as a non-critical prompt for Mr Davidson who had difficulties in maintaining activities and also allowed him to avoid the stigma associated with being picked up by ambulance.
3. Mrs Davidson will receive fortnightly counselling aimed at identifying points of dispute between the couple, helping Mrs Davidson constructively problem-solve, and reducing her level of stress.
4. Mr and Mrs Davidson will reduce their contact time with their grandchildren to 3 days per week (thus reducing the burden they both feel in supporting their son and daughter-in-law).
5. Mr Davidson will henceforth be seen on a 3-monthly basis in the out-patient clinic by the same psychiatrist for an indefinite period (the team consultant, rather than junior doctors who tend to be in post for short periods).

Mr and Mrs Davidson adhered to this plan. Several months later, at the time of writing, they both report being much happier together, Mr Davidson has maintained his activity levels and shouting matches now occur on a fortnightly basis rather than daily. Mr Davidson is no longer depressed and has become actively involved in household tasks. Although they see their grandchildren on a daily basis, it is usually only one or two at a time and for short periods.

rations had to be made. The therapists helping to arrange the couple's daily routine led to more long-term benefits than the attempts to reduce expressed emotion in the household. However, it should be noted that Mr Davidson was, as a consequence of establishing a daily routine away from home, subject to less criticism and hostility. The reduction in stress (resulting from Mr Davidson's behaviour and caring for their grandchildren) then led Mrs Davidson to be less hostile. The maintenance of long-term relationships with hospital staff encouraged Mr Davidson to attend regularly and to report potential problems. A recent study showed that maintenance of relationship with a particular psychiatrist leads to improved use of services by long-term mentally ill people and a more flexible response to patients' needs on the part of the clinician. This in turn leads to a reduction in admissions (Abbati & Oles 1993).

CONCLUSIONS

This chapter provides an overview of schizophrenia in relation to elderly patients. Much of the literature reviewed relates to younger patients because little research has been carried out on the elderly population. Schizophrenia is usually a lifelong relapsing condition characterised by positive symptoms which become most prominent during relapses and are at least partly treatable with appropriate medication. Negative symptoms persist throughout the illness. Elderly people may also suffer from late paraphrenia, a similar but rarer disorder, in which negative symptoms are less prominent.

Underlying the symptoms of this illness are a number of possible neuropsychological deficits. Many patients are also subject to other neuropsychological deficits not specific to these symptoms. This makes detection of organic brain diseases and other psychiatric disorders difficult in elderly patients unless careful assessments are made.

The mainstay of treatment until the 1950s was long-term institutional care where patients were 'protected' from the social consequences of their illness. Since this time, overcrowding and other unfortunate aspects of institutional care, economic considerations and the development of neuroleptic medication has led to the rundown of large psychiatric hospitals. However, this is not to say that smaller institutions 'in the community' will necessarily lead to the end of institutionalism.

Modern treatment is still dependent on the prescription of prophylactic neuroleptic medication, which has a number of severe side-effects to which the elderly are especially prone. Recent developments in the psychological management of schizophrenia, such as the application of family interventions aimed at reducing expressed emotion and individual cognitive behavioural techniques, show promise in supporting the positive impact of medication. In addition, traditional behavioural approaches such as the use of token economies and social skills training are important in maximising patients' social functioning, especially where some form of residential care is required. However, the use of these approaches requires a high degree of training and at present there is a lack of the relevant skills amongst the professions involved in the care of the elderly patient who suffers from schizophrenia. The development of training programmes is essential if this situation is to be remedied.

Given that the needs of the elderly chronically mentally ill are diverse in the domains of residential care, finance, symptomatology, physical health, etc., there needs to be a coherent system for assessing these and providing appropriate interventions. Therefore, effective management will be important in the provision of optimal services for the elderly with schizophrenia.

REFERENCES

Abbati J, Oles G 1993 Continuity of care in serious mental illness. Psychiatric Bulletin 17: 140–141

Abrahamson D 1993 Institutionalisation and the long-term course of schizophrenia. British Journal of Psychiatry 162: 533–538

Almeida O P, Howard R, Forstl H et al 1992 Should the diagnosis of late paraphrenia be abandoned? Psychological Medicine 22: 11–14

American Psychiatric Association 1980 Diagnostic and statistical manual of mental disorders, 3rd edn. (DSM III). American Psychiatric Association, Washington DC

American Psychiatric Association 1987 Diagnostic and statistical manual of mental disorders, 3rd edn. revised. American Psychiatric Association, Washington DC

Anthony W A, Liberman R P 1986 The practice of psychiatric rehabilitation: historical and conceptual research base. Schizophrenia Bulletin 12: 542–559

Archer J, Hay D C, Young A W 1992 Face processing in psychiatric conditions. British Journal of Clinical Psychology 31: 45–61

Arie T, Jolley D T 1982 Making services work: organization and style of psychogeriatric services. In: Levy R, Post F (eds) The psychiatry of late life. Blackwell, Oxford

Barrowclough C, Tarrier N 1992 Interventions with families. In: Birchwood M, Tarrier N (eds) Innovations in the psychological management of schizophrenia: assessment, treatment and services. Wiley, Chichester

Barrowclough C, Tarrier N 1990 Social functioning in schizophrenic patients 1: the effects of expressed emotion and family intervention. Social Psychiatry and Psychiatric Epidemiology 25: 125–129

Barton W R 1959 Institutional neurosis. Wright, Bristol

Bellack A S, Mueser K T 1993 Psychosocial treatment for schizophrenia. Schizophrenia Bulletin 19: 317–336

Bentall R P 1990a The syndromes and symptoms of psychosis: or why you can't play twenty questions with the concept of schizophrenia and hope to win. In Bentall R P (ed) Reconstructing schizophrenia. Routledge, London

Bentall R P 1990b The illusion of reality: a review and integration of psychological research on hallucinations. Psychological Bulletin 107: 82–95

Bentall R P, Kaney S, Dewey M E 1991 Paranoia and social reasoning: an attribution theory analysis. British Journal of Clinical Psychology 30: 13–23

Bentall R P, Haddock G, Slade P D 1994 Psychological treatment for auditory hallucinations: from theory to therapy. Behaviour Therapy 25: 51–66

Birchwood M, Cochran R, MacMillan F, Copestake S, Kucharska J, Cariss M 1992a The influence of ethnicity and family structure on relapse in first episode schizophrenia: a comparison of Asian, Afro-Caribbean and white patients. British Journal of Psychiatry 161: 783–790

Birchwood M, Macmillan F, Smith J 1992b Early intervention. In: Birchwood M, Tarrier N (eds) Innovations in the psychological management of schizophrenia: assessment, treatment and services. Wiley, Chichester

Bleuler E 1911 Dementia praecox or the group of schizophrenia. English translation by J Zinkin 1950. International Universities Press, New York

Brenner H D, Hodel B, Volker R, Corrigan P 1992 Treatment of cognitive dysfunctions and behavioural deficits in schizophrenia. Schizophrenia Bulletin 18: 21–26

Bristow M F, Hirsch S F 1993 Pitfalls and problems of the long-term use of neuroleptic drugs in schizophrenia. Drug Safety: 136–148

Burns B J, Larson D B, Goldstrom I D et al 1988 Mental disorder among nursing home patients: preliminary findings from the national nursing home survey pretest. International Journal of Geriatric Psychiatry 3: 27–35

Burns A, Jacoby R, Levy R 1990 Psychiatric phenomena in Alzheimer's disease. British Journal of Psychiatry 157: 72–76

Campbell P G 1992 Graduates. In: Jacoby R, Oppenheimer C (eds) Psychiatry in the elderly. Oxford University Press, Oxford

Cardin V A, McGill C W, Falloon I R H 1986 An economic analysis: costs, benefits and effectiveness. In: Falloon I R H (ed) Family management of schizophrenia. John Hopkins University Press, Baltimore

Challis D, Davis B 1986 Case management in community care. Gower, Aldershot

Charlesworth G M, Hymas N, Wischik C M, Hodges J R, Sahakian B J 1993 Late paraphrenia, advanced schizophrenic deterioration and dementia. International Journal of Geriatric Psychiatry 8: 765–773

Ciompi L 1986 Review of follow-up studies on long-term evolution and aging in schizophrenia. In: Miller N E, Cohen G D (eds) Schizophrenia and aging. Guildford Press, New York

Clements K, Turpin G 1992 Vulnerability models and schizophrenia: the assessment and prediction of relapse. In: Birchwood M, Tarrier N (eds) Innovations in the psychological management of schizophrenia: assessment, treatment and services. John Wiley, Chichester

Cooper J E, Kendell R E, Gurland B J et al 1972 Psychiatric diagnosis in New York and London. Maudsley Monograph no 20. Oxford University Press, London

Corrigan P W 1991 Strategies that overcome barriers to token economies in community programs for severe mentally ill adults. Community Mental Health Journal 27: 17–30

Cramer P, Weegmann M, O'Neil M 1989 Schizophrenia and the perception of emotions: how accurately do schizophrenics judge the emotional states of others? British Journal of Psychiatry 155: 225–228

Curson D A, Pantelis C, Ward J, Barnes T R E 1992 Institutionalism and schizophrenia 30 years on. British Journal of Psychiatry 160: 230–241

Cutting J 1986 Outcome of schizophrenia: overview. In: Kerr A, Snaith R P (eds) Contemporary issues in schizophrenia. Royal College of Psychiatrists, London

David A S 1994 The neuropsychological origin of auditory hallucinations. In: David A S, Cutting J C (eds) The neuropsychology of schizophrenia. Lawrence Erlbaum, Hove

Davis J M, Andriukaitis S 1986 The natural course of schizophrenia and effective drug treatment. Journal of Clinical Psychopharmacology 6(supplement): 2s–10s

Department of Health 1987 Promoting better health. HMSO, London

Department of Health 1989a Working for patients: CM 555 working paper 6 medical audit. HMSO, London

Department of Health 1989b Caring for people. HMSO, London

Department of Health and Social Security 1986 Statistics of mental illness and mental handicap in England (various years and subsequent booklet series). DHSS, London

Dunkley G, Rogers D 1994 The cognitive impairment of severe psychiatric illness: a clinical study. In David A S, Cutting J C (eds) The neuropsychology of schizophrenia. Lawrence Erlbaum, Hove

Erickson R C 1988 Neuropsychological assessment and the rehabilitation of persons with severe psychiatric disabilities. Rehabilitation Psychology 33: 15–25

Falloon I R H, Boyd J L, McGill C W et al 1985 Family management in the prevention of morbidity in schizophrenia: clinical outcome of a two year longitudinal study. Archives of General Psychiatry 42: 887–896

Fischer P J, Breakley W E 1986 Homelessness and mental health: an overview. International Journal of Mental Health 14: 6–41

Ford M, Goddard C, Lansdale-Welfare R 1987 The dismantling of the mental hospital? Glenside Hospital Surveys 1960–1985. British Journal of Psychiatry 151: 479–485

Frith C D 1992 The cognitive neuropsychology of schizophrenia. Lawrence Erlbaum, Hove

Frith C 1994 Theory of mind in schizophrenia. In: David A S, Cutting J C (eds) The neuropsychology of schizophrenia. Lawrence Erlbaum, Hove

Garety P A, Hemsley D R 1987 Characteristics of delusional experience. European Archives of Psychiatry and Neurological Science 236: 294–298

General Register Office 1964 The registrar general's statistical review of England and Wales for the year 1960. Supplement on Mental Health. HMSO, London

Gierl B, Dysken M, Davis J M, Lesser J M 1986 Neuroleptic use in the elderly. In: Miller N E, Cohen G D (eds) Schizophrenia and aging: schizophrenia, paranoia, and schizophreniform disorders in late life. Guilford, New York

Goffman E 1961 Asylums: essays on the social situation of mental patients and other inmates. Penguin, London

Green M F 1993 Cognitive remediation in schizophrenia: is it time yet? American Journal of Psychiatry 150: 178–187

Greenblatt M, Levinson D, Williams R 1957 The patient and the mental hospital. Free Press, Illinois

Gunderson J G, Frank A F, Katz H M, Vannicelli M L, Frosch J P, Knapp P H 1984 Effects of psychotherapy of schizophrenia, II: comparative outcome of two forms of treatment. Schizophrenia Bulletin 10: 564–598

Haddock G, Sellwood W, Tarrier N, Yusupoff L 1994 Developments in cognitive behaviour therapy for persistent psychotic symptoms. Behaviour Change 4: 200–212

Haddock G, Bentall R P, Slade P D 1995 Focusing versus distraction in the psychological treatment of auditory hallucinations. In: Haddock G, Slade P D (eds) Cognitive-behavioural interventions with psychotic disorders. Routledge, London

Halford W K, Hayes R 1991 Psychological rehabilitation of chronic schizophrenic patients: recent findings on social skills training and family psychoeducation. Clinical Psychology Review 11: 23–44

Hall J 1983 Ward based rehabilitation programmes. In: Watts F N, Bennett D H (eds) Theory and practice of psychiatric rehabilitation. John Wiley, Chichester

Hall J N, Baker R D 1986 Token economies in schizophrenia; a review. In: Kerr A, Snaith R P (eds) Contemporary issues in schizophrenia. Gaskell, London

Hassett A M, Keks N A, Jackson H J, Copolov D 1992 The diagnostic validity of paraphrenia. Australian and New Zealand Journal of Psychiatry 26: 18–29

Hawks D 1975 Community care: an analysis of assumptions. British Journal of Psychiatry 127: 276–285

Herbert M E, Jackson S 1967 Late paraphrenia. British Journal of Psychiatry 113: 461–469

Hirsch S R, Jolley A G 1989 The dysphoric syndrome in schizophrenia and its implications for relapse. British Journal of Psychiatry (Supplement) 5: 123–127

Hoffman R E 1986 Verbal hallucinations and language production processes in schizophrenia. Behavioural and Brain Sciences 9: 503–548

Holden N L 1987 Late paraphrenia or the paraphrenias? A descriptive study with a 10-year follow-up. British Journal of Psychiatry 150: 635–639

Howard R, Levy R 1992 Which factors affect treatment response in late paraphrenia. International Journal of Geriatric Psychiatry 7: 667–672

Howard R, Almeida O, Levy R 1993 Schizophrenic symptoms in late paraphrenia. Psychopathology 26: 95–101

Howe G 1991 The reality of schizophrenia. Faber and Faber, London

Jeste D V, Wyatt R J 1986 Aging and tardive dyskinesia. In: Miller N E, Cohen G D (eds) Schizophrenia and aging: schizophrenia, paranoia, and schizophreniform disorders in later life. Guilford, New York

Johnson D A W, Freeman H 1973 Drug defaulting by patients on long-acting phenothiazines. Psychological Medicine 3: 115–119

Johnstone E C, Owens D G C, Frith C D, Calvert L M 1985 Institutionalisation and the outcome of functional psychoses. British Journal of Psychiatry 146: 36–44

Jorm A F, Korten A E, Henderson A S 1987 The prevalence of dementia: a quantitative integration of the literature. Acta Psychiatrica Scandinavica 76: 465–479

Kaney S, Bentall R P 1989 Persecutory delusions and attributional style. British Journal of Medical Psychology 62: 191–198

Kay D, Roth M 1961 Environmental and hereditory factors in the schizophrenias of old age ('late paraphrenia') and their bearing on the general problem of causation in schizophrenia. Journal of Mental Science 107: 649–686

Kendell R E 1988 Schizophrenia. In: Kendell R E, Zealley A K (eds) Companion to postgraduate psychiatric studies, 4th edn. Churchill Livingstone, Edinburgh

Kingdon D G, Turkington D 1994 Cognitive-behavioural therapy of schizophrenia. Lawrence Erlbaum, Hove

Kottgen C, Soinichsen I, Mollenhauer K, Jurth R 1984 Results of the Hamburg Camberwell Family Interview Study: I–III. International Journal of Family Psychiatry 5: 61–94

Kring A M, Kerr S L, Smith D A, Neale J M 1993 Flat affect in schizophrenia does not reflect diminished subjective experience of emotion. Journal of Abnormal Psychology 102: 507–517

Levene L S, Donaldson L J, Brandon S 1985 How likely is it a district health authority can close its large mental hospitals? British Journal of Psychiatry 147: 150–155

Liddle P F 1987 The symptoms of chronic schizophrenia: a re-examination of the positive–negative dichotomy. British Journal of Psychiatry 151: 145–151

Lindström L H 1994 Long-term clinical and social outcome studies in schizophrenia in relation to the cognitive and emotional side-effects of antipsychotic drugs. Acta Psychiatrica Scandinavica 89(supplement 380): 74–76

McCreadie R G, Robinson A D T, Wilson A O A 1985 The Scottish survey of new chronic in-patients: two year follow up. British Journal of Psychiatry 147: 637–640

McKenna P J, Tamlyn D, Lund C E, Mortimer A M, Hammond S, Baddeley A D 1990 Amnesic syndrome in schizophrenia. Psychological Medicine 20: 976–972

Mahr B A 1974 Delusional thinking and perceptual disorder. Journal of Individual Psychology 30: 98–113

Mann S, Cree W 1976 'New' long-stay psychiatric patients: a national survey of fifteen mental hospitals in England and Wales 1972/3. Psychological Medicine 6: 603–616

Morris R K, Bowie P C W, Spencer P W 1988 The mortality of long-stay patients following inter-hospital relocation. British Journal of Psychiatry 152: 705–706

Murphy E 1992 Setting priorities during the development of local psychiatric services. In: Thornicroft G, Brewin C, Wing J (eds) Measuring mental health needs. Royal College of Psychiatrists, London

Naguib M, Levy R 1992 Paranoid states in the elderly and late paraphrenia. In: Jacoby R, Oppenheimer C (eds) Psychiatry in the Elderly. Oxford University Press, Oxford

Nelson H E, Pantelis C, Carruthers K, Speller J, Baxendale S, Barnes T R E 1990 Cognitive functioning and symptomatology in chronic schizophrenia. Psychological Medicine 20: 357–365

Onyett S 1992 Case management. Chapman and Hall, London

Pantelis C, Nelson H E 1994 Cognitive functioning and symptomatology in schizophrenia: the role of frontal-subcortical systems. In: David A S, Cutting J C (eds) The neuropsychology of schizophrenia. Lawrence Erlbaum, Hove

Paul G L, Lentz R J 1977 Psychosocial treatment of chronic mental patients. Harvard University Press, Cambridge, Massachusetts

Patmore C, Weaver J 1990 A survey of community mental health centres. Good Practices in Mental Health, London

Pearlson G D, Kreger L, Rabins P V et al 1989 A chart review study of late-onset and early-onset schizophrenia. American Journal of Psychiatry 146: 1568–1574

Perkins R E, King S A, Hollyman J A 1989 Resettlement of old long stay psychiatric patients: the use of the private sector. British Journal of Psychiatry 155: 233–238

Quintal M, Day-Cody D, Levy R 1991 Late paraphrenia and ICD-10. International Journal of Geriatric Psychiatry 6: 111–116

Salit S A, Marcos L R 1991 Have general hospitals become chronic care institutions for the terminally ill? American Journal of Psychiatry 148: 892–897

Schneider K 1959 (English translation by Hamilton M W) Klinisch psychpathologie. Grune and Stratton, New York

Schwartz J T, Brotman A W 1992 A clinical guide to antipsychotic drugs. Drugs 44: 981–982

Shepherd M, Watt D, Falloon I, Smeeton N 1987 The natural history of schizophrenia: a five year follow up study of outcome and prediction in a representative sample of schizophrenics. Psychological Medicine Monograph Supplement 15

Slade P D, Bentall R P 1988 Sensory deception: a scientific analysis of hallucinations. Croom Helm, London

Smith J V, Birchwood M J 1987 Specific and non-specific effects of educational intervention with families living with a schizophrenic relative. British Journal of Psychiatry 150: 645–652

Tarrier N, Barrowclough C, Vaughn C E et al 1988 The community management of schizophrenia: a controlled trial of a behavioural intervention with families. British Journal of Psychiatry 153: 532–542

Tarrier N, Lowsen K, Barrowclough C 1991 Some aspects of family interventions in schizophrenia, II: financial considerations. British Journal of Psychiatry 159: 481–484

Tarrier N, Beckett R, Harwood S, Baker A, Yusupoff L, Ugarteburu I 1993 A trial of two cognitive-behavioural methods of treating drug resistant residual psychotic symptoms in schizophrenic patients, I: outcome. British Journal of Psychiatry 162: 524–532

Tarrier N, Barrowclough C, Porceddu K, Fitzpatrick E 1994 The Salford family intervention project for schizophrenic relapse prevention: five and eight year accumulating relapses. British Journal of Psychiatry 165: 829–832

Tobin S 1989 The effects of institutionalization. In: Markides K S, Cooper CL (eds) Aging, stress and health. John Wiley, Chichester

Tran-Johnson T K, Krull A J, Jeste D V 1992 Late life schizophrenia and its treatment: pharmacologic issues in older schizophrenic patients. Clinics in Geriatric Medicine 8: 401–410

Vaughan K, Doyle M, McConaghy N, Blaszczynski A, Fox A, Tarrier N 1992 The Sydney intervention trial: a controlled trial of relatives' counselling to reduce schizophrenic relapse. Social Psychiatry and Psychiatric Epidemiology 26: 16–21

Vaughn C E, Leff J P 1976 The influence of family and social factors on the course of psychiatric illness: a comparison of schizophrenic and depressed neurotic patients. British Journal of Psychiatry 129: 125–137

Vaughn C, Leff J 1985 Expressed emotion in families: its significance for mental illness. Guilford, New York

Walker J, Wynne H 1994 Review: the frequency and severity of adverse drug reactions in elderly people. Age and Ageing 23: 255–259

Warner R 1994 Recovery from schizophrenia. Routledge, London

Willcocks D, Peace S, Kellaher L 1986 Private lives in public places. Tavistock, London

Wing J K 1992 Comment on institutionalism and schizophrenia 30 years on. British Journal of Psychiatry 160: 241–243

Wing J K, Brown G W 1970 Institutionalism and schizophrenia. Cambridge University Press, London

Wixted J T, Morrison R L, Bellack A S 1988 Social skills training in the treatment of negative symptoms. International Journal of Mental Health 17: 3–21

Woof K, Goldberg D, Fryers T 1988 The practice of community psychiatric nursing and mental health social work in Salford: some implications for community care. British Journal of Psychiatry 152: 783–792

Woods R T, Britton P G 1985 Intervention in institutions. In: Woods R T, Britton P G (eds) Clinical psychology with the elderly. Croom Helm, Kent

World Health Organization 1973 Report of the international pilot study of schizophrenia. WHO, Geneva

World Health Organization 1979 Schizophrenia: an international follow-up study. John Wiley, Chichester

World Health Organization 1992 The ICD-10 classification of mental and behavioural disorders. WHO, Geneva

Wykes T 1994 Predicting symptomatic and behavioural outcomes of community care. British Journal of Psychiatry 165: 486–492

Wykes T, Dunn G 1992 Cognitive deficit and the prediction of rehabilitation success in a chronic psychiatric group. Psychological Medicine 22: 389–398

Young J L, Zonana H V, Shepler L 1986 Medication noncompliance in schizophrenia codification and update. Bulletin of American Academic Psychiatry and Law 14: 105–122

Zubin J, Spring B 1977 Vulnerability: a new view of schizophrenia. Journal of Abnormal Psychology 86: 260–266

RECOMMENDED READING

Birchwood M, Tarrier N (eds) 1992 Innovations in the psychological management of schizophrenia: assessment, treatment and services. John Wiley, Chichester. *This book reviews recent developments in psychological aspects of schizophrenia, including assessment, treatment and service development. It is an important introductory overview and is essential reading for those new to the area.*

Kavanagh D (ed) 1992 Schizophrenia: an overview and practical handbook. Chapman and Hall, London. *Kavanagh has drawn authors from a wide range of disciplines in compiling this book. Consulting it is a valuable first step in finding out about some particular aspect of schizophrenia, be it concerned with neuroanatomy, or psychological and social factors.*

Miller N E, Cohen G D (eds) 1986 Schizophrenia and aging. Guildford Press, New York. *The editors summarise the nature course and treatment of schizophrenia and related disorders in the elderly. This is the only book to do this and, in spite of the largely US orientation, it provides an important reference source for those working with this patient group.*

Warner R 1994 Recovery from schizophrenia. Routledge, London. *This book questions prevalent assumptions concerning the nature and management of schizophrenia. It is an invaluable source of information concerning social and historical aspects of the illness and places modern treatment in context.*

14

Struggling with services

David Brandon
Ray Jack

This chapter begins with a case history which is a true story of the difficulties David Brandon and his family faced when his father-in-law became ill (Box 14.1). The remainder of the chapter draws on these experiences.

THE 'BURDEN' OF CARING

The study and description of the experience of informal care has suffered from two preoccupations – listing the effects of the disabilities and needs of the 'cared for' upon the carer, and comparing the relative impact of the different levels of service provision upon carer wellbeing. The first has resulted in a simplistic view of the informal caring relationship as unreciprocal, with only needs coming from one party, identified as the dependant, and care coming from the other – the carer. Thus a very negative depiction of the informal caring relationship has emerged, portraying it as unrewarding and almost inevitably damaging for the carer. Rarely is there any recognition of reciprocity within such relationships or the potential for mutual satisfaction within them; they are, in fact, implicitly regarded as non relationships. As a result, multiply-disadvantaged disabled people are unblushingly referred to as 'burdens' by commentators who in other contexts would claim to be champions of all that is anti-discriminatory in theory and practice. There is an urgent need for new perspectives on these relationships, a need recognised in a recent study of informal caring relationships which asserts that: ' ... one needs to look behind the facade of the voluminous and often repetitive literature on carers, and to see both the diversity of individual caring situations and the broad patterns into which they fall. This often reveals a picture of interdependence rather than the simple carer/dependant model which underlies so much of the thinking in this area' (Gordon and Easton 1992–1993, p. 16).

Box 14.1 Caring for Leslie Donald Mason

My marriage to Althea,* in 1963, brought me a father-in-law – Leslie Donald Mason.* In his youth he had been a considerable chess player – East End of London champion – and linguist. He had worked as an office manager for a London yeast firm for more than 40 years, except for a 5-year break as an inefficient signaller against the Germans during the Second World War. Now his red hair had turned to thinning white on top of his stooped figure. Nervously restless and a heavy smoker, he was rapidly ageing. Although our relationship was not at all easy, he was very generous to his new young son-in-law. For example, he and his wife had paid for our first flat to be built on the top of their bungalow in Buckinghamshire and they later provided us with some money towards a mortgage.

He came home late from his Liverpool Street office each evening, to the house in rural Buckinghamshire which we all shared. By then he was exhausted and overly content with alcohol and mostly dozed in front of the TV with his dinner half finished on a wooden tray. Each morning, on the 8.10 train from Staines to Waterloo, he cascaded inconsequential casual conversation whilst I tried quietly to read the *Manchester Guardian*. He was very difficult to follow. His topics jumped all over the place – from domestic life to sport to current affairs and back again – all washed down with his quick dry wit. I got cross regularly but, uncharacteristically, held my tongue.

In pursuit of my career, our new family (Stewart* had arrived and Toby* would follow not so long after) split from our in-laws and moved, first southwards to Shoreham-by-Sea on the English Channel and then northwards, to Hatfield and to Preston in Lancashire. The in-laws followed us as far as Shoreham and my wonderfully loving mother-in-law died painfully not long after. So the two men – father-in-law and grandfather-in-law (mother-in-law's father) – shared a house, not terribly comfortably, until grandfather went into an old people's home and died soon afterwards.

Leslie got much worse in his early seventies. He had retired early from his job and so given up the commuting which had provided a disciplined framework for the weekdays. He watched TV, smoked incessantly and went out to the pub. His memory deteriorated. He was less able to look after himself and unsuited to living alone. Neighbours had given a lot of support and felt overwhelmed. There was a crisis. It was decided that he should move the 250 miles northwards to Preston – to him an alien land – and share the family home with our two young children, then about 6 and 9 years old. It was a prospect I dreaded.

That was a very difficult experience for all of us for several years. He was extremely forgetful and untidy. It is hard for non-smokers to accept floors covered with ash. Looking after grandpa and the two young children split us in various ways. It was often like having an elderly cuckoo in the nest. Over time, he got even worse and required much greater attention. It was difficult to banish the smell of stale urine from the house. We rarely went out. We almost never invited people to our home. We

became very stressed and our own relationships were extremely strained. We felt isolated.

Eventually, in an attempt at some relief, we moved him into a separate small flat about a half mile away, close to the main road. Surprisingly, he managed reasonably well for nearly a year and the new arrangement gave us all much more space. Althea visited him, usually several times a day, to provide cooked meals, to do the laundry and the thousand practical things like changing light bulbs.

By that time he had developed cataracts in both eyes and had only blurred vision. An operation was arranged in the nearby Preston Royal Infirmary. He was supposed to be in for a few days but things got really bad. He became restless and confused. They transferred him to the geriatric ward where he received the general label of arteriosclerosis. After a few weeks, with the great pressure on beds, he was sent to a nearby convalescent home, really a glorified short-stay facility for elderly people.

When eventually he returned to his flat we faced an immediate crisis. Now he just couldn't manage on his own at all. The situation had worsened considerably. He just wandered around restlessly, not knowing where or even who he was. He lived mostly in previous decades. He related to people and situations that had long since vanished. Sometimes he was doubly incontinent. He could no longer even make a cup of tea.

One morning he had urinated in the lounge and there were stinking faeces all over the hall. I was filled with rage. I stood in front of him and wanted to knock him to the floor with my fist and kick his stupid smiling face in. I wanted to see him disintegrate into ten thousand pieces. I wanted to kill him. I was so completely terrified by the immensity of the emotions inside me. I sat down feeling very sick. I had never felt anything like the power of those huge feelings. I didn't feel I had any right to feel this overwhelming hatred which seemed much bigger and stronger than me.

We were both rapidly losing our dignity and control. We had to call in help. We faced the usual forked and mystifying labyrinth of health and social services. The community psychiatric nurses came and changed light bulbs and made delicious corned beef sandwiches. They seemed to work in partnership, to have joined a sparse team of people supporting a confused and often unhappy old man. They were also supporting us. When the social workers came they were different. They looked at us and examined from a distance. They were like inspectors. They had sheaves of forms and briefcases and were constantly asking questions and filling those forms in. They were minor bureaucrats working for the social services department. They definitely didn't change light bulbs. Mostly they told us what we couldn't have. We couldn't have meals-on-wheels to ease the situation at lunch times – we lived in the wrong area. If only we had lived 2 miles further south. We couldn't have a home help to assist in keeping the flat clean, in keeping an eye on him, in getting the shopping in – here, too, it would have helped everyone if we had lived somewhere else.

Box 14.1   *Cont'd*

We kept ringing up the area social services office to stress the crisis situation and they arrived – usually in couples, but once in a trio – to visit. They were usually 'assessing'. They asked lots of questions, filled in many forms and said 'No' to a lot of requests. They shook their heads gravely many times and said a great deal about the limits of the existing legislation and did nothing. They always said they would contact us again and never did until we ourselves rang the office. Once one social worker recommended we wrote to our MP about the dire situation. It added insult to injury.

I recall vividly one interview where I had to stand in for Althea. I was working at that time as the director of North West MIND, so the issues for confused elderly mentally ill people were very close to my professional as well as my personal interests, although I was rarely able to square them. This youngish, rather officious social worker called at the house. He carried a briefcase full of forms and talked initially of assessment and of the Department's problems. He talked to me at great length.

He spoke of the practical difficulties. Was father-in-law a health or social service responsibility? There seemed to be a substantial battle going on behind the scenes. We talked very practically and politically for something like 15 minutes – about commodes, wheelchairs, lack of home help services, possible admission to old people's homes ... Then I realised that the conversation had turned into counselling. I was being counselled by this professional for whom I had very little respect. I was being given advice on 'better' ways to live my life.

It was a sort of subtle blackmail, sometimes not so subtle. In my role of caring relative, I did not really exist in my own right. I wasn't the client. The single client was and had to be Grandpa, who wasn't a person any more but a series of conditions and syndromes. Both Althea and I were simply adjuncts to him; a means of supporting his infirmity. Althea and I were unpaid members of a professional team which included him and the community psychiatric nurses. Without our agreement or any discussion, we had become 'carers'. No one at all tended to our grief and distress because we weren't clients. We were invisible. We would have to break down psychiatrically and become clients in our own right, to be seen and heard. There was some possibility of real support and help but in order to receive it we had to be seen as cooperative, open and compliant. I had to share fully my wounds and vulnerabilities to compete effectively with many unseen others in the lottery for help.

The third stage in this assessment interview was when the counselling turned into basic homespun philosophy. This pompous young professional ended our interview with a few words about his own devout Roman Catholic faith, which apparently sustained him through the stresses of situations like ours and a lot more. Attending Sunday mass was an enriching experience – he wanted to recommend it. I was really furious but also really guarded and restricted myself to toothy smiles. In a way I was being abused.

Later, this experience spurred me to Old Testament-style vengeance. I rang the area social services officer, whom I knew, and threatened retribution. 'We need some action, not visits', I said, with such great emphasis it hardly needed the phone. He didn't help much at all. We got a scruffy list of rest homes on a single sheet of paper in the post. We began a long round of residential enquiries. We located a seemingly suitable home in Southport. Quickly it proved very unsuitable. Within hours they were asking for his removal. He was too infirm, too disturbed, too restless; he required skills and support that they did not possess. He cost too much; they wanted passive elderly people who could be quietly neglected, not difficult, confused and disturbed old men who demanded expensive attention.

After several false starts, he ended up in the dreadful back ward of a local psychiatric hospital – in the infamous Whittingham, one of the scandal-beset mental hospitals of the early '70s. The standard of facilities was very low and the support patchy and ill-focused. But it was either his admission or ours. We had reached the very end of the line after a long 4 years. We visited dutifully each weekend. Some staff were welcoming and others openly hostile. Carefully, I had made some comment about the radio being very loud so we couldn't converse with the confused old man. The charge nurse responded with a grim smile, all teeth: 'You can always take him home – can't you?'

Now we were abject beggars asking for favours. They had all the power. They owned him. We were never asked about any of his likes or dislikes, anything of his personal character or history. They knew absolutely nothing about him and didn't feel any lack of knowledge. By letting him go we had lost every right. We couldn't get any help so long as he remained in the community, not even meals-on-wheels. When we abandoned him to the total institution, we lost every right to be his closest relatives. He lost his rights of citizenship in becoming a long-stay patient.

That didn't change at all when he went into the Elderly Severely Mentally Ill unit (ESMI), presumably the brain child of some deranged mandarin in the deep Whitehall south. The ESMI unit cost mega bucks and was space age, with staff battle stations covered by electronic switches: it seemed it would take off to Mars at any moment. There was a day service on the ground floor and residential facilities on the first and second floors. Excellent views of the next door cemetery were to be had from every window. It would have been very simple to lift the coffins directly over the stone walls.

It was a sanitised Hell – completely plastic and undomestic in every detail. It had few human comforts. The staff wore crisp nurse-style uniforms although most were unqualified and untrained. Only the senior staff were qualified nurses. Again we were beggars at the gate, had no real status and the information systems were rudimentary. We visited each Sunday and departed as soon as we decently could. It was hard not to be stifled in such an atmosphere.

He lived a sort of quarter-life for several years. He gradually became more and more incoherent with only very brief flashes of his old cockney wit and awareness that were soon overwhelmed once more by the darkness

Box 14.1   *Cont'd*

of confusion. He died amongst strangers although mercifully, at the last, his lovely daughter Althea was with him, far from anything he or we might call home. For us and his grandchildren, he had really died some years before.

The ESMI unit forced us to be strangers to him. We had no status as close relatives and were rarely consulted or involved in any way. The staff, especially those who were senior, took him over; owned the whole of his being. On one level that was a great relief after our years of

suffering; on another, deeper level it was a tragedy for us. Slowly we learned to carry the massive guilt of our effective abandonment of him.

I had met a man with whom I ordinarily wouldn't have spent 5 minutes in conversation and gained some sort of mysterious commitment to him through marriage – a commitment I never properly understood and failed to honour. For me, it was and continues to feel a massive personal failure. It is hard to imagine a way to let down another human being more comprehensively.

* His/her real name – used with permission.

The second preoccupation has been with the effects of the provision of services on the wellbeing of carers. Considerable evidence has emerged of physical and psychological ill health among carers. Despite the fact that most carers are in older age groups where the prevalence of ill health is higher, the assumption is that such ill health is the direct result of the demands of dependants, of the 'burden' of caring. There is often an implicit assumption that the provision of services will mitigate this burden, leading to improvement in the wellbeing of carers. This preoccupation with describing and comparing the provision of services has led to a neglect of the relationship between informal and formal carers. The nature of the professional relationship itself and its effects on carers has been as neglected as that between informal carers and their dependants. It is rarely considered that the form of professional relationship currently offered may contribute to the alleged effects of the so-called 'burden' of caring. The professional relationship may be part of the problem rather than its solution.

In this chapter we attempt to avoid these dual pitfalls. By exploring David's own experience of being a carer, we try to bring together any insights into the nature and effects of the relationship between 'carer' and 'cared for' and the effects on this of the relationship between informal and formal carers, the so-called 'professional relationship'. The focus is social care because that is our professional experience and social care agencies are the lead agencies in community care.

THE 'PROFESSIONAL RELATIONSHIP'

The account David gives of the distressing and ultimately very damaging experience of the declining years of his father-in-law is full of examples of what

innumerable research studies into informal care have found – social isolation of carers, strained marital relationships, guilt and depression about not caring 'enough' or needing to care 'less' or in a different way, and often a dramatic loss of self-esteem (for comprehensive reviews of this literature see Twigg et al 1990, Parker 1990, Unell 1993). Usually it is taken for granted that these carer experiences originate from the disabilities of dependants and the struggle carers have to meet their needs. However, the title David has chosen for our chapter, 'Struggling with Services', suggests another source of anguish and enduring distress found among carers; the failure of professionals adequately to tend the relationship between informal carers and those for whom they care.

Seldom are any benefits of caring recognised, so that the burdensome nature of the task is taken for granted; the potential for growth and development within such relationships is denied and, along with it, the wholeness of not only cared for but carer. The person labelled dependant is reduced to a list of 'needs'; the carer is all too often ignored completely or, alternatively, their vital human investment in the caring relationship is overlooked in the rush to relieve the 'burden' of caring. There are two examples of this neglect and its effects on the wellbeing of carers in David's account.

When describing the social workers' approach to his request for assistance with caring for his dementing father-in-law Leslie, David tells us: 'In my role of caring relative, I did not really exist in my own right. I wasn't the client. The single client was and had to be Grandpa, who wasn't a person any more but a series of conditions and syndromes. Both Althea and I were simply adjuncts to him; a means of supporting his infirmity ... Without our agreement or any discussion we had become "carers". No one at all tended to our grief and distress because we weren't clients. We were invisible'.

The failure to recognise the importance of the caring relationship in the lives of David and his wife, its existence as something more than just a burden, directly leads to its colonisation by 'professionals'; its enforced severance by the later rush to 'service provision', and then to the consequent sense of abandonment and guilt which the carers were left to endure alone. Were the carers any less abandoned than they feared Leslie had become? Further on in David's account of the eventual institutionalisation of his father-in-law this exclusion and abandonment of the carers is painfully evident:

The staff, especially those who were senior, took him over; owned the whole of his being. On one level that was a great relief after our years of suffering; on another, deeper level it was a tragedy for us. Slowly we learned to carry the massive guilt of our effective abandonment of him ... For me, it was and continues to feel a massive personal failure. It is hard to imagine a way to let down another human being more comprehensively.

The interpretation of professionalism by formal carers determines the nature of the relationships between them and informal carers. It is rarely considered that this interpretation and the relationships which it promotes can damage the carer. Due to shifts in government policy, community care services for older adults are increasingly provided by social care professionals. Dementia sufferers who would have previously been cared for by the health service are now the responsibility of social care agencies. Social care professionals – particularly social workers – are still trained to view their primary role as therapeutic. This may not be the avowed objective of courses but the theories and methods which are taught emphasise human growth and development and the assessment and treatment of physical, psychological and relational disorder and the 'needs' which allegedly spring from them. In consequence, they underemphasise the recognition and promotion of health and coping as opposed to the assessment of disorder and dysfunction; the advocacy of rights as opposed to the assessment of needs; the provision of information and education instead of the search for 'insight', and the practice of partnership as opposed to the imposition of treatment.

THERAPEUTIC MYOPIA IN THE PROFESSIONAL RELATIONSHIP

One commentator (Scott 1970) on social work with disabled people suggests that the professional:

... has been specially trained to give professional help to impaired people. He can not use his expertise if those who are sent to him for assistance do not regard themselves as being impaired. Given this fact, it is not surprising that the doctrine has emerged among experts that truly affective rehabilitation and adjustment can occur only after the client has squarely faced and accepted the 'fact' that he is, indeed, 'impaired'. (Scott 1970, p. 280)

This imposition of a definition on service users as in some way inadequate is inherent in the therapeutic model of the professional relationship and is clearly described in David's account of how a discussion with a social worker about practical forms of assistance subtly turned into an unwanted counselling session:

It was a sort of subtle blackmail ... We would have to break down psychiatrically and become clients in our own right, to be seen and heard. There was some possibility of real support and help but in order to receive it we had to be seen as cooperative, open and compliant. I had to share fully my wounds and vulnerabilities to compete effectively with many unseen others in the lottery for help.

This therapeutic model of the professional relationship has shown remarkable persistence in social care in spite of consistent research evidence of consumer dissatisfaction with it (Mayer & Timms 1969, Mullender 1992–1993) and the existence of readily available alternative models. For example, the social pedagogy model adopted widely in European social work which emphasises education rather than therapy (Lorenz 1991), or the advocacy model developed in Britain over the past 2 or 3 decades within the learning difficulties and disability user movements (Oliver 1983). In addition, the relevance of the therapeutic model of social care has been convincingly challenged from sociology and political economy. In relation to elderly people, the political economy approach developed by Phillipson (1982), and Walker & Phillipson (1986) has shown that many of the so-called 'needs' and much of the dependency of old age are the result not of the ageing process but are socially constructed through the financial dependency imposed in the labour market during the years of paid employment, the benefits system throughout the life span and in old age through the effects of professional intervention. All promote dependency rather than alleviate it.

A similar critique was developed in relation to physical disability by commentators like Oliver and Finkelstein who described the disabling effects of social exclusion and financial disadvantage. This disabilist critique emphasises the social origins of disability in contrast to the conventional pathology model which focuses on the physical impairments of individuals. The individually oriented approach of conventional professional practice is identified as instrumental in promoting dependency rather than minimising it (Oliver 1983, Finkelstein 1993).

Despite these alternative models of practice and the convincing radical critiques which underpin them, the individually oriented pathology model and its associated therapeutic orientation to practice still dominate the interpretation of professional practice in social care. Within the therapeutic treatment oriented world view, professionalism is defined by the exclusive possession of expertise by the professional. This requires a client who, by definition, lacks expertise and needs help to overcome the problems – physical, psychological or relational – which stem from these shortcomings and lead to their failure to cope. Within this world view, simply going to an agency for services is seen as symptomatic of inadequate coping skills, and so begins the process of labelling and the paternalistic professionalism which is part of the social construction of dependency. Audrey Mullender (1992) asserts:

All too often disabled people find that going to an agency to seek essentially practical help makes them fair game to be turned into 'clients' by social workers, rather than simply being given the required assistance. The person who has gone along to enquire about housing, income or jobs, is made to feel that the social worker wants to dabble in his or her whole life, asking questions about feelings and relationships, even if the disabled person considers these wholly irrelevant to the barrier or obstacle to daily living which he or she is trying to overcome. Being labelled a 'client' can mean being expected to be a passive recipient of intrusive intervention and required to accept the 'expert's' definition of the problem.   (Mullender 1992, p. 10)

This therapeutic model of the professional relationship has damaging effects on both carers and those for whom they care. Many of the deleterious and long-term effects of struggling with services described by David can be directly attributed to this outmoded and largely indefensible form of professionalism. Despite the rhetoric of participation and partnership in vogue in the health and welfare professions currently, the conventional interpretation of professionalism survives and continues to bestow the expertise exclusively upon the professional. In this model, there are only two roles – client or professional – there is no role for anyone who is neither. Thus the carer is excluded from the 'professional relationship' between client and professional which can lead inexorably to the feelings of failure and guilt of imagined abandonment described by David. As he says, too often the only way to change this exclusive relationship is to become a patient yourself. This may be an attractive option to distressed and over-stressed carers but taking this route does nothing for the dependant

nor the relationship between carer and dependant. It simply reaffirms the preconceptions of the professional and further entrenches them in conventional therapeutically oriented approaches towards not only dependent people but also their carers.

The therapeutic model defines service users as dependent and imposes unwanted and inappropriate counselling services whilst denying the practical assistance which is urgently needed and to which, incidentally, there is often a legal right (RADAR 1993). It also denies services to those who are not defined as dependent, i.e. carers; as David says, the only way to get help as a carer was to become a client: 'No one at all tended to our grief and distress because we weren't clients. We were invisible. We would have to break down psychiatrically and become clients in our own right to be seen and heard'.

This passage opens up a new dimension on the research evidence on mental stress among carers and the inability of professional interventions to reduce it – the possibility that carer stress is actually increased by professional intervention. Perhaps this is another facet of the social construction of dependency depicted by Phillipson (1982, Walker & Phillipson 1986) as the result in many instances of those interventions.

THE IMPOSITION OF DEFINITIONS

The demand, inherent in the therapeutic model, that one party to the 'professional relationship' must be the dependent client is simplistic and damaging. Gordon & Easton (1992–1993), in their study of informal caring relationships, conclude:

Standard labels such as carer or dependant obscure the individuality of people and their relationships. An appreciation of this diversity offers one of the keys to understanding informal care. Good informal care is founded on a healthy relationship, often one developed over very many years, which takes for granted the individuality of the people involved. Good care – informal or formal – is centred on people and their interrelationships, their interdependencies. Poor care centres on their problems and the problems they create for others.
                    (Gordon & Easton 1992–1993, p. 24)

The study identified three patterns of caring:

- mutual/reciprocal
- distinct roles with no element of mutuality or reciprocity
- social services dependent.

None of these relationships conform to the assumptions inherent in the therapeutic model of the professional relationship in social care. For example, within the social services dependent group, the cared for people actually defined themselves as being independent because they were receiving paid care to which they were entitled and thus were not dependent on unpaid informal care on a grace-and-favour basis. Again, one of the carers had difficulty thinking of himself as a carer – he did not perceive caring for his mother as an obligation or burden. These people, involved often in mutually rewarding caring relationships, simply did not see themselves in the way they have been defined within the conventional interpretation of the professional relationship.

Further evidence of the imposition of inappropriate definitions on clients and carers comes from two recent studies of the views people with disabilities have of professionals in health and social services. Ellis's (1992) study of assessments of disabled people discovered that professionals often brought preconceptions to the assessment, including the perception of disability as a solely individual condition rather than a social construction, and an unshakeable conviction of the superior value of their professional judgements leading to a devaluation of those of clients and carers. Secondly, Morris (1993) found that inflexible statutory services based on preconceived ideas about the needs of clients actually created barriers to independence and that often disabled people preferred untrained, non-professional staff to qualified workers because they felt untrained workers had fewer preconceptions and were more able to give an individualised service .

Mullender (1992–1993), quoting a disabled person's views of professional help, proposes that a major shift of perspective is required more appropriately to meet people's needs. The service user felt that the failure of social workers to offer solutions to practical problems such as dressing, using the toilet and cooking was the problem and continued, 'what I need is someone who will help me to achieve these things ... allowing me to preserve my personal integrity at the same time' (Mullender 1992–1993, p. 9).

She concludes that such a shift is proving difficult for therapeutically oriented social care professionals to achieve. She asserts that:

It is important to note that social work help has traditionally not been offered on these terms and that this will require a significant shift of approach ... Assistance in the past has tended to come with an accompaniment of psychological assumptions focusing on adjustment to loss ... It regards the disabled person as lacking something basic which we have and they do not. It ignores the fact that, even without that function, they may still be a more whole or rounded person ... Hence the traditional social work emphasis on therapy for disabled people ... may often be entirely misplaced.
(Mullender 1992–1993, p. 9)

David illustrates this preoccupation with therapy and the imposition of inappropriate definitions and interventions when he describes how a discussion with a social worker about practical forms of assistance slipped into counselling: 'We talked very practically and politically for something like 15 minutes ... Then I realised that the conversation had turned into counselling. I was being counselled by this professional for whom I had very little respect. I was being given advice on 'better' ways to live my life'.

A PROFESSIONAL HIERARCHY OF SERVICES

Another adverse effect of the therapeutic model of the professional relationship in social care is that it has influenced attitudes to particular forms of service not only among formal carers but also among lay people, clients and informal carers. Consumer surveys repeatedly find that practical services such as home help and welfare rights advice are regarded by social workers as less complex and indeed less 'professional' than counselling services.

The reluctance of social workers to engage in practical supportive activities such as those described in David's account was confirmed in a recent study of social workers in social services departments. This found that the practical activities which clients and carers find most helpful are those least valued by social workers who regard them as being less 'professional' than 'therapeutic interventions' (Marsh & Fisher 1992). This clash of perspectives and values between social workers and their clients about the appropriate nature of the professional relationship has been found in consumer research over 25 years (Mayer and Timms 1969, Rees and Wallace 1982, Vernon 1986). Its persistence today is shown in David's account when he compares the activities of the community psychiatric nurses with those of the social workers:

The community psychiatric nurses came and changed light bulbs and made delicious corned beef sandwiches. They seemed to work in partnership, to have joined a sparse team of people supporting a confused and often unhappy old man. They were also supporting us. When the social workers came they were different. They looked at us and examined from a distance. They were like inspectors ... They definitely didn't change light bulbs. Mostly they told us what we couldn't have.

In social work, child care with its emphasis on child and family therapy has been accorded high prestige in contrast to the low status afforded to work with elderly people – conventionally regarded as incapable of change, beyond therapy. A dual system of qualification in social work until recently reflected this – the low status Certificate of Social Services being seen as suitable for elder care workers and the Certificate of Qualification in Social Work as a requirement for the allegedly more complex professional tasks involved in child care. The low status given to residential work with old people both in health and social services reflects this hierarchy and leads directly to the view of institutions as interventions of last resort, quite literally 'the end of the road'. As David graphically recounts, this professional interpretation of elder care institutions is signalled to residents and relatives by the uncanny frequency with which they are placed near cemeteries.

The therapeutic model of the professional relationship adopted by social workers defines institutional care as an undesirable last resort whose main function in relation to old people is to manage dying and death as efficiently as possible. Included in the definition of efficiency is the complete absolution of familial obligations, to the extent that not only are relatives 'relieved of the burden of care' but are denied the right to care once their dependant has been surrendered. In David's account: 'The ESMI unit forced us to be strangers to him. We had no status as close relatives and were rarely consulted or involved in any way. The staff ... took him over; owned the whole of his being'.

Within this interpretation of professionalism and the construction of institutional care which follows from it there can be no role for family relationships, indeed very little role for human relationships: 'It was a sanitised Hell – completely plastic and undomestic in every detail. It had few human comforts ... He died amongst strangers ... '

By defining and constructing institutional care in this way social care professionals have denied to many the opportunity of allowing themselves to accept the only form of care shown to improve the wellbeing of carers. In reviewing the literature on informal care, Parker (1990) describes the results of the Gateshead community care project often quoted as exemplary of the benefits of community care for carers and cared for alike. She reports clear evidence that in all aspects of carer outcomes except mental health problems, the carers whose dependant had gone into residential or hospital care appeared to have made more improvement than those whose dependants received community care. Parker concludes that: ' ... it is not at all clear that any substantial benefit accrued to carers despite improvements in service inputs (through the experimental community care scheme) ... As the figures suggest, admission to residential care might well have been the only option which would have had any real impact on the carer' (Parker 1990, p. 115).

Had institutional care been afforded a higher status by social care professionals, standards would have been higher and its public image more acceptable. This would allow more stressed carers to accept it for dependants, and having done so, not feel the overwhelming sense of guilt and failure described by David. This sense of guilt and failure is not something inherent in institutional care. It results from the way professionals have traditionally defined and constructed residential care. How could one not feel guilty consigning one's loved one to the 'last resort'? 'Slowly we learned to carry the massive guilt of our effective abandonment of him ... For me it was and continues to feel a massive personal failure. It is hard to imagine a way to let down another human being more comprehensively'.

There is some evidence of the further damaging effects of the therapeutically blinkered view of residential care. This comes from research into care preferences expressed by various age groups in the general population. It suggests that the therapeutic myopia of the professional has prevented them perceiving the real wishes of people. For example, Gilhooly (1986) found that, whilst carers valued practical assistance in the home, they would still have preferred residential care for their elderly relative, if they had the choice. In a similar vein, a study by West et al (1984) explored public attitudes to residential care and found that there was overwhelming support for residential care for confused elderly people. Another study reported by Parker found that among middle aged people contemplating their own future care needs: 'A substantial majority had favourable attitudes towards being looked after in nursing homes or residential homes' (Weeks [undated] in: Parker 1992–1993, p. 35).

There are several ways in which the therapy model of the professional relationship in social care may lead directly to the neglect of the informal caring relationship, the devaluing of certain types of formal care and to feelings of guilt and inadequacy in those carers who feel they have abandoned their loved ones to a second rate service. Despite the myopic condemnation of residential care by social care professionals over many years and their apparent confidence in the benefits for the public of community care, Parker (1990) suggests that the evidence shows that community care services, whilst they probably do prevent or delay admission to residential homes: ' ... seem to do so by preventing carers "giving up" rather than by providing what carers actually want. We have no evidence that the quality of caring prolonged in this way is adequate, nor what the long-term effects on the carer may be' (Parker 1990, p. 111).

The alarming reactions David recounts to the incontinence of his father-in-law ('I was filled with rage. I stood in front of him and wanted to knock him to the floor with my fist and kick his stupid smiling face in ... I wanted to kill him') and the sense of massive personal failure with which David was left after the death of his father-in-law is perhaps an indication of what can happen to the 'quality of care' and the type of 'long-term effects' which can result from inappropriate forms of professional relationship and the inadequate response to the real needs of people to which it inevitably leads.

As with the professional relationship itself, there are alternative, more positive models of institutional care, for example from the hospice movement. Here tending is given the recognition it deserves and the holistic approach to the individuality and humanity of both patient and informal carer is the focus of care – not the 'burdens'. To return to Gordon & Easton's (1992–1993) assertion: 'Good care – informal or formal – is centred on people and their interdependencies. Poor care centres on their problems and the problems they create for others' (Gordon & Easton 1992–1993, p. 24).

INTERPROFESSIONAL RIVALRIES

The conventional therapeutic approach to the professional relationship not only directly denies users services they need, but it does so indirectly because of the rivalries it has created between the professions. This has led to difficulties in interdisciplinary working and the integration of care packages from more than one agency. The adoption of therapeutically oriented models of professional care within the social care field was prompted by the success of the medical and allied professions in attaining professional recognition and the accompanying social status. This assisted social work to achieve recognition as a semi-profession but at a cost to its clients, through the imposition of unwanted and unhelpful forms of intervention which other professions either regard as inappropriate in themselves or inappropriately provided by social care workers, who they feel are unqualified to deliver them.

A recent review (Sheperd 1987) of the attitudes of general practitioners to social workers talks of the generally poor relationships between GPs and social workers: 'GPs considered social work services for the elderly and mentally ill to be performed well ... [However,] noticeable minorities ... considered social

workers to perform these tasks badly ... [and] two fifths ... were dissatisfied with the quality of liaison with medical staff' (Sheperd 1987, p. 84).

The enduring nature of these problems was highlighted during the implementation of the National Health Service and Community Care Act, with difficulties in communication between health and social care agencies – not least around the role of GPs in community care assessments.

Those familiar with research in this field will not be surprised that David describes an awareness of undeclared agendas behind the social worker's assessment to do with whether the father-in-law was a health or social services responsibility. He says, 'There seemed to be a substantial battle going on behind the scenes'. Dalley (1993) describes the destructive effects of clashes in professional ideology and what she describes as 'organisational tribalism' disclosed by her own research on inter-professionals working in Scotland. She quotes a GP who refers to competition between medicine and social work over the definition of problems: ' ... doctors and social workers ... vie for whether a problem is a social or a medical problem ... to establish precedence there' (Dalley 1993, p. 34). Again, a social worker from a primary health care setting says that she ' ... felt disappointed in the level of co-ordination ... I mean, dreadful things happen – and people fall between ... I think professional orientation [causes it]' (Dalley 1993, p. 35).

ALTERNATIVE MODELS

Conventional notions of professionalism are being questioned by government, and by consumer and user movements. Alternative models of formal helping relationships are being sought by many involved in social care who are concerned to rid the provision of the paternalism inherent in conventional therapeutic models (Adams 1990, Smale et al 1993, Marsh & Fisher 1992). For example, current government policy encourages health and social services authorities to balance the model of patient/therapist against that of purchaser/provider. This immediately implies a different balance of power in the relationship, allowing patient and carer to retain the control over their relationship which David felt had been usurped by the 'expert' professional.

The policy guidance associated with the National Health Service and Community Care Act urges social service authorities wherever possible to promote the 'user as care manager' model of which there are numerous examples in the disability literature. Research shows this approach to the delivery of services to be empowering for individuals and also cost effective (Oliver & Zarb 1993).

Another model, mentioned earlier, is that of social pedagogy, i.e. an educational as opposed to a therapeutic approach to the caring relationship (Lorenz 1991). Training in the practical skills of physical care is highly valued by informal carers and user-led organisations and groups frequently emphasise training rather than therapy. Assertion and advocacy skills are increasingly a focus as the relationship with professionals and the bureaucracies in which they work becomes ever more adversarial. Chilling evidence for this and an intimation of how far the 'professional relationship' has been corrupted is the account from one 60-year-old carer quoted in a recent report from the Alzheimer's Disease Society (1993): 'The social workers tell me that my husband is my responsibility and not the state's ... As it is I am going to have to sell our home and fund his care for the rest of my life' (Alzheimer's Disease Society 1993, p. 24).

The Alzheimer's Disease Society's report shows that carers want more information from professionals to enable them to plan what they want to happen and to maintain control over their own lives. Doctors are criticised for devoting too little time to this aspect of the relationship. Perhaps this is because within their professional model of diagnosis–treatment–cure there is no need for the patient to know anything. To divert time from the core professional tasks of diagnosis–treatment–cure (even when there isn't one as with Alzheimer's) is not perceived to be in the patient's best interests.

The very low take-up of benefits by elderly people, many of whom are carers, suggests that there is a massive social pedagogy task which currently professionals are failing to tackle, perhaps because it is not regarded as of sufficiently high status within the therapeutically oriented model of professional relationship. The abject poverty of millions of old people and their carers revealed in the report suggests that relieving some of the stress imposed by financial pressures through welfare rights counselling would be at least as therapeutic for carers as affectively oriented counselling designed to alleviate the depression caused, at least in part, by poverty. Parker (1990), in her review of research on informal care, asserts that studies of carers' needs have repeatedly shown that

information is frequently entirely neglected by professionals but ' ... can make a substantial difference to carers' lives and relationships with service providers' (Parker 1990, p. 124).

Much of the research we have described, and all of David's account of his own experience as a carer, suggests that there is an urgent need to relinquish outmoded and unhelpful forms of 'professionalism'. Nonetheless, as the work of Marsh & Fisher (1992) described earlier showed, the construction of the professional relationship in social care seems remarkably resistant to change. Lorenz (1991) in his description of the, at times, conflicting traditions of social casework and social pedagogy in Europe, suggests one reason when he says that: ' ... pedagogical methods within social work were ... ideologically suspect because of their non-individualistic orientation' (Lorenz 1991, p. 74). If social workers continue to cling to irrelevant and outmoded forms of professional relationship they will become increasingly marginalised as other more flexible occupations emerge and user-led organisations increasingly provide the services people want rather than those 'professionals' assess them as needing.

Mullender (1992–1993) gives one example of what the future may bring when she describes how: 'The dissatisfaction with social workers' basically therapeutic approach, rather than practical, needs-led packages of care, was one reason why the Derbyshire Centre for Integrated Living set up its own practical services, including peer counselling' (Mullender 1992–1993, p. 11).

Perhaps one of the most damaging effects of this form of professionalisation in social care has been the way in which the relationship between carer and cared for has been devalued, neglected and sometimes destroyed. It is clear from David's account that the form of relationship offered by social care professionals had personally damaging effects for him, his wife and his father-in-law and for the relationship between them. No further indictment of the inadequacy of this model of professional relationship is needed than the realisation that, after years of committed caring and contact with many different professionals, this particular 'informal carer' was left to struggle alone no longer with services but with a sense of massive personal failure.

REFERENCES

Adams R 1990 Self-help, social work and empowerment. Macmillan, Basingstoke

Alzheimer's Disease Society 1993 Deprivation and dementia. ADS, London

Dalley G 1993 Professional ideology or organisational tribalism? the health service/social work divide. In: Walmsley J, Reynolds J, Shakespeare P, Woolfe R (eds) Health, welfare and practice: reflecting on roles and relationships. Sage, London

Ellis K 1992 Squaring the circle: user and carer participation in needs assessment. Joseph Rowntree Foundation, York

Finkelstein V 1993 From curing or caring to defining disabled people. In: Walmsley J, Reynolds J, Shakespeare P, Woolfe R (eds) Health, welfare and practice: reflecting on roles and relationships. Sage, London

Gilhooly M 1986 Senile dementia: factors associated with caregivers' preference for institutional care. British Journal of Medical Psychology 59: 65–171

Gordon David S, Easton N 1992–1993 Patterns of caring: case studies in informal care. Practice 1: 16–24

Lorenz W 1991 Social work practice in Europe: continuity in diversity. In: Hill M (ed) Social work and the European Community. Jessica Kingsley, London

Marsh P, Fisher M 1992 Good intentions: developing partnership in social services. Joseph Rowntree Foundation, York

Mayer J, Timms N 1969 The client speaks. Routledge and Kegan Paul, London

Morris J 1993 The independent living project©: final evaluation. Spinal Injuries Association, London

Mullender A 1992–1993 Disabled people find a voice: will it be heard in the move towards community care? Practice 6(1): 5–15

Oliver M 1983 Social work with disabled people. Macmillan, London

Oliver M, Zarb G 1993 Personal services. Community Care 4 (3): 22–23

Parker G 1990 With due care and attention: a review of research on informal care. Family Policy Studies Centre, London

Phillipson C 1982 Capitalism and the construction of old age. Macmillan, London

RADAR 1993 Disabled people have rights. Interim Report, RADAR, London

Rees S, Wallace A 1982 Verdicts on social work. Arnold, London

Scott R A 1970 The construction of conceptions of stigma by professional experts. In: Douglas J (ed) Deviance and respectability: the social construction of moral meanings. Bask Books, New York

Sheperd M G 1987 Dominant images of social work: a British comparison of general practitioners with and without attachment schemes. International Social Work 30(1): 77–90

Smale G, Tuson G, Biehal N, Marsh P 1993 Empowerment, assessment, care management and the skilled worker. HMSO, London

Twigg J, Atkin K, Perring C 1990 Carers and services: a review of research. HMSO, London

Unell J 1993 Informal care: the research contribution. In: Day P R (ed) Perspectives on later life. Whiting and Birch, London

Vernon G 1986 Untrained carers are tops. Community Care 628(11): 28–29

Walker A, Phillipson C (eds) 1986 Ageing and social policy: a critical assessment. Gower, Aldershot

Weeks D [undated] Ageism and being alone – a suitable case for prevention? Preliminary Report. Jardine Clinic, University of Edinburgh

West P, Illsley R, Kelman H 1984 Public preferences for the care of dependency groups. Social Science and Medicine 18(4): 287–295

RECOMMENDED READING

Adams R 1990 Self-help, social work and empowerment. Macmillan, Basingstoke. *An extremely useful introduction to the concepts, theories and practice underpinning the self-help movement and its relationship with the social work profession.*

Oliver M 1983 Social work with disabled people. Macmillan, London. *Though now 11 years old, this remains a stimulating and evocative account of the shortcomings of social work with disabled people and how it – and indeed other professional intervention – can be practically improved.*

Smale G, Tuson G with Biehal N, Marsh P 1993 Empowerment assessment, care management and the skilled worker. HMSO, London. *An interesting exposition of how assessment practice may or may not contribute to the disempowerment of its subjects. Practical guidance is offered on how to avoid the type of service-oriented, 'professional' assessment which virtually excludes the real needs of clients as they experience them.*

Walmsley J, Reynolds J, Shakespeare P, Woolfe R (eds) 1993 Health welfare and practice: reflecting roles and relationships. Sage, London. *A book of readings from a variety of different professional perspectives. Critical analyses of professional and inter-professional roles and relationships and some practical examples of how professional practice can connect helpfully with people's everyday lives.*

15

Mental health promotion in old age

Elizabeth Armstrong
Tracey Sparkes

The myths surrounding older people, their wants, needs and abilities, are ever present in society. There is a tendency to view older people as a homogeneous group and to treat them accordingly and this is reinforced by media accounts of a group that is vulnerable, impoverished, ill and confused. Many people are now beginning to challenge these myths and to present a picture of older people as individuals with as diverse a range of interests and needs as any other age group.

There are two particular myths that this chapter sets out to challenge: first, that there is an inevitable link between older people and mental illness, and second, that older people are not able to change or alter their lifestyles to improve their health. In order to deliver the models of health promotion to older people that are illustrated within the chapter, this challenge needs to underlie the beliefs of health and social care professionals.

This chapter considers models of health promotion and prevention, including screening and targeting, and the links that may exist between mental and physical ability, autonomy and control, social support and stress reduction. The opportunities for mental health promotion with carers are also discussed.

WHAT IS MENTAL HEALTH?

The *Concise Oxford Dictionary* defines 'mental' as 'of, in or done by the mind'. A second, colloquial, definition is 'mad' or 'crazy'. This highlights a major difficulty which we have in discussing mental health. Mental health, to professionals as well as the general public, becomes synonymous with mental illness. The situation is further complicated since those who care for the mentally ill refer to themselves as mental health workers.

There seem to be two main views about what health is. One, usually called the medical model, is that health is simply an absence of symptoms of illness. In mental health terms, this view is popular with psychiatrists. Trent (1991) refers to it as the single continuum where health and illness are seen as opposite ends of a line.

The second definition is that of the World Health Organization (WHO), that health is 'a state of complete physical, mental and social wellbeing and not merely the absence of disease or infirmity' (Dines & Cribb 1993). The strength of this view is that it emphasises wholeness. The different aspects interact and are mutually dependent. But life is not all bliss. There are negatives as well as positives, sadness as well as happiness. Perhaps, after all, this definition is just too idealistic. In addition, many people would argue that the lack of a mention of spiritual or emotional health in this model is a serious flaw.

Instead of the single continuum, with health at one end and illness at the other, Trent (1991) proposes two continua, one for health and the other for illness. They are separate, though linked. The medical model is not invalidated but kept in its place, with illness. The person who is ill goes to a doctor to be treated. The person who wants to be healthy acts for herself.

This concept of health includes an idea of autonomy; of the individual as key player.

Separating health from illness, as Trent does, makes it easier to consider all facets of health – physical, mental, social, emotional and spiritual – together. Mental health is part of health as a whole, not something to do with madness.

Missing from the discussion so far has been the effect of culture. Whilst accepting the widely-held concept of health as not merely an absence of illness, Fernando (1991) believes that culture influences the perceptions people have of both continua. Although western culture may place a high value on the control individuals exercise over their social relationships and circumstances, people from other parts of the world may be more concerned with the person's integration into family and community, even extending to the spiritual dimension and including ancestors and god(s).

Nevertheless, it can be argued that health and illness are related in some way in every culture, though not in the same way. For instance, in the Chinese tradition illness is caused by an imbalance between two 'poles of life energy' – the yin and the yang. Many forms of distress which would in western medicine be classified as 'illness' might be seen in the Ayurvedic tradition of Indian medicine as religious or philosophical problems.

Torkington (1991) believes that racism is a factor in the development of mental illness in black people. This is not just that lack of cultural awareness on the part of health workers may lead to misdiagnosis, although this happens. It is also that black people experience, on a day-to-day basis, a society which has deeply ingrained beliefs of the superiority of white cultural norms. It is not hard to understand how this might lead to a lowering of self-esteem, and therefore to mental health problems.

HEALTH PROMOTION

Health promotion is usually seen as including three main activities: disease prevention, health education and health protection. Inherent in this concept is the implication that something is done by an expert to clients to make them healthier. Clients have only a passive role. Yet if the client is an autonomous individual who can make choices, it might be suggested that there is more to health promotion than this.

The First International Conference on Health Promotion, held in Ottawa in 1986 (Dines & Cribb 1993: 205), produced what is now known as the *Ottawa Charter*. Health promotion was defined as the 'process of enabling people to increase control over and improve their health'. Health was seen as something positive which includes personal and social elements, not just physical attributes or abilities. For this reason, health is not simply a matter of healthy lifestyles. Rather it is incumbent upon all who make decisions which affect people's lives to be aware of the likely health consequences of their decisions.

Health is therefore not just the responsibility of the health professionals. An integral part of the *Charter* is the acknowledgement that people cannot reach their health potential without control over the things which affect their health. Factors which influence health may be political, economic, social, cultural, environmental, behavioural and biological. Health promotion action may occur in any of these areas.

That the *Charter* defined health promotion as a process implies some kind of change. In order to improve health there needs to be change at individual, community and government levels. Tudor & Holroyd (1991) consider that the focus of the promotion of positive mental health should be at two levels, individual and community. They quote strategies described by McPheeters (1976) suggesting that, at both levels, action should be directed towards helping people improve their ability to cope better with the vagaries and problems of everyday living.

Whilst the *Ottawa Charter* might set health promotion action in its widest context, it may not be much help in determining what health promotion is at the level of most health and social service workers. Dines and Cribb have suggested that asking what health promotion is might be the wrong question. It may be better to ask of every intervention with patient or client, 'Is this being done in a health-enhancing way?'

The health of the nation

In 1992, the government published its White Paper, *The Health of the Nation,* setting out a strategy for health in England which placed emphasis on disease prevention and health promotion in five key areas (Department of Health 1992). One of these was mental illness.

The document identified national targets for each of the key areas, suggested action which was needed to meet them and put in place a framework for monitoring and review (Box 15.1).

Box 15.1 Mental illness targets in *Health of the Nation*

A. To improve significantly the health and social functioning of mentally ill people.
B. To reduce the overall suicide rate by at least 15% by the year 2000.
C. To reduce the suicide rate of severely mentally ill people by at least 33% by the year 2000.

Within the mental illness key area, older people were identified as a vulnerable group. Severe mental illness is as common in older as in younger people. The prevalence of depression increases with age, and dementia affects mainly older people. *The Health of the Nation* notes that in many cases preventive measures can be just as effective with older people as they are in younger age groups.

In 1993 the follow-up document, the *Mental Illness Key Area Handbook* (Department of Health 1993), pointed to the wide arena in which mental health promotion needs to take place; not just the National Health Service and social service departments, but also voluntary organisations, housing departments and the local media. The document highlights the many opportunities presented to professional contacts to enhance mental health.

PROMOTING MENTAL HEALTH WITH OLDER PEOPLE

Preventing mental illness

Preventive activity is commonly divided into primary, secondary and tertiary. Jenkins (1992) has used this model to describe prevention in terms of mental illness.

Primary prevention implies that a disease is prevented from happening at all. It means either identifying the cause and countering it, which is the rationale behind immunisation, or identifying the risk factors and taking steps to reduce or modify them. For example, carers, particularly elderly carers, are known to be at increased risk of becoming depressed. Adequate support and good information offered early in the caring process might help to minimise this risk by increasing confidence that help will be available should it be required.

Secondary prevention measures shorten the length of an illness, thereby reducing the period during which the individual suffers distress. They also lessen the likelihood of long-term adverse consequences. Depression is common in older people, but it is not a natural consequence of ageing. Blanchard (1992) suggests that although GPs may recognise depressive illness in their older patients, they may fail to offer effective treatment. Treatment, whether by drugs, psychosocial methods or a combination, is likely to be just as effective as it is with younger people, and will undoubtedly improve the quality of the person's life.

Tertiary prevention is mainly to do with limiting the disability caused by chronic illness or injury. It enables people to make the most of residual skills and prevents pre-existing conditions getting worse. Miller (1992) describes a number of initiatives which have tried to improve the functioning of people with dementia. He considers that such patients are responsive to environmental changes, albeit in a limited way, and that quality of life can be enhanced.

Newton (1992) has offered a definition of prevention which seems to overlap the concepts of primary and secondary, or to combine elements of primary prevention and early detection. She suggests that prevention may be seen as anything which is aimed at reducing the likelihood of mental illness occurring amongst people who, though distressed, do not meet the criteria appropriate to diagnosis. This definition is said to avoid the danger of labelling as 'ill' those who are experiencing normal reactions to stressful situations. Work with people who have a small number of symptoms can be considered prevention rather than treatment.

It is normal for those who have lost a loved one to

feel sad, in low spirits, to cry and feel 'depressed'. These feelings are part of the grieving process. But as Parkes (1986) has demonstrated in his famous studies of widows, it is unusual for bereaved people to require psychiatric help. He suggests that knowledge of the factors which influence the grieving process can help to identify those bereaved people who may benefit from supportive interventions early in their loss. These factors include poverty and lack of family support. Information about these factors is often sought during screening programmes (see below) and can be used to target help at those who are most likely to benefit.

Screening

Screening is a method of assessing the wellbeing of older people in order to discover untreated illness and unmet social needs. It may either be 'opportunistic', that is, undertaken whenever the person presents for any reason to a GP or other workers, or universally offered regardless of whether people are in contact with services or not. These methods do not in themselves promote health, but they offer opportunities for such interventions.

The requirement for the annual health assessment of people aged 75 or over (Health Departments of Great Britain 1990) has caused much debate and controversy. As a national initiative which makes explicit the need to assess the functional, social and psychological wellbeing of older people, it has been welcomed by some. Others are sceptical of its value.

Empirical evidence about the benefits of universal assessment of older people is vague. There is evidence to suggest that between 86% and 90% of older people consult their GP at least annually, and that those who do not are fit and healthy (Scott & Maynard 1991). There is also considerable evidence to show that, when they do consult, older people tend to under-report certain symptoms; in particular, urinary symptoms (Perkins 1991, Williamson et al 1987) and problems associated with the feet, dementia and depression (Williamson et al 1987). The early findings of the Elderly Person's Integrated Care Scheme (EPICS) in North Kensington, London (Aylward 1991) found that, although 82% of the people aged 75 and over who were assessed had seen their GP within the previous year and 38% within the previous month, 67% indicated that they would accept additional help if it were offered, and 27% said they wanted help but were not receiving it.

There seems to be consensus from much of the research that the main benefits of regular elderly assessments are increased morale and quality of life

(McEwan et al 1990, Scott & Maynard 1991, Tulloch & Moore 1979, Vetter et al 1984). This has been supported more recently by Tremellan (1992) who found that doctors felt there was no merit in over-75 assessments; nurses felt it was important but wanted more training; and patients found it worthwhile. Barber and Wallis (1978) found that the greatest improvements amongst older people who had been assessed regularly by health visitors were sociomedical.

It seems important to guard against the assumption that those who do not visit their GP must necessarily have many unmet health needs. As early as 1984, Ebrahim et al showed that generally this group enjoyed better health than those who did consult.

It is equally important to recognise that screening may cause anxiety for individuals and for families (Williams 1992). Raising anxiety amongst family members may unwittingly mean the family taking over, leading ultimately to a loss of autonomy and independence for the older person. Screening should therefore be sensitively handled and the choice of the older person whether or not to participate must be recognised.

A further adverse consequence of screening could be that inappropriate reassurance is given to those who are objectively assessed to be at risk (McIntosh & Power 1993).

Whatever the views of professionals, the requirement for the annual assessment of people aged 75 and over remains in the GP contract, despite the fact that the government has neither made clear the reasoning behind it, nor provided specific, national guidelines. Nevertheless, there have been some interesting developments in response to the assessment, notably that of 'linkworking' in the London wards of Kensington and Chelsea, and Westminster (Young et al 1993). These authors describe a scheme in which older people were linked to their general practitioner through a delegated team member who, following specific training, used a structured assessment schedule. The scheme enabled practices to comply with their contractual obligations, and it maximised the effectiveness of the health checks.

The 'linkworker' was a new primary care team member, not necessarily a health professional, who could offer a less medically oriented assessment using a holistic approach. The linkworker also developed an extensive knowledge of local resources and referral agencies and could therefore empower people to improve their own health by passing on relevant information.

The Royal College of General Practitioners has taken the linkwork assessment schedule a stage further in publishing its own version. Describing this, Williams & Wallace (1993) say that if any sense is to be made of the contractual obligation, assessment should not be seen as just a health check. It should include health education, health promotion, review of medication, review of carer's needs and primary and secondary prevention. They also highlight the potential, as in the linkwork scheme, for planning from the information gained.

Whether necessary or not, the universal assessment has provided an opportunity for health promotion with a group previously left out of such initiatives. The ageist concept that older people as a group cannot or will not change unhealthy aspects of their lifestyles, and cannot or will not learn to do so, is beginning to fade.

Screening also provides a means by which people at high risk of developing mental health problems might be identified. A pilot study of a method to identify people at risk of a depression, which could be used by nurses in the course of a general health check at a well person clinic, was acceptable both to the nurses who tried it and to their patients – very few patients refused to answer questions relating to psychological and social health (Armstrong 1993). The assessment was linked to a problem-solving technique for helping people access appropriate community support. It was intended for use with a younger age group but many elderly people participated. An earlier study by Iliffe et al (1991) showed that annual assessments yield much new evidence of depression and dementia and assist in the identification of heavy drinkers.

Linking physical and mental health

Once physical peak is reached in the late teens, there is a decline in the physical capacity of everyone. However, the pace of such decline is variable and generalisations about older people cannot be made. Muir Gray (1991) suggests that there is a critical time for immobility and that the promotion of physical exercise is an important contributory factor in the prevention of disease in old age.

The link between physical health and depression has been acknowledged by many authors. Jenkins & Shepherd (1983) describe the link as complex. On the one hand, depressed people often go to their doctor with physical symptoms. This may be partly due to the stigma which still surrounds mental illness – it is more respectable to have a physical than a psychological symptom – or it may be because people who are depressed often become more aware than

before of bodily sensations. Many authors agree, though, that there is a real association between mental and physical illness which is not explained by these phenomena (Sharp & Morrell 1989, Wright 1993). In particular, depression may often be secondary to chronic, disabling or lifethreatening illness. Older people, who are more likely to suffer from physical illness, sensory deprivation, immobility and social isolation are particularly at risk (Jenkins 1992).

Katona (1993) agrees that the link between physical illness and depression can be connected to poor health affecting function, for example, chronic lung disease, stroke, severe arthritis and dementia.

Jenkins (1992) suggests that the factors involved in the development of mental illness, including depression, operate in three ways: as predisposing factors, precipitating factors and maintaining factors. There are biological, social and psychological components to each factor. In the present context, disabling injury, such as stroke or malignant disease, might be seen as precipitating factors – in Jenkins's words, they determine when the illness starts.

Chronic pain – of arthritis – and disability are maintaining factors. That is, they may prolong an illness and delay recovery. Particularly important are hearing loss and visual impairment since they may predispose to social isolation which is a risk factor in its own right.

It will also be seen that the symptoms of a depressive illness may themselves lead to a loss of function, ranging from the inability to enjoy participating in physical activities to a loss of interest in performing even the most basic daily tasks.

Take, for example, the elderly man who has been used to having a twice-daily walk with his dog. He loses the dog, then subsequently withdraws from his normal activities and begins to find that he can no longer walk as far as the post office to collect his pension. It might be tempting to conclude that he is just getting older, and his family might advise him against having another dog. Cause and effect can be difficult to separate, but it is equally possible that he may be suffering from depression precipitated by the loss of his companion – his dog. Recognise and treat his depression and his physical capacity may improve as well.

Williams (1992) considers that lifestyle, diet, habit and psychological differences all affect the pace of physical deterioration, and that functional ability, rather than morbidity level, is the best measure of health in old age. He has described three levels of physical function, or 'activities of daily living', which an older person should ideally perform effectively:

- 'sociability'
- 'domestic'
- 'personal'.

There is a dynamic link between the levels whereby functional deterioration tends to affect the first level – sociability – initially, then move through domestic to personal.

Williams depicts this model as a set of concentric rings (Fig. 15.1) which illustrate that there is natural decline in all three levels as people age. The time frame of this decline is accelerated by illness. If the progress of illness is prevented or modified, deterioration may be slowed down and quality of life improved.

It is also useful to consider whether this link between functional ability and depression means that there is a link between the avoidance of deterioration and avoidance of depression; whether continuation of physical activity might prevent the onset of a depressive illness. Williams's model suggests that this is so. It seems therefore to be a valuable tool for both physical and mental health promotion in old age.

Kennie (1993) describes studies undertaken by the World Health Organization into health promotion programmes for older people in which participants adopt healthy lifestyles and practice 'body maintenance'. The results of these programmes have demonstrated 'improved psychological wellbeing,

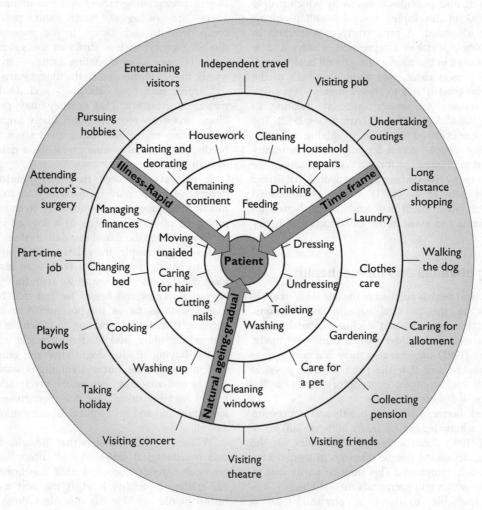

Figure 15.1 Williams's Rings. From: Williams E I. Over 75: Care, Assessment and Health Promotion. Reproduced by permission of the publishers, Radcliffe Medical Press, Oxford.

confidence and some coping skills' (Kennie 1993, p. 5). This seems to provide further evidence of the helpfulness of Williams's Rings as a model for both opportunistic and planned health promotion interventions for older people, which could affect both physical and mental wellbeing.

Linking social and mental health

Autonomy and control

It has been acknowledged that a variety of factors affect health. We have also seen that an effective model of health promotion must take into account the wider circumstances of the individual and community. Kennie (1993) describes the concern in the USA about the emphasis which health promotion has put on the 'responsibility' of individuals whilst ignoring what he calls their 'response-ability'. That is, their power to respond to environmental and social challenges.

There are aspects of health which neither old people nor professionals can easily change such as housing, income and transport. As Newton (1992) acknowledges, there are plenty of good reasons, aside from promoting mental health, for seeking to improve the income and standard of housing of many older people.

La Gaipa (1990) calls attention to the conflict which may arise between the needs of an individual for autonomy and an element of dependence on outside resources. He suggests that there is a trade-off between having a reliable support system and the ability to act independently. Reducing dependency may not necessarily achieve autonomy, particularly if it increases social isolation.

Another consideration regarding autonomy is the idea of reciprocity, or how mental wellbeing is affected by the necessity to be cared for by someone else. A change in status within the family, for example from provider to dependant, can be difficult to face for all involved (Woods 1990). Avoidance of, or failure to acknowledge this issue will make change in health difficult to achieve.

Models of health promotion which seek to empower the individual, such as the *Ageing Well* initiative promoted by Age Concern England, might therefore seem to be the most appropriate. This initiative is a national programme to promote positive health and prevent disability and ill health in later life. After the advent of the *Health of the Nation* strategy, *Ageing Well* concentrated on the specific target areas, including mental health. The key to the approach of

Ageing Well, which was managed by Age Concern England, was the recruitment of 'senior health mentors' – professionally trained older volunteers who support and encourage their peers to adopt healthier lifestyles: '*Ageing Well* recognises older people's value as a health resource to their community and to each other' (*Ageing Well* publicity leaflet, Age Concern England).

Social support

Social support and health, mental and physical, are seen to be closely linked. This suggests that there is a need to link health care and social care. This need is being addressed by the innovative EPICS projects (Aylward 1991) which are designed to integrate primary and social care for elderly people.

Three EPICS projects have been developed by the Helen Hamlyn Foundation in London with health authorities, Family Health Service Authorities and social service departments in the English counties of Derbyshire, Shropshire and in North Kensington, London. They are based on the 'On Lok' model of care developed for the Chinese elderly community in San Francisco, where all-inclusive care operates through a 'consolidated care management' system.

Each of the three UK projects has developed in response to local circumstances, but all are based on four key elements and each has four key principles (see Boxes 15.2 and 15.3).

Box 15.2 Key elements of the EPICS project

- a shared profile of health and social needs
- a generic care worker
- an interdisciplinary operations team
- a joint management board.

Source: Aylward (1991)

Box 15.3 Key principles of the EPICS project

- consumer-led, holistic, putting older people first
- centre-based, providing one-stop shops as access to health and social care and social activities
- all the staff from different agencies work as if from one organisation
- they are adequately resourced to avoid waste and duplication of effort.

Source: Aylward (1991)

Carers

As the chance of having to rely on another person for physical care increases with age, so does the chance of having to care for someone else. The peak age for caring is 45–64 years (24%) but 13% of people aged 65 or over described themselves as carers in the 1990 General Household Survey (Office of Population Censuses and Surveys 1992). However, a survey of 1003 carers, undertaken in the same years by Crossroads Care, found that 53% were aged 60 or over and 14% were aged over 70 (CCETSW 1993).

It has been shown that 'carers' do not always identify themselves as such due to the incipient way caring often creeps up on them (CCETSW 1993). In view of this, it seems possible that the older the carers the less likely they are to identify themselves like this for the General Household Survey, especially if they are caring for a spouse who has gradually grown frail.

The effect of the caring role on physical and psychological health is well documented (e.g. Kennie 1993, Woods 1990). The new legislation in England under which social service departments provide a care management service to all vulnerable residents in their locality, emphasises the need for a separate assessment of the individual needs of carers (Secretaries of State for Health and Social Security 1989). Kennie (1993) considers that meeting the needs of carers also means promoting their health. Newton (1992) suggests that whether or not an individual is able to live independently until death depends mainly on his or her health and support network. Newton criticises the media-induced perception that all old people eventually become dependent and burdensome. Nevertheless, she refers to the 1980 General Household Survey which showed that, at that time, help for frail elderly people living with a spouse or younger relative was limited or non-existent (Office of Population Censuses and Surveys 1982). Anecdotal evidence from carers indicates that there is still a long way to go before appropriate information and support is readily available to them.

Burke (1992) suggests that older carers can benefit particularly from counselling, organising of practical support and befriending offered by a social worker alongside GP services. Burke believes that this might be the only form of help that some older carers will accept.

CONCLUSION

At the beginning of this chapter we set out to challenge two widely held myths about older people and their health. We believe that mental illness in later life is far from inevitable. In particular, much depression is probably preventable by early intervention with those at risk. Moreover, the deterioration in physical function and the reduction in quality of life which accompanies depressive illness can be prevented by recognition and prompt treatment.

We began considering the concept of health. Whilst acknowledging that health and illness are linked, we have shown that health is a distinct, separate concept with values of its own which do not depend on the presence or absence of illness.

Within the idea of health, we have criticised the distinction made between its various aspects, notably physical, mental and social health. We believe that the evidence is incontrovertible that these aspects are linked and that it is not possible to promote one aspect without considering the others. This seems to us to support the argument that health and social care should be integrated and we have described models that show how integration could be achieved.

To be effective, any model of health promotion, including methods of illness prevention, must take into account the rights of individuals and communities to:

- be part of decisions that affect their health
- have sufficient knowledge on which to base informed choices
- have appropriate skills to enable them to act on the choices made.

Although older people may have specific needs which are linked to age, these principles of promoting health – mental, physical and social – are the same for all age groups.

REFERENCES

Armstrong E 1993 Mental health check. Nursing Times 89(33): 40–42

Aylward P 1991 The North Kensington elderly person's integrated care scheme: linkwork project, interim report 3. Helen Hamlyn Research Unit, London

Barber J H, Wallis J B 1978 The benefits to an elderly population of continuing geriatric assessment. Journal of the Royal College of General Practitioners 28: 428–433

Blanchard M 1992 The elderly. International Review of Psychiatry 4: 251–256

Burke M 1992 Counselling in general practice: options for action, B: the social worker's point of view. In: Jenkins R, Newton J, Young R (eds) The prevention of depression and anxiety: the role of the primary care team. HMSO, London

CCETSW 1993 Care management and assessment. Contact-a-Family in conjunction with Carers National, London

Department of Health 1992 The health of the nation: a strategy for health in England. HMSO, London

Department of Health 1993 Mental illness key area handbook. Department of Health, London

Dines A, Cribb A 1993 Health promotion: concepts and practice. Blackwell Scientific, London

Ebrahim S, Hedley R, Sheldon M 1984 Low levels of ill health among elderly non-consulters in general practice: practice observed. British Medical Journal 289: 1273–1275

Fernando S 1991 Mental health, race and culture. Macmillan, London

Gilbert P 1991 An evolutionary approach to the conceptualisation of mental health. In: Trent D (ed) Promotion of mental health, vol 1. Avebury, Aldershot

Health Departments of Great Britain 1990 General practice in the National Health Service: the 1990 contract. HMSO, London

Iliffe S, Haines A, Gallivan S, Booroff A, Goldenburg E, Morgan P 1991 Assessment of elderly people in general practice, 1: social circumstances and mental state. British Journal of General Practice 41: 9–12

Jenkins R 1992 Depression and anxiety: an overview of preventive strategies. In: Jenkins R, Newton J, Young R (eds) The prevention of depression and anxiety: the role of the primary care team. HMSO, London

Jenkins R, Shepherd M 1983 Mental illness and general practice. In: Bean P (ed) Mental illness and general practice. John Wiley, Chichester

Katona C L E 1993 The aetiology of depression in old age. International Review of Psychiatry 5: 317–326

Kennie D C 1993 Preventive care for elderly people. Cambridge University Press, Cambridge

La Gaipa J L 1990 The negative effects of informal support systems. In: Duck S (ed) Personal relationships and social support. Sage, London

McEwan R T, Davison N, Forster D P, Pearson P, Stirling E 1990 Screening elderly people in primary care: a randomised control trial. British Journal of General Practice 40(332): 94–97

McIntosh I B, Power K G 1993 Elderly people's views of the annual health assessment. British Journal of General Practice 43: 189–192

McPheeters H L 1976 Primary prevention and health promotion in mental health. Preventive Medicine 5: 187–198

Miller E 1992 Promoting better mental health in the elderly: the problem of Alzheimer's disease. In: Trent D R, Reed C (eds) Promotion of mental health, vol. 2. Avebury, Aldershot

Muir Gray J A 1991 Preventing disease and promoting health in old age. In: Pathy M J (ed) Principles and practice of geriatric medicine, 2nd edn. Wiley, Chichester

Newton J 1992 Preventing mental illness in practice. Routledge, London

Office of Population Censuses and Surveys 1982 General household survey 1980. HMSO, London

Office of Population Censuses and Surveys 1992 General household survey: carers in 1990. OPCS, London

Parkes C M 1986 Bereavement: studies of grief in adult life. Penguin, London

Perkins E R 1991 Screening elderly people: a review of the literature in the light of the new general practitioner contract. British Journal of General Practice 41(350): 382–385

Scott T, Maynard A 1991 Will the new contract lead to cost effective medical practice. Centre for Health Economics, University of York, York

Secretaries of State for Health and Social Security 1989 Caring for people: community care in the next decade and beyond. HMSO, London

Sharp D, Morrell D 1989 The psychiatry of general practice. In: Williams P, Wilkinson G, Rawnsley K (eds) The scope of epidemiological psychiatry. Routledge, London

Stevenson O, Parsloe P 1993 Community care and empowerment. Joseph Rowntree, York

Torkington N P K 1991 Black health: a political issue. Catholic Association for Racial Justice and Liverpool Institute of Higher Education, Liverpool

Tremellen J 1992 Assessment of patients aged 75 and over in general practice. British Medical Journal 305: 621–624

Trent D 1991 Breaking the single continuum. In: Trent D R (ed) Promotion of mental health, vol. 1. Avebury, Aldershot

Tudor K, Holroyd G 1991 Between psyche and society: the role of the mental health promotion officer. In: Trent D R (ed) Promotion of mental health, vol. 1. Avebury, Aldershot

Tulloch A, Moore V 1979 A radomised controlled trial of geriatric screening and surveillance in general practice. Journal of the Royal College of General Practitioners 29: 773–772

Vetter N J, Jones D A, Victor C R 1984 Effect of a health visitor working with elderly patients in general practice: a randomised controlled trial. British Medical Journal 289: 1522–1542

Williams E I 1992 Care, assessment and health promotion. Radcliffe Medical Press, Oxford

Williams E I, Wallace P 1993 Health checks for people aged 75 and over. Royal College of General Practitioners. Occasional Paper 59, RCGP, London

Williamson J, Smith R G, Burley L E 1987 Primary care of the elderly: a practical approach. Wright, London

Woods R T 1990 Preventing and overcoming psychological problems in retirement. Journal of the Royal Society of Health 3: 85–89

Wright A F 1993 Depression: recognition and management in general practice. Royal College of General Practioners, London

Young E, Wallace P, Bruster, Sparkes T, Jarman B 1993 Linkworking: maximising the potential of health checks for people aged 75 and over by linking them to community care provision. Department of General Practice, Lisson Grove Health Centre, London

RECOMMENDED READING

Dines A, Cribb A 1993 Health promotion: concepts and practice. Blackwell Scientific, London. *This book introduces readers to the wide range of concerns in the theory and practice of health promotion, illustrating both the opportunities and the constraints. It contains an overview of health promotion and nursing practice.*

Kennie D C 1993 Preventive care for elderly people. Cambridge University Press, Cambridge. *An excellent and readable account of all aspects of preventive health care for older people. It discusses the practical implications of introducing preventive measures and looks at the cost implications.*

Young E, Wallace P, Bruster, Sparkes T, Jarman B 1993 Linkworking: maximising the potential of health checks for people aged 75 and over by linking them to community care provision. Department of General Practice, Lisson Grove Health Centre, London. *This practical report chronicles the development of linkworking over its first 3 years. It includes a copy of the linkwork assessment instrument and provides an analysis of the information collected in the first 3 years of linkworking.*

Stevenson O, Parsloe P 1993 Community care and empowerment. Joseph Rowntree, York. *This book describes a project which considers the involvement of users and carers in decisions about their own lives. It provides useful models for assessment and care management that include empowerment and gives practical advice about working with users and carers in a way that empowers.*

Sparkes T 1994 A study of professional attitudes towards older people within an interprofessional context. Journal of Interprofessional Care 8(2): 183–191. *This article presents the results of a qualitative study which considered the perceptions of different groups of professionals in the health and welfare field about the needs of older people. Attitudes towards older people affected perception of need and, in general, older people were perceived by professionals to be passive recipients of care.*

The Ageing Well Handbook 1993 Age Concern England, London. *A practical guide to setting up health promotion activities for older people.*

Ewles L, Simmett I 1985 Promoting health: a practical guide to health education. Wiley, Chichester. *This classic book is an easy to read, practical guide to health education which is divided into three sections: philosophy, planning and practice.*

Therapeutic intervention

16

Counselling: maintaining mental health in older age

Steve Scrutton

COUNSELLING – A DEFINITION

The primary objective of counselling is to involve individuals in a process whereby they can be helped to reflect on, and become more aware of, their current situation and the complexity of their own needs. It seeks to allow them to express their own feelings about their lives, without any attempt to impose our own ideas and views. Thereafter, it seeks to enable them to initiate and develop new and appropriate responses to their situation. (Scrutton 1989, p. 6)

Communication

Counselling involves communication with another person, particularly those who are unhappy, troubled, or finding it difficult to live their lives in harmony with the world. But counselling is more than communication in that it tries to help people to focus on their actual feelings, and to reflect upon their real lives.

The counselling sessions provided Rose (Box 16.1) with the first real conversations she had experienced for a considerable time, and she enjoyed the experience. For Amy (Box 16.2), after being given time and space, she was able to communicate her problems to another person.

A caring or therapeutic technique

Counselling is usually offered from genuine care or concern for an individual, or from a professional responsibility or commitment. But counselling is more than the offer of simple friendship and support. Nor is it just a means of direct help or care (which can be both patronising and disabling); it is more a means of enabling people with problems to help themselves.

This was important for Rose: the counselling session made her a real person again, someone who could converse sensibly. This encouraged other people to talk to her, to be less patronising to a 'senile' woman who

---

Box 16.1 Rose: counselling an older person with dementia

Everyone at the residential home where she lived was attracted to Rose, an amiable, gentle 75-year-old widow. People were beguiled by her welcoming smile, her warmhearted manner, her soft, rounded features, her wise-looking face encircled by curls of grey hair. People responded to her. Rose was everyone's idea of the ideal grandmother.

It was only when she engaged in conversation that people realised that she was suffering from dementia. An initial exchange of pleasantries was inevitably followed by a baffling, bizarre conversation, most often about her 'going home' before her husband returned from work. She had to prepare his tea. When people realised that her husband had died several years previously, they were usually saddened.

Her son and daughter visited regularly, usually briefly. They too were sorrowful that their mother had come to this melancholy condition. Other visitors, after an initial exchange of smiles and 'hellos', moved away and avoided her. The staff had become frustrated with her monotonous conversation. They had heard everything before and bypassed her to continue their work. They were regularly faced with the problem of her late afternoon wandering, often brought back by well-meaning people questioning why staff had 'allowed her out' when she was so clearly confused and a danger to herself. What could they do? Lock her up? They told her in frustration that she lived with them, this was her home, that she no longer had to prepare her husband's tea. She smiled, agreed – and wandered off again.

Rose sought companionship, but was everywhere rejected, spurned by embarrassment rather than intentional hurtfulness. People did not know what to say, or how to respond to her; and they wanted to avoid the pain of witnessing the disintegrating mind of an otherwise charming elderly woman.

Rose loved to sit in her garden chair on warm summer days. Intrigued, I would seek her company, exchange smiles, and try to engage her in conversation. Most people felt I was wasting my time. She attended our 'reality orientation' groups, could identify everyday objects, recall the days of the week, and recognise the weather outside! But the present realities did not seem to impinge on what, to Rose, were the greater urgencies of the past.

So what about the past? Had she always lived in this town? I asked her about her mother and father. Did she have brothers and sisters? What did she do as a child? What games did she play? What school did she attend? Who was her teacher? Did she remember her class friends? How did she spend her weekends?

Rose's responses to these questions were clear and bright. She became animated. She recalled events of 60, even 70 years ago with a clarity that belied her current confusion and apparently dementing brain. Conversations became fascinating history lessons of a young girl who had spent her childhood in the years preceding the Great War. Her recall seemed total, remembering minute details of events with clarity. Moreover, the stories were alive and consistent. She was eager to recall ever more of her past, and always reluctant to finish.

Perhaps her life history could be traced from these childhood memories. Such a journey might unlock the mysteries which surrounded her confused mental state, and gradually bring her to accept her current reality. Her earliest memories of parents and siblings, her play activities, her progress through school, her friends, hobbies and pastimes, even the household chores she undertook, were remembered clearly. Her early boyfriends were recalled with a twinkle in her eyes and demeanour. Here, still present, was the child and the young woman. Old photographs were sought and found, featuring an attractive young girl who would clearly have been a much sought-after companion by the local male population.

'When did you meet your husband?' Memories still flowed from her, perhaps with less animation. 'When did you marry? Do you remember the ceremony, did you have a honeymoon?' Her wedding dress was still vivid in her memory. Her pride in herself, and her parents' pride in her, was evident. But there was also some sadness. 'When were your children born? What were they like as young children?' She spoke of her pride as a mother. Yet progress became more difficult; concentration harder to retain. 'Tell me about your husband. Where did you live? Did you continue to work?'

After this there was nothing, a block; she would not allow further delving into her life. She wished to continue talking about her earlier years; or she became anxious to return home; after all, she had tea to prepare.

I spoke to her daughter. Could she explain this block? She described her mother's unhappy marriage. Her father was often violent towards her. She had little freedom, no life of her own. Tea had to be ready on her father's return from work, or else 'all hell was let loose'. When her father died she thought it would be a release for her. But instead, she began to lose her mind. It was very sad.

It was never possible to delve further into her life, Rose would not permit it. She had locked it away, forever. Her children had grown up, left home, and started families of their own. Perhaps she felt that there was nothing more of value in life for her.

What price sanity within a world she did not want to live in?

But the sessions did bring her happiness by recalling the years of her youth and, by doing so, distracted her from some of her current anxieties. The staff had something to talk to her about. She became a person in her own right, not an empty vessel where once lived a woman.

Perhaps with more time, with greater skill, more would have been possible. Perhaps if the traumas of her life had been counselled contemporaneously her mental decline may have been avoided.

Box 16.2 Amy: counselling an older depressed person

Amy had been in residential care for a year, and was clearly becoming unhappy. Care staff had noticed that in recent weeks she was withdrawing into herself, subject to changing moods, and eating very little. She had complained of boredom, and had spoken several times about 'ending it all'.

This was a transformation from how she had been when she first arrived. She was now saying that she wanted to move to another home, although at the same time she emphasised that she had no complaints about the treatment she was receiving. Nothing anyone could do seemed to cheer her. She seemed to be getting increasingly distant and unapproachable.

She had suffered a series of small strokes before coming into residential care. These had left her with impaired movement and speech. She had recognised that she could no longer cope with living independently and after a brief time with her son's family she had made the decision to move into permanent residential care.

In our initial discussion, Amy confirmed that she wanted to move. She found talking difficult; her speech was slurred and it took her some time to form her words. Often, she would be unable to find the word or an expression she wanted. This would make her very frustrated with herself, angry that she was unable to express herself readily. Amy was an intelligent woman, still bright and aware, but her undulled intellect now appeared to be in advance of her impaired verbal skills.

Unhurriedly, we looked at the options together. We discussed whether she felt that she could live independently in a flat, or in sheltered housing. Amy thought that this was no longer possible and she did not want to cope again with the lonely nights with which she had had difficulty before moving in with her son.

We discussed moving to another residential home. Amy insisted that she had no complaints about where she was, and that another home might be no better. But her daughter lived in the neighbouring town and she wondered whether she would be able to visit more frequently if she moved closer to her. She herself had spent most of her life in the neighbouring town so a return did seem to make some sense. Her son, who lived in this town, had not visited her for some 2 months. We agreed to look at the option but she did not seem happier at the prospect.

At the second meeting Amy was initially quiet. She did not seem interested in discussing the proposed visit. Instead, we talked about her life prior to her strokes. She had lived an active life, involved in many interests and hobbies, as well as her work, to which she was deeply committed. She loved to meet people and travel, and particularly enjoyed writing to the friends she had made throughout the country. She enjoyed being involved with people and said that she had always been happy when helping them with their problems.

Now she felt useless. She was younger than most residents and in less need of support than many. She felt that care staff concentrated on the other residents. She thought that this was correct, she did not want to be critical; but she was obviously hurt by it. Did she feel neglected? Well, a little. She would like an all-over wash every morning but could not manage by herself; and she would like a bath more frequently.

Amy admitted that she was bored. She no longer had a routine and there was no purpose or interest in her life any more. She had accepted that this had to be so. She was, after all, growing old, and she was now disabled. She could not expect to do what she had done as a younger person; but her mind was still active. She had her television and her records, but this was not enough.

In the next session Amy began to talk about her family. She had gone to live with her son when she could no longer cope on her own. It was a disaster. Her grandson was horrible to her and did not want her to live there. So she felt that she had no option but to leave the unpleasantness and, as her home had been relinquished, she thought that her only option was to go into residential care.

Her son had not visited her for some time. Her daughter only came occasionally, living some 10 miles away with a family and a job of her own and no transport. Yet both could visit more regularly if they wanted; they obviously did not want to do so. And she was hurt by this, after all she had done for them over the years.

Amy was worried about losing her temper. She hated the way she felt, and thought it was unlike her to feel so violently angry. She felt that everything had gone wrong during the last year. There were times when she felt suicidal; she said that she would feel like 'walking out' and not coming back. She would not say what she would do, she was uncertain, but she was afraid of what she was intending to do to herself.

Several sessions with Amy followed. Gradually, she began to see that she was too accepting of the limitations of her age and her disability. Both had disabled her more than they should have done, partly because she had accepted that they would and that there was nothing that she could do about them. Her image of old age had always been one of incapacity and dullness; she had accepted them into her life without complaint. We discussed the alternatives, each time challenging and making her examine any 'I cannot' responses.

With Amy's agreement, discussions were opened up to care staff and a new, more detailed care plan was drawn up. She joined the day care group; she re-learnt to write, with her other hand; she joined a local 'exercise' group for stroke victims. She began to live, and to make demands on life again.

could not hold a reasonable conversation. Counselling enabled Amy to express herself, and to understand some of the reasons for her depression. It helped her come to terms with her ageism and disabilities. Eventually, she was able to recognise her underlying feelings, and make decisions about what she was going to do about her situation.

Changing or modifying behaviour

Ultimately, counselling seeks to influence the attitudes and behaviour of another person; but it is more than giving advice, however useful and well-intentioned. The counselling process should enable people:

- to understand
- to come to terms
- to determine their own solutions to their personal problems and situation.

In the time available, Rose was not able to alter her behaviour or attitudes. A tacit decision was taken not to proceed further into the counselling process – to challenge her, or to seek to develop self-awareness. Therefore, it did not lead to noticeable change in her life. But for Amy it began the process of re-examining her life, helping her examine for herself what use she could positively make of her later years.

WHY COUNSELLING IS IMPORTANT IN OLDER AGE

Counselling tasks, that is, the problems addressed by counselling, are not age-specific. They remain the same regardless of a person's age. Moreover, there is no reason why counselling skills cannot be as effective with older people as they are at any other stage of life. The primary counselling objective should be to help maintain and, where possible, to enhance quality of life. This is particularly important in older age which is not normally considered a time in life when satisfaction and fulfilment is either possible or likely. This was certainly so in Amy's case.

Good mental health is intimately linked to life satisfaction and fulfillment. To the extent that people can improve the quality of life of older people, counselling can be a valuable skill and one which is probably much under-used. However, in older age there may be a different emphasis in counselling. This is often associated with an increased experience of loss, and the resulting experience of bereavement. Significant losses may have a powerful impact on mental health in older age unless they are satisfactorily grieved and resolved.

The loss of the parental role

The onset of Rose's distress, and possibly even the onset of her dementia, could probably be traced more to her children leaving home than the death of her husband. This is not an uncommon experience, particularly for those older women who have never worked, or been expected to work in paid employment and for whom child rearing was the principal social role. Yet, because children grow up and move away from parents – an accepted, natural, even a happy event – the impact of such loss on ageing people is often underestimated, unrecognised and remains undiscussed. Many older people have to suffer the loss alone, their feelings of loss often teased and sometimes ridiculed.

Yet if the void is not filled with constructive and fulfilling alternatives, future life can and often does seem to be without value to some older people. They can feel worthless, and suffer a serious loss of self-esteem. For Amy, it was the rejection by her son and grandson that underlaid her depression, allied with the feeling that she was no longer wanted or needed by her family.

Retirement

The loss of the work role is more clearly recognised as a potential problem, perhaps as it is a more male-oriented issue. Pre-retirement counselling courses are now provided by many companies. Rose's husband was not unusual in dying shortly after retirement. Many older men have based their social status, their friendships, and spend the greater part of their time, at their workplace.

The loss of the work role is often thought by others as a gain rather than a loss. Many people fail to recognise the losses involved until it happens to them; many have not prepared themselves for the emptiness, and the feelings of worthlessness that can enter their life. Amy had a fulfilling job, and in part her depression was concerned with the gap that retirement left unfilled in her life.

The loss of financial status

Retirement is often seen as a social reward, but it invariably brings with it a financial cost which, for many older people, severely restricts their social activity and consequently their social engagement. Neither Rose nor Amy had savings and, after the death of their husbands, had to live on state pensions. This merely added to their losses and social isolation.

Loss of social role and involvement, and the increased experience of loneliness

Dominant social attitudes towards old age can disqualify older people from playing a useful social role (McEwan 1990). Age disqualification in employment, even in voluntary work, is common. This remains so regardless of an individual's wishes, abilities and fitness. Older people with the enthusiasm, commitment, acquired wisdom and experience to provide useful social functions are often prevented from doing so, solely on account of their age.

Many older people, including Amy, accept enforced social redundancy and internalise feelings of being worthless and unwanted. It damages their self-esteem, encourages them to opt out and lays the foundation for depression, loneliness, lack of fulfilment and the prospect of a life in older age without meaning or purpose. Even amidst her confusion, Rose clung to her longstanding marital role of having to prepare her husband's tea, long after it had any relevance in her life.

Loss of health

There is no significant correlation between age and health, despite common assumptions. No illness, and no cure for illness, is age-specific. Unfortunately, the idea that old age brings an increased experience of pain, illness and disease often leads older people, and professional medical personnel, to make ageist assumptions about health in older age (Scrutton 1993).

That being said, some older people are subject to increasing pain, illness and disease which can reduce their ability to live fulfilling lives. Often these conditions are considered to be progressively and inevitably degenerative. They are often told there is no prospect of cure.

Good health is important to everyone. In old age, however, ill health is not always recognised as a loss but as a natural and inevitable life event. There is an assumption that older people can accept this without question, distress or regret. This was not so with Amy. No one, including Amy herself, had fully grasped the gap that her stroke had made in her life. There was an assumption, internalised by her, that her strokes had happened, that they were unavoidable, and that all she could do was to accept her disability as a normal part of the ageing process.

Declining physical abilities and dependence

When older people can no longer fend for themselves and when they increasingly have to rely upon other people to carry out basic daily tasks, it can be a depressing, anger-inducing and undignified experience. The emotional impact of dependence is underestimated by carers who, motivated by the best, most caring of intentions, forget the personal loss of esteem and dignity that such help can signify to the individual. When older people have to be dressed, undressed, washed, toileted and fed, carers are undertaking the most intimate functions. They are invading the privacy of other individuals who will almost certainly have feelings about their dependency, feelings which are too often overlooked and rarely discussed.

Counselling was able to help Amy realise that the distress of illness and disability, of becoming dependent on other people, had an important impact on her self-image and therefore on her mental health. This impact could not be discounted or dismissed, regardless of her age.

Loss through death and preparation for death

Survival into old age means that people have outlived many of their peers. As their circle of close friends and relatives declines, each subsequent death can seem more significant. The death of a spouse or longstanding friends can leave an enormous void in the lives of older people. Even the death of media and show-business personalities of their generation, or younger, can appear to be a serious personal loss. For these reasons, bereavement counselling should be an important aspect of the care of older people. However, until 1995 there was no publication which dealt with the subject specifically in relation to older people.

Perhaps one reason for this is that the significance of death in older age is often discounted, considered to be a natural, unavoidable event. This, in turn, can lead to discounting the impact that such loss can have on older survivors. Death may be an inevitable event but it still has to be mourned. It is not uncommon for older people to be denied an opportunity to view the body, or even attendance at funerals, in the belief that they may be too upset; and the tendency to remove bodies rapidly after death seems to be increasing.

Each death not only brings the anguish of bereavement, but the sense of impending personal death. Older people are usually quite aware of their mortality; but younger people either do not want to discuss such matters with them, or they underestimate the importance of doing so.

All these losses, common features of older age, can lead to social and emotional distress, and they are all closely connected with an individual's mental health. They are the legitimate concern of counselling, a process which can help older people come to terms with them as they arise. Thus, effective counselling can not only help older people maintain the quality of their lives but also assist in the maintenance of their mental health.

AGEISM: ITS IMPACT UPON MENTAL HEALTH

Many of the counselling agendas of older age derive, at least in part, from dominant social attitudes about ageing and older people. We no longer value our elders, discounting the wisdom and experience of age in favour of the energy of youth, generally preferring to exchange competence for vigour, loyalty for change, continuity for innovation, and reliability for new ideas and 'progress'. Youth-oriented social preferences lead to discrimination against older people – ageism.

There are two forms of ageism. One arises from genuine concern but becomes patronising when it underestimates the abilities of older people:

- we do not allow older people to work
- we protect them from harm, real or imaginary
- we no longer believe older people can, or should fend for themselves.

This form of ageism, apparently arising out of compassion, can be disabling. We clean their homes, fetch their shopping, ferry them to where they wish to go; and we do all this without thinking that our 'care' might be undermining their independence, even their morale.

The other form of ageism arises from neglect, from discounting the needs of older people. It diminishes social status, reduces social roles, undermines self-esteem, and denies older people a fair share of social resources. Why else do we insist that older people cannot be employed after a certain age? Why else do we ensure that pensions are close to subsistence levels? Why else is the care of frail, dependent older people so frequently inferior to that provided for other social groups?

Both forms of ageism create and foster prejudices about the nature and experience of old age. These usually project unpleasant images of older people which subtly undermine their personal value and worth. Commonly held ideas restrict the social role and status of older people, deny them equal opportunities, structure their expectations of themselves,

prevent them from achieving their potential. The basis of our ageism is deep rooted:

- Capitalism places high value on productivity, and as older people are not (or are not allowed to be) productive, they are undervalued, more often considered to be an economic liability than an asset.
- Religious belief teaches us that the problems of this world are not as important as our place in the next, that closeness to death means closeness to a 'better' world – an attitude that allows us to discount the inferior social status and situation of older people.
- Psychology has taught that the older personality is fixed and unchanging, unable to change and grow. Freud (1905) stated that psychotherapy was not possible after the age of 50 because 'old people are not educable'.
- The medical establishment, a powerful source of dominant social attitudes, informs us that medical skill now enables people to live longer, but when older people become ill there is nothing that can be done to help them; they are ill because of their age.

It is important to understand ageism when counselling older people with mental health problems. It has a powerful influence on how we view older people and, perhaps more important, how older people see themselves. This was certainly true in Amy's case. It produces a stereotype of old age, consisting of a number of different myths (Dixon & Gregory 1987):

The myth of chronology

The idea that elderly people are a homogeneous group by virtue of their age, discounting individuality in terms of need and rates of ageing.

The myth of ill health

That old age automatically involves physical pain, deterioration, and that illness in old age is part of normal ageing, not a disease process, and therefore inevitable and untreatable.

The myth of mental deterioration

That older people automatically lose their mental faculties, slow down and become 'senile'.

The myth of inflexible personality

That personality changes with age to become more intolerant, inflexible and conservative.

The myth of misery

That older people are unhappy because they are old.

The myth of rejection and isolation

That society rejects, and is uncaring towards its older people, and that older people withdraw into themselves and prefer to 'disengage' from life.

The myth of non-productivity/dependence

That older people are not productive members of society; because they are not engaged in paid employment they are inevitably dependent upon others.

To the extent that ageism is endemic within social values, and resides within all of us, these myths are deeply distressing. The stereotype of old age today is perhaps the individual living alone, socially isolated, managing on an inadequate income, suffering from poor health, poorly housed, dependent on younger carers for support and seen generally as a burden. This paints a picture of an old age designed to give rise to mental health problems. Many ageing people believe in and internalise these myths; some may cope with resignation but others become depressed.

Amy had to be challenged about some of the ageist myths that she had internalised. She had been living her life with an acceptance of its dullness, unavoidable because of her age and her disability: myths were preventing her from developing a meaningful life for herself. Counselling was an effective means of asking her to express her understanding of ageing, and for her to reconsider aspects which were not, or which need not be, reality and which might be a cause of her depression, a threat to her mental health.

Professional work with older people – identifying the individual

The importance of good communication with older people cannot be overemphasised. It is central to:

- seeking to enhance the quality of life in old age
- undertaking professional 'needs-led' assessments
- making decisions directly affecting the lives of older people
- developing caring/therapeutic relationships
- the efficient delivery of medical and social services to older people
- constructing programmes of individual care

- developing and maintaining programmes of quality assurance in all professional settings.

Indeed, it is hard to imagine how there can be quality in work with older people unless we are aware of the personal hopes, aspirations, expectations and preferences of the individual. If the six principles on which good-quality residential care of older people should be assessed are considered (Department of Health 1989), the importance of counselling skills can be readily understood:

If the aim is to provide choice

Choice is invariably exercised at a personal level, and relies upon people understanding their potential and limitations, and the implications of choosing each of the options available to them.

If we want to provide privacy

The distance between privacy and loneliness can be minimal. There has to be an exercise of professional judgement, based on a full understanding of the individual, about where the desire for privacy ends and where loneliness begins.

To maintain a person's independence

It is important that we are able to help people feel sufficiently confident, well-motivated and self-assured to continue doing things for themselves. To achieve this, it is often important to understand why an individual becomes discouraged, resigned to dependency, no longer able to cope without increasing help from other people.

To ensure individual rights

Older people must know and understand what their rights are, what they want for themselves, what is possible, what they can aspire to and to what they are entitled. Too often, older people are grateful for what is being done for them, even when it is too little too late, or even grossly inadequate.

To sustain a person's dignity

It is important that we know what people understand as being 'dignified' and 'undignified', the crucial social and emotional factors upon which their self-image and pride are based, and when these factors are challenged in their lives.

To enable an individual to experience fulfilment

In order for people to feel fulfilled, it is essential that we have some idea about what they wish to strive for and accomplish for themselves; what makes a person feel satisfied and content, and what gives someone enjoyment and pleasure.

Counselling, then, is a means – perhaps an essential means –of identifying the individual, and of being able to recognise and bring out that individuality. It should seek to avoid the many global assumptions – many of them stereotypical and ageist – that are made about older people, their needs and their aspirations. This is particularly important when considering the racial and cultural dimensions of ageing. It is often assumed that ethnic minority elders live within supportive extended families, and that their need for professional care and support are invariably reduced because of their family or cultural group. Such stereotypical views oversimplify the diversity of ethnic cultures, and ignore the many complex processes of family dynamics within minority communities.

Many ethnic minority elders living in this country were immigrants who originally had no intention of remaining here for the rest of their lives. They invariably have fewer age-peers than their white compatriots. The process of cultural assimilation has often meant that there has arisen a divergence of cultural values between older and younger generations within families. The result is that many ethnic elders can feel more lonely, more isolated, more alienated than their indigenous compatriots.

When racism is added to the ageist and cultural agendas (including not only the clashes that occur between minority and dominant cultures, but also language barriers, insensitivity to the needs of different ethnic groups, and the provision of 'culture-bound' services and institutions whose policies and practices have been developed in response to the specific needs of the ageing indigenous population) the social and emotional problems faced by many ethnic minority elders can be considerable. This combination of factors have been described by Norman (1985) as 'triple jeopardy', which can lead to distress and to serious mental health problems.

For both Rose and Amy, counselling was able to change their lives. It meant the difference between passively accepting their situation as an inevitable part of growing older, with the caring task merely a matter of 'warehousing' people who no longer had any contribution to make, and taking proactive steps to improve their quality of life in their later years.

THE COUNSELLING RELATIONSHIP

Counselling implies a level of personal intimacy with another person and this has implications for the counselling relationship. In order to facilitate intimate communication, and to make it ethically acceptable, a special commitment is required on the part of the counsellor which is not always present in conventional professional/client relationships. These relationship factors are all aimed to ensure that the process is client-centred, rather than agency-centred – an important consideration in developing 'needs-led' community assessments.

Non-directive

Counsellors cannot enter into a counselling relationship with the intention of directing counsellees to alter their attitudes, to change their behaviour or to take control of their emotions. This remains so even if, as professional people, we feel that this would be 'in their best interests'.

A directive relationship implies that the 'director' knows best, and that the 'directed' are incapable of reaching their own solutions to their own problems. Such an approach would certainly have been unhelpful with Amy who was quite capable of resolving her own problems. But, with older people, directive relationships are common; they are unequal, comprising dominant and submissive parties. These types of relationship only work if the submissive parties can do what they are told, want to do what they are told, and if there are no internal or external restraints preventing them doing what they are told.

Non-directive relationships imply a respect for the worth of older people, which seeks to recognise their individuality, their dignity and their ultimate responsibility. They assume that people have the right to self-determination and the ability to make sound judgements and decisions for themselves. Rose would talk only about those things that she wished to discuss. It would have been counterproductive, not to say unkind, to have pressed her into discussing matters which were uncomfortable for her.

Non-judgemental

When individual attitudes or behaviour are considered immoral or unacceptable, another problem arises in human communication – there is a tendency to 'pass judgement' on people. This is unhelpful in counselling, whose objective is to understand the feelings and motivations which underlie behaviour. Any hint of disapproval or condemnation can erect barriers which can prevent open and honest communication. It would, for example, have been easy to imply to Amy that by wishing to move she was being ungrateful for the care she had received during the previous year, or that Rose really should try to come to terms with the present. If such a message had been given, Amy would have been unlikely to move on towards the real problems that she discussed in later sessions.

Such moral neutrality is an ideal rarely attained. Often, professional responsibilities make it difficult to achieve. Even so, there are ways of avoiding disapproval. Views can be expressed as 'the social view' concerning their behaviour; or concern can be expressed about the impact that their behaviour has on how they may be seen by friends, or within society generally. Or, more honestly, we can present them as our views, but in a way that invites discussion rather than rejection.

Unconditional positive regard

Counsellors should not look upon older people as inferior or abnormal despite the difficulties their emotional condition or social behaviour may present. This was, to an extent, what had been happening to Rose. Her confusion led to her being dismissed as not worth talking to – she had nothing to say that was worth hearing.

The counselling relationship should be based on the belief that ageing people, whatever their problems, have an inherent worth and dignity, and that their right to self-determination is respected. Counsellees should be seen as individuals in difficulty, but who have the capability, through their own inner resources, to overcome their own problems, and to redirect their lives, through their own efforts.

Empathetic understanding

The counsellor should try to view the world as the counsellee sees it: ' ... to perceive the world as the client sees it, to perceive the client himself as he is seen by himself, to lay aside all perceptions from the external frame of reference while doing so, and to communicate something of the empathetic understanding to the client' (Rogers 1951, p. 29).

In this way it becomes possible to understand some of the apparently illogical or self-damaging aspects of social performance. It is vital that counsellors avoid denying the problems and difficulties as they are perceived by the counsellee. Nothing is usefully served by denying the problems and difficulties others feel. It is sufficient that they feel them for us to take them seriously. To deny them is to fail to respond, and leads to the belief that we do not really care how they feel.

Empathy enables the counsellor to form tentative explanations about what is happening and why it is happening, what people are thinking and why they are thinking it, and linking this with their social performance. The ability to empathise with how an individual feels is central to the counselling process.

In counselling Rose I was able to formulate tentative explanations about the social and mental reasons underlying her dementia – an alternative explanation which may, or may not, have had substance. With Amy, I hypothesised that her internalised ageism, her too-ready acceptance of her disability, and the rejection by her family all contributed to her depression. All these were behind her 'presenting' problem of wanting to move to another home. Amy's responses honed these suppositions. She was able to accept and reject them, or apportion importance to each according to how she actually felt.

Genuineness

Counselling is a two-way process, with the counsellor being able to relate honestly and also capable of sharing her feelings when appropriate: 'The more the therapist is himself or herself in the relationship, putting up no professional front or personal façade, the greater is the likelihood that the client will change and grow in a constructive manner' (Rogers 1961, p. 282).

Social distance and assumptions of superiority are unhelpful in counselling relationships. It is important that counsellors present themselves as people rather than as 'doctors', 'psychologists' or 'social workers', or any other professional title. For people in difficulty, or under stress, there is nothing more depressing than being faced by a paragon, someone with no personal difficulties, the person with all the answers. Such people highlight assumed inadequacies rather than ameliorate troubled emotions. The counsellor should try to be a 'real' person in order to be helpful.

When older people are being counselled by younger people, genuineness becomes a bit of a problem. I was unable to experience life in old age as Rose or Amy did. But showing genuine interest in how people feel is usually sufficient.

Trust and confidentiality

In any relationship dealing with issues surrounding personal emotions, trust is essential. No-one openly reveals themselves to people they do not trust. Confidentiality is an essential basis for a trusting relationship. For many people, the sharing of intimate, unknown details of their lives can lead to embarrassment, guilt or anxiety. It took courage for Amy to admit that she had been rejected by her son and grandson. People will not enter into such revelation unless they are sure that it will not be transmitted to other people.

THE SKILLS OF COUNSELLING

Counselling is not just a matter of talking with another person, particularly when that person is distressed, anxious, and preoccupied with personal problems. In such circumstances it is important that the counsellor is able to offer skills which encourage and enable the expression of feelings.

Establishing a relaxed, non-threatening atmosphere

The counsellor should seek to be as warm, supportive and caring as possible. Comfortable seating, discreet lighting, the absence of distracting noise, the avoidance of interruptions, and a relaxing agent such as a cup of tea, can all be aids to a good counselling session.

It is the responsibility of the counsellor to move into the 'difficult' areas of feeling, and to do so as gently as possible. The counsellor needs to be as relaxed and natural as possible because any sign of tension is easily transmitted and can create anxiety within the counsellee.

Listening

This is the most important counselling skill, but one which is not a universal human trait! The tendency to manipulate, exploit, disseminate information, moralise, sermonise, give advice and instructions, is all too common. Moreover, professional people are probably the worst offenders, trying perhaps to cope with too many time and resource constraints, or with too many agency agendas, all of which militate against giving sufficient time to the time-consuming process of listening.

Listening is the starting point of the counselling process. To arrive there the counsellor has to stop talking, perhaps after asking straightforward, answerable questions, preferably those which have been carefully considered before the meeting, and then giving sufficient time and scope to hear the answers.

So often people do not give sufficient time to older people, perhaps feeling that they have more important things to do. It can be of great benefit when someone does listen and appears genuinely interested in what they say. Just spending time listening to both Rose and Amy had an early and demonstrable effect on their morale.

Assisting self-expression

People will discuss their feelings when they feel that there is someone willing to listen to them sympathetically. The counsellor needs to give continuing reassurance of interest and concern – through facial expressions and both verbal and non-verbal gestures of understanding. One technique, 'reflecting back' involves making short 'summaries' of what has been said. And by seeking 'clarification' the counsellor can both demonstrate interest, and develop deeper understanding.

Some older people have communication problems. With Amy it was important to make her feel at ease despite her inability to find her words. Any sense of impatience would have made the problem worse and probably resulted in less openness and honesty.

The focus of counselling should always be on feelings. The counsellor should seek to ask questions which elicit the individual's emotional state rather than to elucidate the facts of any situation. When counselling Rose, I was able to elicit how she felt at each stage of her life – from the joys of childhood, and child-rearing, to the acceptability of work, to the unhappiness of marriage.

Interpretation

The counsellor has to interpret what is said, extracting from the words being used the feelings and meanings which often lie just beneath the surface, and decoding the body language which often more accurately signifies feeling than what is said. Interpretation is made more important by the daily lies of politeness, disingenuous responses by which we avoid the need to talk about difficult subjects. We do this by only saying things we believe others want to hear, or refraining from saying what we believe they do not want to hear. In this way, people often hide from others the pain they feel.

Older people can be particularly adept at this. They can often express feelings of contentment or resignation which do not represent their real emotions as much as their ageist-reduced expectations of life in old age. They may say that everything is 'OK' when it is far from being so. This may be no more than an expression of their perception about what is possible in old age, about what expectations are acceptable or reasonable for older people to have.

When counselling Amy, I never felt that moving to another home was what she wanted. This was the 'presenting problem', the one she felt able to talk about initially. If I had been wrong she would have pursued my offer. Accepting what she said, but giving her time to talk about what I interpreted to be her real feelings – her ageism, disabilities, and her disappointment with her family – she was eventually able to confirm that they were important factors in her depression. With Rose, there was even more interpretation, principally her unhappy marriage, but most remained unconfirmed.

Working hypothesis

After listening to and interpreting what is being said, counsellors will begin to form their own understandings and insights about what they have heard, and about how the counsellee is experiencing life. This understanding should seek to integrate many factors – their interests and aptitudes, their feelings and relationships, their strengths and weakness, the past, the effect of significant life events, and the way they view their future. Patterns of behaviour may emerge which seem to indicate that the individual is likely to react in similar ways in similar situations. Links and connections can then be made between all these factors.

The hypothesis will focus on self-image and self-esteem, and the way that these impinge upon the individual's perception of the world and his ability to act within it. This may help the counsellor to understand why older people do not respond to situations in more logical, less self-damaging ways. If older people see life through helpless, defeated eyes, when they have become resigned to pain, disappointment, loneliness and despair, their reaction to new situations will not be positive. Negative outcomes will, in turn, serve only to confirm the correctness of their negative view of life.

The working hypothesis is not, however, an unchanging phenomenon, nor necessarily a correct interpretation. It was essential to my hypothesis that Amy had taken an 'ageist' approach to her old age, and that the problems Rose faced concerned her marriage. Counselling requires a continuous process of confirmation, clarification and re-clarification to ensure that such hypotheses are reasonable, accurate, and that they remain so.

Challenging – focusing on difficult areas

As counselling progresses, it is often clear that it begins to do more than 'listening', although listening remains vitally important. It seeks to concentrate on areas which are difficult, even painful for the individual. And, when necessary, it should challenge individuals about their personal position in relation to the issues that confront them.

To dwell upon the problem emotions of others is often frowned upon as 'morbid curiosity', likely to lead to highlighting and prolonging problems, and so causing unnecessary pain. Yet problems ignored are rarely problems forgotten; and counselling which seeks to focus on problems does not cause distress directly, but brings out distress which is already present within the individual, perhaps distress which is affecting social performance and mental health.

Often, when mental blocks are met, people need to be challenged. Older people, often lonely, will use counselling sessions as company, a social prop, and this will not necessarily lead to a re-examination of their life and to change and growth.

It may also be necessary for counsellors to confront counsellees with an alternative understanding of the problems they face. People often blame others for their problems, failing to look at their personal role. People may have become 'locked' within feelings of helplessness, no longer prepared to look at options and decisions that they can make to improve their own situation. Older people can so 'internalise' ageist assumptions that they have accepted the pain and difficulty of their situation too readily, or feel unable to tackle their own problems proactively.

Neither Rose nor Amy was challenged. It was not necessary to do so with Amy, and there would have had to have been more certainty of a positive outcome to do so with Rose. At present, there is little evidence that cognitive abilities can be developed in people with dementia. To have made more progress with her, however, she would have had to be gently challenged about her refusal to talk about her married years. Confrontation is often an essential and necessary step to helping older people regain control of their lives, and movement towards some fulfilment and life satisfaction. Yet the way confrontation is handled should not be destructive; it can be done firmly, but gently and sympathetically.

Facilitating decision-making

Helping people make decisions about their lives is the ultimate goal of counselling. The ability of older people to develop and grow through decision-making is often restricted by ageism. There must be some belief that new attitudes and determinations, innovative approaches, fresh behaviours and outlooks and novel challenges are quite possible in old age.

Counsellors can assist decision-making by considering the options that people feel that they have in their situation, the advantages and disadvantages of choosing each option, and deciding on the best option available to them. This then leads to a personal determination to self-action.

Amy was able to move on to make decisions for herself. She had full control of her faculties and, after several counselling sessions, she regained sufficient confidence in herself to make them. Each decision, each piece of progress confirmed her self-image and enabled her to continue. With Rose it was different. She did not have sufficient control of her mind to begin coming to terms with her past life, or making decisions about her future. Perhaps I did not have sufficient skill, or perhaps there was not sufficient time. The counselling process, for whatever reason, did not reach this stage in her case.

THE COUNSELLING PROCESS

Counselling seeks to involve troubled individuals in an experience of transformation or healing. But how is such a process achieved? And what is the nature of the journey through which the counsellee passes?

Social distress

The counselling process invariably starts with troubled, restricted, inadequate or disturbed individuals, whose feelings of worthlessness, inadequacy, fear or vulnerability have affected their social performance in serious, perhaps damaging ways, and whose relationships with others have become difficult, unbearable or have broken down entirely. Such demoralisation can often become self-fulfilling, establishing what Sherman (1981) describes as the 'vicious circle of increasing incompetence'. This can be particularly important in the lives of older people (as with Amy) when ageism can often ensure that they find it difficult to maintain a sense of personal worth, or to retain a belief that their lives can still have meaning and purpose.

It is into this cycle of social distress and related

mental health problems that counselling can seek to enter. Perhaps Amy was declining into this pattern of grief, unhappiness and depression. Perhaps Rose had declined further into this pattern of despair, unable to address the real problems of her real world.

Self-expression

Counselling is often called the 'talking cure' and is believed to work on the basis of 'a trouble shared is a trouble halved'. The emotional release offered by self-expression can often be seen, especially with older people when, after quite brief periods of talking, many pressures and worries appear to be visibly lifted from their shoulders.

Often, older people will need considerable assistance before they fully explain their attitudes, outlook and feelings about their situation. They may need to feel sufficiently relaxed, at ease and feel that the counsellor is interested in them and has time to listen.

Whenever possible, the counsellor should try to elicit their feelings beyond the superficial emotions of anger, hate, hostility. Often, it is these superficial emotions that are presented initially. These can be real and strong, affecting the way people lead their lives, but 'angry' emotions usually have deeper origins, and counselling can help people move towards these more complex emotions, which usually involve sadness, disappointments, inadequacies, fears and grief.

Amy was unable to speak about her anger towards her family at first. Rose was never able to express her anger about the life she had with her husband. Amy was able to move on, Rose was only able to move back in time. Amy's anger and dissatisfaction were pushing her towards depression, perhaps towards suicide. Rose may have chosen not to live in the real world any more. Perhaps these are psycho-mental, as well as psycho-somatic, mechanisms.

Blocks

Self-expression is not always readily forthcoming. Often the counsellor will encounter 'blocks' – areas or issues which the individual will refuse to discuss. Sometimes blocks can be temporary. It was sufficient to allow Amy time to move on from the initial presenting problems. At other times blocks can be deeper, hiding the 'unpleasant' truths of reality from themselves and others, and remain closed. The block Rose demonstrated, her unwillingness to discuss her married life, was more intractable.

A block, a refusal to move into a particular area of discussion, normally signifies that the counsellor has reached the core of the problem. It is therefore important that the counsellor is able to pursue the issue – to challenge – although without alienating the individual by doing so. There also has to be good reason to move on, perhaps lacking in Rose's case where there was no certainty that she would ever be able to cope with the consequences of looking again at her blocked past.

Developing self-awareness

Enabling self-expression and overcoming blocks allows people to explain where they stand in their world at the present time. The picture they draw helps us understand how they feel. It is often a static picture, a snapshot which is not necessarily helpful in explaining why people have arrived where they are, or give any real clue about possible future development. Self-expression is primarily reflective rather than contemplative.

If there is to be change and development in a person's life, it can only come from within the individual. It cannot be effectively imposed through advice or medication, however well-intentioned. The counsellor has to be the enabler rather than the enforcer of change. Helping counsellees achieve greater self-awareness involves many distinct areas, and different levels of understanding, through which the counsellor can transfer to the counsellee the many factors which affect their social performance (Scrutton 1989). Self-awareness can help counsellees to:

- recognise the situations, events or people that provoke stress, and how they react to such stress
- understand how they have coped with similar stress in the past and draw attention to the coping strategies and behaviours that they might re-use in the current situation
- look closely at their emotions in order to decide whether they are necessary or an on-going indulgence over which they could exercise more self-control
- recognise their personal needs and how these can best be fulfilled in the current situation
- make connections between their unfulfilled needs, their emotions and their social performance
- become aware of repeating patterns of relationships and behaviour which may have led to unhappy situations throughout their lives, thereby identifying the part they play in bringing about these recurring patterns

- look closely at their attitudes and beliefs in order to determine the effect these have on their lives and, when necessary, to begin reassessing their value
- make connections between what has occurred in the past and how this affects what they are achieving or failing to achieve in the present
- understand the social factors which affect their ability to lead their lives and, in particular, the impact of ageism on their entire outlook
- make connections between personal expectations and the constraints imposed upon them by ageism
- examine their current self-image to decide how this can be improved, and what has to be done in order for this to be achieved.

It is interesting to note that as Rose was not taken through the former stage (her block), she was unable to move on to this stage of the counselling process. Whether counselling can help people with a dementing brain regain a capacity for self-awareness and insight remains unclear. It would ultimately depend upon whether some dementias arise from a social withdrawal from a too-painful reality (as I suspect), or if it is entirely concerned with brain dysfunction, which is unproven.

Amy did move on and became more aware of herself, the factors which were leading to her depression, and what she could do to improve the quality of her life.

Decision-making – modifying social performance

Self-awareness requires personal recognition and acceptance of some of these factors. Yet, whilst self-understanding is a vital ingredient of the counselling process, what the individual decides to do with these newly discovered insights is equally important if change is to occur.

Any decision in favour of change has to be allied with the ability and confidence to change. Is change possible in older age? It is certainly not always easy. Many older people, like Amy, have accepted their depressed and unhappy status. Ageism may have undermined their confidence in their ability to effect change or to improve the quality of their lives. Yet for change to occur, there has to be the desire for personal change and the confidence that change can take place.

Once change is seen to be possible, as it was in Amy's case, then certain choices can be made about how an individual is going to tackle the problems. The counsellor can assist this process by:

- deciding upon the nature of the task that has to be accomplished
- discussing the available options and the consequences and possible outcomes of each option
- helping the individual make firm decisions about change
- deciding what is to be done and who is to carry out the tasks
- supporting the individual through the process of change.

The eventual goal of counselling is to improve social and interpersonal relationships, to produce people more aware of their situation and the problems they face but who are able to cope with the pressures, strains and disappointments that life entails.

WORKING IN GROUPS

Counselling older individuals does have its limitations, particularly when they have become inactive, lonely and depressed. There are limits to the 'talking cure': it will not generate activity or companionship, nor demonstrate that other people exist who are grappling with similar problems.

There are several levels at which groups can operate, all of which can be useful when working with older people. At their most basic level, groups can be valuable purely as a means of providing social companionship, activities of all descriptions, and for the intellectual stimulation this can bring to the lives of lonely people. Counselling can encourage older people to join such groups which range from day-care groups, luncheon clubs, church or village/community based groups, social clubs and many others.

Groups can also be established and used specifically to discuss the issues of ageing. It is often possible to assemble counselling groups with the specific intention of bringing together older people with similar problems – perhaps retirement, bereavement, or loneliness. Such groups can then serve a useful 'group-counselling' function. Individuals can be encouraged to share their problems with other ageing people, helping them realise that they are not alone in facing problems, a common belief which isolated personal circumstance can encourage. Older people can then exchange feelings, discuss solutions and give each other some insight into how others seek to deal with their lives. Such sharing can help people move out of their own, often closed, world of despair and begin to focus on other people. This can be mutually beneficial.

They can respond sympathetically and be responded to similarly.

Peer counselling takes the use of groups a stage further. Self-help groups seek to recognise and utilise the abilities and insights of older people directly in the counselling process; older people are counselled by older people. These groups can overcome the arrogant ageism which assumes that older people can only be helped by younger people. Indeed, peer groups have specific advantages; people from the same generation have a shared pattern of experiences, beliefs and attitudes which have all arisen within their particular generation. And they face together and share the same social attitudes towards them.

In recent years there has been an encouraging increase in the number of local self-help groups. One example, dealing with bereaved people, is the 'widow-to-widow' programmes developed by Silverman et al (1974) in the USA, which proved to be extremely valuable in providing counselling and practical support. Women who had passed successfully through the mourning process were recruited and trained to offer help and support to recently bereaved widows, with new widows invited to attend group meetings where they were able to meet people in similar situations, and during which a variety of grief-related matters were discussed.

Ultimately, groups can be formed by older people with specific aims of self-help or even self-action. Older people are gradually becoming less passive, more assertive in demanding their social and political rights. Given the constraints of ageism, this is a positive development with ageing people uniting to fight for improvements in medical care, pensions and other factors relating to their social status and their quality of life.

One final group whose importance needs to be emphasised are age-integrated groups. These have the advantage of opposing the social trend towards age segregation which increasingly maintains that older people, as a group, should be treated, housed and considered in other ways as 'separate' from the rest of the population. Not every older person wants to be in the company of peers and many prefer to spend time with younger people. Opportunities to do so can be provided by groups established to pursue specific interests, pursuits or hobbies in which the older person has an interest, such as cooking or photography.

Age-integrated groups can lead to valuable exchanges of feelings and knowledge between the generations. Moreover, older people with time to spare can often fulfil useful roles within the organisation and running of such groups.

REMINISCENCE

Reminiscence is a useful ally to counselling. It is a means to conversation. It can break the ice and lead to more difficult discussions about the present. It can cement the counselling relationship, and demonstrate a willingness to spend time, to listen to, and understand the counsellee. These were all important factors with Rose.

Whilst people of all ages reminisce, old age is, not unnaturally, a time when looking back at our lives, reviewing the failures and triumphs, the joys and sorrows, the pleasures and regrets, is of particular importance. It is now generally accepted that reminiscence is a normal, and often an important aspect of growing old successfully. It can highlight a person's assets rather than weaknesses, it can enhance feelings of self-worth and esteem, it can help people recognise their individuality and identity, it can aid the process of life review and it can be an enjoyable and stimulating experience.

It was certainly important for Rose. Reflecting on her past stimulated and enlivened her, transforming her from a depressed, anxious woman, losing control of her mind, to a lively and interesting companion. As a counsellor, it enabled me to speak to her easily and without coercion, to engage with her in conversation that was valuable in itself but also led to other benefits and areas of work.

Reminiscence can provide the counsellor with a life history. This in itself can indicate that we are engaged with someone who is more than an unhappy, disturbed person, more than an old man or old woman in inevitable and certain decline. We become aware that we are talking to an individual with a past and with experiences. These can bring the person 'alive', transforming an individual from the ageist perceptions of old people that too often dominate our vision. Such insight can also give useful clues about the problems and difficulties which they have faced in the past and how they have coped, or failed to cope, with them. It can give insights into the past mental health of the individual, and can help locate the origins of current problems which may, as with Rose, go back many years.

It is not usually difficult to reminisce with older people. Indeed, it is often easier to do so than to discuss their current reality. Old photographs and other memorabilia can assist the process. It can lead to people producing a life-history in whatever form and with whatever abilities they can muster. Moreover, such a life-review can help older people make sense of their lives, give meaning to them and place them in a wider perspective – all harmonious, beneficial addenda to the counselling process. Chapter 22 provides a more detailed discussion of the value of reminiscence.

CONCLUSION

The ultimate aim of counselling is to achieve improvement in social and interpersonal relationships, to help people become more adaptable and flexible, to live in the real world of the present, able to deal with whatever problems and difficulties it presents.

Counselling seeks to help people recognise their needs and wants, their likes and dislikes, but to help them to be realistic about when such desires are likely and not likely to be fulfilled. It seeks to help people strive for satisfaction, and to help them defend and protect themselves from disappointments and setbacks. It seeks to help people who can accept responsibility both for themselves and others, who can use their initiative to control events rather than to drift aimlessly through life. It can help people come to terms with their present lives, to accept the past for what it was, remembering it with fondness but able also to look at the present and view the future with a degree of optimism and hope.

Counselling may never achieve all this but, to the extent that it can move some way towards it, it is always beneficial. Amy was able to pass through the process, and became a more fulfilled older person as a result. Rose was not able to make the journey in full; but to the extent that she was able to talk sensibly about the past and, whilst doing so, to engage in conversation other people, it was personally helpful to her. Therefore, in terms of mental health, counselling can be seen in two ways.

First, it can be a preventive measure, as in Amy's case, assisting in the maintenance of good mental health by helping older people come to terms with the many violations of living to old age, and to live comfortably as older people within our ageist social context. Rose would certainly have benefited from counselling at three stages: during her years of marriage, shortly after the death of her husband and after the 'loss' (through marriage) of her children. Had she been able to come to terms with these periods in her life, had she been able to retain her optimism, her happiness, a measure of life-satisfaction, her life as an older person may have been a more positive experience. As it was, counselling enabled her relatives and carers to have sensible conversations with her, in which she became more than just a 'dementing old woman'. It brought her happiness, it increased her circle of companions, people willing to spend time with her.

Could it have done more? The second benefit of counselling is in the treatment of mental health problems. It was certainly beneficial with Amy, who was able to redirect and recommence her life. With more time and confidence, counselling might have encouraged Rose to recall the unpleasant years of her life and the purposeless years that followed. It could have helped her give new meaning to life in her old age. If counselling had provided Rose with more understanding of her situation, outlined her options, if it had raised her expectations and reduced her fears, perhaps even the dementia which was destroying her mind may have been avoided.

What would be useful is more experience in attempting such positive intervention with older people rather than routinely assuming that dementia is an unavoidable, untreatable biological disease. To do so would have meant challenging her, with all the upset and distress that can involve, in order to see whether a response can be gained. In Rose's case there seemed no reason for her not recalling the 'unpleasant' events of her life which, after all, post-dated the pleasant times she recalled quite happily and readily. Had she then been able to re-experience some of the pain of those years, and come to terms with it, she might then have been able to accept the reality of her world and re-enter into the business of living.

Rose died. But there are many other Roses, with many other mental health conditions who will continue to exist. What may be required is the confidence, time and skills to pursue the question of why some older people decide to 'switch off' and whether it is possible to help them recommence the process of living again.

Amy went on to make as much of her life as possible, and she continues to do so, positively and with determination. If counselling can counter ageism and give meaning and purpose to life into older age, it should certainly have an increasing role in the treatment of mental health problems with older people.

REFERENCES

Department of Health Social Services Inspectorate 1989 Homes are for living in. HMSO, London
Dixon J Gregory L 1987 Ageism. Action Baseline, Winter edn: 21–23
Freud S 1905 On psychotherapy. Hogarth Press, London
Norman A 1985 Triple jeopardy: growing old in a second homeland. Centre for Policy on Ageing, London
McEwan E 1990 Age: the unrecognised discrimination. Age Concern England, London
Rogers C 1951 Client-centred therapy. Constable, London

Scrutton S 1989 Counselling older people: a creative response to ageing. Edward Arnold, London
Scrutton S 1993 Ageing, healthy and in control. Chapman and Hall, London
Sherman E 1981 Counselling the aging: an integrated approach. Free Press, New York
Silverman P R, MacKenzie D, Pettipas M, Wilson E 1974 Helping each other in widowhood. Health Sciences, New York

RECOMMENDED READING

Department of Health Social Services Inspectorate 1989 Homes are for living in. HMSO, London. *A booklet which informs the function of inspection. It details the factors inherent in the six fundamental components of good care – privacy, choice, independence, dignity, rights, fulfilment. These are very relevant for consideration by any anti-ageist counsellors of older people.*
Rogers C 1951 Client-centred therapy. Constable, London. *The founder of non-directive counselling, this is one of his many books that have become classic counselling texts.*
Scrutton S 1989 Counselling older people: a creative response to ageing. Edward Arnold, London. *Examines the importance of counselling skills to older people, particularly for people who wish to take an anti-ageist stance. It outlines counselling skills, and applies them to work with older people.*
Scrutton S 1993 Ageing, healthy and in control. Chapman and Hall, London. *The book insists that 'to be old is not to be ill', and focuses on how older people and their carers can both prevent and cope with illness in older age. It is critical of conventional medical treatment and of iatrogenic disease in*
older people, and focuses on self-help and the potential of 'alternative' medical therapies. It includes a discussion on the subject of mental illness.
Scrutton S 1995 Bereavement and grief: supporting older people through loss. Edward Arnold, London.
Sherman E 1981 Counselling the aging: an integrated approach. Free Press, New York. *A US text which tends to present counselling as a complicated skill. It outlines a programme for relieving emotional problems through an 'integrative approach' which incorporates client perceptions and understanding of life events, drawing on the capacities and strengths of older people. It applies and adapts cognitive techniques of counselling to the specific needs of older people.*
Silverman P R, MacKenzie D, Pettipas M, Wilson E 1974 Helping each other in widowhood. Health Sciences, New York. *Describes a US programme in which widows were trained in counselling techniques which they then used to help more recently bereaved widows. It emphasises the importance of empathy in counselling relationships.*

17

Speech, language and communication

Niki Muir
Anne Baseby
Liz Cavaglieri

INTRODUCTION

'We don't seem to be able to communicate any more'
is a phrase to be heard across the generations as
relationships change or founder. Our linguistic and
communicative abilities are, in all probability, the
biggest cognitive skill we possess and yet they are the
most undervalued – until something goes wrong.

Changes in communication output signal changes
in mood, in levels of confidence, in educational growth
and in personal development. Our linguistic abilities
inform our thoughts and our memories, and they help
us organise, plan and retain. If one considers the areas
of life that would suffer should communication be
impaired it is actually impossible to think of any area
which would be totally spared. Most of us have
experienced a degree of communication inadequacy at
first hand in our attempts to learn a second language.
We are therefore aware of the fragmentation of
understanding, the slowness to process, the struggle to
respond and the anxiety over grammar and accent.
Underlying all this is fear of misinterpretation, of
failure or of looking foolish and yet few imagine what
it must be like if the language in question is our own
native tongue.

Many factors throughout our lives impinge on
communication. Sensory deficits as well as general
health and wellbeing affect it and social, emotional,
developmental and psychological factors can cause
significant changes both expressively and receptively.
The purpose of this chapter is threefold. First, to
discuss the complexity of language, speech and communication and to make clear the differences between
each of these skills which are uniquely separate, while
together they form the interactive process each part of
a chain which must be intact. Second, to consider the
variety of ways the normal changes in ageing as well
as specific mental health problems and other acquired

disorders can adversely affect these skills. Third, to discuss management techniques for assessment, differential diagnosis and treatment.

THE ROLE OF THE SPEECH AND LANGUAGE THERAPIST

Communication skills are like an intricate patchwork. No health care professional can adequately and holistically work with elderly people without recognising and addressing issues of language, speech and communication function. These do not just relate to the client's level of functioning but also to our own, since our communication skills are possibly the main 'tool' in our armoury to facilitate and maintain the quality of life of our clients and their carers. To quote Clare: 'Our mastery of communication affects our efficacy as clinicians every bit as much as our technical skill and our theoretical knowledge do' (Clare 1992, p. 12).

The role of the speech and language therapist (SLT) in working with elderly people with mental health problems is comparatively recent and coincides with the expansion of psychiatric services for the elderly from the 1970s (Wattis 1988). A survey carried out by the College of Speech and Language Therapists' Dementia Working Party (1990) found that access to speech and language therapy services for elderly clients had increased from 12% in 1981 (Wattis et al 1981) to 30% in 1990. In spite of this increase in service provision, speech and language therapy remains a small profession and demand for services greatly outstrips supply. This highlights the importance of other healthcare professionals having a good understanding of speech, language and communication difficulties in old age psychiatry and of SLTs exploring the most effective ways of delivering their services.

In common with other healthcare professionals working with elderly people, the role of the SLT addresses issues of assessment, differential diagnosis, management and training. The unique skill of the SLT is the ability to decode degraded and deteriorated speech and language (Faber et al 1983); an ability acquired through a training which includes, amongst other studies, linguistics and phonetics. SLTs are interested in the quality, quantity, content and use of language, their work involves identification, diagnosis, observation and treatment of all speech and language pathologies as well as all aspects of communicative disorders and disturbances, thus highly trained listening skills are essential. Seaman (1990) suggests that, in many aspects of work with elderly people with mental health problems, the SLT may be most effective in a training and advisory role. In our experience the consultative role is the most valuable, in the context of the multidisciplinary team; improving communicative strategies for the client, carer and all staff can reduce isolation and restore elements of control in situations which can seem overwhelmingly complex.

THE PHYSIOLOGICAL BASIS OF SPEECH, LANGUAGE AND COMMUNICATION

The neurology of speech and language

The central nervous system is the most complicated within the human body. It comprises the cerebral cortex, the cerebellum and the brain stem as well as the spinal cord to which the 12 pairs of cranial nerves are attached. From these nerves derive the entire sensory and motor supply throughout the body which confirms the importance of the speech and language function; of the 12 pairs, 10 are involved in some aspect or another.

The central nervous system is the human computer – its motor drive, its storage facility, its learning centre and its sensory feedback and interpretative mechanism. MacLean (1970) conceptualises the central nervous system as a composite of reticular, limbic and neocortical systems and motor activity and its control, including that of speech, is dependent on all three of these systems for proper execution. The reticular

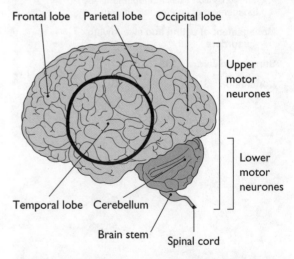

Figure 17.1 Main language/speech centres of the brain (after Russell 1983). Thick line indicates major speech and language areas (Broca's and Wernike's). Upper motor neurones = brain and spinal cord. Lower motor neurones = brain stem and spinal cord.

system is responsible for a general readiness or arousal and for initiating speech. The limbic system provides the drive, motivation and the need to act and the neocortical system serves to execute motor actions.

Along with all other cognitive functions, language and speech are dependent on brain mechanisms which are integrated in and controlled by the two cerebral hemispheres. It has been known since the mid 19th century that of the two hemispheres one – usually the left – is dominant. It used to be thought that speech and language were functions of the dominant hemisphere alone and specifically located within the areas indicated in Figure 17.1, which became known as Broca's and Wernike's after the neurologists credited with their location and the identification of their functions. However, over time, increased capability to localise function has increased awareness of just how widely represented throughout the structures and systems of the central nervous system language and speech are.

The main functions of the lobes of the dominant hemisphere relevant to language, speech and communication are listed in Box 17.1. The role of the right

hemisphere on language and speech has been highlighted by recent research, much of which is based on scanning techniques now possible with magnetic resonance imaging (MRI) and positron emission tomography (PET) (Gardner et al 1983, Bryan 1989, Cutting 1990). Damage within the right hemisphere can impair language and communication in the following ways: deficits in comprehension of connotation, metaphor, humour and inferential thinking, as well as bizarre prosody (rhythm/stress), tangential/disorganised speech, concrete thinking, overpersonalisation and a variety of social use of language deficits.

DISORDERS OF SPEECH, LANGUAGE AND COMMUNICATION

An understanding of the communication chain (Fig. 17.2) is important for SLTs seeking to pin-point the

---

Box 17.1 The main functions of the lobes of the dominant hemisphere relevant to language, speech and communication

Frontal lobe
- upper limb movement (i.e. writing, gesture, etc.)
- personality and self expression
- emotional thought and emotional content of language and speech
- behavioural learning and control (thus communicative appropriateness)
- verbal (reasoning intelligence)
- eye movement (e.g. reading, gaze, eye contact).

Temporal lobe
- memory and word finding
- organising and sending verbal messages
- speech and language comprehension
- perception and interpretation of sound
- interpretation of taste and smell.

Parietal lobe
- sensation and feedback
- perceptual skills (e.g. size, shape, body image, spatial awareness)
- visual perception and interpretation
- some specific abilities necessary for planned movements
- orientation in time, place and person.

Occipital lobe
- vision and visualisation
- maintenance and awareness of both sides of the body in space.

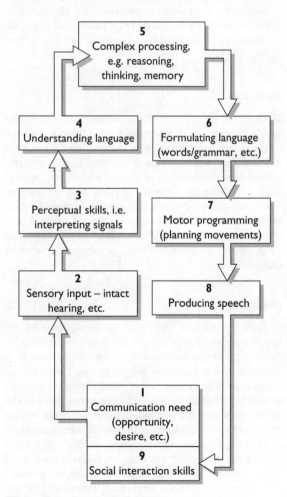

Figure 17.2 Communication chain.

level of linguistic or communicative breakdown in the elderly client. Each of the nine stages shown occur every time we converse and therefore the chain must be intact and functioning for verbal communication to be complete and accurate.

Correct use of terminology is important for assessment and accurate diagnosis. It is relatively easy to identify that someone is having difficulties in communicating but it is difficult to specify the exact nature of the problem as a guide to clear and targeted management.

The first and most important differentiation to make is between speech, language and communication.

Disorders of speech

Speech is the act of talking. It is purely the use of thoracic, laryngeal, pharyngeal and oral structures and musculature to produce respiration and phonation in order to produce voice and to synthesise and sequence a series of recognisable sounds in a fluent and intelligible way.

Dysarthria

If there is damage to the muscles and structures needed for speech or respiration, or if there is damage to the nerves supplying them, the resultant disorder is classified as a dysarthria. This condition is characterised by a combination of slowed and slurred speech with problems of volume, rhythm and intonation. There are different types of dysarthria depending on the site of the lesion(s) (i.e. spastic, flaccid or cerebellar dysarthria) and accurate assessment of the type can help with localisation and accurate differential diagnosis.

Dysphonia

Speech production can also be compromised by specific articulation problems, for example a lisp, or by fluency problems such as a stammer and by disorders of voice. Voice disorders are categorised as types of dysphonia. The causes of dysphonia may be organic, in that the disorder may result from nerve palsy to the vocal cords, or it may be independent of, or secondary to, other neuropathology, with or without concomitant dysarthria. Organic disorder of voice can result from vocal abuse (shouting, smoking, excessively poor vocal technique) which causes laryngeal changes or nodes on the vocal cords, or thickening (keratosis) of the cords, and results in combinations of hoarseness, pitch

changes and disturbances of rhythm (prosody). In the most severe cases there can be complete absence of voice (aphonia).

Dysphonia can also have functional (psychosomatic) causes although, even in the presence of a range of manifest mental health problems, organic causation must be first excluded. When we think of the voice as the instrument for communication we can appreciate that there may be many stress-related reasons for the development of a functional voice disorder. Much can be avoided, or left unsaid, if the voice is impaired and in rare, but severe cases, there can be elective/selective mutism or even a hysterical conversion resulting in hysterical aphonia.

Dyspraxia

A further disorder which can compromise speech is dyspraxia. This is best described as the inability to perform certain purposeful movements, or sequences of movements – speech among them – in the absence of any loss of motor power or of sensation. That is to say that, within the brain, there is a failure of the organisation and sending skills needed to remember how to perform movements with meaning. In terms of its effect on speech, the sufferer will struggle and exhibit many of the characteristics of a dysarthria. But, whereas the dysarthric client will have restricted oral movement at all times, the client with an orofacial or a speech dyspraxia will be unable to perform a movement like opening the mouth on request or following demonstration, but will spontaneously yawn widely showing no evidence of restricted movement. Dyspraxias which affect other voluntary body movements could impair communication by rendering the client unable to use gesture purposefully.

Disorders of language

Language is subdivided into two distinct areas. Firstly, receptive language: our ability to understand and process the words, the meaning (semantics) and the intention of what we hear or read. Secondly, expressive language: our ability to select and formulate words, phrases and sentences and organise them in accordance with correct grammatical rules (syntax) and use this skill meaningfully and responsively. Figure 17.3 shows the discrete cognitive and neuropsychological processes required for receptive and expressive language functions. The upper half of the diagram indicates the processes of receptive language and the lower half of the diagram those of expressive language. Knowledge of these processes can help practitioners

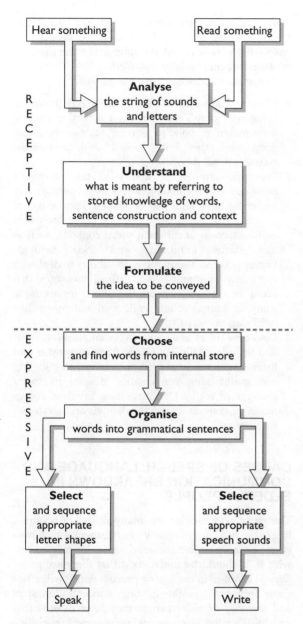

Figure 17.3 The major language processes (Surrey Heartlands Speech and Language Therapy Service 1994).

pin-point the level of breakdown and thus indicate appropriate intervention.

It is important, when assessing language function, to assess the two areas of receptive and expressive language separately, to avoid being misled by an elderly client's well preserved social expressive language skills, into believing that their comprehension is intact. Receptive language can be enhanced by contextual clues as well as by environmental and gestural ones.

Dysphasia

Returning to the analogy of learning a foreign language, many of us will remember how easy it is to guess meanings correctly from the context, situation or a helpful speaker who is using a high level of clear gesture. A totally preserved receptive language ability should be able to function in the absence of clues; if it does not then the language disturbance known as receptive dysphasia exists (aphasia is now used interchangeably with dysphasia). The severity and type of the difficulty will depend on the site and the amount of the damage to the areas of the brain related to the understanding of language and, in small part, to the elderly client's pre-morbid abilities. If the language impairment is retrieving words from the memory store (or lexicon) and organising and sequencing them into meaningful utterances, then the disorder is an expressive dysphasia (or aphasia). Severity depends on the extent and site of damage, and, in some measure, on past attainment.

Dysphasic difficulties, both receptive and expressive, affect oral language (what is spoken and how we speak it) and written language (what is read as well as what can be written). As with so many individualised areas of skills, insight into the dysphasic difficulties will vary from non-existent to total and distressing. Emotional distress is exacerbated because clients do not have an intact verbal mechanism through which to express their fear and frustration. Clients and carers can become locked into an incomplete and unsatisfactory guessing game.

Paraphasia. One type of expressive dysphasic behaviour common in elderly people with mental health problems, particularly those with a diffuse dementia, is paraphasia. Fluent dysphasics have no difficulty in finding words, but the words that pour out are incorrect. Verbal paraphasia occurs when the wrong word is selected from the correct group, for example 'son' instead of 'husband'. Literal paraphasia occurs when the wrong word, but with the correct starting sound, is selected, such as 'I want my car' instead of 'I want my coat'. Words might be invented (neologisms), constantly repeated (perseveration) or unintelligible (jargon). All these difficulties may occur in those with severe expressive dysphasia. Proximity of the brain structures and interrelation of the skills means that most dysphasias are mixed. However, in order to identify areas of need as well as areas of strength, and arrive at individualised management strategies, assessment must separate language skills into receptive and expressive, and distinguish oral from written skills.

Agnosia and other disorders

It is wrong to suppose that all the behaviours of a dementing person are the result of a generalised degenerative process. There are very specific disorders that affect language which may be overlooked. One example is agnosia, which is the failure to recognise, and therefore, to understand and name, familiar objects including people (Sachs 1985). Some classification is inevitable but psychiatric diagnoses may convey relatively little information as to aetiology, symptomatology, treatment and prognosis (Kendall 1988). Knowledge of linguistic skills and cognitive neuropsychological approaches to therapy could add meaningful dimensions to existing classification schemes of disorders. Prediction of specific outcomes might occur as a result and negative 'labelling' of sufferers be avoided. Diamond (1981) points out that in forensic psychiatry, speech content and the linguistic aspects of a client's communication should be considered most important in establishing psychiatric diagnoses. Could not the same be said of the psychiatry of ageing?

Disorders of communication

Communication is the act of interaction between people which is made fully possible by the existence of language and speech together with non-verbal skills. Communication comprises a very subtle and highly complex network of signals and abilities of which language and speech are just a part. Communication skills include eye contact, gesture, posture, proximity, facial expression and attention.

Psychiatric theories are in themselves also theories of communication (Reusch 1987). France (1991), a speech and language therapist working in a mental health setting, states, 'subtle changes in communication may be among the first signs of the onset of a mental illness, thus it is through the way in which people begin to communicate differently that it becomes apparent that all is not well' (France 1991, p. 4). The current practice of breaking communication into its component skills draws upon the theory of pragmatics (Leach 1983) or semantic-pragmatics. This is an in-depth way of understanding and analysing functional communication which considers the social and

contextual use of communication skills and how skilled we are in using communication as a tool. People who have what is now called semantic-pragmatic disorder are therefore functionally unskilled.

Pragmatics addresses three main areas:

1. Communicative intent – the ability to seek attention, to protest, deny, reject, request action or request information, respond to requests, state or comment, greet and use both verbal and non-verbal conversational devices.
2. Presupposition – the ability to take another's perspective in a conversation. This is based on our understanding and use of shared knowledge of people, experiences, the world and the environment and awareness of different social contexts, such as age, status, familiarity and social settings. Presupposition also involves the ability to deal with the many ambiguities and mixed messages that occur in our daily communication, for example irony or idiomatic and colloquial statements like 'well slap my wrist!'
3. Discourse refers to a person's communicative 'flow' and includes skills like taking turns as speaker and listener with minimal gaps or overlaps, so initiating and maintaining conversation despite its many changes of topic. Discourse also involves recognition of conversational breakdown and strategies for its repair.

CAUSES OF SPEECH, LANGUAGE AND COMMUNICATION BREAKDOWN IN ELDERLY PEOPLE

This section focuses on the many causes of acquired linguistic and communicative impairment which may stem primarily from a mental disorder, or may coexist with it. It should be understood that there are many normal changes in the ageing process which will affect these abilities. Eyesight, hearing, concentration span and memory of older people may have deteriorated and with ageing our sensory, neurological, cognitive and physiological systems change (Gravell 1988). Therefore many aspects of language, speech, voice and communication may become less readily accessible and precise in execution. Readers are referred to Espir & Rose (1983) and Hildrick-Smith (1985) for further detail on causation and neurological problems in elderly people.

Cerebrovascular accident

It is important to be conversant with the speech and

language handicaps present in localised cerebral vascular accident (CVA) to better recognise the more pervasive communication handicaps present in the dementias, which result in multiple sites of damage, many of which will be those with linguistic and paralinguistic functions.

CVA localised within the front portion of the dominant temporal lobe in Broca's area will result in a mainly expressive dysphasia, for example, nominal aphasia where word finding is severely compromised. If the damage is localised in the posterior (Wernike's) portion of the main language centre, then the dysphasia will be predominantly receptive, with varying degrees of difficulty being experienced in understanding and processing language anywhere on the continuum from marked difficulty with social and contextual language almost undetectable and occasional difficulty with any highly complex language. Usually, language disturbances will reflect elements of both expressive and receptive dysphasia and there are often allied deficits in varying degrees of visual or auditory perceptual disturbances (agnosias). There can also be difficulties with elements of reading, writing (Benson 1979) or calculation (dyslexia, dysgraphia and dyscalculia) and writing and gesture will also be affected by paralysis or paresis. On occasion, stroke victims may neglect the affected side of the body or be unaware of its existence due to lack of ability to interpret the visual stimuli being received by the brain from one half of the visual field (hemianopia).

It is often the case in CVA that certain aspects of expressive or receptive language are spared. This is most often because these skills are retained in deeper structures of other lobes of the dominant hemisphere or because they are functions of the non-dominant hemisphere of the brain (usually the right).

Clients may display preserved emotional language (e.g. swearing or expostulating). They may, in the absence of little other language, correctly use primitive words which were among the first learned (e.g. yes and no). Automatic speech, such as songs and poems, may remain as may serial speech, like the alphabet or the days of the week and the months of the year. One client we know was only able to produce a particularly ripe expletive. She said the word with appropriate and varied intonation patterns which enabled us to understand what she meant; this helped us all even though the swearing caused her and her carers considerable embarrassment. A further common feature of severe dysphasia is perseveration, which is when the client becomes stuck on a word, phrase or theme. This is most likely in cases where the lesion is frontal (Buckingham 1985). Readers are referred to Code (1991) for details of speech and language deficits in CVA.

Dysarthria can occur in CVA if there has been bilateral damage to the upper motor neurones of the central nervous system which supply the cranial nerves which in turn supply the speech and respiration musculature. This pathology is known as pseudo-bulbar palsy (or suprabulbar palsy) which exists when damage has occurred to both sides of the system. Dysarthria and dysphasia will only coexist with bilateral infarction and when the main language centres of the dominant hemisphere are also involved. Other pathologies in addition to CVA can cause a pseudobulbar palsy, if they occur bilaterally (Espir & Rose 1983), for example motor neurone disease referred to later in this section. Clients with a pseudobulbar palsy may have a history of vascular disease and previous strokes. This type of dysarthria makes speech slow and quiet, with prolongation of sounds and words and delay between sentences. The muscles of the tongue and face have the spastic characteristics of increased tone and reflexes. There is likely also to be some dysphonia with the voice being excessively nasal and altered in pitch. The patterns of phonation (coordination between air and sound) alter and grunts are often made at the end of a sentence. Swallowing may also be affected (dysphagia). Espir & Rose (1983) state that 'the patho-physiology of aphasia (dysphasia) is the most difficult in neurology' (p. 31).

The dementias

The dementias are syndromes characterised by acquired, persistent impairment of language, both expressive and receptive, as neuropsychological skills deteriorate. The effects of dementing illness on language are varied and differences occur between and within the dementia types. Readers are referred to Lubinski (1991) for further details.

Alzheimer type dementia

Probably the most extensively researched of all the dementias is Alzheimer's disease or Alzheimer type dementia (ATD). Language function deteriorates as the disease progresses. Cummings et al (1985) conclude that the areas of language most impaired in these clients are:

- information content of speech
- comprehension of complex commands
- naming
- word list generation

- writing to dictation
- narrative writing
- completion of nursery rhymes.

Their results on tests involving word and number repetition, reading aloud and dysarthria did not show differences between the experimental group of subjects and the control group. Other studies have supported Cummings et al's conclusions. For example, Shuttleworth and Huber (1988) noted anomic (naming) errors which occurred as a result of impaired semantic processes (understanding of meaning). Anomia also results from impaired perception (i.e. the item is simply not recognised) and both types worsen with increased severity of dementia.

Comprehension of language is also compromised by impairment in the semantic processes; the complexity of the command is as important as the length of the command (DeRenzi and Faglioni 1978). Complex linguistic operations like proverb interpretation and working out ambiguities are highly sensitive to change (Bayles & Boone 1982). The structure of language (syntax grammar) is relatively well preserved in ATD but expressive language is often described as vague, empty or tangential. Little propositional content of speech is evident and paraphasias become more frequent as the disease progresses. There is little adherence to conversational rules and speech becomes less coherent with decreased information content. What content there is can be bizarre and irrelevant with increased disturbance of articulation. Mutism can be the end result of the global impairment of speech and language (Benson et al 1990).

Disturbance of reading and writing is common in ATD but the ability to read aloud can be well preserved throughout the course of the illness. Poor comprehension of what is actually being read is the problem and this is impaired in the early stages. Reading aloud deteriorates in the later stages as a result of increasing perceptual, cognitive and semantic changes. Agraphia (the disorder of written language) is evident in ATD and the severity correlates significantly with the degree of cognitive impairment. Code & Lodge (1987) found that written spelling is very sensitive to the effects of ATD.

Disproportionate deterioration in language ability has been claimed to be a distinguishing feature of ATD of early onset, that is before the age of 65. However, Selnes et al (1988) found no significant differences between subjects and language dysfunction correlated positively with the severity of the dementia. Benson et al (1990) cite the work of Kirshner et al (1984) in which it is asserted that isolated aphasia may precede the

onset of deficits in other cognitive areas by several years. Readers are referred to Kempler (1991) for details.

Multi-infarct dementia

Multi-infarct dementia, also known as vascular dementia or, incorrectly, as arteriosclerotic dementia, is referred to by speech and language therapists, among others, by the preferred term of cerebrovascular dementia. This term seems more accurately to cover the group of dementia syndromes that have different behavioural features depending on which structures of the brain are affected together with the size of the blood vessel involved and the underlying disease process. A step-by-step deterioration is typical and speech and language changes occur, with dysphasia, dysarthria and dyspraxia being present, depending on the site of the infarction. Therefore, cortical infarctions in the left hemisphere result in specific dysphasic syndromes and those in the right hemisphere in deficits in comprehension of connotation, metaphor, humour and inferential thinking. Ischaemic damage in the subcortical areas would lead to dysarthria, slowness to respond and monotonous speech which is typical of subcortical dementias.

Subcortical dementia

Subcortical dementia occurs mainly in Huntington's chorea and stages of Parkinson's disease when cognitive impairment is present. It is rare to see Huntington's chorea in the elderly since it is a congenital degenerative disease which strikes young (mainly 35–45) and progresses quickly. However, it can occur and clients will experience considerable speech disorder (dysarthria) along with poor syntax (grammar), decreased phrase length and disruption of rhythm and intonation. Withdrawal from situations that demand communication is common and not surprising considering the nature of the illness. A degree of insight leading to depression and coupled with extreme difficulty in being understood may explain taciturn behaviour. Dysphagia (eating and swallowing disorder) occurs in many cases because of muscular weakness and lack of coordination of the oropharyngeal tract.

On the whole there are differences between speech and language behaviours of people with cortical versus subcortical dementia, primarily because the motor strip of the cortex is spared in a cortical dementia (Obler & Albert 1981). Therefore, there is no adverse effect on speech production nor dysarthria, as occurs for those with subcortical dementia. Language skills, both expressive and receptive, tend to be better in those with a subcortical dementia and inappropriate in those with a cortical dementia. Some detailed examples of this are discussed in Bayles & Kaszinak (1987, Ch. 8).

HIV encephalopathy

As with Huntington's disease, another rare form of dementia which may occur in the elderly is HIV encephalopathy. Speech and language characteristics follow the course of changes in cognitive function. There are initial complaints of impaired reading secondary to poor comprehension of written material. Verbal response is slow and later speech becomes sparse and dysarthric.

An unusual condition called leukoencephalopathy may occur when loss of coating (demyelination) of nerve fibres in the brain takes place, resulting in hemiparesis, visual and movement defects, sensory impairment and sometimes seizures.

Speech and language disturbances exist and resemble those of a subcortical dementia. Lethlean & Murdoch (1993) present a single case study which expands on all of the above. In it they describe a client who had intact auditory comprehension, repetition, reading and writing skills but poor initiation of speech and marked reduction of spontaneous speech in conversation. Naming deficits and impaired performance on high level language tasks, including verbal reasoning, reconstruction of sentences, formulation of inferences and interpretation of absurdities, ambiguities and metaphors were also identified.

Creutzfeldt–Jakob disease

Creutzfeldt–Jakob disease is mercifully rare but people suffering from this transmissible disease develop speech and language changes early in its course. Benson et al (1990) report that most sufferers are dysphasic and dysarthric in the early stages and nearly all progress to mutism following a progressive paucity of spontaneous speech.

Pick's disease

Pick's disease too is rare and also manifests speech and language changes early on. Speech can be stumbling and stuttering in nature. Struggle to articulate sounds is evident. Auditory comprehension, whilst intact in the early stages, becomes impaired later.

Progressive aphasia

Progressive aphasia was first identified by Mesulam (1982) and many cases have been reported since. A slow progressive dysphasia develops in the absence of cognitive and intellectual decline. As the condition progresses, generalised dementia follows. There are, however, variations in the neuropathological changes reported in various studies (Poeck & Luzzatti 1988, Kirshner et al 1987, Golding 1989, Pogacar & Williams 1984). This leads us to conclude that this condition could be a non-specific syndrome with several potential causes.

Parkinson's disease

Parkinson's disease affects the extrapyramidal system, the nuclei of which are in the basal ganglia of the brain. The production of dopamine is ineffective and the results are involuntary movement of musculature or poverty, slowness and stiffness of movement. There is also marked tremor and dysarthria, characterised by slowness and unclear production of sounds. Sometimes speech can get faster and faster until the words run together; this condition is called palilalia. There can also be dysphonia, characterised by weak, feeble and monotonous voice production and drooling which is embarrassing for the client and can indicate swallowing problems.

Facial expression is often severely limited by the 'mask-like' appearance and restricted range of movements of the musculature of the face. Intellectual and cognitive functioning can become impaired in the latter stages and therefore language and the complexities of communication will also deteriorate. It is estimated that overt dementia, of the subcortical type, occurs in about 40% of cases (Cummings et al 1988).

Parkinson's disease can, on rare occasions, occur after encephalitis and may not manifest itself until much later in life. It can also be one of the side-effects of neuroleptic medication. In this case speech changes and the onset of a dysarthria can be the first sign of the need for a case review by mental health care professionals. Readers are referred to Critchley (1981) for further details of speech and language deficits in Parkinson's disease.

Multiple sclerosis

Multiple sclerosis (MS) usually has its onset between the ages of 20 and 45 years but many people over 65 may develop the disease or it may return after remission. The demyelination (loss of coating) in plaques (groups) of nerves throughout the central nervous system results in loss of motor and sensory abilities. Dysarthria also occurs and is exacerbated by fatigue and characterised by slurred and scanning speech, as if the speaker is reading unfamiliar text. Dysphonia, characterised by an often explosive, staccato voice, also occurs and dysphagia (swallowing problems) may develop (Matthews 1978).

It is increasingly recognised that cognitive decline is a feature of MS. Therefore, communication will be further degraded by lowered attentional, memory and psychomotor functioning. Filley et al (1989) suggest that these impairments are greater in MS than in Alzheimer's type dementia but notes that dysphasia has only rarely been documented in clients with MS.

Nerve damage

Damage to the cranial nerves involved with respiration, eating and speech can be caused by trauma (e.g. surgical procedure), tumour, or inflammation of a particular nerve (e.g., polyneuritis, Bell's palsy). In these cases speech can be dysarthric with weakness of production and imprecision rather like the temporary motor and sensory loss brought about by a dental injection. Dysphonia may also occur, characterised by a nasal voice due to a palatal insufficiency. In Bell's palsy the dysarthric features are slurred speech and particular difficulty with 'lip' sounds (p/b/m) because of the one-sided facial paralysis.

Motor neurone disease

Motor neurone disease, or what has been referred to as bulbar palsy, affects the lower motor neurones of the central nervous system which pass through the medulla or bulb of the brain stem. It can also affect the upper motor neurones, in which case it can cause a concomitant pseudobulbar palsy (Rose 1977).

Its cause is unknown and its effects drastic (Perry 1982). There is severe, progressive dysarthria and dysphonia. Speech is very indistinct with all sounds affected due to weakness of tongue, lips and soft palate. There is wasting of the tongue and speech muscles and fasciculation (involuntary movements) of the tongue in this type of dysarthria, although there will be spasticity too, due to the upper motor neurone involvement. There is also dysphonia, in that the weakness of the soft palate also causes the voice to become nasal. Respiration becomes progressively more difficult. The cough reflex disappears and swallowing problems are severe. Along with other cognitive skills,

language for thought is preserved and with it, as many sufferers indicate, painful insight.

Muscle disorders

Muscle disorders, such as polymyositis and myasthenia gravis can all occur in the older person and may cause a dysarthria which renders speech both slurred and slow with imprecise and indistinct articulation of sounds. In myasthenia gravis a weak dysphonic voice and swallowing problems can also occur. These disorders may also affect both communicative gesture and facial expression (Darley et al 1975).

Encephalopathies

Encephalopathies affect language in that they affect memory for words, for people and for situations. Communication is grossly affected in the most severe cases in that it depends to a great extent on stored memories of events and meanings; interaction cannot make progress when, as in the case of true amnesia, every meeting is for the 'first time'.

In meningitis and encephalitis some elements of the amnesia are often irreversible if the viral infection has caused widespread atrophy of brain tissue and structures. Transient memory and language disturbances may result from any severe infection as well as from metabolic disorders (renal failure, chemical deficiency or substance abuse) (Parkin 1987).

Long-term alcohol abuse can result in a Wernicke's encephalopathy, commonly known as Korsakoff's psychosis. Its effects can mirror those of both CVA and the dementias. There are often severe memory problems (particularly for short-term memory), new information cannot be stored and remote memory is often confused, resulting in a tendency by the afflicted person to confabulate. The characteristics of a 'fluent' dysphasia are often present, hence the reference to Wernicke since there is great similarity in language output to a Wernicke asphasia caused by CVA. There may be a lot of expressive language produced but with very little substance and there is likely to be much receptive language confusion and error as well as probable visual and/or auditory perceptual difficulty (Butters & Cermak 1980).

Interventions with Mr Winter, who suffered from severe dysphasia resulting from Korsakoff's psychosis, are discussed in Box 17.2.

Epilepsy

Epilepsy of both grand-mal and petit-mal types can

Box 17.2 Intervention via augmented communication strategies

Mr Winter, aged 65, suffered from severe dysphasia resulting from Korsakoff's psychosis. The history of alcohol abuse was longstanding and appeared to originate from his job as a hotel manager and to be compounded by his divorce, the death of his son, his ex-wife's suicide and his job loss. He had experienced multiple trauma and grief over a period of 10 years.

The assessment showed that his dysphasic difficulties had caused some comprehension deficits for high level language. Simple language was well understood and written comprehension was noticeably better than verbal. There were memory deficits (particularly short-term), but the most significant handicap was a severe expressive dysphasia. This is an uncommon feature of Korsakoff's psychosis, but the damage localised on CT scan was mainly to the anterior part of the temporal lobe (Broca's area), although there was generalised atrophy.

The expressive dysphasia was characterised by extreme, severe word finding difficulties, which rendered Mr Winter virtually unable to respond meaningfully at a verbal level. Most of his spoken responses consisted of a recurrent jargon utterance which he found difficult to bypass by imitation or by other strategies, due to an oral dyspraxia. There was a high level of frustration and often verbal outbursts. Non-verbal communication was pretty much intact, there being no other kind of dyspraxia, and

Mr Winter occasionally used clear gestures to make himself understood.

Therapy consisted of expanding this skill with gesture and teaching him and key staff a wider range of meaningful signs. Also, given the better preserved levels of written skills, he was assessed for and issued with a Canon communicator.® This stored a few regularly used phrases which could be recalled easily and shown on the display or printed on a small piece of paper. It also enabled him to respond to questions and interact socially. Direct therapy was then aimed at improving his reading skills further and this sometimes enabled him to read aloud what he had written. Over time, Mr Winter became less frustrated and more out-going. He left hospital to live in a small residential home, where he had some independence.

In this case, the lesson for the clinical team was the importance of assessment and diagnosis of linguistic competence by the speech and language therapist in elderly people for whom organic language deficit and psychiatric disorder coexist. In the case of Mr Winter, the clinical team was able to use a variety of communication modalities which improved the client's communication abilities. These approaches also empowered the client and the team in a situation where the absence of verbal interaction could have left all concerned feeling helpless.

cause communicative disturbances. There can be inconsistencies of memory functions, attentional deficits and overall lack of interactive awareness. In focal attacks (e.g. temporal lobe epilepsy) there can be transient dysphasia and dysarthria. Hearing may also be affected, along with the other senses, as part of the 'aura' signalling the sudden abnormal discharges of electrical activity and the onset of the fit (Laidlaw & Richens 1982).

Trauma

The incidence of trauma to the brain caused by closed head injury and penetrating or open head injury rises sharply in the elderly population. The range of causes is reflected in the diversity of speech and language symptoms. For example, non-fluent expressive dysphasia is often found in patients with left hemisphere penetrative injury but rarely in those with closed head injury. Recovery of language skills is better than for people with cerebrovascular disease but residual defects in complex receptive language and verbal skills are frequently present. Other post-traumatic speech disorders which may occur include mutism, stuttering, echolalia, palilalia and dysarthria. Repeated head trauma in ex-boxers may lead to

dementia pugilistica, with extrapyramidal (Parkinsonian) speech symptoms. Readers are referred to O'Neil (1989) for further details.

Tumour

Any space-occupying lesion can cause compressive damage to the brain. Tumours produce their effects by destruction or distortion of the brain, or through the effects of raised intracranial pressure and are discussed in detail by Sharr (1989).

The clinical effects produced by destruction of brain tissue are not reversible but paralysis of function caused by raised intracranial pressure is. Tumours occur throughout the central nervous system and usually the speech, language and communication symptoms reflect the site of the lesion. If the tumour has a slow rate of growth, learned compensation of language function can take place. The most common form of intracranial neoplasms (tumour) are gliomas. These are malignant cerebral tumours involving the glia (supporting tissues) but not the neurones (cell bodies), and they can grow to quite a size with surprisingly little language impairment even if sited in the dominant temporal lobe. However, when these tumours are removed, a considerable dysphasia can result since the neurones are going to be removed along with all the supporting tissue.

Tumours of the frontal lobe can lead to an expressive dysphasia if they are sited in the prefrontal (Broca's) area. Progressive dementia, with its attendant disturbances of language and communication function, is also characteristic of a frontal lobe lesion. Pressure on surrounding nerve tracts can cause weakness of the tongue and facial muscles which in turn results in a dysarthria.

A left-sided tumour in the posterior part of the parietal lobe can lead to receptive language disorders and a Wernicke's dysphasia. If there is a tumour on the vermis (median lobe) of the cerebellum, or when lesions involve the cerebellar connections to the brain stem, then a cerebellar dysarthria typified by explosive, staccato speech can occur.

Rare tumours, which will usually be large by the time they are diagnosed in an old person, are acoustic neuromas. The first sign is deafness and the problem is that hearing loss is often accepted as a part of the ageing process and not as a sign of disease. When these neuromas are removed, there is a risk to the facial nerve because it and the auditory nerve run alongside each other. Communication can break down due to hearing loss, sensory problems and deteriorating speech. A mild form of dysarthria similar to that of a Bell's palsy (nerve damage) may also occur. A tumour in the medulla or bulb of the brain stem will produce a bulbar palsy and bilateral tumours and pseudobulbar palsy, both will lead to dysarthria, dysphonia and dysphagia.

The local effects of tumour depend on the site and type of pathological lesion. Lesions to the nerve supply of particular muscle groups will result in muscle dysfunction and corresponding speech deterioration. Tumours occurring in any area of the vocal tract can give rise to all manner of speech problems, whether they affect respiration (lungs), phonation (larynx), nasality (soft palate), prosody or sound production (larynx, soft palate and articulatory organs).

Removal of growths on the tongue may not necessarily affect articulation of speech because compensatory movements occur or can be taught postoperatively. But growths on the laryngeal nerves can cause changes to both voice and phonation, and those in or around the larynx can give rise to marked changes in voice quality.

Deafness

Deafness can be conductive or sensory-neural and both may be congenital or acquired. The amount that they impair language, speech and communication depends on the severity of the hearing loss. Some elderly people with mental health problems may have had a hearing loss from birth and are therefore prelingually deaf in that they have not developed language along 'normal' lines and will have acquired speech problems associated with the hearing loss. Communicative strategies may also be influenced by the perception of self as being part of the deaf rather than the hearing world.

It is possible that a few elderly clients in long stay psychiatric wards who were admitted with behavioural disturbances when young may, in fact, be deaf. Eastwood et al (1986) found that 66% of older nursing home residents had clinically significant hearing loss, most probably due to deterioration in hearing acuity with ageing (presbycusis). Deafness can lead to feelings of isolation and to withdrawal, anxiety and hysteria (Denmark 1985).

The more common of the two types of hearing loss in elderly people is conductive loss (Davis 1983). This may be due to blockage (e.g. impacted wax), to perforation of the ear drum or to inadequate vibration of the small bones of the middle ear through calcification. It is hearing for the higher frequency sounds (1000–8000 herz) that is most affected. Acquired hearing loss in the elderly often begins with sounds between 4000–8000 herz. Speech sounds which fall into this category are consonants like s, z, sh and f. Most vowel sounds are within the lower frequency range. A conductive hearing loss which requires 40–55 decibels of amplification in order for sounds to be heard is considered moderate, whilst a loss requiring amplification of 70–90 decibels would be considered severe by audiologists.

Sensory neural loss results from damage to the inner ear, the auditory nerve or to the auditory interpretative centre of the brain. The hearing loss extends across the frequency range, so all speech sounds may be compromised. Amplification is of less value in severe cases of sensory neural loss than in cases of conduction loss. In many cases of sensory neural loss, speech conservation may be achieved through lip reading and emphasis on maintaining tactile and kinaesthetic sensory feedback (Orlans 1985).

Communicative changes with hearing loss are alterations in the rate of speech, reduced precision of articulation with prolongation of consonant and vowel sounds giving often bizarre rhythm. The voice quality deteriorates with disturbance of nasal resonance, inappropriate volume and reduction in the range of pitch. Interactions are characterised by excessive or very little eye contact. Posture and proximity may change and the elderly person may fail to anticipate turn-taking boundaries.

Two further aspects of hearing loss deserve special mention. The first is recruitment factor, a distressing complaint whereby, below a certain frequency, a sound is not perceived by the elderly person but at, and immediately above that frequency, the sound becomes painful to listen to. This condition is called hyperacusis. The second aspect is tinnitus which is often described as a subjective ringing, roaring or hissing sound in one or both ears (Davis 1983). The increased attentional problems and isolation caused by tinnitus and the effort needed to cope with it cannot be overemphasised. Depression is common in tinnitus sufferers (Harrop-Griffiths et al 1987) and, in the elderly, tinnitus occurring together with depression and other disabilities may be unbearable.

The detection and management of hearing deficit is illustrated by the case of Mrs Dowling discussed in Box 17.3.

Box 17.3 The detection and management of hearing deficit

Mrs Dowling, aged 80, with a diagnosis of vascular dementia, was very quiet and notably confused. Both expressive and receptive language skills had deteriorated, but there was appropriate social communication at a basic level and a willingness to interact.

Assessment was difficult and observation of Mrs Dowling led the speech and language therapist to suspect a marked hearing loss. It was not possible to test accurately with an audiometer, so an auditory trainer was used, which gave bilateral amplification to more than 100 decibels. At full amplification to both ears, Mrs Dowling began to respond verbally and appropriately to basic questioning and to simple structured conversation. Both ears were treated for impacted wax and powerful body-worn hearing aids were issued at the audiology department of the local hospital. Mrs Dowling gained a great deal socially and communicatively during the time she was able to tolerate her hearing aids. As further cognitive deterioration took place she used the aids less often but other amplification which was not as intrusive (Telemik) was used for one-to-one interactions, and good practice strategies for hearing management were practised by the health care team.

In this case, the lesson for the clinical team was the importance of hearing screening for elderly people with mental health problems, even in cases where there is a marked confusional state. Further, that adapting the form of aid to hearing as the client's needs change, and adopting good practices for maximising hearing, increases the possibility of meaningful interaction being maintained for a longer period.

Psychotic disorders

Psychotic illness states, alone or in combination with other mental health problems, can cause a multiplicity of linguistic and communicative impairments. One of the most significant is disorder of thought which can be recognised through a client's expressive language output, both verbally and in writing. A client may show loose association of thoughts or random linking of thoughts and ideas which make their expressive language difficult to predict and follow (APA 1987).

Delusional ideas can prevent genuine linguistic interaction which is often a forum for change. The inability to express thoughts in abstract terms is the major feature of concrete thinking. Attention levels as well as the desire to interact deteriorate with paranoia and hallucinations. Therefore receptive language may suffer. Monologue militates against turn taking and other interactive processes (France 1991).

Every aspect of communication can be affected, with clients showing a range of speech and language abnormality. The voice may change in pitch, volume and quality and there can be bizarre vocalisation (e.g. speaking on inspiration rather than expiration, speaking under one's breath). The rhythm, delivery and fluency of speech may be stilted or pressured and articulation can be affected by dystonic reactions or by tardive dyskinesia (Baldessarini 1988).

Neurotic disorders

Neurotic disorders, whether involving anxiety, panic, hysteria, phobia or obsession/compulsion, can also affect the elderly person's communication. These disturbances may be a direct result of extremely poor social and communicative skills or the anxiety itself may lead to social and communicative incompetence. In both cases the many organic and psychological changes and stresses of the ageing process can exacerbate the underlying cause.

Whatever the aetiology of neurotic disorders, there is marked communicative performance anxiety and, as suggested by Phillips (1984), such people do not comprehend the possibility of gaining pleasure from human interaction. Language can be affected receptively by attentional deficits which result directly from preoccupations and rituals.

Expressive language can be affected by excessive anxiety about causing offence, or by rituals which may involve repetition of words and phrases, or even by pressure of speech. Communication is likely to be disturbed by avoidance mechanisms and the voice may show dysphonic disturbances of laryngeal tension with hoarseness and poor respiration and phonation. We are all aware of the vocal and respiratory changes that extreme tension can bring – the dry mouth, croaky, hesitant voice and shallow breathing patterns. In extreme cases this can cause disturbances of fluency (stammering) or even in rare cases, severe panic attacks, avoiding speech and total voice loss (hysterical aphonia) (Stemple 1984).

Personality disorders

Personality disorders of long standing will signify that communication is often very polarised, negative and manipulative and there is likely to be difficulty in discussion and negotiation techniques and in the ability to genuinely share feelings and information. If this is allied to reticence commonly found in the older, 'stiff upper lip' generation, then it has even more serious implications for care programmes involving counselling. In people with a personality disorder, vocabulary can be limited and gesture and facial expression are often abnormal, either being limited or threatening and aggressive. Research leads Hare (1986) to suggest that there may be subtle deficits or anomalies in the interhemispheric organisation of the language processes.

Depression

Depression can have psychotic or neurotic features and can have devastating effects on communication in all its aspects. We are all familiar with feelings of sadness, hopelessness, conflict and alienation in a reactive and hopefully short-term sense and may be aware that during such times there is a diminution in our wish for social interaction. Clinical depression can result in an intensity of these feelings for the elderly person and language becomes limited and colourless.

Speech becomes slow with frequent pauses and hesitations and, if there is an agitated depression, speech is repetitive and staccato. Breznitz & Sherman (1987) suggest that the long pauses in the expressive output of the depressed client can be due to the interjection of depressed thoughts which interfere with the person's organisation of verbal responses. Voice can be very flat with reduced volume, pitch and intonation and altered resonance, almost as if vocal behaviours are mirroring the underlying state. This is another example of communication, and of voice in particular, providing a window on the soul.

Non-verbal communication too can become very restricted with a withdrawn and/or rigid posture, decreased eye contact and often immobile facial expression. In agitated depression, conversely, there can be restlessness and much tension being shown in fidgeting hand movements and taut and grimacing facial movements.

Even for people with a masked depression, when articulation of speech can be normal and voice and non-verbal patterns quite lively, there are language changes characterised by limited output and short responses containing minimal information, negative content and low levels of description. The complex relationship between speech and depression would benefit from further research, as it opens many theoretical and clinical avenues (Nilsonne 1988).

ASSESSMENT OF SPEECH, LANGUAGE AND COMMUNICATION

This section considers reasons for and the aims of screening and assessment procedures undertaken by the speech and language therapist. It details specific tests and outlines differential diagnoses and the implication for management of clients' communication needs.

Human communication is the most intricate and complex of behaviours, and the underlying aetiologies can be equally complex. The purpose of assessment is to determine, when possible, causation and to devise an individualised programme of management (Chapey 1986). Information sources are the medical and nursing notes, other professionals, the clients themselves and their families, relatives and friends. This is supplemented by thorough observation of communication across the widest range of situations and environments. Communication changes may be linked to a myriad of other factors and both qualitative and quantitative information is used to form a baseline against which to measure future change.

To start with, speech and language assessment will be informal and should be carried out in a familiar environment, often the client's home. Since accurate assessment requires sensory needs to be met, eyesight and hearing should be taken into consideration and any hearing aids or spectacles checked for defects and for cleanliness. A client's overall response, both verbal and non-verbal, at an introductory interview can give a lot of information about their level of functioning. The therapist will note:

• levels of alertness and awareness
• eye contact

- attention span
- social appropriateness
- range and depth of language used
- vocal and articulatory functions.

Any everyday objects to hand, like a newspaper, clothes, items in a bag or on a desk can be used to obtain an informal measure of the client's powers of perception, comprehension and expressive use of language. Assessing the linguistic, physical and social environment in which the client is living, whether institutional or home, can also be revealing.

Most speech and language therapists working with old people with mental health problems will have devised their own checklists for receptive and expressive language, speech, communicative performance and environment. Informal screening of communication highlights areas which require more detailed investigation using a range of specific, standardised tests.

Formal testing

Formal assessment of speech, language and communication of elderly clients with mental health problems is often difficult. Few tests have been standardised for this population and speech and language therapists will therefore select relevant subtests from batteries which assess localised dysphasia or general cognitive neuropsychological functioning. In mental health care settings, the therapist may be the first to assess hearing before the client is referred, if need be, to a hearing clinic. 'Free field' testing of a client's acuity for sounds of varying pitch, including speech sounds, may be carried out or a paediatric audiometer can be used. Closed circuit audiometry using headphones will provide a more accurate picture of the client's hearing in response to pure tones of varying intensity and frequency; the client is asked to respond verbally on hearing a sound. Ear nose and throat (ENT) medical consultants and audiologists are able to carry out bone conduction testing if the client's responses are unreliable and it is likely that amplification via a prescribed hearing aid will be of long-term value for those clients with conduction deafness.

Formal testing of linguistic performance assesses the range of receptive language and expressive language functions. It provides a profile of performance in discrete areas of linguistic ability, thus enabling future management to be demonstrably needs led.

Linguistic tests

In the main, linguistic tests assess expressive functioning in the following areas: the ability to give personal details; naming skills of increasing complexity; verbal fluency; imitation of speech; written copying and writing to dictation; writing spontaneously; reading; drawing; sentence construction; memory; descriptive abilities. Sub-tests for receptive language functions are likely to include: matching; categorisation; sequencing; processing and performing verbal and written tasks of increasing complexity; perception; calculation; implied meaning; and further areas of memory.

Tests of speech

Tests of speech consider: respiration; phonation; strength of facial musculature at rest and in movement; range and accuracy of movement; reflexes; rate of utterance; intelligibility; rhythm; and use of stress. The aim of the assessment is to determine the extent and type of the dysarthria.

Tests for dyspraxia

Tests for dyspraxia address meaningful oral skills (smiling, licking lips, whistling, blowing, etc.); difficulties with these would indicate an oral praxis. Tests also assess meaningful gesture (thumbs up, making a fist, pointing, etc.); difficulties here indicate an ideomotor praxis. Further testing includes drawing representations (shapes and pictures) or making things from matches to detect a constructional praxis.

Tests of voice

Tests of voice investigate posture, respiration, vocal tension, vocal and respiratory coordination, quality, tone, pitch, resonance and the ability to sustain a sound.

Functional communication

An important aspect of assessment with elderly people with mental health problems is functional communication since preservation of this is the central need for these clients. These tests consider the pragmatic skills of social interaction and the level at which the 'rules' of conversation and of non-verbal interaction are maintained. As with other professionals, the speech and language therapist looks for strengths rather than weaknesses and for skills that can be used creatively in therapy or can be helpful in management of communication and the communicative environment for that individual. Box 17.4 lists formal tests commonly used by speech and language therapists with elderly people in mental health care settings.

Box 17.4 Tests of linguistic and communicative ability

Cognitive tests:
- Clifton Assessment Procedure for the Elderly (CAPE) (Pattie & Gilleard 1979)
- Wechsler Adult Intelligence Scales (WAIS) (Wechsler 1981).

Behavioural/mood tests:
- CAPE: Behavioural subtest (as above)
- Beck Depression Inventory (Beck et al 1979).

Linguistic tests:
- Whurr Aphasia Screening Test (Whurr 1974)
- Boston Diagnostic Aphasia Examination (Goodglass & Kaplan 1983)
- Minnesota Differential Diagnostic Test of Aphasia (Schuell 1965): Shortened Version (1973)
- The Revised Token Test (McNeil & Prescott 1978)
- British Picture Vocabulary Scales (Dunn et al 1982)
- Cognitive Neuropsychological Tests (after Coltheart et al 1987).

Speech tests:
- Dysarthria Profile (Robertson 1982)
- Frenchay Dysarthria Test (Enderby 1988)
- Victoria Infirmary Voice Questionnaire (Lockhart & Martin 1987)
- Huskins's Non-Verbal Apraxia Test (Huskins 1986)
- Dabul's Apraxia Battery (Dabul & Bollier 1978).

Communication tests:
- Edinburgh Functional Communication Profile (Skinner et al 1984)
- Communicative Activities of Daily Living (Holland 1980)
- Profile of Communicative Appropriateness (Penn 1988).

Differential diagnosis:
- Middlesex Elderly Assessment of Mental State: Functional versus Organic (Golding 1989)
- Test for the Reception of Grammar (TROG): Dementia versus Depression (Bishop 1983)
- Severe Impairment Battery (SIB): Functional versus Organic (Saxton et al 1993).

Assessment of dysphagia

Assessment of dysphagia (feeding and swallowing) is carried out by the speech and language therapist (SLT) to evaluate the four phases of the swallow. In the first oral preparatory phase, opening of the mouth, lip closure and lip seal are considered. In the second oral phase, the function of the jaw and cheek muscles are assessed as is the hard palate and the tongue, including its ability to assist in the chew and to transfer the food bolus to the back of the mouth. The third pharyngeal phase is the reflex controlled swallow phase and therefore it will be very important to check on the movements of the soft palate and the other protective mechanisms for the airway. The final phase of a swallow is the oesophageal phase, during which food is transported by peristaltic movements to the stomach. An indication that all is not well in this phase would be vomiting after having eaten. If problems are suspected, particularly in the third or final phases of the swallow, referral for assessment using videofluoroscopic X-ray is recommended as a priority.

During the assessment of swallowing attention is given to:

- recent medical history (e.g. respiratory tract infection)
- sound of voice (e.g. 'bubbling')
- weight charts
- posture and head positioning
- general body sensation
- oral sensation
- reflexes (e.g. gag, cough, palatal, etc.)
- oral mobility
- compensatory techniques being used by the client.

A full oral examination is carried out and documented and trial swallows given. These involve giving measured, small amounts of food and fluid of different texture and thickness in a controlled way. The team approach to dysphagia is as important in assessment as it is in management.

The case of Mr Flew who suffered from dysphagia is discussed in Box 17.5.

Differential diagnosis

Differential diagnoses can often be made by considering the elderly person's linguistic and communicative performance. The main distinction that must be made is between dysphasia and dementia. The question here is whether the elderly person is suffering from a localised stroke or from deeper linguistic confusion of a dementing disorder.

A great deal can be determined through the general process of assessment, particularly by noting general performance and the behavioural response to materials and tasks. A column to note 'off test' behaviours can be a valuable insertion into any assessment profile, as

---

Box 17.5 Management of dysphagia

Mr Flew, aged 71, was admitted to the ward of a local hospital unit specialising in the care of elderly mentally ill people, for respite care. This was to provide his daughter with the opportunity for a much needed holiday.

Assessment by the multidisciplinary team 12 months previously had revealed that Mr Flew suffered from dementia, most probably of the Alzheimer type. Following this assessment, speech and language therapy management focused on teaching his carers the nature of his difficulties and strategies which could be employed to alleviate communication problems.

Following his recent admission to the ward, nurses noticed that he had difficulty swallowing food and that he coughed when trying to drink tea. He was referred to the speech and language therapist for a dysphagia assessment. He was seen the following day but his symptoms had disappeared and he had eaten a hearty

breakfast with no problems. The therapist monitored him daily and over the following week; a pattern of dysphagia/ no dysphagia began to appear. A fluctuation in speech intelligibility was evident and he showed signs of orofacial dyskinesia with severe dysarthria.

On admission to the ward he had been very restless and difficult to manage and Haloperidol® was prescribed orally to be taken each evening. The medication was withdrawn. No further episodes of dysphagia took place and his limited communication became intelligible again. He also became more familiar with the ward and settled into his new environment.

In this case, the lesson for the clinical team was the significance of the onset of both the swallowing and speech disorders as a differential diagnosis pointer indicating underlying neurophysiological problems which, in this case, were drug induced.

---

can playing back video recordings of the sessions. Table 17.1 lists some commonly seen differences between the two conditions.

Distinguishing between dementia and depression may also be aided by speech and language therapy assessment. Lezak (1983), in his preface, calls it 'the knottiest problem of differential diagnosis'. The Test for the Reception of Grammar (TROG) (Bishop 1983) is designed to assess the understanding of the grammatical contrasts in English and, although not standardised for this care group, it has been found to

be useful in showing a difference in performance levels between depressed clients and those with a dementia. Bishop (1983) asserts that depressed clients can usually perform the TROG with no marked difficulty.

Verbal fluency tasks are often useful differential diagnostic pointers with depressed clients showing relatively normal function (Kronfol et al 1978) whereas those with dementia show poor functioning (Miller 1984). Close observation and testing of voice can also be of value, in that the client with clinical depression will have less range and volume to their voice as well

Table 17.1 Differential diagnosis pointers (after Stevens 1985)

	Dysphasic	Dementia
1. Social behaviour (social skills)	Tends to be appropriate	Tends to be inappropriate
2. Orientation (time, place, person)	Likely to be intact	Likely to be poor
3. Short-term (recent) memory	Relatively good	Likely to be poor
4. Affect (emotional responses)	Tends to be appropriate	Tends to be bizarre or absent
5. Personality changes	Tend to be fewer	Significant changes likely
6. Level of insight	More insight leading to frustration	Less insight – less frustration
7. Activities	Tend to be more purposeful	Can be purposeless (e.g. 'screaming', 'fiddling', etc.)
8. General behaviour	Likely to be more consistent	Likely to be more inconsistent
9. Initiation of activities	Likely to initiate an activity	Rarely initiates an activity
10. Retention of information (ability to learn)	Remains relatively intact	Tends to be poor
11. Social use of language (pragmatics/functional communication)	More appropriate	Less appropriate
12. Non-verbal behaviours	More appropriate	Less appropriate

Table 17.2 Differences between depression and dementia

The person with depression	The person with dementia of the Alzheimer type
Often complains of poor memory	Is often unaware of memory problems
Will say 'I do not know' in answer to questions which require thought or concentration	Will 'confabulate' or make up answers to questions which require concentration or good memory and appears unaware that the answer is incorrect
Shows fluctuating ability and uneven impairment on cognitive testing	Tends to show consistent, global impairment on cognitive testing
Gives up easily, is poorly motivated and uninterested	Has a go
May be slow but successful in any complex task, aware of errors	Unsuccessful in carrying out tasks which require concentration, appears unaware of errors

From: Stokes & Goudie 1990.

as lowered prosodic features. Some major differences between depression and dementia are shown in Table 17.2, which has been reproduced from Stokes & Goudie (1990).

Broad based assessment of speech, language and communication functioning can add immeasurably to the multidisciplinary mental health care team's understanding of the elderly client's needs and thereby to the formulation of individualised, targeted interventions.

MANAGEMENT OF SPEECH, LANGUAGE AND COMMUNICATION DISORDERS OF ELDERLY PEOPLE

The elderly person with mental health problems is often multiply-handicapped and therefore requires a multiprofessional approach to management. The speech and language therapist manages the client's communication needs either directly or indirectly. Direct management consists of group or individual therapies and indirect management involves work with and through the other members of the team and/or the carers. Speech and language therapists working with elderly mentally ill people have knowledge of and training in psychological approaches to treatment such as reality orientation and reminiscence, validation and resolution therapies (discussed in Chs 20, 21 and 22). These approaches can be used in combination with specific treatment techniques discussed in the remainder of this chapter. These relate to the management of dysphasia (language disorder), dysarthria (speech disorder), dysphonia (voice disorder), communication skills, hearing loss and dysphagia (swallowing disorder).

Management of language impairment

Management of language impairment begins by addressing attentional deficits, since no worthwhile short-term or generalised interaction can take place if the client is unable to concentrate. This is particularly true for those clients with a dementia. The list in Box 17.6 provides useful attention management hints.

Box 17.6 Techniques for gaining the client's attention

1. Ensure that sensory deficits are corrected, i.e. glasses are worn and clean, hearing aid(s) are worn and fitted correctly and the 'better' ear is used.
2. Reduce distracting background noise and activities or, if possible, move to a quieter area.
3. Position yourself directly in the client's line of vision and ensure that your face is well lit and your mouth is not hidden.
4. Use touch to gain and maintain attention, if the client can tolerate it.
5. Use the client's preferred name regularly to preface what you say.
6. Only one person speak at a time, with only one piece of information given or one question asked at a time.
7. Speak slowly and clearly while maintaining the natural flow of the communication.
8. Use clear, appropriate gesture to highlight what you are saying, but beware of using too much.
9. Heighten your use of facial expression.
10. Use the client's personal experiences as topics to maintain attention.
11. Keep conversation in the present.
12. Use visual clues of objects, clear pictures or written words.

Receptive language therapy activities

Attention levels need to be maximised on every occasion to ensure a full response to receptive language therapy activities. These activities vary in complexity depending on the level of need indicated in that part of the language assessment relating to understanding of spoken and written language.

Any person talking to someone with comprehension difficulties can maximise the likelihood of improved understanding by following a few basic guidelines. For example, try not to talk too rapidly or to use sentences that are too long and complex and allow plenty of time for response. Paraphrase what you say, i.e. if you are not understood then express what you want to say in another way. Pause between sentences to check that you have been understood and use this opportunity to ask the person to repeat or précis in their own words what you have said. Avoid using too many technical or 'jargon' words and try not to change the topic of conversation suddenly or with inadequate signalling. Use of clear gesture and signs can be of great help as can using objects, pictures, clear line drawings and the written word.

The only clinical tool that is absolutely essential for interaction to be successful is oneself and one's own communication skills. Common feelings when faced with an elderly person who has impaired receptive language are embarrassment and inadequacy. For communication to thrive there has to be feedback and if it is absent or incomplete because of comprehension problems this can be discouraging. By using a range of approaches, and by being imaginative and creative with our own communication, the skills of the elderly person can be maintained and prevented from further deterioration through disuse.

Speech and language therapy programmes for receptive language skills are based on the theories and premises of cognitive neuropsychology (Coltheart et al 1987, Ellis & Young 1988). Cognitive psychology studies the mental processes which underpin and enable behaviours to occur, among them linguistic recognition and planning. Neuropsychology looks at the behavioural functions of particular brain structures. Cognitive neuropsychology provides models which can explain both what is impaired and what is left intact when a person suffers brain damage, and can be of immense value to health care professionals working with elderly people in that it enables programmes to be tailor-made for individuals. Figure 17.3, discussed earlier in this chapter, is a simple cognitive neuropsychological model of language.

Sorting and matching tasks. These can promote greater recognition within various semantic groupings (e.g. nouns of a certain type – animals, utensils, family). Materials should be chosen based on level of need so that elderly people with the greatest receptive language impairment work first with real objects rather than pictures. Since both coloured pictures and line drawings are two-dimensional and representational they are considered higher level materials. The complexity of sorting and matching tasks can range from simple identical matching (comparing like with like) and simple colour or shape sorting, to more complex tasks involving unidentical matching or sorting tasks based on everyday concepts (e.g. modes of transport). Other sorting and matching tasks can reflect written language, so involving tasks with shapes, letters, numbers, words, phrases and sentences. They can also involve the recognition and understanding of items representing non-verbal concepts (e.g. emotions) with requests to sort/match happy (sad, angry, etc.) faces.

Selection tasks. These can be used in escalating degrees of complexity to access the 'semantic store'; that is, the store of an individual's unique and personalised linguistic knowledge. There is an almost inexhaustible fund of activities which can be cued by the request to 'show me', or 'point to', or 'find', or by the question 'which is?', or 'where is?'. Nouns, verbs, adjectives and prepositions, even mood states, can all be represented visually either with objects, pictures, mime or the written word.

Categorisation tasks. These are valuable in that they explore semantic links between concepts and expand the sorting skill to check a person's understanding of how things relate to each other in linguistic terms; for example with reference to bus, car and plane the client may be asked what makes two of these the same and one different, given they all come from the same general grouping. Categorisation tasks can also reflect non-verbal concepts in that they include items which reflect the client's perception of mood states; for example asking the client to sort photographs of faces into happy and sad categories.

Encouraging clients to follow and carry out instructions of increasing complexity forms the basis of another rich seam of receptive language tasks. In a simple form the task can involve listening, processing and responding appropriately to only one item (e.g. 'give me your hand') but in a more complex form, these tasks can involve sequencing and memory to quite a high degree; for example, 'dial this phone number', or 'bring me a newspaper, a box of matches and a Mars bar'. In these cases the client has to retain, process and organise a response in the correct order to several different items or concepts. Rehearsal strategies may need to be taught, repetition may need to be built in and then limited and gradually phased out. Above all it is important to be sure that there has been genuine linguistic understanding which is unaided by the many environmental clues which, unwittingly, may not have been screened out. For instance, it is easy to guess we are being asked if we want a cup of tea when the kettle can be heard boiling or the cups clinking on the trolley.

Written and pictorial comprehension exercises. These can also be of value. A story read aloud by the therapist or read aloud or silently by the client can be summarised, fully retold or responded to in terms of time, place and person in answer to written or verbal questioning. Implied meanings to pictures and stories can be sought via questions like 'how can we tell?' or 'what does that suggest?'

Expressive language therapy activities

Expressive language therapy activities are also wide ranging and now based on the principles of cognitive neuropsychology.

Cueing strategies. There are many cueing strategies which carers can use to facilitate the verbal output of their clients and their relatives. Amongst the most useful are the following:

- Contextual cueing – using the correct environmental context to alert the client to the correct meaning; for example talk about the kitchen *in* the kitchen.
- Gesture cueing – using and helping the client to use a clear action which may then trigger the word, e.g. forming a hand into the shape of a cup to indicate 'drink'.
- Run-in cueing – starting a phrase that the client completes; e.g. 'let's have a cup of ... ', 'knife and ... '.
- Phonemic cueing – giving the first sound of the word the client is attempting.
- Forced alternative cueing – giving the choice of two very different words; for example 'do you want a drink or a horse?' The number of choices can be progressively expanded and the degree of difference and the unlikelihood of the pairing can be narrowed if and when the client can cope.
- Verbal associative cueing – 'hot and cold', 'head and hair', etc. These associations can also be made by gesture to accompany the spoken word or by writing the association, if writing is the better preserved modality.
- Stereotyped speech and social speech can also act as cues because these are often preserved expressive skills.

Eye contact. Eye contact is often something that as carers we forget to note. Many clients will give the non-verbal expressive response of looking at the item requested or required when they are unable to name it or to form a question or state their need. If this ability remains then it should be noted and cued as often as possible.

Naming activities. These form the basis for many treatment sessions with people who are expressively impaired. Representations of nouns, verbs, adjectives and adverbs can be used to help the client gain access to their lexicon, which may be thought of as the dictionary within the brain. Objects, pictures and mime can all be used in conjunction with the cueing strategies listed above. The aim of naming tasks is for the client to build from the one word level to progressively more complex expressions. That is, from a noun or subject word (e.g. man), to phrases with a subject and a verb (e.g. the man is drinking) and then to sentences containing subject, verb and object (e.g. the man is drinking a cup of tea).

Word-finding activities can be extended from variations on naming to include tasks which involve synonym finding, where the individual or group have to find as many words with the same or similar meanings as possible. Activities can also become more complex and descriptive, involving action pictures, story pictures, discussions and problem solving sessions. All tasks which can be done verbally can also be done by reading and writing. These are often better preserved skills in elderly people and match their pre-morbid level of intellectual functioning (Nelson 1983).

If an expressive language impairment is very severe, then a variety of alternative or augmented communication strategies may be required. These might involve use of a computer with selected software packages, from the ever increasing range, as part of therapy, or assessment of the value of a communication aid. There is now an extensive choice of devices available which range from simple communication charts to complex computerised equipment, some of which have electronic 'voices'. Regional and national communication aids centres can advise on the appropriate aids which take account of the elderly client's level of cognitive and motor functioning, as well as their lifestyle and personal preferences. Gestural systems may be incorporated into therapy and there are several to choose from. These range from sophisticated systems for use with the deaf, such as British Sign Language (BSL) and Paget Gorman (Brennan et al 1980), to more simple and iconic systems like Makaton (Walker 1979) and Amer-Ind (Skelly 1979). These systems can be taught quite easily to elderly people, even those with some comprehension impairment, and use of a gestural system can at least facilitate a degree of functional communication.

Memory deficits

Memory deficits, whether in terms of storage of information or retrieval of words, will often need specific management as part of a speech and language therapy programme for elderly people with mental health problems. Good practices for assisting elderly clients to receive and retain information are 'little and often' therapy interventions and the simplification and reduction of the amount and type of information. It is important to establish which sensory pathway to the brain is most receptive; for example auditory, visual or kinaesthetic routes. Memory retraining activities may include alphabetical searching, first letter prompts, mental retracing, rhymes, mnemonics, visual imagery (e.g. names linked to pictures: 'Bob' = picture of coin), or even the use of external aids like a timer or other sound signal prompt to action or a notebook/diary for event recall. Wilson & Moffat (1984) offer many ideas for the management of memory impairment.

Speech impairment and voice disorder

Management of speech impairment involves many exercises for the alleviation of dysarthric or dyspraxic difficulties. These treatments may, as with expressive dysphasia, involve introducing an augmented communication strategy, if hand/eye motor control or motor organisational skills are adequate. Therapy involves teaching exercises for improving or maintaining respiration and phonation, as well as modification of posture, muscle tone and strength by use of generalised exercises and facilitated stimulation of the oral musculature and specific lip, tongue and palate exercises. Treatment of articulation and prosody (rhythm and stress) is dependent on influencing the client's insight, motivation and potential for sustaining progress. Robertson & Thomson (1982) provide a useful compendium of techniques and exercises.

Management of voice disorder, whether functional or organic in origin, begins with relaxation exercises, both general and specific, to the head, neck and respiratory musculature. Environmental changes aimed at reducing the potential for vocal abuse (e.g. smoking and shouting) can form a valuable part of management. Direct exercises for phonation and voice production can be helpful and a counselling approach is recommended, with opportunities for supported practice (Martin 1987).

Communication skills management

Communication skills management for elderly people involves many elements of social skills training which are often more traditionally used with younger mentally disordered clients (Trower et al 1978).

Non-verbal communication may be improved by focusing sessions on eye-contact, facial expression, body posture, gestures and proximity in interpersonal communication and physical appearance. Therapy sessions may also involve vocal and verbal skills, and emphasising and helping people to maintain the appropriateness of speech and language as well as its production.

Social and communication skills groups help clients to form and, most importantly, to maintain relationships and therefore can prevent the worst extremes of communicative isolation which can accompany old age. The programme should be run slowly and comfortably so that there is time for self-help, reinforcement, modelling and shaping of skills and for social development through spontaneity. Anxiety management may be included and above all the group needs to be flexible, informal and supportive. Social and communication therapy sessions may focus on clients' strengths, offer a forum for discussion and provide an outlet for emotions in a psychotherapeutic setting. To extend these activities to encompass more direct work on the pragmatic aspects of communication is a useful next step if group members have the residual abilities. Burnard (1990) is a source of useful ideas which can be adapted for use with elderly mentally impaired people.

For severely, globally communicatively impaired elderly clients the therapeutic aims are to make the best of residual abilities. This may be achieved through sensory stimulation or sensory integration therapy (Ayres 1972). Sensory information sets the boundaries of conscious experience. However damaged the brain – even in coma – it can register some level of sensory input. Sensory stimulation can be incorporated into most daily activities thereby rendering them therapeutic and genuinely interactive. Texture, colour, smell, taste, sound and temperature are all part of our daily lives and we adapt to them. Some elderly people may not have accurate recognition or adaptation abilities and will benefit from interventions which offer a structured regime of controlled sensory input which is tailor-made to meet individual needs. Sensory integration goes beyond mere stimulation in that it seeks to promote the adaptive response. Therapy interventions include encouraging the client to turn to sounds of different pitch and from different sides and distances, following objects with the eyes and the hands, and experiencing in a structured format different smells, tastes, textures and temperatures. If verbal interaction goes together with sensory stimulation, sensory stimulation can assure ongoing interaction between carers and even the most impaired client long after the point at which speech and language has deteriorated beyond use in speech.

Management of hearing impairment

For the elderly person with a hearing loss, management will vary depending on whether there is also cognitive impairment, and to what degree, and also whether the person can cope with a hearing aid or some other form of amplifier. Even today's small, sophisticated and powerful post-aural (behind the ear) hearing aids can be intrusive because they amplify all sounds and therefore demand tolerance, patience and increased attention from the wearer. One lady we know needed the most powerful of body-worn aids to hear and became increasingly distressed by them. Her distress was worst at mealtimes, which was not surprising since she wore the box under her dress to disguise the aid. Consequently all her own body noises were picked up as well as static from her clothes as she moved. The combined effect of body noises with feedback distortions from the hidden microphone and the noise and clatter of mealtimes was the source of her distress.

Some clients cannot use a hearing aid or do so only in controlled environments. Other forms of amplifier may be considered and can be discussed with a Communication Aids Centre or the local branch of the Royal Association for the Deaf or The Royal National Institute for the Deaf in London. It is important that hearing aids should be well fitting, correctly set and well maintained. The plastic ear mould and the tiny switch and dial mechanisms may be difficult for elderly fingers and confusion may result if the ear piece is placed in the ear incorrectly – even upside down or in the wrong ear. Feedback howl may occur because the ear piece is dirty or incorrectly inserted. Responsibility for changing the batteries and for fitting the aid correctly may fall upon a carer.

Speech and language therapists may assist by offering sessions (for individuals or groups) aimed at establishing auditory competence with the amplification and hearing aid management. Speech conservation exercises aimed at preserving articulation and voice may also be offered in addition to discussion of communication changes, both real and anticipated, and social and communication skills work to enhance

---

Box 17.7 Tips for improving communication with hard of hearing elderly clients
1. Face the person directly and at the same level.
2. Ensure adequate light is falling on the speaker's face.
3. Ensure light is not directly in the eyes of the deaf person.
4. Do not talk from another room!
5. Remember hearing is less good when the person is tired or ill.
6. Speak in a normal fashion but a little more slowly.
7. Don't shout.
8. Keep your hands away from your mouth.
9. Try not to talk too rapidly, or use long, complex sentences.
10. Adopting a slightly lower pitch to the voice may help.
11. Don't move your head around, as a lip reader may find it difficult to see what you are saying.
12. Bright, large earrings and neck attire can be distracting.
13. Lip readers find it very difficult to understand people who have large moustaches and/or beards.

coping, such as increased attention and basic lip reading. Tips for improving communication with elderly clients who have existing mental health and hearing problems are shown in Box 17.7.

MANAGEMENT OF EATING AND SWALLOWING DISORDERS

Management of eating and swallowing disorders is a relatively new but an increasing part of the work of the speech and language therapist working with elderly mentally ill people. It is an important area of work because mechanical deficits, causing problems in feeding and swallowing, are potentially life threatening. A prerequisite of this work is specialist training in the functions of the head and neck and most speech and language therapists working in this area have accredited training and experience. However, a team approach to management is vital and would be improved if diagnostic procedures like barium swallow and videofluoroscopic X-ray were more widely available. Management depends on which phase of the swallow has broken down – oral, pharyngeal or oesophageal as previously discussed.

There are many procedures, some knowledge of which will be of immense benefit to all carers working with this client group. These procedures, as discussed below and taught by the speech and language therapist to key carers, can be seen as good practices towards a measure of prevention even in cases of silent aspiration, where choking is not obviously present and there is no marked activation of the cough or gag reflexes. It is very important to note that it is a myth to assume that because a client has an intact gag reflex they are safe to swallow. Having assessed the client it is most unlikely that the speech and language therapist will be able to personally feed each client at each meal, so equipping other staff to deal with the client is of paramount importance.

The speech and language therapist can help by guiding, demonstrating, training, advising and supporting other professionals and lay carers who help the elderly client with eating. Direct work with the client may take the form of neuromuscular facilitation exercises and stimulation. It may involve applying ice to the facial musculature or gentle brushing and stroking along the line of the muscles to initiate a sensory response which may encourage better patterns of movement during eating.

When possible, clients who need assisted feeding should be served first and one at a time. Correct management of feeding and swallowing is time consuming and often very messy. Meals and drinks should not be too hot and feeding is best done from in front of the client, who should be fully awake and concentrating and encouraged to participate. Eating aids (e.g. plate guards, adapted handles for cutlery, special cups) may be needed so that a measure of independence can be achieved and postural adaptations may also be required, since feeding and swallowing can only be fully maximised if the client is in a symmetrical position, is comfortable and correctly supported. Advice from the physiotherapist may be helpful in these cases.

Clients will need a soft diet if they have chewing problems, or a puréed diet if they are prone to choking or aspiration. A liquidised diet is seldom recommended since it has lower nutritional value and its high water content can increase the likelihood of aspiration.

When feeding the client, the assistant should sit comfortably, offer explanation and be aware of non-verbal communication from the client. Manual stimulation, such as gentle circular massage of the cheeks, may help a client chew. Only small spoonfuls of food or small sips of fluid should be given and if the client does not open his mouth, has a pronounced bite reflex, or is unaware of the spoon or cup, then spreading a little food or fluid on the lips can stimulate opening. Food should be placed centrally on the tongue and clients can be helped to swallow by lowering the chin and making sure the head is tipped slightly forward. Sufficient time is needed for the client to chew and swallow each mouthful before another is offered. A routine of food in the mouth – chew – perform two swallows – clear throat is advised. Drinks should be offered before and after but not during the meal since it will not aid food transport and may cause build up at the level of the pharynx and aspiration caused by spillage into the larynx.

Clients with severe eating problems may need fluids thickened with products such as Carobel®; this makes them go down more slowly and safer to swallow. If little is being taken orally then the dietician may advise on possible supplements such as Complan®, Build-up®, Fortipud® and Fortisip®. In extreme cases medical intervention will be needed for intravenous infusion or nasogastric intubation, or even surgery (gastrostomy). If a change of dietary and feeding regime is necessary, the likes and dislikes of the client should be taken into consideration, as should the colour, texture, temperature, smell and overall presentation of the food. Mixed textures should be avoided, for example minestrone soup, because each type of food requires a different amount of chewing and will be swallowed at a different rate. Stringy textures (e.g. bacon, cabbage, runner beans, etc.), floppy textures (e.g. certain types of lettuce) and foods that are acidic (e.g. lemons) and alcohol should also be avoided. Other potentially dangerous foods are peanuts, peas, broad beans, sweetcorn and chips. Staff involved in feeding elderly clients who may be at risk of choking should be conversant with possible dangers and skilled in first aid procedures.

SUPPORTING CARERS

Elderly people with mental health problems enjoy communicating at whatever level is available to them and relatives and other carers need to be helped to achieve the greatest possible degree of reciprocal communication (Tanner & Daniels 1990). All aspects of the elderly person's communication and programmes being used should be discussed with carers, and implementation strategies devised to enable changes to be made and improvements gained to be retained. The client's home, day care or ward environment should be modified to facilitate improved communication. Changes include labelling and the use of clear signs to promote orientation and ensuring ease of access to items which will aid communication and communicative independence (e.g. pens and paper, remote controls for the TV). It is often important to a family to be involved on a practical level with therapy,

---

Box 17.8 An individualised language programme with environmental modification

Mr Richards, aged 78, started to experience word-finding difficulties. CT scanning revealed a scar on the left temporal lobe. There was gradual deterioration in Mr Richards's condition with increased expressive dysphasia and the onset of night-time convulsions. Multi-infarct dementia with ongoing transient ischaemic attacks seemed the most likely diagnosis.

On language assessment, Mr Richards displayed marked difficulty in carrying out both written and verbal commands, although the latter skill was marginally more intact. Reading skills were poor. His expressive language was by then severely compromised, with serious word-finding difficulties, poor self-monitoring and a speech dyspraxia. Basic social speech was preserved but this was used repetitively and therefore mainly inappropriately. He had insight into his difficulties and there was attendant frustration.

Since assessment had revealed a preserved ability to perform a range of matching tasks, this became a focus of therapy, which was undertaken at home. Tasks involved object/object, picture/picture, word/word matching initially and progressed to combination tasks

(e.g. picture/word) and to categorisation tasks relating to his home, family and interests. These tasks offered an opportunity for success and positive feedback in a situation where there was very little of this, and provided structured formats to involve the client's family at a time when they felt helpless.

Sets of photographs were built up of Mr Richards's household objects, of verbs (posed by his wife or the therapist) and of emotions (posed by the therapist). A velcro-based communication board was devised so the photographs and matching word labels could be constantly re-used and made to relate to any room in the house. This ensured familiarisation and the maintenance of relearning. Mr Richards was also able to indicate his feelings by use of the board. The therapy programme developed to become a family affair, continually undertaken in the comfort of home, thus maintaining skills and ensuring stimulation for Mr Richards and feedback for his family.

This case demonstrates the importance of accessing whatever verbal skills and opportunities for interactive communication are retained and offering the possibility for structured stimulation and positive feedback at home.

---

since this can offer a structured approach to care which can be supportive to them. A home-based programme using photographic aids for Mr Richards is discussed in Box 17.8.

Family therapy and counselling sessions for relatives and carers can be valuable in maintaining communication and motivation to continue. Carers need to know why their partner or parent is behaving in a particular way and good education and advice can alleviate some of the guilt which many people experience as communication becomes more difficult. To maximise rapport, the carer may have to change communication patterns acquired over a lifetime; this is not easy. It is stressful to deal constantly with the repetitive nature of talk from some people with dementia and to cope with deterioration in language and memory. Support groups for carers can be a source of practical advice, information sharing and support. It may be that approaches and adjustments which have worked for one person can help others. Some carers in support groups report that having an opportunity to talk makes them feel less isolated and more accepting of their situation.

We cannot overestimate the sadness and loss experienced by carers as communicative links fade. Mulhall (1988) describes the relationship between a wife and her 69-year-old husband suffering from a dementia. On his admission to hospital for respite care, the wife reported being relieved but felt herself to be a failure and recognised with sorrow that his departure was probably the end of the most important chapter in their mutual lives. As described by a carer we know, 'this gradual loss of our ability to communicate as we used to is like a succession of little bereavements'.

CONCLUSION

This chapter has underlined the importance of speech, language and communication in the lives of elderly people and has discussed principles of management when these skills are affected by a mental health problem in old age. Improving communication personally and professionally as well as for and about our clients can contribute immeasurably to the quality of life of elderly clients. As part of a multidisciplinary approach to care speech and language therapists can help lessen the impact of the 'little bereavements'.

REFERENCES

American Psychiatric Association 1987 DSM III R Diagnostic and statistical manual of mental disorders, 3rd edn. American Psychiatric Association, Washington

Ayres A J 1972 Sensory integration and learning disorders. Western Psychological Services, Los Angeles

Baldessarini R J 1988 A summary of current knowledge of tardive dyskinesia. L'Encephale XIV: 263–268

Bayles K A and Boone D R 1982 The potential of language tasks of identifying senile dementia. Journal of Speech and Hearing Disorders 47: 204–210

Bayles K A, Kaszniak A W 1987 Communication and cognition in normal ageing and dementia. Taylor and Francis, London

Beck A T, Rush A J, Shaw B F, Emery G 1979 The depression inventory: cognitive therapy of depression. Wiley, Chichester

Benson D F 1979 Aphasia, Alexia and Agraphia. Churchill Livingstone, Edinburgh

Benson D F, Webster Ross G, Cummings J L 1990 Speech and language alterations in dementia syndromes: characteristics and treatment. Aphasiology 4(4): 339–352

Bishop D 1983 Test for the reception of grammar. University of Manchester

Brennan M, Colville M, Lawson L 1980 Words in hand: a structural analysis of the signs of British sign language. The BSL Research Project, Moray House, Edinburgh

Breznitz Z, Sherman T 1987 Speech patterns of normal discourse of well and depressed mothers and their young children. Child Development 58: 395–400

Bryan K 1989 The right hemisphere language battery. Winslow Press, Oxford

Buckingham H W 1985 Perseveration in aphasia. In: Stanton N and Epstein R (eds) Current perspectives in dysphasia. Churchill Livingstone, Edinburgh

Burnard P 1990 Teaching interpersonal skills. Chapman and Hall, London

Butters N, Cermak L S 1980 Alcoholic Korsakoff's syndrome. Academic Press, New York

Chapey R 1986 Language intervention strategies in adult aphasia. William and Wilkins, Baltimore

Clare A 1992 The Jansson Memorial Lecture: communication in medicine. European Journal of Disorders of Communication 28(1): 1–12

Code C 1991 The characteristics of aphasia. Lawrence Erlbaum, Hove

Code C, Lodge B 1987 Language in dementia of recent referral. Age and Aging 16: 366–372

Coltheart M, Sartori G, Job R 1987 The cognitive neuropsychology of language. Lawrence Erlbaum, Hove

College of Speech and Language Therapists 1990 Dementia working party survey. Unpublished report, CSLT, London

Critchley E M R 1981 Speech disorder of Parkinson's disease: a review. Journal of Neurology, Neurosurgery and Psychiatry 44: 751–758

Cummings J L, Benson D F, Hill M A, Read S 1985 Aphasia in dementia of the Alzheimer's type. Neurology 35: 395–397

Cummings J L, Darkins A, Mendez M, Hill M A, Benson D F 1988 Alzheimer's disease and Parkinson's disease: comparison of speech and language alterations. Neurology 38: 680–684

Cutting J 1990 The right cerebral hemisphere and psychiatric disorders. Oxford University Press, Oxford

Dabul B, Bollier B 1978 therapeutic approaches to apraxia. Journal of Speech and Hearing Disorders 41: 268–276

Darley F L, Aronson A E, Brown J R 1975 Motor speech disorders. Saunders, Philadelphia

Davis A C 1983 Hearing disorders in the population. In: Lutman M E, Haggard M P (eds) Hearing science and hearing disorders. Academic Press, London

Denmark J C 1985 A study of 250 patients referred to a department of psychiatry for the deaf. British Journal of Psychiatry 146: 282–286

DeRenzi E, Faglioni P 1978 Normative data and screening power of a shortened version of the Token Test. Cortex 14: 41–49

Diamond B 1981 The relevance of voice in forensic psychiatric evaluation. In: Darby J K (ed) Speech evaluation in psychiatry. Grune and Stratton, New York

Dunn M, Dunn M, Whetton C 1982 British picture vocabulary scales. NFER Nelson, Windsor

Eastwood M R, Corbin S L, Reed M, Nobbs H, Kedward H B 1986 Acquired hearing loss and psychiatric illness: an estimate of prevalence and psychomorbidity in a geriatric setting. British Journal of Psychiatry 147: 552–556

Ellis A W, Young A W 1988 Human cognitive neuropsychology. Lawrence Erlbaum, London

Enderby P 1988 The Frenchay dysarthria assessment. NFER Nelson, Windsor

Espir M L E, Rose F C 1983 The basic neurology of speech and language. Blackwell Scientific Publications, Oxford

Faber R, Abrams R, Taylor M et al 1983 Comparison of schizophrenic patients with formal thought disorder and neurologically impaired patients with aphasia. American Journal of Psychiatry 140: 1348–1351

Filley C M, Heaton R K, Nelson L M, Burks T S, Franklin G M 1989 Comparison of dementia in Alzheimer's disease and multiple sclerosis. Archives of Neurology 46: 157–161

France J 1991 Psychosis. In: Gravell R, France J (eds) Speech and communication problems in psychiatry. Chapman and Hall, London

Gardner H, Brownell H H, Wagner W, Michelow D 1983 Missing the point: the role of the right hemisphere in the processing of complex linguistic material. In: Pereaman E (ed) Cognitive processing in the right hemisphere. Academic Press, New York

Golding E 1989 The Middlesex elderly assessment of mental state. Thames Valley Test Company, Hants

Goodglass H, Kaplan E 1983 The Boston Diagnostic Aphasia Examination. Lea and Febiger, Beckenham

Gravell R 1988 Communication problems in elderly people. Chapman and Hall, London

Hare R D 1986 Twenty years of experience with the Cleckley psychopath. In: Reid W H, Dorr D, Walker J I, Bonner J (eds) Unmasking the psychopath. Norton, New York

Harrap-Griffiths J, Katon W, Dobis R et al 1987 Chronic tinnitus: associated with psychiatric diagnosis. Journal of Psychosomatic Research 31(5): 613–621

Hildick-Smith M 1985 Neurological problems in the elderly. Ballière Tindall, London

Holland A L 1980 Communicative abilities of daily living: a test of functional communication for aphasics. Pro-ed Taskmaster

Huskins S 1986 Non-verbal apraxia screening test. In: Huskins S Working with dyspraxics. Winslow Press, Oxford

Kempler D 1991 Language changes in dementia of the Alzheimer's type. In: Lubinski R Dementia and communication. B C Decker, Philadelphia

Kendall R E 1988 Diagnosis and classification. In: Kendall R R and Zealley A K Companion guide to psychiatric studies. Churchill Livingstone, Edinburgh

Kirshner H S, Webb W G, Kelly M P, Wells C E 1984 Language disturbance: an initial symptom of cortical degenerations and dementia. Archives of Neurology 41: 491–496

Kirshner H S, Tanridag O, Thurman L, Whetsell W O 1987 Progressive aphasia without dementia: two cases of focal spongiform degeneration. Annals of Neurology 22(44): 527–532

Kronfol Z, Hamsher K, Digre K, Wazir R 1978 Depression and hemispheric functions: changes associated with unilateral ECT. British Journal of Psychiatry 132: 560–567

Laidlaw J, Richens A 1982 A textbook of epilepsy, 2nd edn. Churchill Livingstone, Edinburgh

Leach G 1983 The principles of pragmatics. Longmans, London

Lethlean J B, Murdoch B E 1993 Language dysfunction in progressive leukoencephalopathy: a case study journal of speech and language. Pathology 1(1): 27–34

Lezak M D 1983 Neuropsychological assessment, 2nd edn. Oxford University Press, Oxford

Lockhart M, Martin S 1987 The Victoria Infirmary Voice Questionnaire. In: Martin S (ed) Working with dysphonics. Winslow Press, Oxford

Lubinski R 1991 Dementia and communication. B C Decker, Philadelphia

MacLean P 1970 The triune brain, emotion and scientific bias. In: Schmitt F (ed) The neurosciences second study programme. Rockerfeller University Press, New York

McNeil M R, Prescott T E 1978 The revised Token Test. Winslow Press, Oxford

Martin S 1987 Working with dysphonics. Winslow Press, Oxford

Matthews W B 1978 Multiple sclerosis: the facts. University Press, Oxford

Mesulam M M 1982 Slowly progressive aphasia without generalised dementia. Annals of Neurology 11: 592–598

Miller E 1984 Verbal Fluency Test. British Journal of Clinical Psychology 23: 53–57

Mulhall D J 1988 The management of the aphasic patient. In: Rose F C Whurr R, Wyke M A (eds) The management of the aphasic patient. Whurr Publications, London

Nelson H E 1983 The New Adult Reading Test. NFER Nelson, Oxford

Nilsonne A 1988 Speech characteristics as indicators of depressive illness. Acta Psychologica Scandinavica 77: 253–263

Obler L K, Albert M L 1981 Language and aging: a neurobehavioural analysis. In: Beasley D S, Davis G A (eds) Aging: communication processes and disorders. Grune and Stratton, New York

O'Neill P 1989 Cranio-cerebral trauma. In: Tallis R (ed) The clinical neurology of old age. Wiley, Chichester

Orlans H 1985 Adjustment to adult hearing loss. Taylor and Francis, London

Parkin A J 1987 Memory and amnesia: an introduction. Blackwell, Oxford

Pattie A H, Gilleard C J 1979 The Clifton Assessment Procedure for the Elderly. NFER Nelson, Oxford

Penn C 1988 The profile of communicative appropriateness: a clinical tool for the assessment of pragmatics. University of Witwatersrand, Johannesburg

Perry A R 1982 What can the speech therapist offer in motor neurone disease? In: Rose F C (ed) Research progress in motor neurone disease. Pitman Medical, Tunbridge Wells

Phillips G 1984 A perspective of social withdrawal. In: Daly J A, McCroskey J C (eds) Avoiding communication: shyness, reticence and communicative apprehension. Sage Publications, Beverley Hills

Poeck K, Luzzatti C 1988 Slowly progressive aphasia in three patients. Brain III: 151–168

Pogacar S, Williams R S 1984 Alzheimer's disease presenting as slowly progressive aphasia. Rhode Island Medical Journal 67: 181–185

Reusch J 1987 Values, communication and culture. In: Reusch J, Bateson G (eds) Communication in the social matrix of psychiatry, 3rd edn. Norton, London

Robertson S J 1982 A dysarthria profile. Winslow Press, Oxford

Robertson S J, Thomson F 1982 Working with dysarthrics. Winslow Press, Oxford

Rose F C 1977 Motor neurone disease. Pitman Medical, Tunbridge Wells

Sachs O 1985 The man who mistook his wife for a hat. Picador, New York

Saxton J, McGonigle K L, Swihart A A, Boller F 1993 Severe Impairment Battery. Thames Valley Test Company, Bury St Edmunds

Schuell H 1965 The Minnesota Test of Differential Diagnosis of Aphasia. University of Minnesota Press

Schuell H 1973 The Shortened Schuell Test. University of Minnesota Press

Seaman 1990 Key issues in understanding and caring for elderly mentally infirm people. Speech Therapy in Practice 6(6): viii–ix

Selnes D, Carson K, Rorner B, Gordon B 1988 Language dysfunction in early and late onset: possible Alzheimer's Disease. Neurology 38: 1053–1056

Sharr M 1989 Tumours of the nervous system. In: Tallis R (ed) The clinical neurology of old age. Wiley, Chichester

Shuttleworth E C, Huber S J 1988 The naming disorder of dementia of the Alzheimer type. Brain and Language 34: 222–234

Skelly M 1979 Amer-Ind gestural code, based on universal American Indian hand talk. Elsevier, New York

Skinner C, Wirz M, Thompson I, Davidson J 1984 The Edinburgh Functional Communication Profile. Winslow Press, Oxford

Stemple J C 1984 Clinical voice pathology theory and management. Charles C Merrill, Oxford

Stevens S J 1985 Dementia checklist. Hammersmith Hospital, London

Stokes G, Goudie F 1990 Working with dementia. Winslow Press, Oxford

Tanner B B, Daniels K A 1990 An observation study of communication between carers and their relatives with dementia. Care of the Elderly 2(6): 247–250

Trower P, Bryant B, Argyle M 1978 Social skills and mental health. Methuen, London

Walker M 1979 The Makaton: in perspective. Apex 7: 12–14

Wattis J P, Wattis L, Airie T 1981 Psychogeriatrics: a national survey of a new branch of psychiatry. British Medical Journal 282: 1529–1533

Wattis J P 1988 Geographical variations in the provision of psychiatric services for old people. Age and Ageing 17: 171–180

Wechsler D 1981 The Wechsler Adult Intelligence Scale. Psychological Corporation, Sidcup

Whurr R 1974 An Aphasia Screening Test. Whurr Publications, London

Wilson B, Moffat N 1984 Clinical management of memory problems. Chapman and Hall, London

RECOMMENDED READING

Bayles K A, Kaszniak A W 1987 Communication and cognition in normal aging and dementia. Taylor and Francis, London. *Few speech and language therapists working with elderly people could manage without this book. It is the result of years of detailed research and information gathering in the field of elderly care. It provides clinical guidance and can be used by all as a vital reference book.*

Benson D F 1979 Aphasis, alexia and agraphia. Churchill Livingstone, Edinburgh. *A useful text which relates syndromes to their neurological bases. The definitive text on cortical localisation.*

Code C 1991 The characteristics of aphasia. Lawrence Erlbaum, Hove. *Easy to read. No jargon without accompanying clear explanations. A definitive overview of aspects of aphasia.*

Ellis A W, Young A W 1988 Human cognitive neuropsychology. Lawrence Erlbaum, Hove and London. *A splendid and accessible book leading the reader through the otherwise complex maze of cognitive neuropsychological theory and practice. Comprehensive and practical.*

Espir M L E, Rose F C 1983 The basic neurology of speech and language. Blackwell Scientific Publications, Oxford. *At last an intelligible book on the neurology of speech and language! Straightforward, pocket-sized and to the point. An excellent guide to the neurological aetiology and pathology of speech and language.*

Gravell R 1988 Communication problems in elderly people. Chapman and Hall, London. *Written by a speech and language therapist working with elderly people this book is accessible to all health care professionals. It contains many practical ideas, emphasises the role of the speech and language therapist in the multidisciplinary health team care team and details the many communication changes which may be experienced by elderly people.*

Logemann J 1983 Evaluation and treatment of swallowing disorders. College Hill Press, San Diego, California. *The definitive book on dysphagia management. A vital resource for all health care professionals likely to become involved in the management of feeding and swallowing problems.*

Lubkinski R 1991 Dementia and communication. B C Decher, Philadelphia. *In four sections, this book addresses the bases for communicative changes in dementia, the social impact of dementia, language changes and dementia and issues in rehabilitation. All contributors are researchers or practising clinicians. A detailed but accessible book.*

Sachs O 1985 The man who mistook his wife for a hat. Picador, New York. *Case studies of neurological disorder which bring the reality for the clients to life.*

The 'Working With' Series. Winslow Press, Oxford

Fawcus M, Robinson M, Williams J, Williams R 1986 Working with dysphasia. Winslow Press, Oxford

Martin S 1987 Working with dysphonics. Winslow Press, Oxford

Robertson S J, Thomson F 1982 Working with dysarthrics. Winslow Press, Oxford

Stokes G, Goudie F 1990 Working with dementia. Winslow Press, Oxford

This series of books is a constant source of ideas and therapeutic inspiration and they contain a wide range of practical activities for speech and language therapists and for other professionals.

18

Reducing challenging behaviour of elderly confused people: a behavioural perspective

Catherine Wells
John Wells

INTRODUCTION

The goal of behaviour therapy is to increase desirable behaviour, reduce undesirable behaviour and/or produce new behaviour. Behaviourists have been reluctant to engage in the study and treatment of the problems of the older adult. This reluctance, supported by the erroneous belief that older adults were unlikely to gain benefit from psychological interventions (Morris & Morris 1991), was based on the belief that experiences such as urinary incontinence or aggression were the inevitable and irreversible consequence of biophysical and cognitive degeneration due to ageing (Carstensen 1988). This chapter looks at interventions, based on instrumental learning, which are used to address challenging behaviours exhibited by the older adult. A consideration of the development of behaviourism, its principles and involvement with older adults, is followed by discussion of behavioural assessment and interventions. Two examples of challenging behaviour (aggression and urinary incontinence) are drawn upon to illustrate the therapeutic interventions and techniques commonly employed.

There are a number of terms which are used interchangeably to describe behaviour therapy, such as behaviour modification and behavioural psychotherapy. These do, however, carry specific clinical meanings or connotations. Therefore, throughout this chapter, behavioural interventions are described in the context of behaviour therapy, defined here as a body of knowledge, based on learning theory, which aims to assist individuals, through training modalities, to overcome behavioural problems.

Behaviour therapy, it has been claimed, addresses only the problems identified by others (for example relatives and carers) as opposed to those identified by older people themselves. In other words 'socially significant' behaviours are addressed such as incontinence, which pose difficulties for carers, rather than 'clinically significant' problems, such as intrusive imagery, which are important to the individual (Richards & Thorpe 1978, Bradbury 1991). However, socially significant problems can also cause older people personal distress because they have a negative effect on interaction with their environment. The behaviour therapist is committed to the alleviation of individual suffering by increasing the independence of individuals through improving their level of skill functioning within their immediate environment. In this endeavour the therapist is guided by an agreement with the client in which goals and techniques of treatment are explicitly defined. In this way the therapist attempts to ensure that the client's priorities and best interests are at the heart of the therapeutic relationship.

BEHAVIOUR THERAPY AND OLDER PEOPLE

Although behaviour therapy broadened its scope and theory as it developed, it focused on young populations or on those within a broad diagnostic category, such as learning disability. The problems of older people were largely ignored. There were a number of reasons for this neglect, prominent amongst which was the belief that this group was cognitively unsuited for therapy, as decline in old age was irreversible, and a traditional lack of clinical interest in the problems of older adults. This attitude began to change in the early 1970s when research demonstrated that speech in elderly psychiatric patients could be reinstated using reinforcement (Richards & Thorpe 1978, Burgio & Burgio 1986). Baltes & Lascomb (1975) used reinforcement successfully to treat an elderly person who screamed incessantly, whilst McClanahan & Risley (1975) were able to increase the socialisation and interaction of residents of a nursing home by modifying the environment, for example opening a shop. Interest in the behavioural management of incontinence with older adults also grew at this time, although results of studies were mixed (Pollock & Liberman 1974). What this limited work served to do was to dispel the myth that decline and inability to learn were intrinsic features of the ageing process.

After this initial interest there was an apparent return to the status quo. Between 1973 and 1980, on average only 11 articles per year were published on behavioural interventions with older people (Burgio & Burgio 1986, cited in Carstensen 1988). What appeared to hamper professional interest and, to some extent

continues to do so, was the lack of a journal specifically devoted to the development of behaviour therapy with older people, reinforced by an apparent anti-age bias by the behavioural journals and an anti-behavioural bias by gerontological journals (Carstensen 1988).

The late 1980s saw an increase in interest in the use of behaviour therapy with older adults, possibly connected to the rhetoric of the impending demographic time bomb of ageing (Carstensen 1988). Bradbury (1991), in a review of the literature, noted that this upsurge in clinical attention has tended to ignore people living in the community and remains focused on institutionalised groups. Nevertheless, behavioural gerontology is an area of increasing interest if largely underdeveloped.

THE BEHAVIOURAL APPROACH

Key issues in the development of behavioural theory

Behavioural approaches to human problems have a long history and may be traced to the writings of John Locke in the 17th century, who advocated the use of exposure to cure a child's fear of frogs, and to the systematic use of contingency rewards in controlling prisoners in the 1800s (O'Sullivan 1992). Towards the end of the 19th and first half of the 20th century, the foundation of the modern behavioural approach to clinical problems was laid through the development of learning theory. Within this field the work of Watson, Pavlov, Thorndike, Skinner and Wolpe was seminal.

The US psychologist Broadus Watson (1878–1958) was the first to expound a systematic behavioural interpretation of human action. His advocacy of the use of objective methods, described as methodological behaviourism, and view that the interaction of individuals within their environment was central to the learning process, set the pattern for the future of behavioural investigation (Watson & Rayner 1920, BABCP 1993).

The Russian physiologist, Ivan Pavlov (1849–1936), developed a theory of learning centred on reinforcement. In *Conditioned Reflexes*, published in 1927, he described this theory as classical conditioning. He noticed that dogs salivated when they heard specific sounds before being fed. Pavlov rang a bell (a neutral stimulus) immediately before the dogs were presented with food (an unconditioned stimulus) and they in turn salivated (an unconditioned response). After this procedure had been carried out a number of times, Pavlov rang the bell without presenting the food. The dogs continued to salivate on hearing the noise. The bell had become a conditioned stimulus and the salivation a conditioned response. If the bell continued to be rung without presenting food, salivation at the sound of the bell gradually disappeared or became extinguished. Subsequent work also demonstrated that emotional reactions, such as fear, could also be conditioned. Classical conditioning, in part, helps to explain the development of phobias (BABCP 1993).

Lee Thorndike (1874–1949) developed an alternative framework of learning. He placed cats in a box from which they could only escape through a panel, held in place by a catch, in order to get food. Thorndike observed that the cats, through a process of trial and error, learned to operate the catch. As the cats became familiar with the catch they took less time to open it between sessions. He called this the 'law of effect' – a correct response is established whenever it leads to a satisfying reward. Again, once the food was removed the behaviour was gradually extinguished (O'Sullivan 1992, BABCP 1993).

Thorndike's theory was controversial because it postulated an internal process, satisfaction, not open to observation and flew in the face of the contemporary behavioural view that internal subjective processes were unimportant in relation to behaviour. However, B F Skinner (1904–1990) reconciled Thorndike's work with mainstream behaviourism through the development of the concept of reinforcers within a learning model termed operant or instrumental conditioning. He found that animals could learn behaviours as a result of their effect on their environment. Rats were placed in a box with a lever. When the lever was depressed food was dispensed. The rat learned that by interacting with its environment (the lever) via a specific behaviour (pressing the lever) it received food (a reinforcer). If a behaviour was reinforced then the probability of the behaviour being repeated increased. Skinner also discovered that if reinforcement was used intermittently, rather than every time, it actually strengthened the association between the behaviour and the response, making it more difficult to break. During the 1950s, Skinner effectively employed operant conditioning techniques with various patients suffering from chronic psychiatric conditions.

Josef Wolpe, in the 1950s, hypothesised the development of neurosis on the basis of classical conditioning. Wolpe observed that fear responses could be reduced by simultaneously presenting an individual with a reciprocal inhibitor of anxiety, leading to a weakening of the link between the stimulus and the anxiety. He taught patients to use progressive muscle relaxation whilst proceeding through a hierarchy of anxiety-provoking situations in imagination initially and then in real life (in vivo). This treatment, called systematic desensitisation, became the main behavioural intervention for phobias and anxiety, although later work refined it so that both the imagery and muscle relaxation elements were not considered necessary for the efficacy of treatment. Currently the dominant treatment method is in vivo exposure alone.

Throughout the 1950s and 1960s the application of learning-based theory for the treatment of a whole range of difficulties began to be designed and used. This led to the development of behavioural medicine, aversion therapy to treat addictions and deviant behaviours, exposure therapy for phobias and the treatment of obsessional disorders. Therapists such as Allyon, utilising instrumental conditioning developed 'token economies' in institutional settings (BACP 1993). In the 1970s, as empirical evidence for success grew, treatment expanded and widened, leading to the development of new behavioural therapies such as biofeedback and social skills training.

Principles and assumptions

As discussed above, a major assumption of the behavioural approach is that a person's behaviour is shaped by their experiences and is learned, either through classical or instrumental conditioning. If that experience can be changed or influenced, people can learn new behaviours or unlearn maladaptive ones, thereby enhancing their wellbeing and empowering them to achieve their personal goals (O'Sullivan 1992). For learning to be said to have taken place, there must be a relatively permanent change of behaviour that is demonstrably attributable to prior experience.

The behavioural approach defines behaviour broadly as all actions carried out by an individual, including passive activities such as sitting motionless. In addition, the approach views individual behaviour as occurring not in a vacuum, but within a contextual setting. Individual behaviour is therefore shaped by the immediate environment, involving place, time, persons and objects present and their activity and/or relationship to the individual and the behaviour they display (McBrien & Felce 1992). An essential feature from the therapeutic standpoint is 'specificity'. As Richards & Thorpe (1978) put it, 'how may which behaviours in what individual be most effectively and efficiently altered by whom?'

It follows that the behavioural approach is

concerned with what is overt and observable in behaviour and the environment. The behavioural therapist is not concerned with the individual's subjective 'internal world', or underlying unconscious motivations. This does not necessarily deny that these things exist, or that they are not important to the individual; it is merely that in terms of objective evaluation they are hard to measure (Cautela & Kearney 1990). It is argued that the overtness of behaviour makes it comparatively susceptible to effective intervention and treatment and that autonomic responses, cognitions, motivations, etc. are so inextricably linked, that influencing behaviour inevitably affects these other areas (Richards & McDonald 1991). Having said that, a number of behaviour therapists have developed a strong interest in the development and application of techniques which change cognitions and thus behaviour. Others have argued that the internal world of thoughts and feelings may be seen as behaviours in their own right and thus susceptible to behavioural analysis and intervention (Cautela & Kearney 1990).

As we have said, the approach focuses on behaviour in relation to context and in particular the consequences of behaviour. Consequences are characterised as one of the following:

- Positive reinforcement – a pleasing consequence that results from a behaviour, thus increasing the likelihood of the behaviour being repeated. For example, washing one's face is reinforced by a feeling of comfort and cleanliness.
- Negative reinforcement – the ending of an unpleasant situation through the behaviour. For example, passing urine to relieve a full bladder.
- Positive punishment – a behaviour results in a disagreeable consequence, likely to result in that behaviour subsequently declining. For example, a small child pulling the cat's tail and receiving a scratch.
- Negative punishment – the taking away of something that the individual finds pleasant, as a consequence of a behaviour, eventually making it unlikely that the behaviour will be repeated. For example, an employer deducting earnings for lateness (McBrien & Felce 1992).

Through consequence, individuals learn to do things which, overall, give greatest benefit, and learn to stop or avoid doing things which, overall, result more in punishment than benefit. McBrien & Felce (1992) stress that reinforcement and punishment are defined in terms of the effect they have on behaviour. They should not be thought of as subjective value

judgements such as nice/nasty. Poorly trained therapists may, for example, confuse negative reinforcement with the lay person's understanding of punishment, leading to its misapplication. Such confusion will inevitably lead to a failure in achieving goals and cause unnecessary distress to the client.

There are advantages of the behavioural approach for older clients. Therapy is relatively short (time being an increasingly precious commodity as one ages), more cost-effective and more obviously relevant to the problems experienced than more psychotherapeutic or psychoanalytic approaches. Church (1983) argues that changes in the ability to think abstractly as a consequence of the ageing process, point to the use of less interpretative interventions such as behaviour therapy. However, others have taken issue with this, arguing that older adults are perfectly able to engage in abstract thinking (Bradbury 1991).

The behavioural emphasis on the active role of the therapist is an important consideration for older clients. Older people may want the therapist to be more directive within the therapeutic relationship, as they become less physically and intellectually effective in controlling their environment (Richards & Thorpe 1978). The development of a strong therapeutic component is of primary importance in a directive relationship. Keijsers et al (1991) found that a successful behavioural treatment outcome correlated with the client's assessment of the quality of the therapeutic relationship. An accepting relationship based upon empathy and support, as perceived by the client, was found to be particularly important.

In summary, therapists adopting the concepts and techniques of the behavioural approach have a commitment to objective methods of investigation and analysis; precise identification, and treatment, of specified behaviours within their environmental context; allegiance to experimental psychology; exact methods of intervention explicitly formulated; and empirical evaluation techniques, behaviours and goals (Walker 1982).

BEHAVIOURAL ASSESSMENT OF ELDERLY PEOPLE

Older people, as with younger, present a variety of problems and difficulties. Before any form of treatment or intervention can be planned or implemented, a thorough assessment of the problem or situation must be carried out. The assessment can fulfil different purposes:

- to make a diagnosis
- to enable the professional to choose the most appropriate intervention or treatment
- to establish baselines and set goals of treatment
- to evaluate changes in condition or circumstances
- to calculate the possible outcome of treatment or intervention or care
- to plan care and identify where such care might best be delivered – e.g. home or hospital (Sturmey 1994).

As mentioned earlier, behaviour therapy has evolved from within the field of experimental psychology, with its emphasis on measurement and evaluation. It is not surprising, therefore, that behaviour therapy in the clinical setting incorporates these principles in assessment and treatment. This emphasis on measurement is primarily to facilitate understanding of the problem and assist in planning the most suitable intervention and measure its success.

A full assessment will comprise physical, psychological, social and environmental factors. Following this there may be a need to appraise behavioural facets of the individual in more detail (Brooker et al 1993). This is because most behaviours are complex and vary in frequency, intensity and duration.

The first step in assessing a behaviour problem is to describe it in very specific terms. This requires behavioural data to be collected through one or more methods, such as rating scales or direct observation and behavioural analysis of the specific behaviour. We will consider each of these in turn.

Behaviour rating scales

There are a variety of rating scales which have been tested extensively for reliability and validity, and are in widespread use for measuring the behaviour of older adults. These scales vary in their content, application, administration and method of evaluation. Thus the therapist's choice of rating scale will depend on a number of factors such as the type of assessment required; the type of behaviour to be assessed; who will administer the rating scale, especially with regard to whether or not there is a need for qualified personnel; the method of evaluation and how this is to be carried out (e.g. statistical analysis of the data).

Sturmey (1994) analysed the constraints within behaviour rating scales designed for older adults using factor analysis, and he examined their robustness in clinical trials. He found that most of the scales contained items in nine categories: orientation, activities of daily living, speech and language, extra

personal maladaptive behaviour, social behaviour, sensory deficits, psychiatric disorders, learning and memory and intrapersonal maladaptive behaviour.

Authors of most of these scales had grouped items into relevant sub-scales and there was a wide variation in the number of items used to measure any specific behaviour. Sturmey (1994) found the three most robust factors were adaptive behaviour, extrapersonal maladaptive behaviour, and memory and orientation. He also noted that the population samples studied were drawn from a variety of settings but that almost all the studies excluded a community sample. This, as he points out, does not reflect the level of disability amongst older people living in the community (OPCS 1988).

The choice of scale should be informed by a clear understanding of what the scale purports to measure. When developing treatment plans and observing change more detailed, precise and individual scales may need to be devised, for example to examine the level of agitation displayed by a particular client. The use of scales allows extensive measurement of behaviour to be made and provides essential data for comprehensive knowledge and accurate understanding of a problem.

Carers need training and instruction in the use and value of rating scales and scales should be selected that do not involve excessive extra work for them, particularly for family carers who may already be overstretched. It is important to note that the results of rating scales should be interpreted in a global context and include an evaluation of the older adult's social environment in which the behaviour occurs (Woods & Britton 1985).

Direct observation

Direct observation involves the active scrutiny of a client in either a structured setting, such as a hospital or residential facility, or a natural setting, such as a person's own home or familiar environment. The individual is directly observed by a staff member or carer. There are problems carrying out this type of observation in a structured setting which may bias the data collected. For example, elderly people who have a problem with incontinence may exhibit more difficulties in an unfamiliar environment because they cannot find the toilet. Therefore, direct observation in a person's natural environment is preferred whenever possible. It will provide rich, individual and accurate information upon which to plan and implement interventions and care (Woods & Britton 1985).

Two of the most frequently used methods of direct

observation are time sampling and event recording. Time sampling is used to overcome some of the complications in recording high frequency behaviours and involves recording behaviours at given moments of time (e.g. every 15 seconds). The observer records the behaviour at the specified time so building up an accurate description of an individual's behaviour over a period of time. Event recording is used to count the frequency of a particular behaviour. It is often combined with duration recording. For example, behaviour such as shouting would be recorded every time it occurs within a specified time, such as every hour. The duration of the shouting on each occasion would also be noted (McBrien & Felce 1992).

Direct observation can be used to analyse a person's behaviour in depth in order to define a 'problem' and to plan to reduce or eliminate it altogether. It can also be used to provide data on a service as a whole or on a particular care environment. For example, Bowie & Mountain (1993) used direct observation to find out how elderly patients in a long stay care setting spent their day.

Problems can arise when using direct observation. It can produce a huge amount of data which need to be managed efficiently for a comprehensive analysis. The data may be biased by the actions of staff who change their behaviour during the data collection process. There may also be difficulty in recording specific behaviours when other behaviours are excluded, for example a violent behaviour may be recorded whilst an accompanying pacing is not. Or there may be confusion when behaviours are ambiguously defined (Woods & Britton 1985), for example 'disturbed behaviour' could mean verbally aggressive, violent or crying.

Behavioural analysis

Behavioural analysis is often used for specific problem behaviours, usually referred to as challenging behaviours. They present carers with considerable difficulties and demands on their time and abilities, and are described as 'extrapersonal' in that they have a profound effect on the lives of those directly involved in the care. Restlessness and aggression are examples of challenging behaviours often seen in elderly care settings. To assess these problems thoroughly it is necessary to find out what maintains the behaviour and what its consequences are. A behavioural analysis concentrates on three aspects of the behaviour, termed the ABC :

- Antecedent: the catalyst for a behaviour, that is the stimulus or circumstance which triggers the behaviour.
- Behaviour: what the individual says or does.
- Consequence: the reinforcer, that is the reward the individual receives as a consequence of the behaviour, thus making it likely for the behaviour to be repeated in response to a similar antecedent.

These three components provide an understanding and an insight into why the behaviour is occurring and what purpose it accomplishes or fulfils. By establishing the antecedent and the consequence the function should gradually be uncovered.

Behavioural analysis can be performed by a therapist or appropriately trained carer personally observing and recording the behaviour; this is necessary with behaviours which may have many possible reasons or effects that need to be disentangled. Alternatively, an elderly client's behaviour can be described at interview by a carer or someone who knows the client well. This approach is less satisfactory in uncovering the function of complex behaviour because it relies upon description and partial interpretation by a third party. For example, an elderly person who hits a specific individual regularly is exhibiting a simple problem behaviour and therefore circumstances and activity are more likely to be accurately described by a third party. However, a client who hits a number of people apparently randomly but only some of the time is exhibiting a more complex problem behaviour, influenced by numerous variables, which may not be identified by a third party.

The usual way to carry out a behavioural analysis is to record the defined behaviour on an ABC chart (see Table 18.1). This yields information which can be interpreted by the assessor or by the care team. The ABC chart is used to assess sporadic behaviours which occur usually no more than a few times a day. If the behaviour happens more frequently than every half hour, staff may collect behavioural data through direct observation. The ABC chart is designed to analyse the environmental factors which may be affecting the behaviour and discover a pattern to the behaviour to facilitate understanding and inform the plan of care or treatment. The chart is especially useful for collecting information on fairly discrete behaviours which serve only one purpose and which have a discernible antecedent. In such cases the chart may need to be used only for a short time to identify a pattern. However, the chart will often be used to study complicated behaviour and will therefore need to be completed over a longer time scale for a pattern to emerge.

Table 18.1 Example of an ABC chart

Date and time	Antecedents	Behaviour	Consequence	Signature
10th April 1995 8.30 a.m.	At dining table eating breakfast	Hit Sally (nurse) with fork and swore at her	Sally told him off, other staff helped him with his breakfast, spreading jam on toast and cut it for him	S. Turner
10th April 10 p.m.	Getting ready for bed	Slapping night staff on the head	Left to himself and later put to bed by 2 staff	P. Davey
12th April 3 p.m.	Visited by wife, Mrs Gayle	Shouted at Mrs Gayle and swore at her	Mrs Gayle left. Staff spoke to him about the episode	T. Smith
13th April 11 a.m.	Sitting in lounge with other residents	Shouting and swearing at staff nearby	Removed from the lounge and sat in the dining area	P. Conway
13th April 12.45 p.m.	Asked to come to the dining room for lunch	Hit Mary (nurse) and swore at her	Left alone. Meal brought into lounge	P. Conway

As illustrated in Table 18.1, an ABC chart is usually divided into five sections:

Date, time and place

It is essential that this information is completed accurately as it alone may furnish data regarding the pattern of behaviours.

Antecedents

This section records information about:

- the activities of the elderly person immediately preceding the target behaviour, for example, had any people been interacting with the older person (e.g. relatives) or been in the vicinity?
- the form of interaction that took place
- a description of the environment at the time; for example was it busy or noisy, was the TV on or was it very quiet?
- whether the person just finished or been engaged in a particular task or activity, or was sitting in the day area with a spouse after just being out for a walk.

Behaviour

The behaviour should be well known already to the carer or care team and be recorded on the chart. This section should include an accurate, precise factual description of the behaviour (subjective interpretation and opinions should be avoided). For example: 'Albert got out of his chair and went over to Mr Spencer, who

was watching TV, and hit him on the upper arm with his clenched fist. He then went and sat down by his wife. He said nothing'.

Consequence

This section should include information regarding the immediate events following the target behaviour, incorporating data about the exact action by both the person observed and by those who witnessed the behaviour. Additional information should be recorded concerning the continuation or cessation of activity or intervention following the behaviour and supplementary details about the consequent action of staff, for example whether medication was given or the elderly client moved to another room. Particulars about the conversation or verbal requests made by the individual should also be noted, for example, 'wife became concerned about Mr Spencer and told her husband, Albert, off, saying that she would not visit again. He did not respond and refused to talk to staff about the behaviour'.

This element of the analysis is particularly important in relation to behaviour because it strengthens learning, and is a focus for both analysis and intervention. This is not to deny that antecedents are also important but they are not necessarily amenable to change, because particular precipitating circumstances may be unavoidable. If antecedent factors cannot be changed the therapist will want to empower the elderly client to behave in a different way in a similar situation; thus the consequence of the behaviour needs to be changed. For example, the elderly person living at home with a carer becomes very agitated (behaviour) every time the carer leaves the house to go shopping for food (antecedent). Therefore the carer does not leave the house and the older adult stops feeling agitated (consequence). Here the therapist would not want to change the antecedent, because it is necessary for the carer to leave the house. The aim of therapy must be to change the consequence by affecting the behaviour.

Signature

It is essential to have the name of the member of staff who witnessed the behaviour because further details may be needed.

The chart should always include the above five sections as a minimum and should record only essential information; completion of lengthy charts can be difficult in a caring situation. However, other sections may be added depending on the behaviours to be observed, for example the intensity or duration of a target behaviour, or the precise description of the consequence over a period of time depending upon the needs of individual clients.

PLANNING BEHAVIOURAL MANAGEMENT

Houts & Scott (1976, cited in Garland 1991) describe a goal-planning framework for planning and implementing behavioural management of older people, based upon the following principles:

Involve the client from the beginning

This principle is of paramount importance as it forms the basis of the therapeutic relationship between client and therapist through which the planned programme is implemented. The older person should be informed of the reasons for referral and what the therapist has to offer and consultation should be sought even if it appears that the person cannot understand or communicate effectively. If this is the case, the client's primary carer or advocate should be approached and asked to endorse every stage of the programme. Involvement of the client has very obvious advantages for the success of the intervention; it will help to ensure compliance with the care offered and help to detect and evaluate areas of difficulty, particularly if the programme is less effective than had been hoped. The client will be able to appraise elements of the programme and influence its direction and progress. Involvement will also help to strengthen the therapeutic alliance, so facilitating future intervention if required.

Use the elderly person's strengths to set goals which help to meet her needs

This element of the goal-planning framework is central to ensure a balanced approach in the care programme. Identifying strengths means that they are acknowledged and developed by the client and by those delivering the care. Thus positive and constructive characteristics of the client can be used when addressing challenging behaviours. Sometimes clients' strengths are masked by challenging behaviours or they may seem insignificant or taken for granted by others. For example, the ability to enjoy a television programme, taking a keen interest in their hair or clothes, their ability to knit, sew, tidy or clean, straightening pictures or their interest in what the staff are doing. These capacities are a resource which may be of value in therapy.

Set reasonable goals

There can be a tendency in the planning stage to aim for complete extinction of a problem. This is usually unwise because most goals are far-reaching and ambitious and often difficult to achieve. Unrealistic goals can have a negative effect since failure to achieve them may make the client and also staff disheartened and lose faith in the programme. Unrealistic goals can also appear to reduce progress already achieved. Realistic goals are those that are moderately difficult, are seen as beneficial to the elderly person and their carer and test out the effectiveness of the approach. For example, a percentage reduction in aggressive behaviour over a time period is likely to be a realistic goal, whereas absence of aggressive behaviour is not.

Spell out the steps necessary to reach each goal

Having agreed the goals we can indicate the stages required to reach them. This is best done explicitly and in detail, should be agreed by those involved and documented so that all those concerned have access. Stages should be evenly spaced, allowing time for each one to be implemented and accomplished before the next is attempted. Some goals will need a number of stages and others relatively few depending upon the complexity of the problem and the number of people involved. An example of a problem which would require a number of stages would be when an aggressive behaviour was extreme, such as physical attacks on staff and other residents of a nursing home. One of the goals may be to ensure the safety of staff and residents and there may be several steps along the way; for example, first protect residents, then protect staff, then protect the older person before moving to the various interventions to be used when aggressive behaviour occurs and to more specific interventions to prevent or predict its occurrence, intensity or frequency.

State clearly what the patient will do, what the staff will do, and when you expect to reach the goal

It is critical that all those committed to the treatment know what their contribution entails. This ensures consistency in the approach and its implementation and thus accuracy in evaluation. If this element is unclear, those involved will interpret what they should do on an individual basis. This will give rise to confusion and disagreement, and result in a half-hearted commitment to the planned care, which may be terminated before it has been given an adequate trial.

INITIATING CHANGE

Preconceived ideas of what constitutes a successful outcome may need to be reconsidered when treating elderly people. For example, improvements in the behavioural problems of physically frail elderly people may stop if their health deteriorates and sometimes maintaining baseline levels of behaviour functioning may be an appropriate goal of therapy (Carstensen 1988).

The reinforcement strategies most commonly used when treating older adults are token economies, shaping, prompting and fading, extinction, and modelling:

Token economy

This is a systematically planned programme of reinforcement in which elderly people are trained to develop new behaviours by receiving a token when a desired behaviour is demonstrated. These tokens can then be exchanged for positive reinforcers. Token economy is oriented towards specific problems rather than populations and typically is applied in an institutional setting. Richards & Thorpe (1978) report a number of studies in which this method was used successfully with elderly people, for example to increase social interaction. However, token economies demand a complex and all-encompassing environment to be most effective. This was previously provided by the large mental hospitals, but as these have declined so has the use of token economy as a therapeutic

intervention. Indeed, token economy is seen by some as an institutionalising intervention rather than an empowering one.

Shaping

Involves developing a new behaviour by progressively reinforcing behaviours that approximate to the behavioural target. Take, for example, an elderly person who has become anxious about her gait and therefore refuses to walk. The target behaviour would be 'walking'. Reinforcement would therefore be given when the client stands up, takes one step, takes two steps and so on. The main disadvantage of shaping is that it is time-consuming and difficult to use for complex behaviours. However, Flannery (1974) successfully treated a 77-year-old man for physical and social problems, perceived as a consequence of an unresolved grief reaction, using shaping as part of a multifaceted behavioural approach to encourage the discussion of grief-related topics.

Prompting

Involves some form of physical activity by the therapist to initiate an activity, for example a verbal instruction or reminder, or the use of a visual aid. Prompting has been extensively used in the treatment of urinary incontinence (see below). Linked to prompting is fading, in which the prompt is gradually withdrawn so that the behaviour continues without relying on the prompt. For example, the therapist prompting an older adult to wash will gradually lower his or her voice to a whisper, then mouth the instruction and eventually say nothing at all. Thus the prompt fades.

Extinction

Involves the lack of a reinforcement which eventually leads to the behaviour disappearing. A commonly experienced example is the person who loses his watch. He will continue to automatically look at his wrist whenever he wants to know the time. However if, over time, the watch is not replaced he will gradually look less and less at his wrist until eventually he stops altogether. The behaviour is then said to have been extinguished.

Modelling

Involves the therapist demonstrating a behaviour and

encouraging the individual to imitate it. For example, the therapist might demonstrate the simple movement of pointing at an object and the client is then reinforced every time she makes a similar gesture. Modelling is particularly useful in social skills and self-help skills training. Downs et al (1988) report experiments conducted with elderly patients in a nursing home to reduce avoidance of whirl-pool bathing. Clients were assessed for behaviours they exhibited to avoid bath time, for example leaving the bedroom or leaving the lift chair after a bath, and these were placed in a hierarchy of difficulty. Distress ratings were obtained by nursing aides who asked participants to rate their distress by pointing to a scale of six facial expressions, from very happy to very sad. The patients were divided into groups and participated in four 1-hour sessions during which a therapist modelled bath time activity, broken down into 36 separate steps. This demonstration was accompanied by a verbal explanation for patients to copy. Participant modelling proved superior in terms of behavioural improvement at 4 week follow-up compared to both the control group, which received no intervention, and a group which received a film to demonstrate procedures.

Having identified some of the main ways of changing behaviour we now consider two problem behaviours encountered in clinical practice which have important implications for interpersonal relationships and wellbeing of elderly people and are amenable to behavioural analysis.

AGGRESSIVE BEHAVIOUR IN THE ELDERLY PERSON

The terms aggression, violent behaviour, agitation and disruptive behaviour are used frequently by researchers and carers, and can give rise to misunderstanding and confusion. Patel & Hope (1993) recommend the following as a working definition of aggressive behaviour: 'Aggressive behaviour is an overt act, involving the delivery of noxious stimuli to (but not necessarily aimed at) another object, organism or self, which is clearly not accidental' (p. 453).

Nasam et al (1993) found that 65% of patients in long term care exhibited one or more of six distinct types of such behaviour: escape, aggression, restlessness, wandering, regression and verbally disruptive behaviours. Cohen-Mansfield & Marx (1990) identified three different types of agitation exhibited by nursing home residents: aggressive behaviours (hitting, kicking, cursing); physically non-aggressive behaviours (restlessness, pacing, inappropriate robing

or disrobing); and verbally agitated behaviours (complaining, negativism, repetitive phrases).

Aggressive, violent or disruptive behaviour is a significant and exacting problem in the care and treatment of the older person, both in the community and in residential care settings. Aggression is one of the most frequently used reasons for referral to psychogeriatric services and for admission to nursing homes and other residential facilities (Patel & Hope 1993, Eastley & Mian 1993) and is a prevalent and particularly demanding problem in the care of people suffering from dementia. Indeed, disturbed and aggressive behaviours are recognised as dominant and pervasive problems for carers, particularly those who are care sole caregivers, and who receive little support from outside agencies (Ware et al 1990, Hallberg & Norberg 1990). Barnes & Raskind (1980) found that behavioural disturbance was the most common reason for carers seeking help from their physician. Whall et all (1992) found that disruptive behaviour was exhibited by 36% of elderly nursing home residents, 85% of whom were memory impaired. Amongst the most commonly cited behaviours were hitting or slapping, identified by more than 70% of nursing staff as being the most disruptive behaviour. Verbal aggression (60%) and screaming (50%) were the next most disruptive behaviours described by nursing staff. These types of behaviour demand a high staff–patient ratio and may also lead staff to emphasise medication regimens and the use of physical restraints (Teri et al 1992).

Aggressive behaviours are overt and are thus open to scrutiny and observation; making them amenable to behavioural interventions. Aggression impacts mainly on the wellbeing of the caregiver rather than the aggressive person, although the effect on the interpersonal relationships of the aggressor is detrimental to that person's wellbeing too. Thus the aim of behavioural intervention is usually to reduce the behaviour and increase the caregiver's ability and skill in managing it (Pinkston et al 1988).

The behavioural approach to the management of aggressive behaviours has two important strands. Firstly, an assessment of the elderly person's aggressive behaviour in relation to the environment in an effort to understand the reasons for the behaviour. Secondly, a plan of intervention, based on the assessment, is incorporated into an individualised care package. To illustrate these points we now discuss individual assessment, the presenting problem(s), the planning of care interventions and possible behavioural techniques and their application. Following this is a case report.

Common causes of aggression

There are a number of factors facing elderly people that may predispose them to aggressive behaviour. Common factors include:

- Frustration associated with failing physical abilities.
- Problems of perception which cause elderly people to believe that their personal space is being invaded by others, especially unknown caregivers, whom they fail to recognise.
- Memory difficulties which lead elderly people to believe that someone has stolen or hidden their possessions.
- An inability to make themselves understood.
- The need to attract the attention of the carer. This is especially likely in residential or institutional settings where there are great demands on the care staff.
- An attempt to cover up a mistake.
- A reaction to feelings of humiliation, embarrassment or degradation.
- Poor care practices which result in elderly people being neglected or ignored. Thus aggressive behaviours become the only means of self-expression.

Assessment

Assessment is usually carried out over a period of time and includes a behavioural analysis of the aggressive behaviour, a history of the presenting problem, a medical history and an assessment of the environment. We now describe these components of assessment in detail.

As previously discussed, the use of behavioural analysis (incorporating the ABC approach) provides abundant data on the behaviour which forms a baseline from which to begin to plan intervention. Aggressive behaviours are usually sporadic in nature, occurring at most a few times daily and are usually discrete and distinctive. In that the behaviour involves other people or objects, it is observed wholly or in part by carers who can provide a description. The use of an ABC chart can ensure that the most relevant description is recorded in an ordered and objective manner. Before the chart can be used the exact behaviour to be observed must be defined, for example 'any episode of disturbed behaviour which involves harming others or causing harm to the environment'.

Apart from the specific assessment of the problem behaviour it is necessary to assess the individual on a more general level. It is valuable to acquire a history of background, childhood, education and relationship history in an attempt to understand a person's previous adjustment to stress and adversity. A history of the problem needs to be collated by the assessor. This is usually done through interviews with clients, their primary carer and significant others as deemed necessary by the assessor. A description of similar episodes is important because it provides information about the development and pattern of the problem and what, if anything, eased or eliminated it. Current management of the behaviour needs to be assessed and can be done by interviewing people who are in regular contact. The aim is to get a true picture of what happens and it is important not to pass judgement on the rights or wrongs of current management. This information is then taken into account when devising a treatment plan, helping to avoid any pitfalls and the use of methods that were previously unsuccessful.

The person's physical and mental state should be assessed to rule out any such causes for the disruptive behaviour. For example, paranoid delusions may result directly from the belief that other people are out to harm them and the behaviour may be an attempt to protect themselves; or it may be that their eyesight or hearing is impaired and the behaviour of others is consequently misinterpreted, resulting in a defensive or offensive aggressive response.

An assessment of the environment will determine the part it plays in causing or maintaining the undesirable behaviour. This is best done by observing the person's interaction with the environment and by discussing the environment with the prime caregiver. Components of the environment, such as rigid meal times, residential or institutional rules and regulations or other restrictions of daily living that may give rise to feelings of frustration or powerlessness (for example, a ban on pets, poorly maintained lifts, an absence of garden areas, dim lighting, inadequate public transport) should be considered. As can be seen, some environmental difficulties can be addressed directly and others cannot. The object of assessment is to establish the impact of the environment and later to consider what action can be taken to minimise its negative effects.

Planning and intervention

Behavioural intervention for aggressive behaviour should be used as an adjunct to the overall planning and delivery of individualised care. It should complement the broader objectives and goals of care that are offered to the older person. Because the individual presents with an undesirable behaviour, the treatment plan should incorporate strategies and approaches that are aimed at improving the quality of life and not solely at reducing undesirable behaviour. It is important to remember that reducing the behaviour is not the end result but rather, as a consequence, old people will be able to live where they choose, be able to take part in chosen activities, be in a position to maintain existing relationships and foster new relationships, so improving the quality of their life.

Analysis of the assessment data

The aim of the behavioural interventions is to reduce the aggressive behaviour and increase appropriate behaviour and a prerequisite is analysis of information gathered from the assessment process. As previously discussed, the assessment tool that provides detailed information about the target behaviour is the ABC chart. The first step is to add up the number of aggressive episodes that have occurred within the allotted timeframe (it may be useful to calculate these on an average daily basis). Then the specific components of the antecedents and consequences can be examined in an effort to elicit a pattern to each of these elements and to organise them into comparable groups. For example, the antecedents may be concerned with a certain activity such as meal times or the level of attention being given, or with the kind of demands being made such as bathing, dressing, medication. The same procedure should be followed for the consequences. Then proceed to look for a link between the antecedents and the consequences. For example, the antecedent may be that an elderly man is asked or encouraged to dress himself and the consequence is that he does not do so. It is then necessary to analyse the function of the behaviour and to identify this in a clear and succinct format. In this example where demands are made of the elderly person, the aggressive behaviour is sustained by negative reinforcement (i.e. he does not act on the request to dress himself).

Behavioural techniques for aggressive behaviour

Having analysed the assessment information, the range of treatment interventions can be explored to determine the most appropriate and effective for each specific situation. The intervention strategy will consist of a package of different techniques aimed at helping the client achieve defined goals. The strategy should be positive and be concerned with improving the quality of life of the older adult.

To decide on the content of the strategy it is necessary to investigate what might be reinforcing the aggressive behaviour; recall, our assumption is that behaviour continues to occur if it is reinforced. This reinforcement can be either positive or negative. As we have said, positive reinforcement means that there is a pleasing outcome, such as attention from staff or carer, whereas negative reinforcement refers to the removal or avoidance of something the individual perceives as undesirable. Therefore, if behaviour is occurring then reinforcement is also likely to be occurring if we accept the theory behind the behavioural approach. To the untrained carer the meaning of the consequence is not always obvious; for example, being forcibly taken to bed or given injections by nurses because of being aggressive must look to the untrained eye as 'punishment' but may in fact be a positive reinforcer for the socially isolated elderly person who may not get any attention from one end of the day to the next. Thus the interest of behavioural analysis.

The treatment package will comprise strategies aimed at the reinforcer and the antecedents of the aggressive behaviour, and will also provide the carer with a specific plan of intervention to implement when the aggressive behaviour occurs.

If the aggressive behaviour occurs when there are particular antecedents then the intervention will deal directly with this aspect of the behaviour. So, for example, if the behaviour happens when there is undue noise or when a particular person is in contact with the elderly client, then the intervention will be directed at reducing this antecedent. This is fairly straightforward and can usually be carried out with little effort by the carer. However, if the antecedents of the behaviour form only a part of the problem then directly intervening with the antecedent will not succeed in reducing the behaviour, and a more multifaceted approach will be required.

If the antecedent is necessary, such as prompting to wash, the focus of the intervention would be to modify the antecedent to reduce the maladaptive behaviour, whilst retaining the primary purpose. For example, alterations to the prompt to wash might include changing voice intonation or content, or offering a choice of when, where and how.

Differential reinforcement

Differential reinforcement is always used to correct aggressive behaviour which is being positively reinforced. This strategy involves the carer or staff reinforcing some other aspect of the client's behaviour and is sub-divided into 'differential reinforcement of other behaviours' (DRO), 'differential reinforcement of incompatible behaviours' (DRI) and 'differential reinforcement of adaptive behaviour' (DRA). We examine each of these techniques in turn.

In 'differential reinforcement of other behaviour' (DRO) the elderly person is reinforced for any behaviour which is not the targeted aggressive behaviour. To do this it must be known what is reinforcing the undesirable behaviour; for example time and attention from the carer or added help in completing a task. The elderly person receives this reinforcer when behaving in all other ways except aggressively. The aggressive behaviour is never reinforced. If the reinforcement is attention from staff but, because of the need to protect others, staff need to give attention when an aggressive outburst occurs, then this attention needs to be delivered in a neutral, distant manner and staff need to adhere to a predetermined procedure.

'Differential reinforcement of incompatible behaviour' (DRI) involves reinforcing behaviour which is inconsistent or incongruous with the aggressive behaviour. Take, for example, an elderly woman whose aggression involves hitting or slapping others. In this case the incompatible behaviour might involve the person using her hands for another purpose such as knitting, dressing, writing, drawing, cooking. The incompatible behaviour can be reinforced with the client's favoured reinforcer.

'Differential reinforcement of adaptive behaviour' (DRA) involves reinforcing behaviours that are adaptive, appropriate and unlikely to occur at the same time as the undesired aggressive behaviour. For example, the individual could be watching television, reading a newspaper or conversing with others. All such behaviours would be reinforced by the carers.

The characteristics of differential reinforcement are that clients still have access to their preferred reinforcer and are never reinforced for inappropriate behaviour. Thus they learn not to use the aggressive behaviour and suitable and adaptive behaviours are encouraged.

Extinction

Another widely used strategy is 'extinction', which involves intentionally withholding reinforcement from the client. Extinction is often used when the reinforcer is attention from staff. The withdrawal is usually done by ignoring the aggressive behaviour, but can only be carried out if the behaviour does not threaten the safety of the individual or others. Because of this it is more usual to use extinction when the aggressive behaviour

takes the form of verbal insults or abuse. Withdrawal of reinforcement can be stressful for the elderly person, especially if the behaviour has been reinforced for many months or years. This stress may give rise to an increase in the aggressive behaviour initially but with commitment and perseverance from the carers such behaviour will gradually diminish.

Activity diversion

Activity diversion is used when the antecedent of aggressive behaviour is identified as the client not being engaged in meaningful activity or in any activity at all. This, unfortunately, is all too common in residential settings and is sometimes also a feature of domestic or community settings where the elderly person is not engaged in the daily routine of the household. Activity diversion aims to include people in the normal operation of the setting in which they find themselves. This can be any activity such as washing dishes, ironing, gardening, dusting, making beds, cooking, serving meals, shopping, socialising, reading, watching television.

Changing the environment

Changing the environment is directed at deflecting the onset of aggressive behaviour. This could include aspects of the residential routine, such as the timing, serving or content of meals or aspects of the physical environment, such as the furniture, lighting or the use of colour to project tranquillity or stimulation. Also beneficial is to encourage staff to treat the elderly clients as individuals for whom the enhancement of dignity, self respect and privacy are paramount.

The case of Mr Gayle, described below (Box 18.1), illustrates the application of the behavioural techniques discussed here to manage aggressive outbursts in an elderly person living at home with his wife.

URINARY CONTINENCE TRAINING

Behaviour therapy has long been active in the area of continence training of children and those with learning difficulties, achieving a high degree of success (Chanfreau-Rona et al 1986). During the 1970s and 1980s, behaviour therapists adapted a number of the techniques developed with these groups to assist older people with urinary incontinence. Although results in the early years were mixed, more recent research studies have shown promising results (Engel et al 1990). In this section the general issue of urinary

---

Box 18.1 Behavioural management of aggression: the case of Mr Gayle

---

Background

Mr Gayle, aged 76, was recently admitted to a nursing home for the elderly. Before this he was living with his 74-year-old wife in their own house on a large council estate in an inner city area. Mr Gayle's wife asked her GP to assess him because she felt that she could no longer look after him at home.

The main reason she gave for this was that she could not manage his aggressive outbursts, which had resulted in physical injury to herself. The GP, having assessed the home situation, recommended that Mr Gayle be admitted to a local nursing home for further assessment. After admission, Mr Gayle displayed aggressive episodes almost daily. These outbursts usually involved hitting or slapping staff with his hand or any object that was nearby. He was also verbally abusive to staff, calling them obscene names and being generally uncomplimentary and derogatory towards them. The manager of the home requested an assessment from a behaviour therapist because the care staff did not know how to handle this aggressive behaviour and Mr Gayle was becoming isolated within the home.

The behaviour assessment was carried out over a period of 2 weeks. It comprised: an analysis of the aggressive behaviour itself; an analysis of Mr Gayle's strengths, abilities and preferences; his medical, social and personal history; a mental state assessment; and an assessment of Mr Gayle's environment.

Analysis of Mr Gayle's aggressive behaviour

Care staff and Mr and Mrs Gayle were interviewed separately. These interviews produced useful information but there was a lot of inconsistency in the data supplied. The behaviour therapist therefore asked care staff to keep an ABC chart for 2 weeks to collect more specific information about the aggressive behaviour (see Table 18.1).

The number of aggressive incidents recorded on the ABC chart were totalled over the 2-week period and then the average was determined. There were 26 outbursts, with an average of 1.8 per day. The antecedents were of three particular types: Mr Gayle not being involved in any form of activity; having difficulty in carrying out a task; and a lot of activity going on within the home. The behaviours were mainly concerned with hitting, slapping, swearing and abusive language. The consequences of the behaviour usually resulted in attention from staff or removing Mr Gayle from difficult situations. The behaviour therapist concluded that Mr Gayle's behaviour was positively reinforced by attention and assistance from staff and negatively reinforced by removing him from difficult situations and the absence of meaningful activity.

Mr Gayle's strengths, abilities and preferences

This assessment was done in order to find out more about Mr Gayle's behaviour in general. It was compiled by talking to the staff and to Mr and Mrs Gayle about what kind of activities Mr Gayle liked to be involved in, what he used to do for recreation, his hobbies and the things he liked to talk about to his wife and others. The

therapist also discussed what Mr Gayle could do independently for himself. Apart from his work as a welder, Mr Gayle was a keen gardener, enjoyed DIY, liked watching and betting on horse racing and sport in general, enjoyed having a drink at his local pub and at the British Legion club where he socialised with other old soldiers. He could manage most self-care activities himself but required assistance with dressing, bathing and, to a lesser extent, with some activities which involved manual dexterity.

Medical history

The therapist talked to the Gayles' GP about Mr Gayle's medical history with particular emphasis on recent medical problems. This revealed that Mr Gayle had suffered a stroke 18 months before his admission which had left him with a mild paralysis of one arm, hand and leg. He was mobile but only with the aid of a frame and could not manage steps or long distances. He also had mild to moderate cardiac problems but was stabilised well on medication.

Social and personal history

Interviews with Mr and Mrs Gayle, both individually and together, revealed that Mr Gayle had been a welder all his working life and had been made redundant at 60 years of age. They had been married for 43 years and had three children and six grandchildren. All the children lived nearby and were in regular contact. However, since Mr Gayle's aggressive behaviour had become prominent these visits had become less frequent. Mr Gayle was reported always to have been a strict disciplinarian within the family. He had been aggressive at times but only outside the home and this always involved other men.

Mrs Gayle reported that her husband was always the breadwinner and refused to let her take on a part-time job, even when they were having financial difficulties. He always saw himself as a 'man's man' and had very definite and fixed ideas about his role as provider and her role as homemaker.

Mental state assessment

This assessment showed that Mr Gayle was mildly depressed and had mild cognitive impairment. His short-term memory was slightly impaired which resulted in forgetfulness and attempts to conceal these episodes by confabulating; his long-term memory was very good.

Environmental assessment

During this part of the assessment the therapist looked for any aspects of Mr Gayle's environment that might contribute to his aggressive outbursts. The nursing home was well staffed and the majority of residents were women, who were physically well but cognitively impaired and required a lot of attention from the staff. The home was fairly noisy and most of the residents watched television or listened to the radio for much of the day. There was a very limited range of activities on offer.

The intervention

Mr Gayle wanted to do things he had enjoyed previously, such as going to the 'bookies', the British Legion club and

Box 18.1 *Cont'd*

gardening. The therapist attempted to incorporate Mr Gayle's expressed desires and those of his wife and carers into the goals of treatment. These were:

- to reduce the frequency of aggressive episodes, particularly those involving actual physical harm
- to reduce the frequency of abusive language
- to increase involvement in desired activity
- to increase social contact.

The behaviour therapist planned a programme of interventions to help Mr Gayle to achieve these goals as follows:

- Differential reinforcement of adaptive behaviour (DRA) was used to ensure that Mr Gayle was positively reinforced with staff attention for appropriate behaviours. The expectation was that this reinforcement would lead to an increase in appropriate behaviour and it would be unnecessary to use maladaptive behaviours to achieve the same result. The staff were instructed in the use of this technique and the written directions were accessible to all of them (see Box 18.2).
- Extinction was used to ensure that Mr Gayle's aggressive behaviour was never reinforced. Again the staff and visitors, particularly his wife, were instructed in its use and written instructions were accessible to all concerned.
- A daily timetable was drawn up to ensure that Mr

Gayle's time was usefully and desirably employed with different activities planned for each day. These activities were based on Mr Gayle's strengths, abilities and interests. A timetable is vital especially when reinforcing adaptive behaviours. Because activities are preplanned, staff become quickly familiar with them and associated appropriate behaviours are immediately positively reinforced. An extract from Mr Gayle's daily timetable is shown in Table 18.2.

The programme was reviewed daily with care staff for the first week to identify and tackle any problems immediately and ensure that everyone was clear about how to implement the programme consistently. It was then reviewed on a weekly basis with the behaviour therapist and staff using ABC charts to assess aggressive behaviour. Initially there was a slight increase in aggressive behaviour. This was expected since extinction was used and Mr Gayle had to learn to gain attention from staff by other means. After 3 weeks, the aggressive behaviour had reduced substantially. The actual physical assaults dropped to one episode and verbal assaults to six a week. 2 weeks later the physical assaults were eliminated and the verbal assaults had reduced to two each week and appeared to be a response to frustration with physical limitations. Mr Gayle was referred to an occupational therapist who helped him to overcome some of his difficulties with manual dexterity.

Box 18.2 Extract from Mr Gayle's treatment plan

Treatment plan
Intervention to be used: differential reinforcement of adaptive behaviour.
What to do:
1. When you notice that Mr Gayle is involved in any form of appropriate activity go to him and chat in a friendly and interested manner.
2. When Mr Gayle talks in a fitting and suitable manner, answer him and attempt to engage him in conversation.
3. Be aware of Mr Gayle's timetable and encourage his involvement in it.

Intervention to be used: extinction.
1. If Mr Gayle shouts or swears IGNORE HIM.
2. If Mr Gayle throws objects (and they cause no harm) IGNORE HIM.
3. If Mr Gayle hits a member of staff, other resident or visitor DO NOT SAY ANYTHING OR SHOW ANY REACTION in facial or bodily expression. Tend to the person injured and remove them from the scene.
4. Having ignored the aggressive behaviour, go back later and encourage involvement in his timetable.
5. Record incident on ABC chart.

---

continence is examined and the behavioural approach and interventions described. Finally a short case history will illustrate how a programme can be implemented.

The problem of urinary incontinence in old age

Urinary continence is associated with a sense of self control and independence. Its loss leads to lowered

self-esteem, social isolation, inability to concentrate, anxiety and depression (Grimby et al 1993). Its prevalence in the community amongst older adults ranges from 10–20%. This is likely to be an underestimate as many people are unwilling to report incontinence because of a sense of shame and a stereotypical view that it is a normal part of ageing (Newman & Smith 1989). In residential settings prevalence ranges between 38% and 82%. Significantly it has been reported by 89% of family care givers as an

Table 18.2 Extract from Mr Gayle's daily timetable

Daily timetable

Name: Mr Gayle

Date: May 21st 1995

Time	Activity	Place	Who is responsible
8–10 a.m.	Up, wash, shave, dress, breakfast	Bedroom, bathroom, dining room	Tom
10–11.30 a.m.	Re-potting plants and watering plants indoors	Kitchen and lounge	Sarah
11.30–11.45 a.m.	Coffee and chat	Kitchen	Sarah
12.30–1.30 p.m.	Lunch and watch TV news	Dining room and lounge	Mary
1.30–3.30 p.m.	Trip to bookmakers and listen to racing on radio in dining room	Outdoors and dining room	Tom
4–5 p.m.	Rest and chat, wife visiting	Lounge	Mrs Gayle
5–6 p.m.	Supper	Dining room	Mary
7–9.30 p.m.	To pub to watch football on TV	Pub	John
9.30 p.m.	Bed when ready	Bedroom	Pauline

important factor in affecting whether or not they would seek to place an older adult in an institution (Burgio et al 1988). Thus, incontinence is a problem which has profound implications for the psychological wellbeing and future life setting of many older people.

Continence learning

Urinary incontinence may be defined as the involuntary voiding of urine, in response to urge, at inappropriate times and in inappropriate places. Newman (1962) subdivided incontinence into 'true' incontinence, the result of dementia, neurological or bladder neck dysfunction, and 'apparent' incontinence, being circumstantial, such as precipitancy (cited in Chanfreau-Rona et al 1986). Continence learning is associated with the maturation process, the development of the central nervous system and socialisation. Behaviourism views this process in terms of the action of operant behaviours and negative reinforcement. Thus a sense of bladder fullness and the urge to void leads the individual to constrict the urethral sphincter to control voiding until a suitable receptacle is found. These behaviours are reinforced through childhood and adulthood as a way of avoiding punishment or disapproval and embarrassment. For the older person, incontinence may arise from physical and/or mental degenerative processes

disrupting these behavioural controls and leading to either motivational problems or response costs outweighing the previous reinforcers. Cognitive impairment can lead to either an indifference to the social consequences of voiding in socially unacceptable places or forgetting the previously learned behaviours (usually a result of central nervous system disease). Physical impairment can mean that the physical effort to void is so great that it outweighs the previous reinforcers in terms of cost. Thus the previously established behaviours decrease and ever more powerful reinforcers have to be used to maintain them (Heller et al 1989).

Behavioural management

The usual methods of managing urinary incontinence include the use of pads, catheters and condom drainage. However, these methods are associated with a high incidence of urinary tract infection which not only cause physical discomfort but also exacerbate incontinence (Morris et al 1992), and play a large part in increasing mortality.

Medication, such as anticholinergic agents or beta-adrenergic antagonists to increase bladder capacity or increase sphincter resistance, may be recommended (Wein 1990). The problem with drug therapy is over-use and unwanted side-effects. The difficulties associated with more established methods, potential cost-effectiveness, coupled with the behavioural commitment to increase individual autonomy, indicate that behaviour therapy is an approach worth investigating as an alternative to more traditional methods of continence management.

Assessment and planning

Assessment of the older person's incontinence problems is crucial if behavioural interventions are to be successful (Garland 1991). Holden & Woods (1988) state that inadequate assessment of the problem, particularly in relation to environmental factors, coupled with setting over-ambitious goals, such as independent toileting, often explain why behavioural interventions for urinary incontinence fail. Thus the rule governing assessment must be to make assessment thorough and take into account the capacity of the individual when setting targets.

During the process of assessment the type of urinary incontinence will be identified. There are four main types for which behavioural intervention may be beneficial:

- Stress incontinence is an involuntary voiding of urine which occurs during activity, such as rising from a chair or when sneezing or laughing. Usually caused by weak pelvic floor muscles, it is particularly common in women (Norton 1986).
- Urge incontinence occurs when perceived urgency leads to almost immediate involuntary contractions of the bladder, and loss of urine, before the person can get to the toilet (Newman & Smith 1989). This type of incontinence is particularly common in elderly people and people who have suffered cerebral cortex damage. Other symptoms associated with urge incontinence are frequency and voiding at night (Norton 1986).
- Overflow incontinence is characterised by a constant dribbling of urine due to incomplete voiding and a gradual build up of residual urine in the bladder. It is commonly caused by an obstruction, such as an enlarged prostate, or nerve damage to the bladder muscle impairing its function.
- Functional incontinence occurs when the elderly person cannot get to the toilet once an urge to void has been perceived. It is usually caused by environmental obstacles, cognitive or physical impairment, depression or demotivation (Newman 1989).

Assessment does not take place in one session, but usually involves a process of evaluation over a period of days or weeks. It should be carried out with tact and understanding and include: a history of the urinary problem, a comprehensive medical history, mental state assessment, and a functional and environmental assessment.

History of the problem

The therapist needs to determine how long the sufferer has been experiencing the problem and its signs and symptoms such as burning sensations on micturition or haematuria. These are important in formulating differential diagnoses, for example urinary tract infection, for which behaviour therapy would be inappropriate. Current dietary intake is also important in this regard; for example, it is known that certain types of artificial sweetener can irritate the bladder (Newman & Smith 1989).

The pattern of the behaviour associated with the incontinence episodes should be analysed, for example whether the client urinates when sneezing or when getting up from a sitting position. This helps to identify the type of incontinence. In addition, the frequency and time the episodes occur should be charted as a means of identifying usual voiding patterns. This can be done either by the therapist, the client or, more usually, the care giver, completing a bladder record chart. This chart (illustrated in Table 18.3 below), notes the voiding time, both intentional and accidental, place where voiding occurred, reason for any accidental voiding, and a record of fluid intake. The chart identifies problem areas for the therapist and provides both a baseline measurement and evaluation of progress as therapy proceeds.

Medical history

A comprehensive history will address current and past events. Particular attention should be given to the genitourinary history, for example the number of births a woman has had, urinary tract infections and genitourinary surgery all affect bladder function and sphincter strength. Any current problems and, in particular current medication, need to be identified. If taking diuretics, urgency is common which may exacerbate or be the cause of the incontinence, whilst some antihypertensive medication can lead to stress incontinence. A physician or nurse should carry out a physical examination to determine any physical causes and test for sphincter strength and control (see biofeedback below).

Mental state

Cognitive function needs to be assessed with an instrument such as the Mini Mental State Questionnaire (Baigis-Smith et al 1989). This assessment is important, not only because the degree of cognitive dysfunction often correlates with the severity of the incontinence (Heller et al 1989), but also because this information is needed to shape the behavioural programme towards the individual's ability to learn and retain information.

Functional and environmental analysis

Older clients' ability to function independently is not only an issue in terms of the cause of incontinence, but also in terms of their ability to respond to a behavioural programme. The assessment covers their ability to manage self-toileting activities, such as undoing and fastening buttons on clothing, and how mobile they are. In addition, functional dependence on a carer has been shown as a possible cause for urinary incontinence, through inappropriate reinforcement; the carer responds to the older adult when wet but not when dry or when managing successfully without help (Garland 1991).

Environmental assessment focuses on factors in the older adult's usual living circumstances that enhance or impede the ability to maintain continence. For example, location or size of the toilet, light, position of furniture.

One purpose of this aspect of the assessment is to identify individuals who are likely to benefit from behavioural interventions or who may need a different type of approach. Garland (1991) identifies motivation and the ability of sufferers to see themselves as able to take control of their problems, rather than as passive victims of urinary incontinence, as important predictors of suitability for treatment. However, motivational issues are difficult to assess when the person is cognitively impaired. Schnelle (1990) developed a 3-day assessment model for distinguishing between cognitively impaired older adults who are likely to benefit from behaviour therapy from those who are not. The model involves checking elderly clients for incontinence on the hour over 12 hours on day 1 and changing their clothing accordingly. On day 2, clients are encouraged to void urine on the hour and are checked hourly as well. On day 3 the interval between prompts is increased to 2-hourly. Schnelle found that older adults unlikely to respond to behavioural intervention have appropriate toilet rates of less than 45% on day 2, and either do not respond to prompts to void or respond but fail to void when sitting on the toilet. This analysis is supported by Chanfreau-Rona et al (1986) who found that older adults with lower levels of incontinence responded best to behavioural interventions.

When planning interventions an essential element is to clarify the desired response (targets/goals) and communicate these to the older adult and/or carer. This is important within the therapeutic relationship because it defines the parameters of measurement and the agenda for success or failure between the therapist and client. Burgio et al (1988) identify four response definitions to use in continence training:

- Wet/dry: dampness of garments or pads should be scored wet. No dampness should be scored dry.
- Appropriate toileting: voiding into a receptacle designed for receiving urine, e.g. toilet or bedpan.
- Self-initiation: a request from the older adult for assistance to the toilet.
- Independent toileting: using toilet facilities independently.

Of these four the most likely to succeed as targets are the first three for cognitively and physically incapacitated older adults (Burgio et al 1988). It is important to remember that the setting of achievable goals is in itself a therapeutic reinforcer of success whereas unrealistic goals which end in failure may result in a decrease in motivation on the part of client and carer to address the problem.

Intervention

Having assessed the difficulty and identified targets, the next stage is to select the intervention, the choice of which is dictated by the outcome of assessment, and particularly the targets that have been set in relation to the client's environment.

Scheduling and prompting

Scheduled voiding involves assessing the incontinence in relation to the person's voiding pattern and developing a programme to encourage the client to go to the toilet at set times, usually every 2 hours, regardless of whether or not the urge to void has occurred. Clients who have difficulty can be stimulated to urinate, for example by turning on the water tap or instructing them to constrict their urethral sphincter. Clients should be encouraged to remain on the toilet until they have passed urine.

Scheduled voiding aims to keep sufferers dry rather than help them to reassert self-control over their bladder function. For this reason it is most appropriate for cognitively impaired people, and its success depends on the availability of a committed carer to provide encouragement; feedback and praise are particularly important. All too often programmes that rely on the participation of a carer start off well and then fail because of loss of interest or patience on the part of the one charged with its daily implementation. Continence maintenance itself is not a sufficient reinforcer (Schnelle et al 1990). Thus, after training is complete, the therapist has a responsibility to maintain motivation and give support through regular contact and dialogue.

The problem with scheduled voiding is that it does little to increase the sense of autonomy and self-esteem of elderly people, and so they may have little incentive to remain dry. This is less of a problem with prompted scheduled voiding which involves the carer giving regular prompts, as in scheduled voiding, but also encouraging the older adult to go to the toilet independently. In addition the carer gives the elderly person feedback on whether or not they have remained dry, and praise when voiding has been successful without prompting or assistance. As periods of remaining dry increase in length the frequency of the prompting schedule is decreased.

Relaxation and exercise

Through the use of relaxation exercises the elderly client can be taught to increase the length of time period between passing urine. The client is taught to breathe slowly and deeply when sensing the urge to urinate and also to think of a distracting and calming image, such as walking the dog, to reinforce the sense of being relaxed. The purpose of relaxation is to reduce the physical sense of urgency experienced, provide time for the elderly person to get to the toilet, gradually increase the time periods between voiding and restore a sense of self-control.

Exercise, such as taking walks, can be useful in promoting a general sense of wellbeing and is particularly valuable for people used to long periods of inactivity. A decrease in mobility has been linked with incontinent episodes. Baltes (1988) found that nursing home staff tended to reinforce physical disability by failing to recognise the efforts of older residents to be independent. Burgio et al (1986) increased continence in nursing home residents by praising them when they attempted to walk to the toilet. Jirovec (1991) postulates that exercise plays a part in improving the motivation of older adults to attempt self- or seek assistance when needed.

Biofeedback and pelvic floor exercise

Biofeedback is used to increase older people's awareness of their physiological responses to urgency and teach them to regulate the voluntary responses over which they have lost control. This is achieved by enabling clients to observe the results of their attempts to control bladder, sphincter and abdominal tension (Burgio & Engel 1990). Monitoring can be done either with electronic devices, such as a perineometer, an intra-vaginal balloon linked to a sensor, or with exercises, such as interrupting the urinary stream or resting the hand on the abdomen to monitor abdominal tension. Exercise is preferred; using technical aids can exacerbate emotional distress.

Biofeedback is used primarily to treat stress incontinence and urge incontinence, although goals of treatment are different for each. For the former the goal is to train the older adult to increase pelvic floor muscle strength whilst, for the latter, it is to keep abdominal muscles relaxed and to control the sphincter muscle to prevent urine loss. Biofeedback is not recommended for cognitively impaired people because it demands attention and concentration. Research into its efficacy has been promising; Willington (1978, cited in Baigis-Smith et al 1989) reports that 62% of elderly urge incontinence sufferers were cured after the use of biofeedback, and Burgio & Engel's (1990) review of 10 biofeedback research studies addressing urinary incontinence in elderly people conducted between 1978 and 1989 concludes that it is a promising intervention.

Pelvic floor exercises are linked to biofeedback and involve the exercise and strengthening of pelvic floor muscles to increase bladder-sphincter control. The person is taught to identify the pubococcygeal muscle used when urinating by attempting to stop the flow midstream. Once identified, the client is encouraged to exercise the muscle, by contracting it to a count of 10 and then relaxing to a count of 10, 50 times per day, over the course of three sessions of 15, 15 and 20 days. Baigis-Smith et al (1989) report a decrease of urinary accidents at 6 month and 1 year follow-up, in a sample of 54 people, with an average age of 60, who were taught these exercises. As in biofeedback, clients need to be cognitively intact for a programme to be successful.

Environmental change

Changing the environment is often a crucial element in an effective behavioural programme. For example, poor light can cause problems for the older person who has failing eyesight. This can be addressed by checking that the older person has the correct spectacle prescription and improving light sources. Large sofas or a bed close to a wall may mean that the older person finds it hard to manoeuvre to get to the toilet or the toilet may be at the top of the house or some distance from the bedroom; a commode might be the solution.

Within institutional settings a common environmental factor is location and size of signs indicating where the toilet is. Signs should be large, prominently displayed in distinctive colours, using unambiguous and easily understood words. The case of Mrs Parker, described below (Box 18.3), illustrates the use of behavioural techniques with an elderly woman living at home.

Box 18.3 Behavioural management of urinary incontinence: the case of Mrs Parker

Background

Mrs Parker is an 84-year-old frail, housebound but mobile widow, living with her 56-year-old unmarried daughter, Alice, in a large three-bedroom second-storey flat. Mrs Parker had become progressively incontinent of urine over recent months. Her daughter had been coping alone with her mother's incontinence. Mrs Parker was independently minded, though forgetful.

On a routine domiciliary visit by the family GP, Alice became tearful and distressed, and asked for help with her mother's incontinence. She said she had reached the end of her tether with her mother and felt like a prisoner in her own home. The GP referred Mrs Parker to the community nurse for assessment and treatment of the urinary incontinence and to provide Alice with support.

The nurse arranged a home visit to meet both women and carry out an assessment. The nurse gathered information about the history of the incontinence problem and its current effect on both parties. However, it was difficult to collect accurate details of the incontinence such as time, frequency, awareness of urgency, functional and environmental difficulties, degree of continence/incontinence and the effects of the incontinence on both women. As a result the nurse decided to draw up an individually tailored diary to record the missing details and establish baselines. Mrs Parker and Alice were asked to complete a daily diary over a 2-week period (see Table 18.3) during which time the nurse continued with other aspects of assessment.

Assessment

Mrs Parker's medical history was reviewed in conjunction with her GP, and her mental state and relationship with her daughter assessed. The nurse asked Mrs Parker and Alice to show her around the flat, to assess Mrs Parker's ability to mobilise and manoeuvre, and to identify environmental impediments to her reaching and using the toilet. The nurse also observed Mrs Parker's manual dexterity, with particular emphasis on dressing and undressing.

The daily diary showed that Mrs Parker had urinary incontinence as a result of her inability to respond in time to the urge to urinate, due to her physical frailness and the location of the toilet. On average, Mrs Parker experienced five incontinent episodes per day, and managed to use the toilet independently between one and two times per day.

The mental state assessment discovered mildly deteriorating cognitive functioning, particularly in relation

to information processing and short-term memory. It also identified relationship difficulties between Mrs Parker and her daughter, which had deteriorated as both had become socially isolated. This was exhibited in periods of tension and animosity between the two, resulting in long periods of silence.

An environmental difficulty was the location of the toilet, whilst functional problems were difficulty with balance and unsteadiness. Mrs Parker's medical history was unremarkable.

Goal planning and management

After discussing the results of the assessment with Mrs Parker and her daughter, the nurse explained the rationale for behavioural interventions and what this might entail. She stressed the need for commitment to the regime if it was to be successful, but reassured them that she would provide instruction and support. They agreed the following goals:

- reduce the number of incontinent episodes
- increase the number of times Mrs Parker uses the toilet on her own.

The behavioural programme consisted of the following techniques:

- prompted scheduling
- positive reinforcement
- pelvic floor exercises
- environmental alterations.

A behavioural training programme was established to instruct Mrs Parker and her daughter in these techniques (Fox & Azrin 1973). The nurse visited for 3 hours every day for 14 days. 2 hours before the nurse arrived, Alice was asked to give her mother a cup of tea every half hour to facilitate training, and reduce her fluid intake 2 hours before bedtime. The sessions were structured around review, planning and instruction. The review involved looking at how the previous day's programme had gone and discussing any queries and concerns. This was followed by direct instruction to Mrs Parker and her daughter, with the nurse modelling and shaping behaviour through action, praise and feedback on performance. Then problem solving activities (such as what to do if visitors arrived during the programme), planning the rest of the day and the following day were carried out.

Prompted scheduling was chosen because the number of incontinent episodes were frequent and irregular but,

Box 18.3 *Cont'd*

on occasion, Mrs Parker did manage to reach the toilet independently. Prompted scheduling aimed to establish a regular habit at the same time as promoting independence. The programme was based on 2-hourly reminders to use the toilet. This was done by posting large notices of the set times for toileting around the house and buying a large clock for the sitting room, where Mrs Parker spent most of her time. Mrs Parker was encouraged to request help when she felt the urge to urinate. Alice was trained to ask her mother every 2 hours to go to the toilet but only to offer assistance when absolutely necessary. Alice was also instructed in how to give positive verbal reinforcement without being patronising when her mother urinated appropriately, requested help or went to the toilet independently. It will be noted that although the prime focus of this intervention was Mrs Parker's behaviour, it also had the effect of changing and reinforcing her daughter's as well.

In addition to the prompted scheduling and positive reinforcement, Mrs Parker was taught pelvic floor exercises to strengthen her sphincter control. She practised initially with the nurse and then with her

daughter, 15 times in the morning and 15 times in the evening. When mother and daughter reported back pain, the nurse realised that Mrs Parker was tensing her stomach muscles by mistake. The nurse went through the exercises regularly until this mistake was corrected. Environmental alterations were made to the flat. A handrail was installed in the toilet so that Mrs Parker could maintain her balance when lowering herself onto the toilet. In addition, she moved to the bedroom closer to the toilet.

Results
This programme had good results; the frequency of urinary incontinence decreased after 2 weeks. Incontinent episodes (goal 1) dropped by 50%, and self-toileting (goal 2) increased by an average of 40%. After the 2-week period the nurse visited the Parkers once a week for 3 months, during which time they were encouraged to continue with the programme (including the diary), and adjust it according to need. The results were maintained at 3-month follow-up, with self-increasing in frequency.

Table 18.3 Extract from Mrs Parker's bladder record chart

Diary of urine output: Edith Parker

Instructions: Fill in the boxes every time you pass water. Ask your daughter to help you fill in the diary if necessary

Date: 22.03.95

Time	Place	Continent/ Incontinent	How much water passed? (little, moderate, a lot)	What were you doing before passing water? (e.g. sitting, sneezing)	Did you feel the urge to pass water? (yes/no)	What and when did you last drink?	How much did you drink? (cup, mug, glass)	What took place after passing water
9 a.m.	Bedroom	Incontinent	A lot	Getting out of bed	Yes	Tea 8 a.m.	Cup	Got dressed. Alice changed sheets
11.30 a.m.	Toilet	Continent	Moderate	Sitting on toilet	Yes	Tea 10 a.m.	Cup	Went to sitting room
3.15 p.m.	Sitting room	Incontinent	Moderate	Walking to the door	Yes	Tea 3 p.m.	Cup	Changed pad
6.40 p.m.	Sitting room	Incontinent	A lot	Opening the door	Yes	Tea 6 p.m.	Cup	Changed pad, underwear and clothes
8.30 p.m.	Hall	Incontinent	Moderate	Walking to the toilet	Yes	Tea 7.45 p.m.	Cup	Changed pad
10 p.m.	Toilet	Continent	A lot	Sitting on toilet	Yes	Tea 9.30 p.m.	Cup	Went to bed

The importance of carers

Most evidence for the efficiency of behavioural approaches to urinary incontinence comes from studies carried out with cognitively impaired elderly people in institutional care settings. The extent to which these interventions are also successful for elderly people living at home alone or with unpaid carers is less certain. It has been found that institutional staff, such as care assistants, given instruction in behavioural techniques, fail to apply these consistently unless they are systematically managed (Burgio et al 1990). How much more difficult then for some lay carers, subject to stress and isolated at home, to use institutionally developed behavioural interventions with a relative suffering from early dementia. Burgio et al (1990) demonstrated the importance of training in self-monitoring and performance feedback in maintaining the staff's consistency in performing prompted voiding with a group of older adults suffering from dementia. The practicalities of implementing such supervision for lay carers may need to be considered by community psychiatric nurses if incontinence in older adults living at home is to be successfully managed with behavioural intervention.

CONCLUSION

As a number of behavioural studies demonstrate, even when degenerative processes are present, behaviour therapy can contribute to alleviating associated behavioural problems. The behavioural approach to therapy has, at its heart, the client's priorities and best interests if founded upon a thorough assessment of the older adult's problems and situation. The ABC chart is a simple tool for both assessment and ongoing measurement and is frequently used with regard to specific problem behaviours. Interventions based on this assessment are systematically designed, with an emphasis on measurement, to facilitate understanding of the problem and assist in planning the most suitable treatment or care and measure its success.

Behaviour therapy has been demonstrated to be effective in managing behaviour problems in cognitively impaired older adults. If therapy is to be successful, however, behaviour therapists must adjust their perception of successful outcome to the particular life circumstances of older people.

One of the great strengths to commend behaviour therapy to older adults facing challenging problems is its accessibility. Treatment techniques can be taught to non-professional personnel and carers. This gives the approach great flexibility in terms of where and how it may be employed compared to other interventions.

The goal of behavioural intervention is not solely concerned with reducing undesirable behaviour but also with improving the older person's quality of life. Informal and formal carers too can be supported and empowered in their vital contribution to the wellbeing of many older persons. By reducing or eliminating the problem behaviour, older people will be in a better position to choose where they live, participate in activities as they choose, maintain significant relationships, and develop new social contacts and friendships.

REFERENCES

BABCP 1993 Behavioural and cognitive psychotherapies: past history, current applications and future registration issues. Behavioural and Cognitive Psychotherapy Supplement 1

Baigis-Smith J, Smith D A J, Rose M, Newman D K 1989 Managing urinary incontinence in community-residing elderly persons. The Gerontologist 29(2): 229–233

Baltes M M 1988 The etiology and maintenance of dependency in the elderly: three phases of operant research. Behaviour Therapy 19: 301–319

Baltes M M, Lascomb S L 1975 Creating a healthy institutional environment for the elderly via behaviour management: the nurse as a change agent. International Journal of Nursing Studies 12: 5–12

Barnes R, Raskind M 1980 Strategies for diagnosing and treating agitation in the aged. Geriatrics 3: 111–119

Bowie P, Mountain G 1993 Using direct observation to record the behaviour of long-stay patients with dementia. International Journal of Geriatric Psychiatry 8: 857–864

Bradbury N 1991 Problems of elderly people. In: Dryden W, Rentoul R (eds) Adult clinical problems: a cognitive-behavioural approach. Routledge, London

Brooker D J R, Sturmey P, Gatherer A J H, Summerbell C 1993 The Behavioural Assessment Scale Of Later Life (BASOLL): a description, factor analysis, scale development, validity and reliability data for a new scale for older adults. International Journal of Geriatric Psychiatry 8: 747–754

Burgio L D, Burgio K L 1986 Behavioural gerontology: application of behavioural methods to the problems of older adults. Journal of Applied Behaviour Analysis 19: 321–328

Burgio K L, Engel B T 1990 Biofeedback-assisted behavioral training for elderly men and women. Journal of the American Geriatrics Society 38(3): 338–340

Burgio L D, Burgio K L, Engel B T, Tice L M 1986 Increasing distance and independence of ambulation elderly nursing home residents. Journal of Applied Behaviour Analysis 19: 357–366

Burgio L, Engel B, McCormack K, Hawkins A, Scheve A 1988 Behavioural treatment for urinary incontinence in elderly inpatients: initial attempts to modify prompting and toileting procedures. Behaviour Therapy 19: 345–357

Burgio L, Engel B, Hawkins A, McCormack K, Scheve A, Jones L T 1990 A staff management system for maintaining improvements in continence with elderly nursing home residents. Journal of Applied Behaviour Analysis 23: 111–118

Carstensen L L 1988 The emerging field of behavioural gerontology. Behaviour Therapy 19: 259–281

Cautela J R, Kearney A J 1990 Behaviour analysis, cognitive conditioning and covert conditioning. Journal of Behaviour Therapy and Experimental Psychiatry 21(2): 83–90

Chanfreau-Rona D, Wylie B, Bellwood S 1986 Behaviour treatment of daytime incontinence in elderly male and female patients 1986. Behavioural Psychotherapy 14: 13–20

Church M 1983 Psychological therapy with elderly people. Bulletin of the British Psychological Society 36: 110–112

Cohen-Mansfield J, Marx M S 1990 The relationship between sleep disturbances and agitation in a nursing home. Journal of Aging and Health 2(1): 42–57

Downs A F, Rosenthal T L, Lichstein K L 1988 Modeling therapies reduce avoidance behaviour of bath time by the institutionalized elderly. Behaviour Therapy 19: 359–368

Eastley R, Mian I 1993 Physical assaults by psychogeriatric patients: patient characteristics and implications for placement. International Journal of Geriatric Psychiatry 8: 515–520

Engel B T, Burgio L D, McCormick K A, Hawkins A M, Scheve A S, Leahy E 1990 Behavioural treatment of incontinence in the long-term care setting. Journal of the American Geriatrics Society 38(3): 361–363

Flannery R B 1974 Behaviour modification of geriatric grief: a transactional perspective. International Journal of Aging and Human Development 5: 197–203

Fox R M, Azirin N H 1973 Toilet training the retarded. Research Press, Champaign, Illinois

Garland J 1991 Behaviour management. In: Evans J G, Williams T D (eds) The Oxford textbook of geriatric medicine. Open University Press, Oxford

Gilleard 1984 Assessment of behavioural impairment in the elderly: a review. In: Hanley I, Hodge J (eds) Psychological approaches to the care of the elderly. Croom Helm, London

Grimby A, Milsom I, Molander U, Wilkund I, Ekelund P 1993 The influence of urinary incontinence on the quality of life of elderly women. Age and Ageing 22: 82–89

Hallberg I R, Norberg A 1990 Staff's interpretation of the experience behind vocally disruptive behaviour in severely demented patients and their feelings about it: an explorative study. International Journal of Geriatric Psychiatry 31(4): 295–305

Heller B R, Whitehead W E, Johnson L D 1989 Incontinence. Journal of Gerontological Nursing 15(5): 16–23

Holden U P, Woods R T 1988 Reality orientation: psychological approaches to the 'confused' elderly. Churchill Livingstone, Edinburgh

Houts P S, Scott R A 1976 Individualized goal planning in nursing care facilities. Department of Behavioural Science, Pennsylvania State University College of Medicine

Jirovec M M 1991 The impact of daily exercise on the mobility, balance and urine control of cognitively impaired nursing home residents. International Journal of Nursing Studies 28(2): 145–151

Keijsers G, Schaap C, Hoogduin K, Peters W 1991 The therapeutic relationship in the behavioural treatment of anxiety disorders. Behavioural Psychotherapy 19(4): 359–367

McBrien J, Felce D 1992 Working with people who have severe learning difficulty and challenging behaviour: a practical handbook on the behavioural approach. BIMH Publishing, Kidderminster

McClannahan L E, Risley T R 1975 Design of living environments for nursing home residents: increasing participation in recreation activities. Journal of Applied Behaviour Analysis 8: 262–268

Morris A, Browne G, Saltmarche A 1992 Urinary incontinence: correlates among cognitively impaired elderly veterans. Journal of Gerontological Nursing October: 33–39

Morris R G, Morris L W 1991 Cognitive and behavioural approaches with the depressed elderly. International Journal of Geriatric Psychiatry 6: 407–413

Nasam B, Bucht G, Eriksson S, Sandman P O 1993 Behavioural symptoms in the institutionalised elderly – relationship to dementia. International Journal of Geriatric Psychiatry 8: 843–849

Newman D K, Smith D A J 1989 Incontinence in elderly homebound patients. Holistic Nursing Practice 4(1): 52–60

Newman J L 1962 Old fold in wet beds. British Medical Journal i: 1824–1828

Norton C 1986 Eliminating. In: Redfern S J (ed) Nursing elderly people

Norton C 1988 Incontinence can be prevented at all ages. The Professional Nurse October: 22–26

O'Sullivan G 1992 Behaviour therapy. In: Dryden W (ed) Individual therapy. Open University Press, Buckingham

OPCS 1988 Disability in the UK: adults. HMSO, London

Patel V, Hope T 1993 Aggressive behaviour in elderly people with dementia: a review. International Journal of Geriatric Psychiatry 8: 457–472

Pavlov I 1928 Conditioned reflexes: an investigation of the physiological activity of cerebral cortex. Translated and edited by Anrep G U. Oxford University Press, Oxford

Pinkston E M, Linsk N L, Young R N 1988 Home-based behavioural family treatment of the impaired elderly. Behaviour Therapy 19: 331–344

Pollock D, Liberman R 1974 Behaviour therapy in incontinence in demented patients. The Gerontologist 14: 488–491

Richards D, McDonald B 1991 Behavioural psychotherapy: a handbook for nurses. Heinemann Nursing, Oxford

Richards W S, Thorpe G L 1978 Behavioural approaches to the problems of later life. In: Storandt M, Siegler I C, Elias M F (eds) The clinical psychology of aging. Plenum Press, New York

Schnelle J F 1990 Treatment of urinary incontinence in nursing home patients by prompted voiding. Journal of the American Geriatrics Society 38(3): 356–360

Schnelle J F, Newman D R, Fogart T 1990 Management of patient continence in long-term care nursing facilities. The Gerontologist 30(3): 373–376

Sturmey P 1994 Behaviour assessment of older adults: a review of factor analytic studies and a proposed model. International Journal of Geriatric Psychiatry 9: 107–114

Teri L, Rabins P, Whitehouse P 1992 Management of behaviour disturbance in Alzheimer's disease: current knowledge and future directions. Alzheimer's Disease Associated Disorders 6: 77–88

Walker L G 1982 The behavioural model. In: Haldane J D, Alexander D A, Walker L G Models for psychotherapy. University of Aberdeen, Aberdeen

Ware C, Fairburn C, Hope R A 1990 A community based study of aggressive behaviour in dementia. International

Journal of Geriatric Psychiatry 5: 337–342

Watson J B, Rayner R 1920 Conditioned emotional reactions. Journal of Experimental Psychology 3: 1–14

Wein A J 1990 Pharmacologic treatment of incontinence. Journal of the American Geriatrics Society 38(3): 317–325

Whall A, Gillis G L, Yankou D, Booth D E, Beel-Bates C A 1992 Disruptive behaviour in elderly nursing home residents: a survey of nursing staff. Journal of Gerontological Nursing October: 13–17

Willington F L 1978 Urinary incontinence and urgency. Practitioner 220: 739–747

Woods R T 1992 Psychological therapies and their efficacy. Reviews in Clinical Gerontology 2: 171–183

Woods R T, Britton P G 1985 Clinical psychology with the elderly, 1st edn. Croom Helm, London

RECOMMENDED READING

Bradbury N 1991 Problems of elderly people. In: Dryden W, Rentoul R (eds) Adult clinical problems: a cognitive-behavioural approach. Routledge, London. *One of two good reviews of the literature on behavioural and cognitive-behavioural work with the older adult. It covers conceptual literature dealing with the process of ageing as well as assessment and intervention studies with older adults suffering from a variety of problems.*

Burgio L, Engel B, McCormack K, Hawkins A, Scheve A 1988 Behavioural treatment for urinary incontinence in elderly inpatients: initial attempts to modify prompting and procedures. Behaviour Therapy 19: 345–357

Burgio L, Engel B, Hawkins A, McCormack K, Scheve A, Jones L T 1990 A staff management system for maintaining improvements in continence with elderly nursing home residents. Journal of Applied Behaviour Analysis 23: 111–118

These two articles should be read in tandem. Although both are research reports, they provide a clear description of the treatment interventions and techniques for the management of urinary incontinence in a nursing home. The second article provides a useful analysis of the role of the co-therapist in maintaining long-term goals.

Patel V, Hope T Aggressive behaviour in elderly people with dementia: a review. International Journal of Geriatric Psychiatry 8: 457–472. *An informative discussion of the conceptual issues surrounding what constitutes aggressive behaviour in this group, followed by a comprehensive review of the literature on aetiology, epidemiology, methods of assessment and management of aggressive behaviour in older adults with dementia.*

McBrien J, Felce D 1992 Working with people who have severe learning difficulty and challenging behaviour: a practical handbook on the behavioural approach. BIMH Publishing, Kidderminster. *Although aimed at professional carers dealing with individuals with the combined problems of learning disability and challenging behaviour, this excellent manual is also valuable for care of older people more generally. It takes the reader step by step through theory, functional assessment and various interventions, explaining all of these in an accessible and precise form. In addition, the authors have*

included a series of forms (supplemented by comprehensive instruction) that can be used to direct assessment, treatment, process and outcome.

Newman D K, Smith D A J 1989 Incontinence in elderly homebound patients. Holistic Nursing Practice 4(1): 52–60. *This is a comprehensive and lucidly written review of what urinary incontinence is and its different manifestations. It takes the reader through the means of assessment, and nursing followed by a general description of nursing and behavioural management.*

Pattie A H, Gilleard C J 1981 Manual of the Clifton assessment procedures for the elderly (CAPE). Hodder Stoughton, Sevenoaks. *This widely used assessment tool in residential and hospital settings, is well worth examining. It enables a systematic consideration of the individual to be made from various perspectives in relation to self and environment.*

Stokes G 1987 Aggression. Winslow Press, Telford. One of the few available books that deals with this subject in the context of the older adult, it is one in a series entitled 'Common Problems with the Elderly Confused' edited by U P Holden. *This book is accessible to professionals and non-professionals. It explains some of the techniques that can be employed when dealing with the aggressively confused older adult although it is less helpful in this respect than McBrien & Felce (1992). The book's value lies in helping to explain to lay carers the behavioural approach to the management of aggression.*

Thompson C (ed) 1989 The instruments of psychiatric research. John Wiley, London. *This book is for those interested in rating scales. It provides a comprehensive review and critique of the major rating scales used in psychiatry, including those used in behavioural work. Its final chapter specifically covers those scales most commonly used in functional and cognitive assessment of the older adult.*

Woods R T 1992 Psychological therapies and their efficacy. Reviews in Clinical Gerontology 2: 171–183. *Dealing with a wide range of therapies, this review, though perhaps not as comprehensive as Bradbury (1991), is well written and up-to-date. It focuses more on cognitive therapies but does cover work in the behavioural field.*

19

Cognitive therapy with older people

John Wells
Catherine Wells

Distressing life events, for example failing eyesight or the loss of a spouse, are common in old age (Yost et al 1986) and the older adult has to adjust to altered physical capabilities and changing social roles. Since ideas of self-esteem are founded on such capabilities and roles, their alteration or loss can lead to negative thinking patterns and behaviour; for example 'I can't catch that bus, I'm not able anymore'. The thoughts that accompany and interpret these circumstances can sometimes lead to sadness and depression.

Cognitive therapy is based on the supposition that individuals can learn to identify, challenge and alter their thoughts and the underlying assumptions on which they are based, and that, by this process, they will eventually dispel their symptoms of depression and become equipped to prevent future relapse. It is a treatment approach that is structured, goal directed, focused, time limited and patient centred and aims to train individuals in the use of particular skills, as a means of coping with circumstances that can lead to depression. These elements make cognitive therapy particularly appropriate as a therapeutic intervention for use with the depressed older adult (Morris & Morris 1991). Elderly people require an intervention that is flexible and deals with current life issues. As cognitive therapy concentrates on current difficulties, with development of relevant, applicable skills, short-term goals and a focus on reducing cognitive distortions, its therapeutic relevance has immediate value for elderly people whose life circumstances can change rapidly (Yost et al 1986). In addition, the approach enables them to challenge stereotypic values and beliefs about the ageing process which may often act to reinforce a sense of disability and low self-esteem.

Habitual negative thoughts are a major focus of cognitive therapy. Elderly people have had many years to develop and fix cognitions and assumptions. Now, with more time on their hands than in the past, they have the chance to reflect upon and mull over past experiences or are exposed to habitual thoughts from which work might have been a distraction. If these thoughts are unpleasant they can become distressing and disabling, especially if the individual has limited opportunity for physical activity or social contact (Yost et al 1986). For example, some older adults remember things from the past which they regret or for which they feel guilty (Morris & Morris 1991). As time passes these memories can increase in intensity yet it is unlikely that anything can be done to change the events upon which the memories are based. Similarly, some elderly people find themselves unreconciled to their present environment, believing that they can only be happy if things could be like they were 'in the good old days'. Thus the future can look bleak and without hope (Morris & Morris 1991). The cognitive approach can be used to assist these people to develop a more objective and rational assessment of such issues, by encouraging flexible thinking and constructive rather than unhelpful negative thoughts. Thus depressed older people can be helped to view their future in a more positive and balanced way.

This chapter briefly surveys the development of cognitive therapy, describes the most commonly used cognitive model of depression and considers principles of treatment as applied to the individual, together with predictors for outcome and efficacy. Cognitive group therapy is briefly examined and other problems encountered by the elderly person for which a cognitive approach can be useful are discussed.

THE BACKGROUND TO COGNITIVE THERAPY

Cognitive therapy was initially developed in the USA in the 1960s and 1970s. Within the UK it became widely known and used from the 1980s. The work of Ivy Blackburn, John Teasdale and Melanie Fennel established its efficacy in the treatment of depression and showed it could be used in the NHS environment as well as the private practice setting of the USA (Moorey 1990).

It has been claimed that cognitive therapy can trace its roots back to the Stoics and Epicureans of Classical Greece (Mahoney 1993), although perhaps a more recognisable cognitive philosophy was that of the 18th and 19th century 'mind cure' movement. This emphasised the importance of positive thinking, through practical exercises, based on a framework of Christian thought, in the development of a healthy personal psychology.

In more modern times, cognitive therapy, as an explicit method of treatment, appeared in the 1970s. This was as a consequence of a growing dissatisfaction with the applicability, and efficacy, of pure behavioural approaches as the treatment of choice for a number of conditions (Foa & Emmelkamp 1983). It can be argued that its development as a separate treatment approach grew from the synergy of four strands of thought derived from the work of Kelly, Rachman and Lang, and Ellis and Bandura.

In the 1930s, Kelly, one of the founders of modern constructivist psychotherapy, developed a treatment approach based upon the idea of clients cultivating alternative identities. They would then surreptitiously 'rehearse' these alter-egos in their everyday lives, discussing with their therapist the resultant changes they observed in their regular activities and social relationships (Neimeyer 1993). Though Kelly denied the cognitivist connection, his *Psychology of Personal Constructs* (1955) had an inspirational influence on many subsequent cognitive therapists (Mahoney 1993).

The work of Rachman and Lang in conceptualising psychological problems as a three systems response consisting of behavioural, cognitive/affective and physiological systems (British Association for Behavioural and Cognitive Psychotherapies (BABCP) 1993) facilitated the identification of specific results of treatment in each of these domains. Thus it became possible to analyse how each of these systems responded to different approaches, and demonstrate that the cognitive aspects of a problem did not change in the same way, or at the same time, as the behavioural and physiological.

The third strand was Ellis's (1962) work on reason and emotion in psychotherapy, and his resultant rational-emotive therapy (now identified as a cognitive therapeutic approach), which demonstrated that the feelings and actions of individuals were mediated by their concealed beliefs and values. In other words, certain situations activated dysfunctional beliefs which impacted on behaviour and emotions. This idea still underpins all cognitive therapies (Yost et al 1986).

Finally, there was Bandura's work on learning theory and, in particular, his model of self-efficacy. He suggested that in order to achieve behavioural change, based on the acquiescence of the client, the client had to believe that they were capable of executing the new activity (BABCP 1993). This helped to establish the importance of individual cognitions in effecting behavioural change in therapy (BABCP 1993). This was combined with the idea of self-control, consisting of self-observation, self-evaluation and self-reinforcement.

These ideas can be seen to have culminated in the development of Meichenbaum's (1977) self-instructional training in cognitive behavioural modification, based around the idea of self-efficacy; and Beck's cognitive therapy, based upon the concept of the modification of automatic negative thoughts and dysfunctional assumptions. Indeed, a recent report on the development of the behavioural and cognitive approaches identified these last two, plus Ellis's rational-emotive therapy, as the main cognitive therapies currently in use (BABCP 1993).

BECK'S COGNITIVE MODEL OF DEPRESSION

Depression gives rise to a variety of symptoms which can leave the older adult in a state of despair. These symptoms (discussed in detail in Ch. 8) can be many and affect people in quite different ways. The pattern of depressive symptoms seen in clinical practice is distinct from those which are experienced in normal life by most people when they are confronted by loss. A normal reaction to loss is characterised by a resultant low, but transient, mood. In a depressive state, however, duration and intensity of feeling are far more extensive. One of the commonest symptoms is feeling intensely sad, accompanied by tearfulness. This may lead to irritability, agitation and anxiety. Other symptoms, which are often related, are those of guilt, difficulties with interest in or enjoyment of normal activities and feeling that everything is an effort. As the depression worsens it may lead to biological disturbances of sleep, appetite, concentration, memory and sexual desire. These symptoms, when combined, can lead to a growing sense of hopelessness and helplessness and, in some cases, to suicidal ideation and intent.

Negative cognitions have been shown to be present in older adults (Lam et al 1987) and are linked to depressive illness. A number of therapies attempt to relieve depression by changing negative cognitions and, of these, Beck's cognitive-behaviour therapy (Beck 1967) is the most widely accepted and used. Beck provides a theoretical and conceptual paradigm of the disorder of depression and describes the structure and process of treatment.

Beck's model suggests that depressed people maintain and intensify their depressive disorder through a distorted perception and interpretation of themselves, the world and the future; the so-called cognitive triad. It is proposed that this pattern of thinking can be changed by cognitive therapy, with a resultant positive effect on mood and behaviour. The therapeutic approach, based upon Beck's model of depression, is illustrated by the case of Mrs Turner, described in Box 19.1.

Box 19.1 Cognitive therapy with a depressed elderly person living at home: the case of Mrs Turner

Background
During a 1 year follow-up appointment with her general practitioner, following a heart attack, Mrs Turner, a married woman aged 70, became tearful and upset. She had made a good recovery from her heart attack and was physically stable. However, her general practitioner thought she was depressed and referred her for cognitive therapy, so that she could talk to someone about her problems and explore ways of coping with them.

Mrs Turner had been married to her husband for 42 years and they had three children, all of whom were married and living away from home. Before her marriage Mrs Turner had lived with her parents in a poor working class neighbourhood and had unhappy recollections of her childhood. Mr Turner, aged 80, was a retired bricklayer, who had always relied on his wife to run the home and organise the family. Mrs Turner had always seen herself as an accomplished housewife and mother and the decision maker within the family. Her children, even as adults, had always relied upon her for counsel and she was an active influence in the life of her grandchildren.

During the year before her heart attack Mrs Turner had found it increasingly physically demanding to carry out her usual day-to-day tasks around the house as well as shopping and her hobby, gardening, but had carried on regardless of her feelings of tiredness. Mrs Turner's heart attack came without warning and she found the experience of severe ill health and hospitalisation difficult and disempowering. On her return home from hospital, and even when fully recovered, fear of a second heart attack stopped Mrs Turner getting back into her usual routine. She also voiced regrets to her family about her past life and the total commitment she felt she had given to her husband and family. She became convinced that she only had a short time to live, despite reassurance to the contrary from the doctors, and this reduced her level of physical activity and adversely affected her relationship with her family; for example, every time one of her grandchildren visited she became tearful and said that she would not see them again. She also said that she was a burden to the family, describing herself as a 'cardiac cripple' who had outlived her usefulness, since she could no longer do what she had previously done.

On assessment by the cognitive therapist Mrs Turner described signs and symptoms of depression.

Box 19.1 *Cont'd*

These included feeling sad almost all the time, being tearful, especially when she thought of her grandchildren, and finding it difficult to fall asleep at night, often lying awake for hours. She also described a lack of interest and pleasure in the things that she had previously enjoyed and perceived the future as threatening and filled with more dangers. She described feeling tired and had lost her appetite, whereas previously she had enjoyed cooking and eating.

Formulation

Beck argues that depressed people operate upon the basis of dysfunctional schemata or assumptions which have been formed by past experience, childhood, education and background. For example, Mrs Turner's poor social background in childhood, and the subsequent importance she placed on work and physical fitness, played a major part in the way that she evaluated her situation and her role as carer and provider. The schemata are the means by which information is perceived, coded, stored and recalled and explain why an individual will sustain the same attitudes and beliefs about self, the world and the future, despite objective evidence to the contrary (Moorey 1990). The schemata incorporate beliefs, attitudes and assumptions which people hold about their abilities, attributes, the way others view them and their worth and self-esteem. Thus they structure an individual's picture of the world and the part they play in it both currently and in the future. Normally, an individual operates on the basis of this framework with no problems. Schemata are considered 'dysfunctional' when they are fixed, excessive and difficult to change (Fennell 1991). An older person has a vast store of life experiences, which might be informed by fairly entrenched attitudes and beliefs that may never have been challenged. From our case example, it can be seen that Mrs Turner's schemata developed from her need to be the active provider of care and nurture to her children and husband. Examples of her assumptions, formed as a result of this schemata included, 'I am only worthwhile if I can work and look after my husband', 'unless I can do everything as I have always done it, then everything will go wrong'.

Dysfunctional schemata or assumptions remain relatively dormant until they are activated by an important event which acts as a catalyst. The event can be anything from a major life event, such as illness or death of a close relative, to something relatively minor such as an argument with a neighbour. Beck et al (1979) argue that the person will seek to make sense of such an event by utilising a matrix of schema. In Mrs Turner's case the critical event was her heart attack which was particularly distressing to her because she had always valued herself in terms of her ability to be physically active and found being cared for humiliating. These feelings, coupled with her physical weakness and the possible threat of another heart attack, lowered her mood.

As a result of the activation of the schemata the individual produces negative automatic thoughts which in turn produce negative emotions such as anxiety. Beck describes these thoughts as automatic (spontaneous) and not a result of conscious reasoning. They are habitual, involuntary, extensive and plausible to the individual and are persistent and judged as true, leading to a lowering of mood and other symptoms of depression. They increase in frequency and displace more rational thoughts. Mrs Turner experienced frequent, intrusive negative thoughts. In her case they centred around her future and present circumstances; for example, 'I will never be of any use to anybody ever again', 'there is no use in trying to do anything because I will probably not be able to do it properly', 'I will probably end up as a cardiac cripple and become a burden to my children'. These thoughts led to a further lowering of Mrs Turner's mood and activity. Other symptoms of depression such as lethargy, sleep disturbance and poor appetite increased her belief in the validity of her negative thoughts.

A cognitive model of depression for Mrs Turner is represented in Figure 19.1. From this we can see how Mrs Turner's past experiences shaped her dysfunctional schemata or assumptions but, in spite of these, she was able to lead an ordered life with no apparent psychological difficulties until they were activated by her heart attack. This event produced negative automatic thoughts, which increasingly dominated the way she perceived and interpreted her wellbeing and roles within her family and society. When her negative automatic thoughts were associated with other symptoms, such as lethargy, lowered activity levels, disturbed sleep and difficulty concentrating, a vicious circle of helplessness and hopelessness ensued and she became clinically depressed; this vicious circle is illustrated in Figure 19.2.

ASSESSMENT

Assessment is discussed in detail in Chapter 6. Prior to

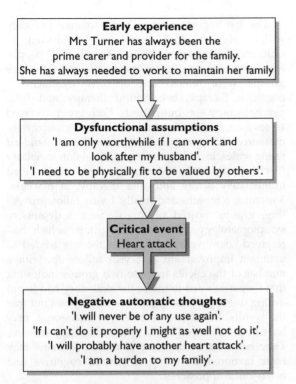

Figure 19.1 A cognitive model of depression for Mrs Turner.

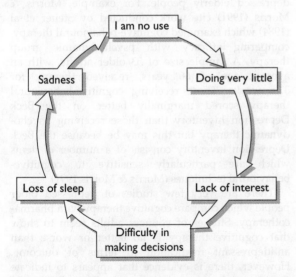

Figure 19.2 Mrs Turner's vicious cycle of helplessness and hopelessness.

cognitive therapy, assessment will include both specific and general information about the person and the presenting problem. Specific data about the history of the current problem should include details regarding

onset, with particular reference to precipitating events, duration of the problem, specific and general effects on the patient, his family/significant others and activity level (Emery 1981). The assessment should attempt to elicit information about any negative automatic thoughts and other symptoms of depression. It should also include general data about the patient's life, i.e. family, background, education, occupational history, relationships, sexual history, previous emotional difficulties, medical history (including alcohol, medication and drug use), previous treatment and any family psychiatric history. Assessment should be carried out by a qualified therapist who can diagnose depression and eliminate other possible causes, such as psychosis.

If cognitive therapy is thought an appropriate treatment, the next step is to provide a treatment rationale for the client (Fennell 1991). The therapist explains the general plan of treatment, why cognitive therapy is the intervention of choice and the role of the client's thoughts in the illness and, therefore, in recovery. The therapist will discuss the terms used in therapy and explore with clients the relationship between their feelings and the way that they think.

One of the most commonly used assessment instruments is the Beck Depression Inventory (Beck et al 1961) which was designed to be administered by an interviewer but today is usually used as a self-rating scale. The scale comprises 15 items on psychological symptoms and six on somatic ones, all scored 0–3. It provides a quantitative assessment of the intensity of depression and a rapid method of screening and assessment. The Beck Depression Inventory has a greater degree of cognitive bias than other scales used to measure depression (Thompson 1989) and this bias could be seen as a limitation for its utility as an assessment tool. Its other limitation is that it cannot be used for severely depressed individuals who may not be able to give meaningful answers or choose between responses. However, the scale is straightforward and quick to administer, usually taking less than 10 minutes. Scores are summed to provide an overall rating of depression. Because of its relatively undemanding length, the scale can be administered regularly without engendering boredom or resentment in the client and is a useful instrument in monitoring the progress of therapy. In addition, because it is client-rated it is compatible with the therapeutic philosophy of a collaborative partnership between therapist and client, with the client cast as a 'scientist' measuring and monitoring the problem and treatment.

One of the main questions to ask when deciding whether or not to use cognitive therapy with an older depressed person is 'will it help this particular individual?' In other words, how likely is therapy to succeed in alleviating or curing the depression. To answer this question two issues need to be considered: evidence for the success of cognitive therapy with elderly people and predictors of a likely successful therapeutic outcome.

THE EFFICACY OF COGNITIVE THERAPY FOR DEPRESSION IN OLD AGE

Writing in 1959 Rechtschaffen, having reviewed the literature on psychotherapy for the elderly, declared, 'systematic, controlled studies of the effectiveness of various treatments of older people are still lacking. Ultimately, there must be empirical grounds for predicting which type of treatment will work best for which type of patient' (cited in Weiss & Lazarus 1993, p. 95). Although there has been development in this area, his comment remains relevant as far as cognitive therapy for the older adult is concerned. There are few studies that specifically compare cognitive treatment efficacy for depression in the older adult against other interventions.

Hollon et al (1993), looking at the overall efficacy of cognitive therapy for depression, conclude that it appears to be effective as a treatment. However, they state that this opinion is tempered by a number of criticisms concerning the methodology of published studies. They point out that a number of psychosocial comparative studies lack clinical representativeness, and that those that compare pharmacotherapy to cognitive therapy fail to include pill-placebo controls. They therefore conclude that the evidence is promising with regard to cognitive therapy, but not yet conclusive. However, Weiss and Lazarus (1993) argue that within psychosocial therapies, double-blind, placebo-controlled research is fraught with difficulty. Not only is it more dependent on subjective judgement than biological investigations but the treatment process is less quantifiable. In addition, the study of an older population has a number of variables that may affect outcome, such as coinciding medical problems, using rating instruments originally designed for younger populations and the need to train therapists to be specifically sensitive to the changes brought about by advancing age. This is, in their view, the reason why so few studies in this area have been conducted. Yet, in spite of this, research exists which appears to indicate that the approach can benefit the depressed older adult.

The first important research into treatment efficacy with depressed older people was conducted by Gallagher & Thompson (1982). A sample of 30 people, with an average age of 68.3 years, divided into three groups, were offered one of three treatments – cognitive therapy, behavioural therapy and brief psychotherapy – as out-patients. Each group received 16 sessions, lasting 90 minutes. All three groups were measured for depression using a number of standard rating scales, including the Beck Depression Inventory (Beck et al 1961). Measures were administered immediately before and after therapy, at 6 weeks, 3 months, 6 months and finally 1 year follow-up. All three groups showed an improvement in depressive symptomatology. However, the groups which had received cognitive and behaviour therapy tended to maintain improvement at 1 year follow-up, with a number of the clients in these two groups indicating that they continued to utilise the skills they had learnt during therapy. Weiss & Lazarus (1993) point out that the results, in relation to brief psychotherapy, may have been influenced by the length of therapy sessions. They believe that the long 90-minute sessions may have favoured the more structured cognitive and behavioural approaches.

There have been some comparative studies of therapy, which used a cognitive component, with depressed elderly people. For example, Morris & Morris (1991) cite work conducted by Steuer et al (1984) which examined cognitive-behavioural therapy, comparing efficacy with psychodynamic group therapy. A sample size of 53 older adults, with an average age of 66 years, received therapy for 37.5 weeks. Those receiving cognitive-behavioural therapy scored marginally better on the Beck Depression Inventory than those receiving psycho-dynamic therapy but this may be because the Beck Depression Inventory consists of a number of items which are particularly sensitive to cognitive-behavioural techniques (Morris & Morris 1991).

There are very few studies of depressed older people which compare cognitive therapy with pharmacotherapy. Studies of younger adults seem to show that cognitive therapy is no better or worse than antidepressant medication in terms of outcome. However, there is evidence that appears to indicate that it might be superior to both modalities of treatment used alone (Hollon et al 1991, Hollon et al 1991).

One of the few studies of pharmacotherapy and cognitive therapy with depressed elderly people was by Beutler et al (1987) who compared the effectiveness of group cognitive therapy to Alprazolam. 56 subjects, with an average age of 71, who were diagnosed as having major unipolar depression, were subjected to one of four treatment conditions: cognitive therapy and a placebo; cognitive therapy and Alprazolam; a placebo and support; and Alprazolam and support. Treatment was given for a period of 20 weeks. Subjects who received cognitive therapy and a placebo showed the greatest improvement at 3 month follow-up and were less inclined than those in other groups to drop out of treatment. However, this study has methodological limitations; in particular, subjects were not randomised, with those entering the study earliest being assigned to one of the cognitive therapy groups. In addition, Alprazolam is a benzodiazepine, and not a usual pharmacological intervention for depression (Hollon et al 1991).

Predictors of success with elderly people

The most important question that the person recovering from depression wants answered is whether the depression will return. We do not know of any research which has looked beyond a year at long-term follow-up for depression in older people. However, studies of younger adults with depression (who were treated with cognitive therapy) at 2 year follow-up, report a reduction in risk of symptom return of 64%. This is the greatest reduction reported for an intervention for depression after treatment withdrawal. The best result for pharmacotherapy has been 26% (Hollon 1990), whilst interpersonal psychotherapy has yet to be definitively shown to be effective in the long term once therapy has finished, although there are some indications that it may reduce relapse (Hollon 1990).

Studies have tried to identify the significant factors which can affect outcome of depression in older people (Thompson et al 1988, Marmar et al 1989, Hartley 1985 cited in Weiss & Lazarus 1993). These found that unipolar depression, accompanied by personality disorder and low expectations for treatment, led to a poor outcome. In particular, client motivation and commitment to therapy were significant factors in the success of cognitive therapy.

Teri & Lewinsohn (1986) found two factors to be strong predictors of successful outcome of cognitive therapy: a low number of stressful life events and a low score for the initial level of depression as measured on the Beck Depression Inventory (Beck et al 1961). However, this study was not specific to elderly people and other studies have cast doubt on the value of initial symptomatology as a predictor of outcome with older

clients. For example, Gaston et al's (1988) study of a sample of 60 elderly depressed out-patients found little association between the level of initial symptomatology and the level of client participation in the therapeutic alliance which, as mentioned previously, has been found to be a predictor of success. Teri and Lewinsohn identified several other factors associated with successful outcome which are relevant to elderly people. For example, they found that subjects were more likely to improve if they were physically active and had high expectations of success.

Yost et al (1986), in discussing selection criteria for group cognitive therapy for the depressed older person, stress the importance of the individual's potential for establishing meaningful interpersonal relationships. The importance of this factor was highlighted in research by Teri and Lewinsohn (1986) and by Gaston et al (1988) who found a positive correlation between the extent of social and emotional support available to the older person from her family and the individual's willingness to engage in the therapeutic process. This relationship was supported by Jarrett et al's (1991) finding that clients who were married and had fewer dysfunctional attitudes, responded best to cognitive therapy.

Another important consideration, in the case of the older person, is the differentiation of organic brain disease from functional mental disorder (Yost et al 1986). For example, someone experiencing Alzheimer's disease is likely to have a less successful outcome in therapy than one who is experiencing a depressive reaction to a bereavement. It should be noted, though, that the use of cognitive therapy with those suffering from Alzheimer's disease may be valuable, particularly in the condition's early stages (Teri & Gallagher-Thompson 1991).

Fennell (1991) lists several issues which need to be considered when attempting to assess whether or not cognitive therapy will be beneficial for the individual. In particular, evidence of the cognitive triad is important since therapy will directly focus on this. She also emphasises how important it is to accept the treatment rationale. Gaston et al's (1988) study, referred to earlier, found that the older person's degree of defensiveness about their problem was associated with their lack of commitment to therapy.

Fennel (1991) also states that the range of behavioural and cognitive coping competencies the individual possesses, or possessed, are important predictors of successful outcome. This appears to be supported by Jarrett et al (1991) who found that individuals with fewer dysfunctional attitudes responded well to cognitive therapy. They speculate that such individuals have a faculty for 'cognitive flexibility', that is, the capacity to view the self, the world and the future from alternative perspectives.

From the above it is plain that no one elderly person is ever likely to meet all the predictive criteria for the most positive outcome. Most will fall somewhere in the middle. It would be a poor therapist who refused to treat individuals because they did not meet most of the criteria. However, analysing the older person's suitability for therapy is an important exercise, not only to ensure that she is offered appropriate assistance but also to ensure that alternative, and perhaps more beneficial, therapies, specific to the circumstances, are not excluded.

In sum, the short term efficacy of cognitive therapy for depression in older people has not been conclusively demonstrated as superior, compared to other treatments. However, cognitive therapy seems to be as effective as other psychosocial and behavioural interventions and, in combination with pharmacotherapy, possibly better, than antidepressants alone. As far as recurrence of depression is concerned, once therapy has finished, whilst no research has been specifically targeted at the older population, results from general studies are very positive and promising.

PRINCIPLES AND PROCESSES OF TREATMENT

Aims of treatment

In broad terms the aims of treatment are to:

- alleviate the depressive symptoms
- assist clients to modify their underlying assumptions
- provide clients with a broader repertoire of coping skills. (Moorey 1990)

Within these broad aims the client and therapist proceed to define specific goals for each session related to individual homework exercises.

The therapeutic relationship

The relationship between therapist and client in cognitive therapy is based on collaboration in which both parties actively participate in the treatment process, effectively joining forces to defeat the depression. Through this collaboration the notions of problem-solving and self-efficacy are fostered and encouraged. In this joining of forces the symptoms, thoughts and assumptions are viewed in a detached

and objective fashion and the client is asked to be a 'scientist' (Moorey 1990). In this role the client is encouraged to put forward hypotheses and then to initiate experiments to test them, so testing the validity of their thoughts, beliefs and assumptions. Through this process of testing, experimenting and applying the results to the dysfunctional schemata, the negative automatic thoughts become less frequent and are substituted by more rational thoughts. As a result of this change in thought process, and the continuous challenging of negative thoughts, the depressive symptoms gradually lessen in intensity. This is the fundamental process of therapy.

Within the therapeutic relationship there are specific issues that need to be recognised. Therapist and client are exposed to the influence of the social stereotyping that can accompany growing older as much as anyone else. Effective therapists are aware of their own attitudes, beliefs and assumptions about older people and recognise that these can negatively influence their expectations of treatment and outcome. For example, the therapist may patronise the client through tone of voice or be overly directive in therapy, ignoring the essential collaborative nature of the cognitive approach.

Equally, the elderly client may believe that they need to be told what to do by the 'all knowing therapist', which can result in over-dependence. Also, clients may strive to maintain their independence by being obstructive or overly argumentative in the therapeutic process. In a constructive therapeutic relationship the therapist examines issues of independence and dependence and avoids the struggle for dominance by acknowledging the difference in age between the two participants.

Summary of the treatment process

Treatment sessions are structured and focused. The first session is spent jointly agreeing priorities for treatment and thereafter each session is conducted on the basis of these priorities. The agenda is set and agreed by both therapist and client at the beginning of every session. Although flexible it will contain some consistent elements:

- a review of the previous session
- feedback regarding the last week and homework
- today's problem(s)
- setting homework.

When these are completed, time is spent concentrating on the main focus of the session (Beck et al 1979).

Table 19.1   Extract from Mrs Turner's thoughts diary

Date and time	Emotion How bad is it? (0–100)	Situation What were you doing or thinking about?	Thoughts How much did you believe them? (0–100)	Rational response What are your answers to the thoughts? How much do you believe them? (0–100)
June 13th 9 a.m.	Feeling sad – 60	Burnt toast making breakfast	Everything is an effort – 80	Apart from the toast, I managed to prepare a cooked breakfast – 50
			I'm always making mistakes – 90	
	Feeling tired – 80	Thinking about the day ahead	I'm too tired to do all that I have to do today – 90	I am tired, but I have already achieved something by getting up, washed, dressed and making breakfast – 40
				I could decide to do one or two particular things today, which I could achieve – 45
June 14th 4 p.m.	Feeling sad – 50	Walking around the garden	I don't know what to do – 75	I have enjoyed walking around the garden – 35
	Feeling hopeless –60		I will never be able to keep this garden the way I used to – 95	I have started to think about what needs to be done – 30
				I could decide to do a little weeding every day – 30

The sessions are characterised by questioning and enquiry which is achieved by giving and receiving feedback and checking for understanding. This process is used to develop and form links and trends in thought to facilitate identification of negative automatic thoughts. The therapist and client then proceed to challenge these negative thoughts and their underlying assumptions.

During the session the therapist and client conceptualise the specific problems (Beck et al 1985). This conceptualisation is based on the client's present difficulties, past experiences and vision of the future. From this conceptualisation the client is asked to identify any automatic negative thoughts. This is usually achieved by asking the individual to monitor and record them on a daily basis together with any accompanying feelings and activities/situations in which the thoughts occurred. This is illustrated by an extract from Mrs Turner's thought diary shown in Table 19.1.

Following on from this, the client is invited to modify these thoughts by using various means. This is often achieved by encouraging the client to view their thoughts in a different way, for example by setting up experiments to test out their validity, looking for supporting and contradictory evidence or by examining the advantages and disadvantages of such thoughts. During this process the client is asked to record a rational response to the thoughts and is then helped to identify underlying assumptions and to recognise the functioning of faulty cognitive processes or systematic errors in thinking (what Beck terms 'faulty information processing', Beck et al 1979) which include:

- over-generalisation – which involves drawing broad conclusions from a specific event or situation (e.g. 'I always make mistakes')
- selective abstraction – consists of picking out only the negative, even when this is taken out of context, or disregarding the positive (e.g. 'nothing went right today')
- magnification and minimisation – involves judging the relevance or significance of an event to an extreme (e.g. 'this is the end of our relationship it can never be the same again')
- dichotomous thinking – comprises thinking in extremes (e.g. 'if I can't get it right first time, there is no point in doing it at all')

- personalisation – refers to the way a person will attribute an event or situation to themselves (e.g. 'it's all my fault. I've made him feel upset')
- catastrophising – refers to attributing dire consequences to experienced events (e.g. 'if I exert myself too much I will definitely have a heart attack and die').

Therapeutic interventions

The therapeutic interventions used in cognitive therapy broadly fall into two groups – cognitive and behavioural.

Cognitive interventions

Distraction. This technique gets clients to focus on events, situations or objects other than painful or distressing issues. This can be achieved by asking them to remember a pleasant event in detail, to use their senses and explore the situation in depth, to read or to concentrate on some engrossing subject or to carry out some cognitive activities, e.g. mental arithmetic. Distraction is used mostly in the early stages of therapy when the client has yet to acquire competence in identifying negative thoughts and the appropriate skills in dealing with them. It can help the client to engage in therapy and is a pragmatic and easily employed technique to reduce distress.

Distraction provides the client with a temporary positive coping strategy. This helps to engage older adults in therapy and keep them in touch with difficult situations that produce negative automatic thoughts which can be worked on in treatment. Distraction is not an appropriate intervention in emotionally stressful situations since the client will be unable to utilise it efficiently. However, distraction helps some clients to carry on with their lives by providing temporary respite from their negative thinking.

Monitoring negative automatic thoughts. Monitoring thoughts in the early stages of therapy is essential to the progress of treatment. Clients are taught to monitor their thoughts and emotions, and to record the event or situation in which the thought occurred. The style of monitoring varies from problem to problem. Examining and inspecting these thoughts can be therapeutic in itself, helping to reduce their frequency through enhancing self awareness.

Modification of negative thoughts. The modification of negative thoughts is achieved through confrontation and challenge. The process is active and carried out in an objective and enquiring fashion. The basic strategies involve looking for alternatives to the thought by brainstorming ideas, helping the client to see the situation through somebody else's eyes, examining the evidence to either support or refute the thought, and deliberating on the advantages and disadvantages of viewing the thought in its present form. Another strategy is to ask the client to consider the basis of the thought in very specific detail and then to re-attribute the cause or the responsibility for the thought in a more realistic and wider context.

Socratic questioning. This procedure helps depressed clients to identify and challenge their negative thoughts through questioning which assists them in producing the responses necessary for recovery. The therapist phrases enquiring questions in such a way that clients discover the ineffectual and futile nature of their thinking patterns for themselves. It is important that they identify their own resolutions and challenges so that they can develop the necessary knowledge and skills to enable them to combat relapse and so further enhance the therapeutic gains made. An extract from one of Mrs Turner's therapy sessions illustrates this:

Mrs Turner: I feel useless. I can't do what I used to be able to do anymore.

Therapist: So what is it you're not able to do?

Mrs Turner: I can't do the housework or the gardening the way I used to.

Therapist: So what is so bad about not being able to do it as well as before?

Mrs Turner: Well, unless I can do it properly it is not worth doing at all. I might as well leave it altogether.

Therapist: I see. So if you can't do it perfectly then you would rather leave it altogether. OK. Well how does leaving it altogether make you feel?

Mrs Turner: Well, then I feel awful and useless because I've not done anything and it all builds up and it just gets worse.

Therapist: Do you ever try to do a little bit of the housework?

Mrs Turner: Yes, I do something every day, but I'm not satisfied with what I can do.

Therapist: So, is it the housework with which you are dissatisfied or with everything in general?

Mrs Turner: Actually, I feel useless altogether.

Therapist: It seems to me that the way you feel good about yourself is by the amount of housework you can do.

Mrs Turner: Well, yes I suppose that's right.

Therapist: You cannot see that doing a little bit of housework regularly is an achievement?

Mrs Turner: Well it's still not getting everything done is it?

Therapist: You seem to be discounting the fact that doing a small amount could be worthwhile. Do you feel this way of thinking about yourself is helpful?

Mrs Turner: Well, now you put it like that I'm not sure.

Behavioural interventions

Activity scheduling. This is a behavioural technique that is used at the beginning of treatment to provide structure and purpose to daily activities. Many depressed people gradually reduce their activity level and find that their lives are spent contemplating their negative thoughts. Activity scheduling involves the therapist and client agreeing on tasks to be scheduled on an hour by hour basis throughout the day. The aim initially is to monitor activities and to test out the schedule and its usefulness.

In activity scheduling the therapist will usually attempt to organise activities into those which will give the client a sense of 'mastery' and those which will provide 'pleasure'. This mixture is thought to be effective at helping clients fight dichotomised thinking because it allows them to enjoy activities which give varying degrees of pleasure and mastery (Beck et al 1979).

Graded task assignment. Clients are encouraged to break down tasks into small manageable parts and then carry them out as homework. The tasks become more demanding and difficult as the client achieves success. This builds on the client's existing skills and attributes and develops them further in order to boost self-esteem and confidence.

Behavioural tests (experiments). As previously discussed, the client is asked to act like a scientist, to formulate hypotheses and test them through experiments. The tests are graded so that clients can experience some success and can challenge and test the validity of their negative thoughts. An example of a behavioural test is given in sessions six and seven of Mrs Turner's treatment process which is summarised in the next section.

Behavioural skills acquisition. At assessment, a skills deficit may be identified or this may become evident in the course of treatment. Role play, social skills training, assertiveness training and role rehearsal are all employed on an individual basis in order to meet the specific client's needs (Liberman et al 1975). All of the above can be used in therapy, or the therapist can choose the most appropriate intervention based upon the difficulties of the older person and the presenting problems.

MRS TURNER'S TREATMENT PROCESS

We turn now to summarise Mrs Turner's treatment process to demonstrate use of some of the possible strategies that may be used in cognitive therapy for the older person who is moderately depressed.

Session 1

This session was spent identifying the problems to be addressed in treatment. These problems were listed by Mrs Turner in order of priority as:

1. Feeling tired and that everything is an effort all the time.
2. Feeling no longer of use to anybody.
3. Fearful that she will no longer be able to keep the house and garden to the standard that she had done before her heart attack.
4. Feeling lonely and isolated because of her inability to go out for fear of having another heart attack.

The therapist was able to elicit negative thoughts and conceptualise Mrs Turner's problems in terms of Beck's model (Fig. 19.1) thereby providing a rationale for her treatment. Mrs Turner's distorted thinking was assessed as contributing to her negative feelings and interfering with her ability to carry out her usual activities which, in turn, exacerbated her tiredness and social isolation. This formulation was diagrammatically represented (Fig. 19.2) and used as a focus for discussion. In addition, the therapist recommended that Mrs Turner read *Coping with Depression* by Ivy Blackburn (1992), a short self help book written for clients.

Sessions 2 and 3

In these sessions the therapist explained the process of identifying and monitoring negative automatic thoughts by using the diary (see Table 19.1). Activity scheduling was also discussed and implemented, a schedule of activities being planned and agreed. This was done by scrutinising how Mrs Turner spent her day and asking her to increase gradually her level of activity. The scheduled activities were arranged around those which were to do with mastery (i.e. tasks of everyday living such as dusting, bed making and personal care) and pleasure (e.g. watering indoor plants, baking an apple pie and reading her women's magazine).

In these sessions Beck's thinking errors were explained to Mrs Turner. The errors of 'catastrophising' and 'selective abstraction' were those which the therapist considered to be most relevant in Mrs Turner's case. In addition to explaining the types of errors, the therapist addressed how they might interfere with the way that Mrs Turner filtered or processed information in a negative or unhelpful way. Homework was set around monitoring and identifying negative automatic thoughts and thinking errors and carrying through the activity schedule.

Session 4

In this session the homework diary was examined. The therapist explored other ways of interpreting Mrs Turner's negative automatic thoughts and went on to challenge them. This was done by asking Mrs Turner to provide evidence for the thought and then asking her to consider other ways of viewing the same situation. Mrs Turner was asked to contemplate how she might have perceived her situation before she had the heart attack and how others, particularly her friends, might evaluate her situation and to consider advantages and disadvantages of thinking in these ways. Mrs Turner was then asked to complete the 'alternative thoughts' section of her diary as homework for the following week. The activity schedule was also reviewed and extra activities discussed and added as appropriate.

Session 5

During this session Mrs Turner expressed difficulty in recording her negative automatic thoughts. She felt that recording them was making her feel worse. She reported that she had been crying at home because she was focusing on her regrets and felt hopeless about them. As a result she had stopped her homework and had felt superficially better. She cried continuously throughout the session and said that she could not see how cognitive therapy could make her feel better. The therapist explained that her feelings were a common problem at this stage of treatment and that they were temporary and short term. The importance of addressing and challenging the negative automatic thoughts as they arise, thereby avoiding storing them up for the session itself, was explained. Regular and consistent confrontation and challenging the thoughts was much more likely to result in a successful outcome to therapy. Homework was agreed and set for the following week.

Session 6

Mrs Turner had done well since the previous session,

in monitoring negative thoughts and challenging them. She had carried out her activity schedule successfully and had surprised herself that she was able to do this. She was also feeling less tired. Mrs Turner continued recording her thoughts during the session and at home. At this point the therapist helped Mrs Turner form links between her thoughts and her assumptions about herself, current events and the future. It became clear that 'selective abstraction' and 'over generalisation' errors in her thinking pattern were now the prominent features. These were recorded in her diary, examined and analysed in the session.

Mrs Turner was also encouraged to use a problem-solving approach in relation to her high standards, especially with regard to her gardening. This involved considering a variety of options in a systematic and detailed way; for example, growing more shrubs rather than plants that required a lot of attention would still make the garden attractive and colourful but require less effort. Mrs Turner agreed, as part of her homework, to find out about possible shrubs and plants that she might use in her garden.

Sessions 7 and 8

Mrs Turner's treatment was progressing well. She was beginning to feel able to do more and was getting pleasure from this. She was able to challenge and find alternatives to most of her negative thoughts but she was still unable to challenge the thought that she would have a heart attack if she was far from home for any length of time. This was discussed in the context of her progress so far and it was agreed that she should put her thought to the test. It was acknowledged that this would not be easy for her, but could be done gradually. A behavioural experiment was set up to test the prediction that if she were to spend 30 minutes on her own in town, whilst shopping with her daughter, she would experience the symptoms of a heart attack. She was asked to monitor and challenge negative automatic thoughts whilst she was on her own and to record these later.

In session 8 Mrs Turner gave feedback on the test. She had not had a heart attack and was pleased that she had managed to carry out the test successfully. Mrs Turner decided to extend the length spent alone away from home. She continued to complete her diary and extend her activities at home.

Sessions 9 and 10

These sessions were spent reviewing the progress of treatment and planning for the future. Mrs Turner was encouraged to become her own therapist. She reviewed the components of the therapy that she found most useful and examined how she might be able to use them in future. She was asked to write a plan of how she might reach goals that were not fully attained in treatment. She was also asked to predict future problems and when an exacerbation of negative automatic thoughts might occur and write a contingent strategy for action to prevent deterioration in her mood under these predicted circumstances.

THE OLDER PERSON AND COGNITIVE THERAPY IN GROUPS

As we mentioned earlier, older people may share common experiences and exploring these in group therapy has some advantages over individual treatment. Group therapies include resocialisation groups, pre-placement groups (Yost et al 1986), and other psychotherapeutic groups including cognitive therapy, cognitive behavioural groups and psycho-educational groups (Free et al 1991). Treating older people in groups has the practical advantage of helping more people at one time and thus being cost effective. It also allows older people to be treated promptly because more people are accepted for treatment at the same time, thus reducing waiting lists. According to Yost et al (1986), therapeutic benefits to groups rather than individual therapy for older people include opportunities for socialisation, the chance to express altruistic needs, and recognising how common their problems are (Yost et al 1986).

However, there are some difficulties that older people face which could impede the therapeutic value of groups. Cerella et al (1980, cited in Yost et al 1986) found that older people are less able than young to examine and synthesise concepts and also they find it

difficult to attend for long periods, which can make some forms of group processes demanding. These problems are exacerbated by difficulties ordering thoughts and problems and in remembering information. However, the structure and process of cognitive therapy can largely combat these difficulties (Ford & Pfefferbaum 1980, cited in Yost et al 1986). For example, through the use of an agenda, the formulation of concepts, the consistent use of feedback, structured homework and the logical sequence of the therapy, the therapist and older client can identify and modify these difficulties. The format for group therapy seems to relate well to Beck's cognitive model of depression. Although researchers have emphasised one particular component or another, the key principles of individual cognitive therapy would appear to have been adopted by most. As illustrated in Table 19.2, there is usually a four stage approach to the cognitive therapy group (Yost et al 1986).

The first stage, 'preparation', involves identification of individual problems, establishing rapport and providing initial information about cognitive therapy. The second stage focuses on identification of dysfunctional thoughts and establishing a collaborative relationship between therapist(s) and the group. It may also include some elements of activity scheduling and graded task assignment. The third stage is concerned with challenging and modifying negative thoughts and the acquisition and practice of skills. The last stage is the termination and consolidation stage which is aimed at self-management, continued self-help and integration into the world beyond the group. The group also offers the opportunity for socialisation and for interaction and collaboration between group members. This facet of group therapy is especially important to older people who are isolated from their peers. The process whereby members relate their individual

Table 19.2 Four stages of the cognitive therapy group

Stages	1st	2nd	3rd	4th
Beutler et al 1987	Information and collaboration	Identification of dysfunctional thoughts	Implementation of methods to modify thoughts	Termination and future planning
Free et al (1990)	Orientation to cognitive therapy	Identification of dysfunctional thoughts	Disrupting thoughts and challenges	Techniques for changing beliefs
Yost et al (1986)	Preparation and individual problems	Identification of thoughts and collaboration	Change and practice	Consolidation
Zerheusen et al (1991)	Preparation, rapport and education	Activity scheduling and graded task assignment	Recording dysfunctional thoughts and testing out	Termination and reinforcement of practice

thoughts and beliefs to the group stimulates extensive discussion, reflection and challenge to such thoughts and beliefs. Thus group members are both recipients and contributors to the cognitive therapeutic process.

Effectiveness of cognitive therapy groups

The effectiveness of cognitive therapy groups is difficult to establish as their use is not widespread and they are not consistent in their content or form. From examining the research, however, it is possible to draw some conclusions.

Zerheusen (1991) compared group cognitive therapy with group music therapy and a control group, who received a variety of different types of nursing care in a group setting. The subjects were all nursing home residents. The group who were part of the cognitive therapy process showed a significant improvement in their level of depression compared to the music therapy and the control groups. The cognitive therapy group improved by on average 12.63 points on Beck's Depression Inventory (Beck et al 1961) compared with an improvement of 1.53 for the music group and 2.63 for the control group.

Zettle et al (1989) compared three groups who received complete cognitive therapy, partial cognitive therapy and comprehensive distancing (i.e. an intervention based upon the view that thoughts are facets of behaviour rather than explanations for behaviour; thus behaviour is emphasised as the focus for change rather than the negative cognitions). Clients from all three groups improved in their level of depression over a period of 12 weeks. The two groups which received cognitive therapy showed a reduction in negative thoughts. Another study by Free et al (1991) looked at the effectiveness of group cognitive therapy for 35 subjects who had minor or major depression. They found that group cognitive therapy was clinically effective. However, their results are questionable, as levels of depression varied between subjects and some were also taking medication, which may have affected the results.

A comparative study of treatment efficacy, contrasting a course of group therapy based on a social learning model of depression with individual behaviour therapy and the variables that predicted successful treatment outcome was conducted by Teri and Lewinsohn (1986). They found no significant difference in depression outcome between group and individual treatment. Both treatment conditions showed significant improvement in depression levels over time. This study suggests therefore, that a group

approach is as efficacious as individualised cognitive therapy but with the added advantage of treating a number of people simultaneously and cost-effectively.

In sum, it seems that group cognitive therapy is effective in the treatment of depression in older people. It also provides a sociable forum for a group of people who are prone to isolation and a safe milieu in which fixed beliefs and values, that cause distress, can be challenged.

OTHER APPLICATIONS

The application of cognitive therapy to problems, other than depression, in the older adult is not well developed (BABCP 1993). However, a few studies indicate that cognitive therapy, sometimes reinforced with behavioural techniques, does have a beneficial outcome for a range of psychophysical problems which can confront older people. The more significant conditions in which a cognitive therapy component may be utilised in treatment are discussed below.

Anxiety

Anxiety in late life is discussed in detail in Chapter 7. Studies on the use of cognitive therapy and the older adult with an anxiety state are almost non-existent (King & Barrowclough 1991). However, in clinical practice cognitive therapy is used to treat anxiety in some elderly people and also in the carers of elderly people living at home.

Everyone experiences some degree of anxiety in situations that they perceive as personally threatening. However, for some this sense of anxiety is not restricted to specific situations and can become disabling. The two main types of this sort of anxiety are generalised anxiety disorder, consisting of unreasonable and extreme worry about various personal situations and conditions, and panic disorder, in which there arises unexpectedly acute fear and a sudden experience of distressing physical sensations (BABCP 1993).

Cognitive theory offers two explanations as to how generalised anxiety and panic disorder occur (Clark 1991). It is hypothesised that people with generalised anxiety develop beliefs and dysfunctional assumptions about themselves which make them likely to interpret a wide range of circumstances as threatening. In particular, cognitions around acceptance, responsibility, control and the symptoms of anxiety appear to be central. In panic disorder, individuals have a propensity to catastrophise physical sensations, particularly those associated with anxiety such as palpitations, breathlessness and dizziness, and interpret them as portending an immediate physical or mental calamity.

Treatment for generalised anxiety usually involves a cognitive-behavioural approach which aims to educate clients how to identify, evaluate, control and modify negative and danger-focused cognitions and resultant behaviour. Treatment involves a general cognitive approach for the treatment of depression with particular emphasis on the use of behavioural experiments. This takes the form of behavioural homework for clients to check out the validity of their negative thoughts (Butler et al 1991).

Chambless and Gillis (1993) surveyed nine clinical trials which adopted this approach. They found that cognitive-behavioural methods had a consistently substantive impact on generalised anxiety, with treatment effects being maintained between 6 to 12 months at follow-up. In particular, they report the study conducted by Butler et al (1991) which compared clients treated with cognitive-behavioural therapy against those treated with behaviour therapy. This study found, at 24 month follow-up, that significantly more behaviour therapy treated clients sought additional help compared to those treated with cognitive-behavioural techniques (Chambless & Gillis 1993).

The aim of therapy for panic disorder is to modify catastrophic interpretations of the physical feelings experienced during panic attacks. However, a particular difficulty with this client group is that they will only internalise such modifications if the benefits can be proved to them. This is because they experience real bodily symptoms, for example breathlessness, upon which to base their catastrophic interpretations. Thus the use of behavioural experiments, for example encouraging them to hyperventilate voluntarily as a means of reproducing symptoms and thus provide them with an alternative interpretation, can be crucial within the overall treatment strategy (Clark 1991).

Results for cognitive therapy alone indicate that this approach is making a major contribution to the treatment of panic disorder (BABCP 1993). Chambless & Gillis (1993), reporting on six trials conducted in four countries, found an average of 85% of clients were panic free immediately after therapy increasing to 88% at follow-up. Beck et al (1992) reported cognitive therapy as superior to supportive psychotherapy, whilst Clark et al (in press) report a study showing that cognitive therapy was found to be superior to imipramine and applied relaxation at both short- and long-term follow-up (BABCP 1993).

In a pilot study of cognitive-behavioural therapy for anxiety disorders King & Barrowclough (1991) treated 10 older adults, with an average age of 73 years, for panic disorder and anxiety using Clark's approach. The average number of therapeutic sessions was eight. Using self-report and the Beck Depression Inventory they found that six clients showed improvement at immediate follow-up, and three at 6 month follow-up. The positive results from these few studies suggest the need for further research into cognitive therapy with anxious elderly people.

Insomnia

Insomnia affects 25–35% of people over the age of 65 years (Morin et al 1993, Brabbins et al 1993). For the older person it affects sleep maintenance, whereas for younger people it is sleep initiation that is difficult. When left untreated chronic insomnia, and its consequent debilitating psychological effects, can enhance the propensity to depression (Morin et al 1993). Morin et al (1993) have pointed out that if no cause can be detected then interventions need to be focused around the perceptions and anxieties that insomnia can generate. Therefore the identification of non-pharmacological therapy is of some importance.

Cognitive therapy for insomnia focuses on anticipations of sleep. The main aim of therapy is to change peoples' belief that they are passive sufferers from a disorder – insomnia – to one in which they believe themselves capable of managing the difficulty (Bootzin & Perlis 1992). In order to do this the client is given information about sleep and sleep loss. In addition, irrational beliefs about sleep are identified (for example 'I did not sleep last night so I won't sleep tonight. So there's no point in going to bed') and this information may be supplemented by such interventions as paradoxical intention (instructing someone to stay awake) or thought stopping (i.e. disrupting a thought by shouting 'stop' or using a physical disrupter, such as twanging an elastic band on one's wrist) techniques. It has been found that, although cognitive therapy is effective in treating late life insomnia, it is less effective than behavioural techniques (Morin & Azerin 1988). More recent studies have favoured combining the two approaches in a cognitive-behavioural approach.

Morin et al (1993) examined the use of cognitive-behaviour therapy for late life insomnia in a group of 24 adults over 60 years old. These researchers argue that, when medical factors are excluded, there is evidence that maladaptive behaviour and dysfunctional cognitions about sleep, such as irregular sleep patterns or excessive concerns over sleep loss, significantly affect the older adult with sleep problems. The researchers used a combination of behavioural and cognitive therapy. The behavioural element consisted of sleep restriction (staying in bed only whilst asleep) and stimulus control (a number of instructions as to when and how to sleep).

The cognitive element focused on altering beliefs and assumptions around sleep, such as 'I must have 8 hours sleep'. The therapeutic approach involved distinguishing specific dysfunctional cognitions, challenging the dysfunctional thoughts and implementing methods for substituting the irrational thoughts with reasonable ones. The therapists utilised cognitive restructuring methods which aimed to help clients identify normal pathological changes and relieved the concerns they had about reduced sleep. In addition, they taught clients about the effects of such things as alcohol and caffeine on sleep. The results of the approach were significantly positive, both in terms of objective and subjective measurement and most of the clients voiced greater satisfaction with sleep. At the 12 month follow-up, no subject was using regular medication (of the 24, 13 had used regular medication before therapy), although three used it intermittently.

These studies suggest that a cognitive-behavioural approach, when compared to the use of medication, may be highly cost-effective in terms of duration and outcome but also carry virtually no risk to physical health.

Chronic pain

Chronic pain associated with physical problems can affect elderly people severely. For example, in the USA approximately 5 million older adults suffer from rheumatoid arthritis (Appelbaum et al 1988), and Bergman (1982) found that physical ill health in older people was closely related to depression (cited in Morris & Morris 1991). Indeed, by its very nature, the impact of chronic pain on psychological functioning is significant, with dysfunctional thoughts, such as catastrophising, playing an influential part in the development of subsequent depression. Cognitions around attention, attributions, appraisals and self-statements are believed to play an important role in the individual's adaptation to her state (Turner & Jensen 1993). In particular it has been found that people's judgements of their capability to exercise control over pain, rather than believing that external factors exert an influence, influences the degree of chronic pain experienced (Keefe et al 1992).

The use of purely cognitive techniques for chronic pain has not been widely reported, as most work tends to utilise a cognitive-behavioural approach. An exception is work by Turner & Jensen (1993) who compared the efficacy of cognitive therapy with relaxation techniques in a group of 102 subjects, ranging in age from 22 to 62 years. Within the cognitive therapy group, clients were taught to identify negative emotions related to pain and stressful events. They were then taught to identify linked maladaptive cognitions and develop adaptive thoughts as a means of countering automatic negative thoughts. Although both groups improved the study found no significant difference between the efficacy of each therapy at 12 month follow-up.

More typically, Appelbaum et al (1988) used cognitive-behavioural therapy with a group of rheumatoid arthritis sufferers (ranging in age from 47 to 70 years). Therapy consisted of relaxation techniques combined with teaching the clients to monitor stressful situations and modify maladaptive self-statements by focusing on what they could do rather than what they could not. In addition problem-solving homework was given and this formed the basis of discussion with the therapist. Post-treatment follow-up found significant improvements in pain perception and pain control.

Grief reactions

Loss of loved ones, grief and mourning are a progressive part of life for the older adult. However, sometimes grief and mourning can take on a pathological dimension – the famous example of Queen Victoria mourning Prince Albert being a case in point – characterised as chronic grief. In addition, the loss of a long-term partner may trigger major changes in life circumstances for the older person. For example, the survivor may have to move from the family home into an institutional setting.

A cognitive model to explain the process involved in chronic grief reaction likens it to an emotional feedback loop (Kavanagh 1990). This loop involves exposure to a sustained experience of profound melancholy (such as the death of a loved one), which precipitates negative thoughts, behaviour and physiological processes. These then facilitate the maintenance and intensification of a depressive mood.

Kavanagh (1990) argues that the most effective model of grief for therapeutic purposes is a combined anxiety/depressive one which suggests that bereavement has components of anxiety (for example, physical symptoms such as panic and having anxious thoughts, such as 'how will I cope') coupled with avoidance (for example, an inability to confront the reality of the loss) and depression (for example, bouts of sadness and social withdrawal). Kavanagh therefore recommends a cognitive-behavioural approach to therapy involving controlled exposure to bereavement cues, as a means of habituation to bereavement stimuli, and graduated involvement in roles and activities, as a means of initiating moments of pleasure and thus controlling sadness. The prime cognitive component, based on Beck et al (1979) involves identifying negative thoughts and challenging their validity through Socratic questioning. In particular, attention is focused on hopelessness about the future and thoughts of guilt for being the survivor. Overall the aim of therapy, in Kavanagh's words is, 'to maximise survivors' achievements and minimise the pain they suffer to gain them' (Kavanagh 1990, p. 381).

CONCLUSION

Freud held the view that older people lack the capacity to engage in therapy as a result of cognitive changes consequent to the ageing process. He believed being old makes them inflexible in their thinking processes (Morris & Morris 1991). This may go some way to explain why the use of psychotherapy in general, and cognitive therapy in particular, with older adults has not increased as fast with this group as with younger people. However, if the therapist takes account of the influence of ageing on cognitive and physical processes, for example by reducing the conversational

flow to the speed at which the client can process information, and discussing goals relevant to the older adult's emotions, physical abilities and health status, older adults can make just as much progress as their younger counterparts (Emery 1981). In other words, therapists need to put aside their own stereotypical views of old age.

Much of the evidence for the efficacy of cognitive therapy is drawn from studies of young populations rather than those of older depressed people. This needs to be borne in mind, but does not rule out the value of studies of younger populations for helping us understand the problems and reactions of older people to cognitive therapy (Morris & Morris 1991). Specific studies of the efficacy of the approach with older adults are few, though promising, and those which address grief, pain and insomnia, as well as depression, are particularly pertinent to elderly people.

As one gets older, time becomes an increasingly precious commodity. Cognitive therapy focuses on problems in the here and now. It is of short duration when compared with other available therapies, yet provides the individual with skills that are of immediate use and relevance. In addition, the relationship between client and therapist is one of partnership. Cognitive therapy reinforces the self-esteem of clients and empowers them and challenges the sense of increasing disability that can afflict some older people.

REFERENCES

Appelbaum K A, Blanchard E B, Hickling E J, Alfonso M 1988 Cognitive behavioural treatment of a veteran population with moderate to severe rheumatoid arthritis. Behaviour Therapy 22: 489–493

Beck A T 1967 Depression: clinical, experimental and theoretical aspects. Harper and Row, New York

Beck A T, Ward C H, Mendelson M, Mock J, Erbaugh J 1961 An inventory for measuring depression. Archives of General Psychiatry 4: 561–571

Beck A T, Rush A J, Shaw B F, Emery G 1979 Cognitive therapy of depression. Guilford Press, New York

Beck A T, Emery G, Greenberg R L 1985 Anxiety disorders and phobias: a cognitive perspective. Basic Books, New York

Beck A T, Sokol L, Clark D, Berchick B, Wright F 1992 Focused cognitive therapy of panic disorder: a cross-over design and one year follow-up. American Journal of Psychiatry 147: 778–783

Bergman K 1982 Depression in the elderly. In: Isaacs B (ed) Recent advances in geriatric medicine, vol. 2. Churchill Livingstone, Edinburgh

Beutler L E, Scogin F, Kirkish P et al 1987 Group cognitive

therapy and Alprazolam in the treatment of depression in older adults. Journal of Consulting and Clinical Psychology 55(4): 550–556

Blackburn I 1992 Coping with depression. Chambers, Edinburgh

Bootzin R R, Perlis M L 1992 Nonpharmacologic treatments of insomnia. Journal of Clinical Psychiatry Supplement 53(6): 37–41

Brabbins C J, Dewey M E, Copeland J R M et al 1993 Insomnia in the elderly: prevalence gender differences and relationships with morbidity and mortality. International Journal of Geriatric Psychiatry 10: 473–480

British Association for Behavioural and Cognitive Psychotherapies 1993 Behavioural and cognitive psychotherapies: past history current applications and future registration issues. Behavioural and Cognitive Psychotherapy Supplement 1: 1–75

Butler G, Fennel M, Robson P, Gelder M 1991 Comparison of behaviour therapy and cognitive behaviour therapy in the treatment of generalised anxiety disorder. Journal of Consulting and Clinical Psychology 59: 167–175

Cerella J, Poon L W, Williams D M 1980 Age and the complexity hypothesis. In: Poon L W (ed) Ageing in the 1980s: psychological issues. American Psychological Association, Washington DC

Chambless D L, Gillis M 1993 Cognitive therapy of anxiety disorders. Journal of Consulting and Clinical Psychology 61(2): 248–260

Clark D M 1991 Anxiety states: panic and generalised anxiety. In: Hawton K, Salkovskis P M, Kirk J, Clark D M (eds) Cognitive behaviour therapy for psychiatric problems: a practical guide. Oxford Medical Publications, Oxford

Clark et al (In press). Cited in British Association for Behavioural and Cognitive Psychotherapies 1993 Behavioural and cognitive psychotherapies: past history current applications and future registration issues. Behavioural and Cognitive Psychotherapy Supplement 1

Ellis A 1962 Reason and emotion in psychotherapy. Lyle Stuart, Secaucus NJ

Emery G 1981 Cognitive therapy with the elderly. In: Emery G, Hollon S D, Bedrosian R C (eds) New directions in cognitive therapy. Guilford Press, New York

Fennell M 1991 Depression. In: Hawton K, Salkovskis P M, Kirk J, Clark D M (eds) Cognitive behaviour therapy for psychiatric problems: a practical guide. Oxford Medical Publications, Oxford

Foa E, Emmelkamp P 1983 Failures in behaviour therapy. Wiley, New York

Ford J M, Pfefferbaum A 1980 The utility of brain potentials in determining age-related changes in central nervous system and cognitive functioning. In: Poon L W (ed) Ageing in the 1980s: psychological issues. American Psychological Association, Washington DC

Free M L, Oei T P S, Sanders M R 1991 Treatment outcome of a group cognitive therapy programme for depression. International Journal of Group Psychotherapy 41(4): 533–547

Gallagher D E, Thompson L W 1982 Treatment of major depressive disorder in older adult outpatients with brief psychotherapies. Psychotherapy: Theory Research and Practice 19: 482–490

Gaston L, Maramar C R, Thompson L W, Gallagher D 1988 Relation of patient pretreatment characteristics to the therapeutic alliance in diverse psychotherapies. Journal of Consulting and Clinical Psychology 56(4): 483–489

Hartley D 1985 Research in the therapeutic alliance in psychotherapy. In: American Psychiatric Association Psychiatry Update 4. APA, Washington DC

Hollon S D 1990 Cognitive therapy and pharmacotherapy for depression. Psychiatric Annals 20: 249–258

Hollon S D, Shelton R C, Loosen P T 1991 Cognitive therapy and pharmacotherapy for depression. Journal of Consulting and Clinical Psychology 59(1): 88–99

Hollon S D, Shelton R C, Davis D D 1993 Cognitive therapy for depression: conceptual issues and clinical efficacy. Journal of Consulting and Clinical Psychology 61(2): 270–275

Jarrett R B, Eaves G G, Grannemann B D, Rush A J 1991 Clinical cognitive and demographic predictors of response to cognitive therapy for depression: a preliminary report. Psychiatry Research 37: 245–260

Kavanagh D J 1990 Towards a cognitive-behavioural intervention for adult grief reactions. British Journal of Psychiatry 157: 373–383

Keefe F J, Dunsmore J, Burnett R 1992 Behavioural and cognitive-behavioural approaches to chronic pain: recent advances and future directions. Journal of Consulting and Clinical Psychology 60(4): 528–536

Kelly G 1955 The psychology of personal constructs. Norton, New York

King P, Barrowclough C 1991 A clinical pilot study of cognitive-behavioural therapy for anxiety disorders in the elderly. Behavioural Psychotherapy 19(4): 337–346

Lam D H, Brewin C R, Woods R T, Bebbington P E 1987 Cognition and social adversity in the depressed elderly. Journal of Abnormal Psychology 96: 23–26

Liberman R P, King L W, De Risi W J, McCann M 1975 Personal effectiveness. Research Press, Champaign, Illinois

Mahoney J 1993 Theoretical developments in the cognitive psychotherapies. Journal of Consulting and Clinical Psychology 61(2): 187–193

Marmar C R, Gaston L, Gallagher D, Thompson L W 1989 Alliance and outcome in late life depression. Journal of Nervous Mental Disorders 177(8): 464–472

Meichenbaum D 1977 Cognitive-behaviour modification: an integrated approach. Plenum, New York

Moorey S 1990 Cognitive therapy. In: Dryden W (ed) Individual therapy: a handbook. Open University Press, Buckingham

Morin C M, Azirin N H 1988 Behavioural and cognitive treatments of geriatric insomnia. Journal of Consulting and Clinical Psychology 56(5): 748–753

Morin C M, Kowatch R A, Barry T, Walton E 1993 Cognitive-behaviour therapy for late-life insomnia. Journal of Consulting and Clinical Psychology 61(1): 137–146

Morris R G, Morris L W 1991 Cognitive and behavioural approaches with the elderly depressed. International Journal of Geriatric Psychiatry 6: 407–413

Neimeyer R A 1993 An appraisal of constructivist psychotherapies. Journal of Consulting and Clinical Psychology 61(2): 221–234

Rechtschaffen A 1959 Psychotherapy with geriatric patients: a review of the literature. Journal of Gerontology 14(1): 73–84

Steuer J L, Mintz J, Hammen C L 1984 Cognitive-behavioural and psychodynamic group psychotherapy in treatment of geriatric depression. Journal of Consulting Clinical Psychology 52: 180–189

Teri L, Gallagher-Thompson 1991 Cognitive-behavioural interventions for treatment of depression in Alzheimer's patients. The Gerontologist 31(3): 413–416

Teri L, Lewinsohn P M 1986 Individual and group treatment of unipolar depression: comparison of treatment outcome and identification of predictors of successful treatment outcome. Behaviour Therapy 17: 215–228

Thompson C 1989 Instruments of psychiatric research. John Wiley, London

Thompson L W, Gallagher D, Czirr R 1988 Personality disorder and outcome in the treatment of late life depression. Journal of Geriatric Psychiatry 21(1): 133–146

Turner J A, Jensen M P 1993 Efficacy of cognitive therapy for chronic low back pain. Pain 52: 169–177

Weiss L J, Lazarus L W 1993 Psychosocial treatment of the geropsychiatric patient. International Journal of Geriatric Psychiatry 8: 95–100

Yost E B, Beutler L E, Corbishley M A, Allender J R 1986 Group cognitive therapy: a treatment approach for depressed older adults. Pergamon Press, New York

Zerheusen J D, Boyle K, Wilson W 1991 Out of the darkness: group cognitive therapy for depressed elderly. Journal of Psychosocial Nursing 29(9): 16–21

Zettle R D, Rains J C 1989 Group cognitive and contextual therapies in treatment of depression. Journal of Clinical Psychology 45(3): 436–445

RECOMMENDED READING

Beck A T, Rush A J, Shaw B F, Emery G 1979 Cognitive therapy of depression. The Guilford Press, New York. *The essential manual for the treatment of depression with cognitive therapy, setting out a theoretical model of depression and the techniques of therapy in great detail. By far the most used approach in the treatment of depression with cognitive therapy.*

Emery G 1981 Cognitive therapy with the elderly. In: Emery G, Hollon S D, Bedrosian R C (eds) New directions in cognitive therapy. The Guilford Press, New York. *Although relatively old, this chapter still gives a useful overview of some of the issues that can present in therapy, utilising a number of case examples to illustrate points.*

Gallagher D E , Thompson L W 1982 Treatment of major depressive disorder in older adult outpatients with brief psychotherapies. Psychotherapy: Theory Research and Practice 19: 482–490. *Though relatively old, this remains the most quoted comparative study for the use of cognitive therapy with older people.*

Hawton K, Salkovskis P M, Kirk J, Clark D M (eds) 1991 Cognitive behaviour therapy for psychiatric problems: a practical guide. Oxford Medical Publications, Oxford. *This book is a practical guide to the cognitive treatment of a wide range of problems from anxiety and phobias to somatic problems and marital difficulties. Accessible and easy to read.*

Hollon S D, Shelton R C, Davis D D 1993 Cognitive therapy for depression: conceptual issues and clinical efficacy. Journal of Consulting and Clinical Psychology 61(2): 270–275. *A wide ranging and, some might say, controversial review of the literature with regard to efficacy.*

Teri L, Gallagher-Thompson 1991 Cognitive-behavioural interventions for treatment of depression in Alzheimer's patients. The Gerontologist 31(3): 413–416. *This paper discusses specific cognitive and behavioural strategies to be used in reducing negative cognitive distortions with older adults in the early stages of Alzheimer's disease.*

Yost E B, Beutler L E, Corbishley M A, Allender J R 1986 Group cognitive therapy: a treatment approach for depressed older adults. Pergamon Press, New York. *A guide to the treatment of the depressed older person in a group setting using a cognitive approach. Covers such issues as client screening and cognitive change and is illustrated with case examples of group interventions.*

20

Reality orientation (RO) in the 1990s

Una Holden

INTRODUCTION

Reality orientation (RO) has been one of the positive approaches in use for the past 30 years or so to assist 'confused' elderly people; in fact it was the first structured, positive intervention for older people ever provided. When it was christened by Folsom in the United States and began to gain popularity, there was a protest from several sources complaining that it was simply an attempt to provide hope for those working in a field where there was *no* hope. The growth of intervention and therapeutic methods and the increase of information regarding organic and functional conditions, plus improved understanding of ageing processes and behaviours, have justified the introduction of more positive approaches to care.

Taulbee and Folsom (1966) were the first to publish information on RO. Stephens (1969) stated that: 'The process [RO] can reawaken unused neural pathways and stimulate the patients to develop new ways of functioning to compensate for organic brain damage that has resulted from injury or progressive senility, or from deterioration.' (Stephens 1969, p. vi). Unfortunately, such a statement lacked neuropathological foundation – the exact process of recovery remains far from clear and is subject to much controversy. However, the aim of RO was to provide individuals with the opportunity to use retained ability, to strengthen weakened skills and to relearn others as far as possible. It could act even as a means of holding back, or slowing down, the deterioration process for as long as possible. Several studies supported this aim as they identified a continued ability to learn new material, even if a dementing process was present, although the degree of learning was limited (e.g. Johnson et al 1981, Hanley et al 1981). Initially it was thought that various forms of repetition and updating would be the most appropriate method of assisting the relearning process, so this was stressed when teaching staff to use the RO technique.

A flood of articles and studies followed the publications from the USA, most of which are reviewed in Holden and Woods (1988). Critical reviews (Powell-Proctor & Miller 1982, Miller 1987) claimed that there was little evidence of generalised change, there was too varied a methodology for proper evaluation and that the main effect was to improve staff morale and practice. Degun (1976) provided the first controlled study of RO and showed positive changes for the subjects in group sessions. Other studies showed definite improvements that were not simply due to social attention (e.g. Woods 1979). Furthermore, it also became clear that some patients were not as severely impaired as previously imagined and, with encouragement, were able to become much more independent and alert. The various studies have concentrated on different aspects of relearning and retraining and although they cannot be said to clarify exactly what RO can do, many of them cite improvements and changes in the functioning of many of the subjects involved (e.g. Holden & Sinebruchow 1978, Merchant & Saxby 1981).

RO has continued to be a basic approach in practice, but it has changed considerably in step with the increase of knowledge and information. Bowlby (1991), in an excellent review, concluded that today a 'broader based, eclectic understanding of RO is emerging', providing a reassuring foundation in reality and employing informed responses to behaviour through 'a high level of clinical judgement, understanding of the individual's history and personality, and mediated by empathy and flexibility'.

Even in the early days, the different levels of disability were emphasised. Some patients were found to be suffering from depression or withdrawal rather than a severe dementia and soon responded to a stimulating and empathetic atmosphere. Others who were confused also responded by showing interest and they slowly learned to retain more information. It became difficult to elicit change according to the degree of dementia present, but even small improvements were worth seeing and could occur.

The format originally introduced intended formal or classroom RO to be secondary to a 24-hour RO. The formal RO became the focus of practice and research and, unfortunately, the 24-hour aspect became submerged, possibly because of difficulty in evaluating it. The history and details of the technique and many studies attempting evaluation can be found in Holden and Woods (1988).

A BRIEF OUTLINE OF FORMAL RO

This is the group format, limited to five or six members with two therapists or leaders. It lasts for no more than 1 hour, occurs at least five times a week and was originally divided into three levels – basic, standard and advanced. A social setting is important for all groups and includes many possible forms, e.g. a simulated pub, a comfortable living room, etc. Although relearning of temporal aspects continued to be seen as important, social behaviour became equally important and a means of assisting any relearning process.

The basic group

In the basic group, very simple material is used to establish relationships and to encourage people to think. The day, date, weather, whereabouts as well as members' names are the main topics. Various aids are used – weather boards, calendars, seasonal fruit and flowers, pencil and paper, pictures – anything to help the members concentrate. This group rarely lasts for longer than a week or two and members are moved into the standard group as soon as there is evidence that they are beginning to respond. Initially each session lasts for about 30 minutes, although it can continue for the usual hour. The patients most suitable for such a group are those thought to be quite severely impaired, those who might not even recall their own names.

The standard group

The standard group lasts the full hour and the topics cover a wide range of subjects. The therapists' imagination and specific interests and experience of the members are important. Senses are stimulated, interpersonal relationships are fostered and humour is encouraged. Reminiscence plays a major role and the use of a store of relevant materials is essential. The majority of patients fall into this group. Even those who seem severely damaged will be ready to join at this level after a few days in the basic group.

The advanced group

The advanced group was intended for those who had shown considerable improvement, who were attending a day unit or were in a ward or residential home for older people with only minor cognitive impairment. The members would decide on the topics, activities and outings. Staff would advise and assist, but also keep a watch for signs of deterioration or problems. In practice, this group did not really materialise. It became a maintenance system and is the usual method for RO practice in larger settings such as day units and active residential homes or wards. This group level does not require a day-to-day programme. Obviously the more frequently it can be offered the better but, with a degree of independence, it is not necessary to provide input on a daily basis.

In the USA the setting was usually a classroom and 'graduation' ceremonies were employed to move patients from one group to another. This is not a suitable system for elderly people in the UK because they are likely to resent being sent back to school. Recent thinking in the USA suggests that therapists are also becoming concerned about patients feeling demeaned and patronised by being placed in a 'classroom'. It is essential to seek the most suitable setting and atmosphere for the group members: this will vary from culture to culture and place to place. It may even vary from one group to another. The needs and comfort of the individuals involved are of paramount importance.

THE 24-HOUR RO

Even in the early stages the 24-hour approach was meant to be an essential feature of the intervention, though it was often forgotten in practice and rarely evaluated by research.

Attitudes to ageing which ignored the individual, treated older people as objects or failed to recognise abilities, feelings and needs were seen as unacceptable. Staff were advised to become aware of ways to repeat or provide information which would encourage independence and self-esteem. Modifications of the environment such as improved furniture arrangement, direction signs and the use of colour coding were all gradually introduced.

Environmental assessments were used to help staff improve the care settings (Moos & Lemke 1980, Holden 1984). Guides on handling confused speech, scales to evaluate levels of involvement or engagement as well as improvement were also developed (Holden & Woods 1988). Staff were advised to watch for situations in which a person would feel undervalued, such as the incident in Box 20.1.

This kind of assault on dignity and lack of common politeness is still encountered by older people. The 24-hour RO approach stresses the need to prevent denigrating ageing people and to seek ways to

---

Box 20.1 Example

A small group of elderly people were sitting together and talking. A tall, well-dressed man appeared, went straight to one of the men in the group, produced a cut-throat razor and began to shave him. There was no introduction, no word to the patient and no apology to the group. Instead the man continued to scrape away and told a joke to a nurse who was making a bed further up the ward.

---

recognise their 'personhood', abilities, retained knowledge and experience. A depression may give the impression of deterioration but in a positive, encouraging atmosphere it may become apparent that the person is much more able than previously supposed. Recognising that respect for others and preservation of dignity are the right of all people can make a considerable difference to attitude and response. Furthermore, relearning is not achieved simply by verbal repetition; it requires the use of non-verbal methods as well – in fact these are often more effective. Active and helpful environments can provide other methods of assisting memory and skills relearning. Although the introduction of signs, calendars, correct time clocks and information notices are aids to orientation and learning, they are valueless unless a person is taught and reminded to use them.

THE REAL 24-HOURS

Originally, the informal aspect of RO was limited to about 8 hours – the daytime. It was during the day that most changes were made in the environment and in activity levels. Efforts were made to provide elderly people in care settings with an atmosphere which was more appropriate to their needs. Living areas were made more homely, colour was used more effectively, people were asked questions and allowed to choose designs and help with plans. Patients and residents were encouraged to have their own possessions about them and to do more for themselves, and interests and hobbies were made available as the need for activity and stimulation was recognised (Reeve & Ivison 1985, Williams et al 1987). However, only vague mention was made of the evening and night-time – usually 'can the person recognise his own bed?', or queries on the time of retiring, the degree of privacy or the level of noise.

Evenings in care settings leave a great deal to be desired; they are boring, little changed from daytime and have fewer staff available to take part in any activities. People doze for hours and then are expected to go to bed to sleep. There is little comparison with normal evenings which provide a total change from a working day and different levels of activity. Furthermore, the bedrooms in care settings lack the very personal nature of bedrooms in private homes. It is here that the loss of independence is amplified and normal living is most at risk. Recent literature has provided information on changes in sleep patterns with ageing (Morgan 1987, Morgan & Gledhill 1991) and advice on treatment procedures. Useful assessment scales and ways to examine the environment for unwanted influences and omissions in appropriate practice have also been produced (Holden 1991). Individual needs for different levels of heat, time for sleep, visits to the toilet, levels of illumination and tolerance of noise or interference should be taken into consideration. Suitable facilities, support for night staff and their knowledge of interventions and involvement in daytime-oriented plans (see Box 20.2) are other matters which have been neglected for too long.

Box 20.2 Example

Clover ward had 26 beds. The patients were old and infirm. Half the beds were screened; the others were open. Beside the last beds there was a lift which could open at any time even when a patient was sitting on a commode without a screen. The heating was always so high that staff were unable to work without sweating. On each bedside cabinet was a stuffed toy; each one was different so that if someone wanted to visit a patient at night it was possible to say 'She's the third on the left, the stuffed hippopotamus will tell you which one'. During the day an RO programme was a regular feature, although the night staff had not been informed or consulted.

Staff in units where training and knowledge is consistently updated will find it hard to believe that such situations as the one given in Box 20.2 still exist: unfortunately they do. Sometimes, because one patient has chosen to have a stuffed toy to hug, it is assumed that all old people will enjoy such a possession. It is important to stop and ask: 'Would I find it dignified to be recognised at the age of 80 by some toy animal at my bedside?' Even more relevant, how many people would find it acceptable to be washed, dressed and toiletted in public?

INDIVIDUALISED APPROACHES TO RO

As knowledge of the ageing process progressed, a major change in approach to the care of old people occurred. The longstanding attitude that all elderly people could be treated in a similar way became untenable. The need to seek out the individual and gear treatment and management strategies to meet the needs of each person rather than the group became the focus of care. What might prove suitable for one person might be totally useless for another – a basic piece of common sense, but sense is rarely common. Even in group settings it is important to provide a proper assessment of the individuals involved, to know something about their history, personality, intellectual level, routines, interests and experience. Without such knowledge serious errors can result, as in the example given in Box 20.3.

Box 20.3 Example

The day centre in a rural community served a population which included many retired professional and executive members. On one occasion the leaders of a group asked the patients to think of vegetables beginning with the letter 'M'. One member replied 'mange tout'. The two staff leaders looked at each other; one leant forward towards the patient: 'Vegetables, dear, vegetables beginning with "M", that's what we're asking'.

The experience and ability of each group member in the example given in Box 20.3 was obviously underestimated and the level of stimulation was not made available, thus putting the person in a vulnerable, threatened situation.

Hanley (1988), amongst others, has provided examples for plans for single cases which use retraining and relearning techniques with an RO emphasis. An example is given in Box 20.4.

In the example of Mrs Hilliard given here in Box 20.4, we can see that the daughter needed counselling,

---

Box 20.4 Example

Mrs Hilliard was recently bereaved. After her husband's death she ceased to take care of herself properly, she neglected her home, her intake of food and her personal care. As a result her daughter took over, made her mother leave her home and go to live with her and her family. The daughter dressed Mrs Hilliard, did all the housework and left her mother to sit on her own all day. Previously the husband and wife had been active members of a local club, members of the Church Guild and socially very active. Mrs Hilliard had played the piano, driven less able members to meetings and run most of the services.

Mrs Hilliard required bereavement counselling and the whole situation needed reassessment. Using an RO approach, Mrs Hilliard's abilities could have been used to regain her self-esteem. At first, she should have been referred to a day hospital or day centre where staff would have slowly rebuilt her confidence in group situations. Her piano playing would have been praised, her ability to help in many situations would have been employed and success reinforced by praise and recognition. Then, with the help of other members, she would have been encouraged to rejoin the clubs she used to frequent where her previous organisational abilities would be reinforced. By being placed in the centre of attention as the piano player she would have regained an interest in her appearance and eventually, with her place in her previous social circle re-established, she might have been capable of returning to her own home.

Even in care settings an individualised approach is necessary. Many residents are unable to find their way around a home and so demand help from staff members, thus becoming dependent. If, on arrival, a simple environmental awareness strategy is employed this would not be a problem. The person should be escorted around the area, clues to route-finding pointed out and each room carefully identified. This should be repeated several times, and then the person could be asked to lead the instructor. When mistakes occur, the person can be reminded of the necessary clues and another trip attempted until the entire layout is remembered. This could allow residents familiarity with a large area of the home and enable them to take responsibility as escorts for new arrivals – another form of independence and relieving staff of another 'duty'.

ERRORS IN PRACTICE

RO has been criticised on several grounds, most of which occur because the purpose and practice of intervention are misunderstood:

'They are happy as they are'

Are they?

To force someone to join a group is denying choice. To never offer a choice is to deny opportunity to choose.

'It doesn't work'

Why not?

- Is the group made up of members with different levels of impairment, or members from different cultures? Not only would this make it more difficult for the staff, but it would put added pressure on the members. One could feel demeaned, another threatened.
- Does the group include someone who is disruptive or doubly incontinent, or a person who is suffering from receptive dysphasia and so cannot understand what is happening and is therefore placed in a vulnerable and threatened position?
- Has there been sufficient planning?
- Has the programme begun to operate without adequate preparation?
- Do the staff involved know what to do?

Other matters to consider are:

Is progress being carefully monitored?

It will prove impossible to note small changes, or the need to introduce relevant changes without careful record keeping.

Are staff bored?

If staff are bored it is hardly surprising if their motivation is low.

Gubrium and Ksander (1975) and Buckholdt and Gubrium (1983) provide excellent critiques showing how poor practice and planning give rise to error. An example of such poor practice is given in Box 20.5.

If Nurse Grey (Box 20.5) had received relevant training and if those responsible for organising group activities had been aware of potential boredom and ways to avoid it, the situation outlined would not have occurred (Bender et al 1987). Boredom can affect staff and group members adversely. If staff do not

---

Box 20.5 Example

Nurse Grey was told to run a classroom RO session. She gathered the group together, leant against the weather board and used the pointer. 'Now John, what day is it today?' 'Tuesday.' 'Good. OK. Fred, what is the month?' 'February.' Nurse Grey is thinking about her forthcoming evening and sighs, 'Good. Mary, what is the weather like?' Mary looks out of the window: 'It's sunny', she replies. Nurse Grey taps the pointer on the weather board statement impatiently, 'No, no Mary, read what it says please'. 'It is raining', responds Mary in confusion.

understand that there comes a point when day, date, weather, etc., are nothing more than means to open up relationships and there is some urgency to move forward, boredom will occur. Without progression it is likely that the sessions will add to confusion and deterioration rather than minimising them. It is important to place a time limit on an approach, to monitor it and then spend some time planning the next move:

Once group members have progressed satisfactorily, what happens?

Are they returned to a negative environment or an active, positive one? If the former, deterioration will occur quickly. It is essential to maintain improvement for as long as possible.

How often are common sense and sensitivity employed in staff–patient relationships?

Validation therapy articles have pointed to confrontational situations where RO has been blamed for the ensuing catastrophic reaction (Feil 1967, Dietch et al 1989). It is true that RO aims to keep people in touch with the present but it does not recommend the insensitive response that might occur in the example in Box 20.6.

The type of response of the care staff in the example below (Box 20.6) is not RO-based. It signifies a lack of empathy on the part of the staff member and is not to be recommended. To help people come to terms with life problems, to try to understand the meaning behind apparently incorrect statements are matters which go hand in hand with any intervention or therapeutic approach. There are ways to help a person keep abreast of day-to-day happenings and events and it is also important to help with specific problems or needs. It is essential to listen carefully to what the person is saying, to appreciate that a statement or request can have several meanings. The frequently heard 'I must go and make my mother's tea', when the mother died

years ago, may imply many things – a poor memory, a politely expressed wish to escape boredom or threat, a wish to be away from the present unhappy situation and back with people who knew and loved the person, or a need to be recognised as a person in one's own right and not as an object. To ignore these feelings is to guarantee an unwelcome reaction.

Is there a structure?

It was established in early studies that to hold a social group whose members just talked without any structure was actually dangerous (Woods 1979). If confused talk is allowed then confusion is being reinforced. It is not acceptable to forcibly correct rambling talk, but in order to minimise it materials, pictures, objects or whatever is relevant to the topic under discussion are essential. Using the senses is a valuable method of holding attention, e.g. something to touch, smell or see. Gentle touch and eye contact also help a confused person to respond appropriately.

Are expectations realistic?

To expect miracles is a common mistake. They do happen; for instance, a depressed and withdrawn individual who has not received any personal acclaim for years can surprise everyone by the level of retained ability that has been hidden away. Usually goals are set too high and expectations are never met. It is more reasonable to set very simple goals initially; it is much easier to move up a ladder of achievement than to be forced to descend it.

Are baseline levels of ability being recorded?

Baseline levels of ability must be recorded so that the very small changes that can occur from week to week can be discerned. When they are recorded it is satisfying to see an increasing improvement. Who goes on a diet without first being weighed?

Is the approach sufficiently flexible?

Just because a book, article or guide suggests a particular plan it does not follow that staff should adhere to it unwaveringly. Being rigid might well prove fatal to a programme. The needs of the individuals are paramount; it is their interests and abilities that must be sought and used. The approach must be flexible and the individual must take priority.

Box 20.6 Example

Mrs Keynes was crying for her mother. The care staff said, 'Come on June, you know your mother is dead, we keep telling you that again and again, she died 3 years ago'. Mrs Keynes burst into violent tears and became extremely upset.

Is everyone using the same approach?

Training in the use of strategies is important; everyone must work together using the same approach. However, this is not enough without:

- good leadership
- good communications
- good support
- good work schedules
- positive feedback – both to staff and group members
- improved understanding
- reasonable facilities.

To start a programme of any kind without knowledge of the technique required, with staff who are on poor terms with each other, with no appropriate facilities or equipment and without responsible leadership guarantees failure.

Is the method suitable for all group members?

Problems have also arisen due to a mistaken belief that RO and other interventions are antagonistic. RO is a backdrop, a starting point and not always suitable for every patient. For instance, a person with receptive dysphasia would be very threatened by not understanding the happy chatter of the members of a group session. A person with double incontinence could be a distraction for others and a person who has a hermit-like personality should not be persuaded to join in a group against his or her wishes. In such cases a one-to-one system, or the general use of 24-hour RO, is preferable.

KEY COMPONENTS OF RO

Various studies have shown that other techniques work happily together with RO. Reminiscence, for instance, was always seen as useful in the standard group setting and one study (Baines et al 1987) showed that RO was necessary as a starting point in order to make the reminiscence sessions more effective. The idea behind validation therapy and resolution therapy (Stokes and Goudie 1990) emphasises that remarks made by patients do not always mean exactly what is said, but have a deeper meaning which requires empathy and understanding by the carer. Such an empathetic approach is important in RO too. Exercise is important and music very helpful, and these and other approaches are in no way antagonistic to RO, or vice versa.

In keeping with the above, it is important to remember that RO is an approach which lasts for 24 hours, focuses on the individual and aims to help him or her to live as normal a life as possible. It should seek out knowledge, experience and ability, even if there are impairments, recognise the personhood of the individual and find ways to assist in maintaining this.

In the light of recent research, some of the long-held beliefs about dementia need to be challenged. It is often believed that dementia is an illness which damages all brain function, resulting in global damage. If this were the case the person would be dead, or a zombie. In fact, dementia is caused by a number of conditions, some of which can be reversed. When the illness is reversed so is the dementing process. With all these conditions the damage to brain function varies, so certain systems are damaged and others remain intact, except possibly in the very late stages of the disease. It is this variability in brain damage that makes an intervention such as RO relevant. Unfortunately not all organic conditions are reversible but parts of the brain in most cases remain intact. It is often extremely difficult to identify such retained ability, but it is important to attempt to do so. Positive approaches such as RO play an important part in searching for abilities and putting them to use. It is also true that in many instances these abilities are not hard to find and after a short time in a stimulating atmosphere an individual can demonstrate surprising skills and an unexpected level of independence.

Figure 20.1 represents most of the factors that should be included or considered when employing an RO approach, or any other positive approach for that matter. In order to provide a relevant programme for an individual it is vital to be aware of the normal ageing process, factors that play a part in a person's life, the most relevant assessments, time spent on careful planning and goal setting, taking account of retained abilities and using them. It is also important to investigate and modify other influences such as environmental aspects. The variety of available forms of stimulation and retraining strategies have increased over the years and can be used by all levels of staff who have received some training.

CHANGING TIMES

The use of the basic group sessions is valuable in assisting those who are becoming increasingly confused. If, after several sessions, patients become more alert and involved, they may benefit from joining a larger group of more independent people. Most day

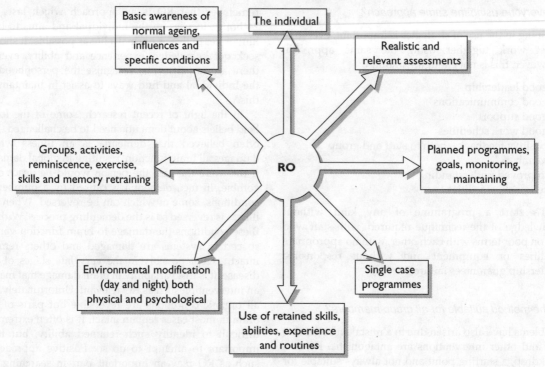

Figure 20.1 RO in the 1990s: the wider scope.

units provide care on only a few days of the week for each person: in this situation the use of concentrated RO is inappropriate because it will all be forgotten by the time the person returns. If a person is so confused, probably a day centre is not appropriate and more sustained assistance is necessary. It is, however, rare to have an extremely confused person attending such a unit. The more confused are usually found in residential settings and it is here that basic RO is more frequently in operation.

Day units provide a wide range of activities which fit in with the standard and advanced group processes. When staff are highly trained, the programmes for individuals will focus on retraining specific impairments or on finding ways to compensate for such problems as language difficulties, agnosias, apraxias and problems caused by frontal damage or specific conditions to which dementia is related. Strictly speaking, this is not conventional or formal RO, but an example of the broader use of RO which incorporates, or works alongside, other appropriate retraining approaches (Holden & Woods 1995).

It is the 24-hour version which is becoming more common in practice. Group work has changed, although the need to help people 'catch up' remains,

but aspects such as modifying the environment to suit the person, instead of the other way around, and providing appropriate activities to meet a person's needs remain the main process. Furthermore, if the circumstances in which someone is presently living are uncomfortable, threatening and demeaning, it is not surprising if that person does not wish to accept them and prefers to withdraw and live in the past. For this reason environmental modification is essential and has become part of the 24-hour RO programme. People need a reason for living, they need to feel useful, loved, valued and respected and reasonably independent amongst familiar things and people. An active, social and homely environment has a major role to play in this.

Many criticisms have been directed against the emphasis on bringing people up to date, usually at all costs. The constant reminders of day, date, weather and whereabouts are regarded as means to become reoriented and have led to many errors and misinterpretations of behaviour, with the result that a catastrophic reaction has been provoked – the antithesis of RO purposes. Although living in the present is one of the aims, the means to attain this and the nature of 'the present' are also matters to be considered. If present circumstances are distressing, then it is understandable if a person chooses to live in the past. If the methods employed to make someone aware of the present are insensitive then, on both counts, criticism is justified.

Unfortunately, a number of critics see RO as simply a verbal reorientation process. The belief that temporal orientation is the sole purpose of RO is outdated. If that is what RO really is, then RO is outdated too. Most studies have shown little evidence of memory improvement being generalised outside the group. Other studies have shown that people without any intellectual deterioration often forget the day and date, unless they have some tag to remember it by. The value of such temporal orientation is limited in comparison with a person's ability to socialise and use his or her retained skills adequately. For this reason simple day-to-day information is only employed in the early stages of RO, in order to develop a good relationship and establish a group. Confused people are as capable of being bored as anyone else.

Perhaps RO should be renamed now that the conventional format is so different (Bowlby 1991). 'Positive reality' is a possibility which would convey RO as a positive approach.

To look back on wards and residential homes operating some 10–15 years ago and compare them with those today will demonstrate whether the technique has been successful in bringing about change. Even today there are units where people are left to sit around the walls with nothing to do and no effort made to offer any aid to retaining some independence, where staff are busy doing things other than working with their clients and where the level of dependency is extremely high. The introduction of an RO programme can promote changes within a short period of time. The staff become aware of the individuals in their care and obtain satisfaction from seeing responses. The patients or residents become more active, more involved and more independent. It can be a struggle to introduce new approaches. It is sometimes hard to encourage staff to adopt different working practices, to persuade dozing, withdrawn patients to take an interest in new events and activities or to obtain the support of authorities to rethink policies and introduce modified environments. But there are innumerable examples around the country and the world which demonstrate achievements resulting from careful planning and a change in attitude regarding ageing people (Holden & Woods 1995).

RO may be getting as old as some of its clients, but it is having a face-lift, a new personality and a wider more active application. Whatever its name should be after distinguishing it, rightly, from simple verbal re-learning, staff should take another look and researchers should re-examine RO in the light of all the changes.

REFERENCES

Baines S, Saxby P, Ehlert K 1987 Reality orientation and reminiscence therapy. British Journal Psychiatry 151: 222–231

Bender M, Norris A, Bauckham P 1987 Group work with the elderly. Winslow Press, Oxford

Bowlby M C 1991 Reality orientation 30 years later: are we still confused? Canadian Journal of Occupational Therapy 58(3): 114–122

Buckholdt D R, Gubrium J F 1983 Therapeutic pretence in reality orientation. International of Aging and Human Development 16: 167–181

Degun G 1976 Reality orientation: a multidisciplinary therapeutic approach. Nursing Times 72: 117–120

Dietch J T, Hewett L J, Jones S 1989 Adverse effects of reality orientation. Journal of American Geriatrics Society 37(10): 974–976

Feil N W 1967 Group therapy in a home for the aged. Gerontologist 7: 192–195

Gubrium J F, Ksander M 1975 On multiple realities and reality orientation. Gerontologist 15: 142–145

Hanley I 1988 Individualised reality orientation. Winslow Press, Oxford

Hanley I G, McGuire R J, Boyd W D 1981 Reality orientation and dementia: a controlled trial of two approaches. British Journal of Psychiatry 138: 10–14

Holden U P 1984 Thinking it through. Winslow Press, Oxford

Holden U P 1991 Day into night. Winslow Press, Oxford

Holden U P, Sinebruchow A 1978 Reality orientation therapy: a study investigating the value of this therapy in the rehabilitation of elderly people. Age and Ageing 7: 83–88

Holden U P, Woods R T 1988 Reality orientation: psychological approaches to the 'confused' elderly. Churchill Livingstone, Edinburgh

Holden U P, Woods R J 1995 Positive approaches to dementia care. Churchill Livingstone, Edinburgh

Johnson C H, McLaren S M, McPherson F M 1981 The comparative effectiveness of three versions of 'classroom' reality orientation. Age and Ageing 10: 33–35

Merchant M, Saxby P 1981 Reality orientation: a way forward. Nursing Times 77(33): 1442–1445

Miller E 1987 Reality orientation with psychogeriatric patients: the limitations. Clinical Rehabilitation 1(1): 231–233

Moos R H, Lemke S 1980 Assessing the physical and architectural features of sheltered care settings. Journal of Gerontology 35: 571–583

Morgan K 1987 Sleep and ageing. Croom Helm, London

Morgan K, Gledhill K 1991 Managing sleep and insomnia in the older person. Winslow Press, Oxford

Powell-Proctor L, Miller E 1982 Reality orientation: a critical appraisal. British Journal of Psychiatry 140: 457–463

Reeve W, Ivison D 1985 Use of environmental modification and classroom and modified informal reality orientation with institutionalised confused elderly patients. Age and Ageing 14: 119–121

Stephens L P (ed) 1969 Reality orientation: a technique to rehabilitate elderly and brain-damaged patients with moderate to severe degree of deterioration. American Psychiatric Association Hospital and Community Psychiatric Service, Washington DC

Stokes G and Goudie F (eds) 1990 Working with dementia. Winslow Press, Oxford

Taulbee L R, Folsom J C 1966 Reality orientation for geriatric patients. Hospital and Community Psychiatry 17: 133–135

Williams R, Reeve W, Ivison D, Kavanagh D 1987 Use of environmental manipulation and modified informal reality orientation with institutionalised confused elderly subjects: a replication. Age and Ageing 16: 315–318

Woods R T 1979 Reality orientation and staff attention: a controlled study. British Journal of Psychiatry 134: 502–507

RECOMMENDED READING

Baines S, Saxby P, Ehlert K 1987 Reality orientation and reminiscence therapy. British Journal of Psychiatry 151: 222–231. *A most valuable article showing that it is necessary to use RO first before introducing reminiscence. Better relationships are established and reminiscence flows more satisfactorily if it follows an RO programme. This controlled study also showed that staff greatly increased their knowledge of individual residents as a result of the programme.*

Bender M, Norris A, Bauckham P 1987 Group work with the elderly. Winslow Press, Oxford. *This is a most useful guide to setting up group work. It covers how to plan, organise, run and monitor any intervention involving several patients or residents. It provides warnings on possible pitfalls and tips on how to manage awkward situations and clients.*

Bowlby M C 1991 Reality orientation 30 years later: are we still confused? Canadian Journal of Occupational Therapy 58(3): 114–122. *Excellent overview of RO, its history and changing character. Although critical of several early studies and the different methods that have been employed, it notes the changes to positive environments and more stimulating procedures introduced in recent years that are ensuring that RO keeps in touch with progressive approaches.*

Buckholdt D R, Gubrium J F 1983 Therapeutic pretence in reality orientation. International of Aging and Human Development 16: 167–181. *Critique of RO practice. Full of examples of misuse and poor applications, written in amusing, cynical style which, unfortunately, does reflect many of the situations that can be found in operation.*

Degun G 1976 Reality orientation: a multidisciplinary therapeutic approach. Nursing Times 72: 117–120. *The first controlled study, improvements in functioning shown by the subjects in an RO group working in a structured, social setting. Details on group or formal RO with psychogeriatric patients.*

Dietch J T, Hewett L J, Jones S 1989 Adverse effects of reality orientation. Journal of American Geriatrics Society 37(10): 974–976. *The authors give examples of bad practice in returning people to reality and provoking a catastrophic reaction. They demonstrate how validation can prove a more effective approach. Unfortunately, they do not state that the methods employed in their RO examples are not acceptable in RO practice.*

Feil N W 1967 Group therapy in a home for the aged. Gerontologist 7: 192–195. *The first appearance of validation therapy, an alternative to RO. Stress is placed on the idea that there is a meaning behind an individual's behaviour and remarks.*

Gubrium J F, Ksander M 1975 On multiple realities and reality orientation. Gerontologist 15: 142–145. *Specifies the misapplied methods and dangerous errors that can increase a person's level of confusion. An early critical account of errors noted in clinical practice – rigidly following directions in a book, being bored and overlooking real facts, stressing correct dates verbally with calendars showing wrong date, etc.*

Hanley I 1988 Individualised reality orientation. Winslow Press, Oxford. *This small book concentrates on the individual. It provides details on how to create a good physical environment, presents RO as a form of therapeutic communication and a psychotherapeutic tool, and it outlines strategies for helping behavioural changes.*

Hanley I G, McGuire R J, Boyd W D 1981 Reality orientation and dementia: a controlled trial of two approaches. British Journal of Psychiatry 138: 10–14. *This group found cognitive abilities improved, but no behavioural changes. However, they outlined a ward orientation programme which proved successful and had potential for cost effectiveness and management purposes.*

Holden U P 1984 Thinking it through. Winslow Press, Oxford. *Basic psychology of ageing, a simple starting point to aid new staff to think about their approach and attitudes towards older people. Offers suggestions on modifying environments to meet needs. It introduces the ORIF scale (Orientation Facilities) which can be used as both an assessment of the physical and psychological environment and a guide to assist in appropriate modification of it.*

Holden U P 1991 Day into night. Winslow Press, Oxford. *24-hour RO usually means daytime; the evenings and nights are forgotten. The hours between 7 p.m. and 7 a.m. are every bit as important for both patient/resident and staff and various influences can add to problems. This small book identifies some of the differences between normal home life during the evening and night and that experienced in care settings. There is a Night Scale which can be of assistance for both assessment and ideas to improve conditions.*

Holden U P, Sinebruchow A 1978 Reality orientation therapy: a study investigating the value of this therapy in the rehabilitation of elderly people. Age and Ageing 7: 83–88. *A two-fold aim was investigated – a controlled study to examine the effectiveness of RO and to see if it would attract the interest of nursing staff. 40% of the subjects in the RO group were discharged as against none of the controls, and staff interest was attracted.*

Holden U P, Woods R T 1988 Reality orientation: psychological approaches to the 'confused' elderly. Churchill Livingstone, Edinburgh. *This standard text in its first part covers a review of studies, the history of RO, methods of assessing intellectual, behavioural and neuropsychological functioning, provides an overview of other positive approaches such as reminiscence, behaviour modification, environmental modification and group living. In the second part it gives detailed accounts of how to use RO, both formal sessions and 24-hour RO. A re-written and up-dated edition is now available (Holden U P, Woods R T 1995. Positive approaches to dementia care. Churchill Livingstone, Edinburgh).*

Johnson C H, McLaren S M, McPherson F M 1981 The comparative effectiveness of three versions of 'classroom' reality orientation. Age and Ageing 10: 33–35. *RO was provided for one group once a day, another group twice a day and once daily individually. All three improved cognitively in comparison to an untreated control group, but there was no value found by increasing the number of daily sessions. It produced changes in all levels of deterioration.*

Merchant M, Saxby P 1981 Reality orientation: a way forward. Nursing Times 77(33): 1442–1445. *A study demonstrating not only improvement in the subjects' cognitive ability, but also showing that staff learned much more about those in their care and about how to improve interpersonal relationships with better insight.*

Miller E 1987 Reality orientation with psychogeriatric patients: the limitations. Clinical Rehabilitation 1(1): 231–233. *A critical overview. Points out the limitations and difficulties caused by varying views of RO. Suggests that the main value is an improvement in stimulating atmospheres and attitudes of staff.*

Powell-Proctor L, Miller E 1982 Reality orientation: a critical appraisal. British Journal of Psychiatry 140: 457–463. *The first real critique of RO. The writers point out the varying methods employed, the lack of generalised response and the limited nature of the intervention, viewing RO simply as a temporal retraining programme.*

Reeve W, Ivison D 1985 Use of environmental modification and classroom and modified informal reality orientation with institutionalised confused elderly patients. Age and Ageing 14: 119–121. *An excellent article demonstrating changes as a result of more comprehensive form of RO. One of the articles demonstrating the modern, broader based use of RO.*

Stephens L P (ed) 1969 Reality orientation: a technique to rehabilitate elderly and brain-damaged patients with moderate to severe degree of deterioration. American Psychiatric Association Hospital and Community Psychiatric Service, Washington DC. *The original account of reality orientation from the USA, containing various articles by Folsom, Taulbee and others concerned with programmes in operation. Unfortunately, the early studies were anecdotal and contained no controlled studies.*

Stokes G and Goudie F (eds) 1990 Working with dementia. Winslow Press, Oxford. *A useful basic coverage by a number of authors on the various psychological findings and approaches in current use. It includes chapters on dementia, RO, reminiscence, introduces resolution therapy as distinction from validation therapy, covers activities, challenging behaviour, etc. and is presented in an easy to read format suitable for a wide range of staff.*

Taulbee L R, Folsom J C 1966 Reality orientation for geriatric patients. Hospital and Community Psychiatry 17: 133–135. *This is another of the early articles from the USA introducing RO methodology.*

Williams R, Reeve W, Ivison D, Kavanagh D 1987 Use of environmental manipulation and modified informal reality orientation with institutionalised confused elderly subjects: a replication. Age and Ageing 16: 315–318. *A further study following the Reeve et al article, continuing to demonstrate changes elicited as a result of a broader scope RO programme.*

Woods R T 1979 Reality orientation and staff attention: a controlled study. British Journal of Psychiatry 134: 502–507. *One of the controlled studies demonstrating the essential need for a structured approach rather than a simple relaxed social gathering. Showed that the unstructured group could reinforce confusion by allowing patients to talk in a rambling manner.*

21

Beyond validation

Ian Morton

INTRODUCTION

There is a sense in which it was inevitable that a 'person-centred' approach to dementia care would come into being and gain a following amongst both professional and family carers. Any future historian who charts the history of thought and ideas in the latter half of the 20th century will be witness to the spreading influence of 'person-centred' principles to many fields of human activity, throughout the western world. First articulated by the US psychologist and therapist Carl Rogers (Rogers 1959) those ideas, variously described as 'person-centred', 'Rogerian', 'humanistic' and 'phenomenological', have permeated way beyond the field of mental health in which they originally grew: education, business consultancy, staff supervision and training, and international relations have all been affected, as has every conceivable speciality and discipline within the field of mental health.

This chapter aims to look at the particular way in which the person-centred approach has become a key component of many of the major developments in the psychological care of people with dementia. 'Validation Therapy', 'Resolution Therapy', the work of Tom Kitwood and the Bradford Dementia Research Group and the latest arrival on the scene, 'Pre-Therapy', are all strongly influenced by the person-centred tradition. In fact I shall argue, at least with regard to the first three, that it is precisely when they depart from this tradition that they become most vulnerable to criticism.

WHAT DOES 'PERSON-CENTRED' MEAN?

Before proceeding further, it is important to clarify what we mean by the term 'person-centred'. I mentioned above three other words which are usually seen as being interchangeable: Rogerian, humanistic and phenomenological.

Rogerian. 'The central truth for Rogers was that the client knows best. It is the client who knows what is hurting and in the final analysis it is the client who knows how to move forward.' (Mearns & Thorne 1988, p. 1). This stance clearly involves a shift in traditional power relations away from the therapist and towards the client. The therapist ceases to give direction, advice or offer insight and takes on a facilitative role, enabling clients to get in touch with, and use, their own inner resources.

Humanistic. 'An approach to psychology which emphasises feelings and emotions and the better understanding of the self in terms of observation of oneself and one's relationship with others.' (*Collins English Dictionary* 1986).

Phenomenological. 'Literally, the description or study of appearances. Any description of how things appear, especially if sustained and penetrating, can be called a phenomenology.' (Lacey 1976, p. 175). Rather than dealing with objective facts, or our insights into the workings of clients' conscious or unconscious minds, we must start with how they see things, their perceptions, how reality appears to them.

Although the validity of this Rogerian, humanistic or phenomenological approach is now unquestioned when applied to certain client groups, its application to people with dementia inevitably invites controversy and disquiet. How, it is asked, can we set ourselves the task of working with an individual's perception of reality, when it is that very perception that is being damaged by disease? How can 'the client know best' when they no longer know some of the most basic facts about themselves – such as where they are or who they are with?

The therapies and approaches outlined in this chapter attempt to address these questions. Their founders and advocates insist that, when we are concerned with people with dementia, there is no other way of working that will meet the most fundamental need for genuine human contact, acceptance and warmth. As medical science has so little to offer, the person with dementia is reliant on those around her to assist in maintaining an acceptable quality of life. Partners, family, friends, nursing staff, care staff and the other people with whom the person with dementia spends a significant proportion of each day are the only potential 'treatment' that we have to offer.

A NOTE ON LANGUAGE

The 'everyday' use of language carries within it a host of assumptions, stereotypes and images which are oppressive to certain groups. An intrinsic part of any attempt at self-liberation by those groups is a challenge to, and reform of, that everyday use of language. Part of the articulation of the struggle of the women's movement, the anti-racist movement and, more recently, the lesbian and gay movement and the movement of people with disabilities has been this refusal to accept everyday language. If this has led to feelings of awkward discomfort, perhaps a sense of resentment, amongst those who have had to look at, and alter, their own use of language then a sense of generosity would suggest that this is a small price to pay, perhaps even a debt that we owe.

We might hope that the awkwardness which surrounds the selection of terms to identify people with dementia reflects a similar process. Certainly the old terms which littered the textbooks – the demented, the dotards, the senile, the feeble minded – speak more to the modern ear about the prevalent attitudes of those writing than they do about the people they were intended to denote. In this chapter I shall use the terms 'people/person with dementia' and 'dementia sufferer' throughout.

The choice of terminology to identify those people without dementia who may be considered to be the 'user' of the approach or therapy being described demands almost equal consideration. Whichever term is chosen – 'therapist', 'carer', 'worker' and 'family carer' – it will exclude certain groups who may find it appropriate to use the approach. Suffice to say that whichever term is used, I do not mean to imply that anybody who is caring for a person with dementia, in whatever setting, should not consider adopting those aspects of the approaches described here which he deems to be useful.

VALIDATION THERAPY: ORIGINS AND DEVELOPMENT

The origins of Validation Therapy (VT) can be traced back to 1963, the year that Naomi Feil returned to the Montefiore Home for the Aged in Cleveland, Ohio to work as a group therapist. This was a return to the home in which she had spent her childhood – where her father worked as the administrator and her mother as a social worker – until 1950 when she left as an 18-year-old to study psychology and social work.

Early writings

Feil's earliest available paper was a presentation to the New York meeting of the Gerontological Society in

November 1966, published the following year under the title *Group Therapy in a Home for the Aged* (Feil 1967). In it she describes her attempts at therapeutic group work with two sets of residents. The first group consisted of eight members who were socially isolated within the home but who were, 'still very aware of reality.' (Feil 1967, p. 193).

The second group consisted of six members, 'all [of whom] had lost ego contact with reality. Suffering from severe arteriosclerosis accompanied by other physical illnesses – strokes, tumours, gastric disturbances, circulatory and organic brain syndromes, and urinary disturbances – they had regressed to an almost infantile level of behaviour' (Feil 1967, p. 194).

Feil found after 3 years building relationships with the individual members of this second group, that they were much more able to express their feelings than the earlier, cognitively intact, group. In fact it was only by exploring subjective feelings that these members could be stimulated. Presenting them with orientating material was ineffective because each group member was: 'trapped in a world of fantasy' (Feil 1967, p. 194).

This conceptualisation of gross and global disorientation as 'fantasy' is an early indication of the psychoanalytic influence on Feil, an influence which became an important element in her understanding of disorientation and dementia. It signals her belief that disorientation is not merely a process whereby a person comes to make misjudgements about time, place and person, etc. Rather it is a process in which the ego loses contact with objective reality and retreats to an inner, subjective reality. A reality which, like our dreams, is inhabited by psychologically significant material and people. Thus confused and seemingly unintelligible speech and behaviour is likely to have meaning, a meaning which would be revealed if it could be viewed in the context of the subjective experience. It is only our lack of ability to see the world as the disorientated person is seeing it which leads us to label them as confused. Feil sums this up as the belief that, 'all behaviour, no matter how bizarre, had a rational explanation' (Feil 1967, p. 194).

Feil and reality orientation

It is clear from this early article that Feil is rejecting the use of Reality Orientation (RO) with this group of disorientated residents. RO, she argues, is inappropriate for those beyond the early stages of disorientation, not only because of the inability of the group to become or remain orientated but also, more importantly, because to attempt to orientate would be to miss an opportunity to uncover the true 'reasons' behind disorientated speech and behaviour.

In her address to the 1972 meeting of the Gerontological Society, Feil is more explicit in her attitude to the use of RO: 'I came to realise that the goal of reality orientation was itself unrealistic. After 6 years of failure to bring about awareness of time, place, age, recognition of staff, or family relationships' (Feil 1972, p. 3).

Feil was by now convinced that the use of RO with this group not only represented a waste of effort and a missed opportunity, but that it also had a more negative impact: 'sudden insight into reality brought about pain, withdrawal, and increased dependency' (Feil 1972, p. 3). This is a viewpoint with which Una Holden takes issue in Chapter 20.

Enter Rogers

Whilst Feil conceded that people in the earlier stages of disorientation can benefit from reality orientation, for her there came a point at which the use of RO became destructive and a new approach was required – an approach that was later to become VT. This approach required the group worker to conduct extensive research into the past lives of the disorientated group members, in order to gain insight into the content of the 'fantasy' or 'inner reality' of the person they are working with. A sufficient knowledge of the psychologically significant characters from the group members' past would enable the therapist to understand apparently confused or bizarre behaviour and speech. This understanding would convey to group members a 'feeling of gratification, of being understood, and a sense of self in the knowledge that their world was meaningful and acceptable' (Feil 1972, p. 6).

A willingness to meet with disorientated elderly people 'on their own ground' requires the therapist to be able to empathise with the feelings, perceptions and experiences of the group members. The use of empathy, later identified as the key requirement of the validation therapist, and the acceptance of the disorientated persons' subjective experience as both valid and valuable, were both radical departures from the prevailing ideas and practices of those working with people with dementia. Both RO and Remotivation Therapy, the other popular psychological treatments for dementia at the time, were based on the assumptions that 'confused' speech and behaviour are the unfortunate symptoms of the disease process of dementia, and as such are to be discouraged whilst any remaining coherent and orientated behaviours are to be reinforced at every opportunity.

This debate between supporters of validation and those who favoured the use of RO was a reflection of the growing rivalry between the rapidly growing Rogerian school and the established traditions, hitherto dominant in mental health, which represented analytical, behaviourist and psychiatric ideas. (Indeed RO, with its emphasis on improved functioning and use of the principles of operant conditioning, could be said to belong within the behaviourist tradition.)

The characteristic which most clearly distinguished Rogers and his supporters was the primary position which they accorded to both the subjective experience of the individual and the sense that each individual makes of their own experience. Each of the other traditions makes some claim to being 'scientific', at least to the extent that they are concerned with making objective 'explanations' of psychological phenomena. Subjective experience is for the analyst, the behaviourist and the psychiatrist, an effect – and they are in the business of uncovering the causes. Once those causes are uncovered, then measures can be taken, with the cooperation of the client yet fundamentally under the direction of the therapist/psychiatrist and their expertise, to modify, or treat, them as required. This 'treatment' might mean a dose of insight, major tranquillisers or positive reinforcement (or a cocktail of all three) which will, hopefully, then lead on to an improved quality of subjective experience.

Rogerians do not treat subjective experience as an effect, and deny that the role of 'expert' on the mental world of any individual can be held by anyone other than that person themself. Rather, each person is their own best expert and the role of any therapist in a truly therapeutic relationship would have to be as an enabler and a facilitator. No amount of science or pseudo-science could alter this reality, as any attempt to 'objectify' human experience in this way was intrinsically misguided.

Feil's application of this viewpoint to her work with people with dementia meant that she became the first person to take the apparently confused and disorientated speech and behaviour of dementia sufferers seriously in their own right. She developed her approach over the following 15 years with a growing emphasis on the need to establish trust and empathy as well as a host of communication skills designed to counter the dual impediments of dysphasia and sensory deficit.

Feil did not allow the great theoretical differences which separated the Rogerian from the Freudian tradition to prevent her from utilising aspects of both in her elaboration of the theory of validation. Feil's method was initially known as 'fantasy therapy', reflecting the persistence of the earlier idea that in severe disorientation there is a, 'Denial of reality [which] has become a coping mechanism for these aged' (Feil 1978b, p. 2).

By the end of the 1970s, then, Feil perceived severe disorientation as a fantasy, the primary purpose of which was to deny a bleak present reality. Her description of 'tuning-in therapy' in the 1978 video *Looking for Yesterday* (Feil 1978a) contains many of the ideas and techniques which were to emerge as validation some 4 years later. There were two ingredients still to be added: the four-stage theory of disorientation and the addition of a final life stage and task to Erikson's developmental model. These later additions claimed to identify another purpose behind the fantasy that is severe disorientation – a fantasy which now not only protected the ego from an unbearable present reality, but also formed a key part of the final developmental life task. A task which, tackled successfully, would prevent deterioration to the later stages of disorientation.

Validation therapy in 1982

The term 'validation therapy' appears to have first been used to describe Feil's approach around 1980. When the first edition of her book *V/F Validation: the Feil Method* was published in 1982 the 'V/F' of the title was an abbreviation of 'validation/fantasy' and the title page proclaimed that the work 'encompasses Fantasy Therapy'. The use of 'fantasy' appears to have ceased, however, and for simplicity and consistency I shall use the term validation therapy (VT) throughout.

Feil's 1982 book was the first attempt at a complete description of the theory and practice of VT. Since its appearance there has been some modification to the theory but the guidance on how to use VT as an interpersonal skill and as a group therapy remain largely unchanged.

INDIVIDUAL VALIDATION

For the validation therapist the essential ability is to empathise with the disorientated person; to understand and imaginatively enter into their feelings and perceptions. Empathy is as central to VT as it is to Rogerian person-centred counselling; in its absence the therapeutic process cannot begin. Whilst we have not ourselves been old and disorientated, we can empathise with the feelings evoked by loss and will have had momentary experiences of disorientation. In Feil's words: 'We share human feelings with the disoriented old-old.' (Feil 1982, p. 6).

In addition to our use of empathy we can, perhaps more importantly, suspend our dismissal of the disorientated person's interpretation of reality as false and, therefore, worthless. Validation does not ask us to behave as if disorientated and confused speech were in fact accurate and true. Rather it insists that we take the account seriously and do not let the factual inaccuracies inhibit the possibility of meaningful interaction and psychological contact. If the therapist is taking the seemingly confused speech and behaviour seriously, and responds to it in an encouraging – rather than a correcting – manner, then new possibilities are opened up for meaningful dialogue with the disorientated old-old. Feil illustrates this with examples of interactions in which a warm, understanding and encouraging approach elicits hitherto unseen meaning in 'confused' speech and behaviour. More often than not, this involves the therapist discovering that the dementia sufferer is enacting significant life events from the past, often in a highly symbolic way:

Therapist: What makes a person crazy?

Mrs G: Having nothing to do. Get me my rubbers. I have to go to work. The company will pay the fare.

Therapist: You miss the company don't you, Mrs G? Was it a big company?

Mrs G: Middle size. A Fendall company. Like the Simofile curtains. (She points to the curtains.)

Therapist: How do you mean? Simo-file?

Mrs G: I file everything in the company. (She pats her purse and stuffs napkins in each compartment.)

Therapist: (Patting the purse with Mrs G.) You are acting like a very efficient File Clerk. (Feil 1982, p. 80)

If the disorientated person's 'inner reality' is populated by emotionally significant characters and scenes from earlier life, then the therapist will need to research into their personal history in order to be able to elicit whatever meaning lies behind seemingly unintelligible speech or behaviour. The knowledge gained will also be helpful in deciphering the meaning of the neologisms and the grammatically incorrect speech which will increase as dysphasia progresses and speech becomes more difficult to comprehend.

As verbal communication declines to the point which Feil describes as the third stage of disorientation, the therapist will increasingly have to rely on non-verbal clues to discover the meaning behind confused speech or behaviour. She argues that the way in which the client uses certain objects can be interpreted in symbolic way to reveal the meaning behind their actions, making a neo-Freudian claim that certain 'universal symbols' will offer us almost a new language of behaviour. For example, people in stages two and three in Feil's four-stage model of disorientation will use a hand to symbolise a baby; a fork or knife to symbolise anger; a sock or shoe to symbolise a child; a purse to symbolise a female sex symbol, vagina, identity; a cane or fist to symbolise a penis, potency and power.

Once the correct interpretation has been made – and acknowledged – the therapist can begin to 'validate' the factual and emotional content of the confused speech or behaviour. If an incorrect interpretation has been made, then the client will simply not respond.

The use of empathy to explore the disorientated subjective experience of past reality is the key distinctive feature of VT.

FEIL'S STAGES OF DISORIENTATION

In order to overcome the obstacles to empathy which communication difficulties erect, Feil developed a range of interpersonal and group techniques which combine adapted Rogerian counselling methods with her own, developed in her work as an outstanding practitioner with people with dementia. The techniques are specific to each of the four discrete and progressive stages of disorientation, and are summarised in Table 21.1.

Stage one – malorientation

It is a characteristic of people in the first stage of disorientation, 'malorientation', that they deny their confusion and tend to blame others in order to explain the effects of their short-term memory loss. Whilst this group will continue to attempt to comply with socially accepted standards of behaviour, they will attempt to deal with significant events from their past by using transference; projecting attitudes and feelings held towards significant others from their earlier lives onto people in the present. Feil believes that people in this first stage of disorientation can benefit from reality orientation and individual validation but are too threatened by an open expression of feelings to be appropriate members of validation groups.

Individual validation in stage one involves the following techniques:

Table 21.1 A summary of Feil's four stages of disorientation

	Stage One Malorientation	Stage Two Time Confusion	Stage Three Repetitive Motion	Stage Four Vegetation
Cognitive features	Some short-term memory problems. Language skills maintained. Usually continent.	Comprehensive disorientation. To retain factual information. Ability to form sentences maintained but uses words in unusual way. Severe short-term memory damage but long-term memory preserved. Is aware of incontinence.	Complete disorientation. Unable to talk in sentences but use words and noises in repetitive and/or musical ways. Some early memories retained. Is unaware of incontinence.	Total disorientation. No verbal expression or other social contact. No evidence of any memory. Makes no attempt to control continence.
Typical reactions to deficits	Deny deficits, blame others. Continue to follow social rules of behaviour.	Do not try to hang onto reality. Retreat to inner reality and memories. Use objects as symbols for past events and people. No longer adhere to social rules.	Use repetitive sound and constant movement in order to stimulate self. Attempt to resolve unfinished conflicts through movement.	Completely withdrawn and inactive.
Helpful approaches	Appreciate orientation. Reject physical contact and dislike talking about their emotions. Will not benefit from validation groups.	Resist orientation. Able to deal with emotional, rather than factual, issues. Use individual and group validation. Appreciate touch.	Beyond orientation. Use individual and group validation with emphasis on physical and musical contact as opposed to verbal interaction.	Use music and sensory stimulation. Beyond the reach of either orientation or validation.

Careful questioning

Exploring (although not correcting) the factual content of their speech, using 'who', 'what', 'where' and 'when' questions. The use of 'why' questions is discouraged as the maloriented person may no longer have the intellectual capability to work out causal or rational explanations. (It could be argued that the use of 'when' questions is as likely to expose a deficit in the early stages of dementia – especially if it makes demands on the short-term memory.)

Rephrasing

The Rogerian techniques of reflection – either summarising or paraphrasing – as those key words which the dementia sufferer accentuates are repeated.

Use of the preferred sense

An idea which appears to originate with neurolinguistics, that individuals have a 'preferred sense' – sight, hearing, touch, etc. – which is indicated by their habitual use of phrases. Thus a 'visual' person will tend to employ words such as 'notice', 'imagine', 'picture', etc. The validation worker identifies the preferred sense of the individual and uses the same sense at every opportunity.

Polarity

Invitations to imagine extremes and opposites: 'When is it worst?'; 'What if it stopped happening?'.

Discussion of feelings is not initiated by the therapist in stage one and touch is only used when a relationship of trust has been built. This relationship may lead to insight into 'the reason behind his blaming and anger' (Feil 1982, p. 49).

Whilst the techniques she outlines will help begin such a relationship, Feil is insistent that no techniques can be a substitute for an empathic, genuine and honest approach.

Stage two – time confusion

In this stage some verbal skills are still maintained

whilst disorientation – in time, place and circumstance – is comprehensive. Reality orientation ceases to be of any benefit during stage two and may be a cause of psychological pain and distress. Members of this group are 'returning to the past' and have reduced concern about present day reality or maintaining socially expected standards of behaviour. Short-term memory is poor but early memories grow stronger and eidetic in form, so that remembered characters and scenes are superimposed onto – and perceived as being part of – present reality. There is little concern for the factual accuracy of speech, which becomes a 'poetic' vehicle for the expression of feelings. Emotions are expressed much more freely. The following techniques are suggested for use with time-confused people, in addition to any of those used in stage one that are still found useful:

Observing, matching and expressing emotion

The main difference in the validation approach to people in stage two is that there is a greater emphasis on the non-verbal elements of communication. The use of touch is encouraged whilst eye contact and voice tone are modified to an exaggerated degree. Validating the emotional content involves observing, matching (i.e. physically reflecting) and expressing their emotions. This is not a problem if one accepts Feil's assertion that there are only four human emotions:
Love/pleasure/joy/sex
anger/rage/hate/displeasure
fear/guilt/shame/anxiety
sadness/misery/grief (Feil 1992a, p. 70).

One can envisage difficulties with this approach if the emotion being expressed is, say, alarm or panic – which is a common emotional companion of disorientation. When I am gripped by panic I do not want the person I am with to mirror my emotion, rather the opposite; I want them to display a reassuring calm.

In other situations, however, this 'non-verbal' reflection can be very useful in communicating to the disorientated person that we are aware of, and accept, their emotional state and are prepared to join them in its expression. Interestingly, Christine Bleathman reports finding the technique of 'expressing their emotion, with emotion' as helpful in interactions with younger sufferers – in the earlier stages – of Alzheimer's disease who are highly frustrated by their inability to express their thoughts and feelings verbally (Bleathman 1994). Expressing that frustration with the appropriate behavioural display of frustration can serve almost as a 'cathartic release by proxy',

enhanced, no doubt, by the sheer relief of witnessing an unambiguous demonstration that someone is aware of how you are feeling.

Using vague pronouns

When unable to understand the speech of time-confused people it can be helpful to use pronouns to explore possible meanings. In response to a statement such as, 'There's what a beauty', the therapist would reply, 'Is he a beauty?'

Entire conversations can take place about a 'he', 'she', 'it' or 'they' without the therapist knowing to whom, or what, the pronouns refer. The important point is not to press for identification, but rather to keep the interaction going – listening for clues for identification – and concentrate on the emotional tone of what is being said.

Identifying needs

Given Feil's belief that disorientation fulfils a need which is not being met in 'present reality', it follows that the identification and expression of that need can facilitate a partial, perhaps temporary, return to present reality. Thus, when an apparently disorientated person is expressing a desire to go home and look after her young children, it may well be that this desire is really a failed attempt to describe a need to return to a period when she felt useful, needed by others and had whatever social esteem is associated with being a parent of young children – in other words it may be an expression of grief at the loss of the 'role' of being a parent of young children. If we are able to articulate this need to be, or feel, useful then it both validates the original expression and again shows the time-confused person that the therapist has an understanding of these feelings and perceptions.

Stage three – repetitive motion

Feil holds that sufficient validation may prevent a progression towards the third stage of disorientation – during which verbal communication ceases to be recognisable as speech. Actions, movements and the use of objects or symbols take over as the means of expression. If people in stage two are said to use language poetically, then those in repetitive motion use language as music – for the sound it makes rather than for its content. Humming, clucking and moaning noises accompany repetitive actions – banging, tapping, buttoning, rubbing. These actions may be for self-stimulation purposes, or the playing out of their 'inner reality' in which everyday objects become symbols, taking on the roles of psychologically significant figures from the past.

Non-verbal communication

Non-verbal techniques from stage two are used along with a method of replicating – through touch – the sensations evoked by fathers, mothers, lovers, friends, siblings and children.

The other technique which is specific to stage three is mirroring – a physical reflection of the movements, posture, etc. of the person in repetitive motion. This is the non-verbal application of the reflective techniques described for stage two, intended to 'build bridges' between the dementia sufferer and the other person.

Stage four – vegetation

The fourth stage is characterised by an absence of responsiveness and can be avoided if the person receives sufficient validation in stages two and three. By the fourth stage it is too late for validation to be of any demonstrable benefit, although Feil suggests that we should still use some of the methods, along with music, in the hope that some contact might still be possible.

The point of it all – resolution versus vegetation

The arrival of the disoriented person at Feil's fourth stage of disorientation represents a failure in the final 'life task', in which they were striving to achieve resolution and avoid vegetation.

We heard earlier of Feil's belief that all apparently confused behaviour, speech and experience had meaning. She also believes that it had purpose: that it was the final part of a lifelong developmental process which had its own goal – to resolve past conflicts and justify having lived. Disorientated old-old people who are receptive to validation, those she describes as being in the first three stages of disorientation, are said to be in the 'resolution versus vegetation' stage of development. Here Feil is elaborating on the theory constructed by Erik Erikson whose model divided psychosocial development – from birth to old age and death – into eight 'stages', each of which involves a psychosocial crisis, or 'task' which has to be dealt with (Erikson 1964) (see Chs 2 and 4 for further elaboration of Erikson's model). The degree of any individual's

success will depend upon the part played by those occupying the significant social relations relevant to the stage, and also upon the degree of success achieved at earlier stages. Thus, for example, the crisis of the adolescent stage of development is known as 'identity versus confusion'. Significant social relations during this stage are peer groups and role-models and a successful outcome would be a person who entered the next stage (early adulthood) with a clear, integrated self-identity. An unsuccessful outcome would be a confused young adult with a poorly formed self-image.

Erikson's model involved eight stages to which Feil added a ninth in which the crisis is 'resolution versus vegetation'. Here the old-old person, in stage two or three of disorientation, is struggling to avoid moving into stage four (vegetation) and seeking to 'resolve' past crises and 'unfinished life tasks'. Thus the seemingly confused speech or behaviour not only has meaning (which the therapist must attempt to decode) it also has a purpose in that it is part of an attempt to complete the final life task, to resolve past conflicts. The past scenes which are being enacted, the significant characters who populate these scenes – long dead parents, relatives, lovers and friends – are not chosen at random. They are chosen as being the key to resolving past crises, the 'unfinished business' from earlier stages which need to be dealt with now, through fantasy and validation.

The early influences on Feil's theoretical development, Rogers and Freud, had been joined by Erikson by the time of publication of the validation 'manifesto' in 1982 (Feil 1982). Feil lists many other influences in addition to this eclectic mixture: the idea of universal feelings owes something to Jung (1964); the value placed upon highly personalised reminiscence reflects the views of Robert Butler (1963); and she was keen to declare support for any studies or reports which sought to discredit the link between observable (post-death) physical changes in the brain and the disorientation – and other symptoms of dementia – which is observed during life. She is understandably eager to play down the degree to which the rate of decline through her four stages is determined by neurological changes in the brain. Her theory and practice rest upon the assumption that it is the way in which people interact with the disorientated person that is the crucial factor in determining whether further deterioration will occur. Implicit in her arguments is the belief that a good deal of validation may outweigh physical damage to the brain and prevent further decline, or even reverse it to some extent. This is possible, the argument would go, because disorientation, together with its associated loss of skills, is not simply a matter of a biochemical process producing certain cognitive and behavioural effects; it is rather a psychological process, in which the biochemistry acts as one factor – even a trigger – which may loosen 'ego contact with reality'. This loss of ego contact is the result of a host of physical, social and developmental factors and is, as we have seen, not entirely negative. The ego has important work to do, a developmental task to complete, and for this reason it is being drawn towards 'inner reality' at the same time that it is being pushed away from 'external reality'.

VALIDATION GROUPS

My first encounter with validation was as a group therapy, the form in which it was first developed by Feil. When Christine Bleathman and I gained funding for a research project into methods of groupwork with people with dementia, we were fortunate in making contact with Gemma Jones, currently one of only four certified validation therapists in Europe, then working in the Institute of Psychiatry in London. She trained us to run validation groups and supervised our work over the 40 weeks of the project. The research method and results of the project are described elsewhere (Morton & Bleathman 1991).

The guidelines on running validation groups which follow are based partly on our own experience and the guidance we received from Jones, and partly on the writings of Feil.

Selecting group members

I will describe later some of our objections to Feil's description of the four stages of disorientation. Suffice to say here that we did not find helpful her descriptions of people in stages two and three – those who are held to be suitable – when selecting group members. The six original members of our group were chosen as being grossly disorientated – unaware of time, place, person and situation – yet retaining a large degree of their expressive and receptive communication skills; they could speak in a reasonably coherent manner and understand the majority of what was being said to them. As such, Feil would probably describe them as being in stage two. They retained their verbal skills despite the absence of opportunity to practise them, our extensive observations of members outside the group showing that their daily lives inside the residential home involved minimal social contact.

Ideally each group should have two workers and between six and eight members.

Setting

A relatively small room is preferable, with comfortable chairs arranged in a circle which is tight enough to allow each person to comfortably hold the hands of those on either side. The room should be 'homely' but without too many distractions such as pictures or ornaments. The chairs should be comfortable but without the 'wings' which can prevent eye-contact with people on either side. The group leader and co-worker should sit opposite each other in order that the co-worker has a clear view of the members to either side of the leader, whose non-verbal cues he is most likely to miss.

Time/length

It has been suggested that cognitive and social functioning are at their peak during the late morning. We began our groups at 11 a.m. and they were over at noon. Whilst we were only able to meet on a weekly basis, I would suggest that groups should be held far more frequently – even daily – to reach their full potential.

Structure – staff roles

One of the two staff members, or 'co-workers', takes the role of group leader. There are many aspects to this role: ensuring the group structure is adhered to, inviting contributions from more withdrawn members, drawing together conclusions, pointing out similarities and shared experiences or feelings, and preventing individuals from dominating the group. Many of the techniques described earlier as appropriate to stages two and three in individual validation are used and the group leader is far more directive than would be usual with a group of cognitively intact people. This may involve asking each group member a specific question in turn, or simply making sure that group members are aware that a particular group member wishes to speak. In our own groups, we found that the amount of control the leader had to exercise diminished as each group went on. Once the group had gained some momentum and a theme had developed then members would often take the lead in discussion themselves and the group leader merely kept a hand on the tiller, as it were, as opposed to pulling the oars.

The co-worker's role is to assist the group leader with any practical tasks and to draw the group leader's attention to members who may wish to speak, are becoming distressed, looking bemused or are in need of attention. The degree of differentiation between the group leader and co-worker roles is largely determined by the relative experience and confidence of the pair. As we were both new to validation, and alternated taking the group leader role, it would not be uncommon for the co-worker to take over the lead role for periods during a group.

Structure – group members' roles

A distinctive feature of validation groups is the allocation of roles to group members, a device which gives each individual a position of status within the group. The exact roles may vary from group to group, our own members' roles being fairly typical: a 'welcomer' who would make a short speech of welcome at the beginning of the group, a 'songleader' who would start off the singing, a 'thanker' who made a short speech at the end of the meeting, and a host who handed around the refreshments after the group meeting had finished.

It is important that group members are comfortable with their roles and preferable that they 'grow into' them as opposed to their being allocated by the staff. It may take until the second or third group before staff can feel confident that an individual would be confident in, and suited to, a particular role.

Whilst the short-term memory damage would prevent members from describing or naming their roles, after a few sessions we found that they required little or no prompting to carry them out. Indeed, after 15 or so meetings our 'songleader' – a woman who showed no evidence of being able to retain new information for more than a few minutes and who was grossly disorientated – would start us off on the appropriate song ('when you're smiling') despite it having been a full week since she had last performed the role.

Group structure – the protocol

Perhaps the most important single feature of a validation group is the emphasis on keeping as rigid a routine a possible, with any variation to either the environment or the format of the groups being kept to an absolute minimum. This rigidity is designed to assist group members in forming a kind of impressionistic memory, or association, of the group

and its environment which, in turn, provides a kind of continuity between the weekly group meetings. It appears to be remarkably successful.

10 minute warning

About 10 minutes before the group began we would approach group members in the lounge of the residential home and, taking care to smile and shake hands as we introduced ourselves, let them know that we would shortly be returning to take them to the group meeting. Although we would usually be greeted with a degree of bemusement and were clearly not recognised, it did increase the possibility that there was some recollection of our faces a few minutes later when we returned to take them to the group.

With the trusting compliance common to so many disorientated people who have adapted behaviourally, if not emotionally, to residential institutions, our group members would agree to our requests for them to accompany us to 'this week's meeting'. Only Flo would, more often than not, turn down this invitation to accompany a stranger to whatever this 'meeting' may be: 'Very kind of you to offer dear, but not today thank you. I've got this terrible "zizzing" noise in my ears you see and that sort of thing doesn't help. Kind of you to ask, dear, but no thanks'.

Ah! We're here!

After a few weeks of running the groups, we began to witness a noticeable moment of recognition as members were led through the door into the small room in which the meetings were held. It was quite remarkable how demeanours would change; from being a compliantly confused older person, unsure of where she was being led by this young stranger, the group member would visibly brighten on entering the room. Now they were in a place with which they were familiar, with people whom they knew and felt comfortable with. Group members who sat near each other in the home and hardly ever spoke would strike up conversation. An air of expectation could be felt. They knew this situation. It was as if the group had a life of its own which ended at noon each Wednesday and was recreated at 11 a.m. the following week.

Welcome

Group members would be guided to sit in the same chairs each week whereupon the group leader would approach each individual in turn, shaking their hands and thanking them for coming. This welcome involved the leader getting close to each person in turn and would assist in gaining their attention which would then be passed over to the welcomer: 'Edith, would you like to thank everyone coming to the group this morning?'

Oh I would. I missed not coming. I came up here once, I've met you once so its twice that I've come up here because its something I look forward to very much. I'll most probably cry before I get to the finish. It's so nice to see you all again so soon after Christmas and I hope everyone here had a nice Christmas, the best one they've ever had. [The date was 2 December, the Christmas decorations were up in the home.]

Opening song

Next comes the opening song. 'When you're smiling' was selected by group members and later led to the group christening itself 'The Wednesday Morning Smilers'. Betty, the songleader, starts us off and the familiarity of the songs means that the (large print) song books are probably only of value to the co-workers. Starting with a song gives an opportunity for each group member to vocalise early in the meeting, as even people with quite severe dysphasia are often able to sing familiar songs without difficulty. After several weeks, Betty no longer needs to be reminded what the opening and closing songs are.

The meeting

By the end of the opening song the group often felt themselves to be in sufficiently familiar company to be able to talk. Discussion often began quite spontaneously, prompted by the song and the memories it evoked. On one occasion, for example, the group elected to sing a second song and turned the page to sing 'In the Shade of the Old Apple Tree', at the end of which Reg remarked, 'Now that reminds me of my father, he used to drink in a pub called "The Old Apple Tree"'.

In the weeks that follow the same sequence is repeated twice, and we had noticed numerous other 'jovial' references to his father's drinking. On the second occasion the group leader invites Reg to share his reminiscences further. What follows is the traumatic account of Reg as a 7-year-old boy being charged by his mother with the responsibility for escorting his alcoholic father, in a vain attempt to keep him out of the public houses that he inhabits with his colleagues from the printing industry. We hear of young Reg's long waits outside the pub and of his

having to assist his barely conscious parent back home to the despairing anger of the mother. Three-quarters of a century later he dwelt alone on his failure to discharge this impossible duty until he felt safe enough to share the experience within the validation group. Likewise Flo with her bitterness towards her unfaithful husband, Win with her disappointment at the lack of passion in her marriage and Edith with her fictional adopted infants compensating for her inability to have children of her own.

We would prepare an idea for a theme for discussion for use when the group did not set off on a course of its own choosing. In the earlier groups we found members readily discussed their childhood years yet rarely referred to their adult years and, in particular, to their partners and spouses. We attempted to move on to this area by opening the discussion with a question, asking each member in turn: 'Can you tell us a little bit about how you met your husband/wife?'

The response was disappointing, there was a lack of either motivation or ability (or both?) to go into any depth. On the advice of Gemma Jones, we later tried a more circuitous route: 'Edith, what advice would you give to a young couple who were thinking of getting married and setting up home together?'

This approach put the group member in a position of status and respect which is part of being asked advice, as well as providing a much wider range of options for possible responses. Taking more readily to this indirect route, the group eventually arrived at the point of sharing their own experiences of courtship and marriage, not as a response to a direct enquiry, but as a by-product of a more generalised discussion.

Similarly a question such as, 'Betty, can you tell us how you feel about living in an old peoples' home? Do you miss your own home?' would meet with a polite correction: 'I'm sorry my dear, I don't actually live here. I'm just visiting my sister. I expect my son will be along shortly to take me home, he's the doctor here'.

To ask our question was to ask Betty to acknowledge her present situation, something she had neither the ability nor the motivation to do. But a lively discussion followed when the group was asked: 'What advice would you give to someone thinking about leaving their own home and moving into an old peoples' home?'

By this stage the degree of the disorientation that group members experienced would often fluctuate within each meeting. Past and present tense became interchangeable. Interestingly, as our own lack of interest in the factual accuracy of each comment became habitual, this fluctuation had little or no effect on the course of the group. We were far more concerned with the emotional tone of the groups, with the feelings that were being expressed.

When the group was not able to find its own way, the group leader would revert to asking the same question of each person in turn, almost in an attempt to 'kick-start' the group before members began again to address each other directly.

Closing the meeting

As with any therapeutic group work, it is important to end the group with a minimum of emotional 'loose ends' being left undealt with. When time became our enemy, this would often mean simply acknowledging any emotionally loaded comments with a reference to a future opportunity to share them further: 'Edith, I'd very much like to talk about that with you further, but time is against us just now. Could we start off next week by discussing that with you?'

After Betty has led us in the final song ('Side by Side') it's time for Reg to make his closing 'thank you all for coming' speech. The meeting is then formally closed and individual conversations break out whilst Win, the 'hostess', passes round the lemonade and biscuits, assisted by the co-worker. It was always at this time that I was struck by the fact that this group of older people with severe disorientation and a considerable degree of cognitive impairment had just sat for some 40 minutes holding each other's attention in a group setting just as well as any other group might. They had listened to each other, stuck to the theme, been supportive, made pertinent and relevant comments, asked each other questions and concentrated throughout. Prior to starting these groups we had, along with most of our professional colleagues, held assumptions that led us to believe that this type of group work was simply not possible with people suffering from this degree of dementia: they would not be able to concentrate, would interrupt each other, become too easily distracted, were too trapped in their own individual worlds.

Our research involved us in 40 hours of direct observation of each member outside the group and during those hours we saw no evidence to counter such assumptions. Yet once inside that room, as the group developed and matured, each individual's social functioning was improved beyond recognition. Dormant social skills thrived in the (artificially created) atmosphere of safety and respect. As a result, whenever we show video footage of our groups on study days etc., the audience protest that we were clearly working with a group of relatively unimpaired individuals. That their patients/clients/residents could

never participate in such a way. The reality is that as professionals and carers we tend to hugely underestimate the latent social abilities of people with dementia. Validation groups are just an indicator of the potential for the design of artificial social environments which will allow the benefits of such skills to be realised.

CRITIQUE OF VALIDATION THEORY

When *Validation: The Feil Method* in was first published (Feil 1982) the author claimed that the approach was then being used in 523 homes throughout the USA and Canada. A decade later she claimed that 'the validation approach is now practised in over 6000 long-term facilities, community-based support groups, adult treatment centres, and hospitals in the United States, Canada, the Netherlands, Norway and Australia' (Feil 1992b, p. 199).

This 10-fold increase and internationalisation of validation requires us to look closely at both the practice and the underlying theory. It has to be said that the theoretical base of validation appears particularly weak when closely scrutinised. This weakness is being addressed, largely by Feil's daughter, Vicki de Klerk-Rubin, whose revision of *Validation: The Feil Method* for the second edition (Feil 1992a) has significantly reduced the scope for criticism. Problems remain, however, and I shall attempt to identify some of them here.

I outlined earlier my belief that the approaches being described in this chapter become more vulnerable to criticism as they depart from the goal of applying the person-centred approach to dementia care. This is particularly true of validation, the theoretical base of which is an unlikely amalgam of influences, many of which begin from mutually incompatible starting points or first principles. The attempt to marry the approaches of Rogers and Freud, for example, is unlikely to succeed as they have such contrasting views on the nature of the relationship between therapist and client, between the helper and the person requiring help.

The Freudian influence

We saw earlier how Feil felt the need to use neo-Freudian ideas to support her theoretical assumption that 'there is a reason behind the behaviour of disoriented very old people' (Feil 1992a, p. 12). This is itself an echo of one of her earliest statements that 'all behaviour, no matter how bizarre, had a rational explanation' (Feil 1967, p. 94).

Whilst we may applaud Feil's insistence that we take the content of disorientated people's speech seriously, we do not have to share her beliefs in order to do so. It would be better to rephrase the statement as 'it is wise to respond, at least initially, to all confused behaviour and speech as if it has meaning'.

This allows us to acknowledge that some confused speech and behaviour may simply be scrambled activity, devoid of content and reflecting a (possibly transient) stuporous state. Whilst we may support Feil's reaction against the tendency to label all confused speech and behaviour as meaningless, we have to acknowledge that her response – labelling all such speech and behaviour as meaningful – is something of an over-reaction.

This brings us on to a second criticism of the Freudian influence on Feil, first elaborated by Goudie & Stokes (1989) who accuse her of being over-reliant on psychodynamic interpretations in her search for meaning. Although it may be true that some disorientation involves a return to developmentally significant scenes from long ago, it is surely dangerous to assume that all confused speech and behaviour has its explanation rooted in the past. Feil's examples of the use of validation are dominated by scenes in which people with dementia are clearly imagining themselves to be back in some previous time – resolving past crises. Yet those who work in this area are aware that for a large part of the time people with dementia are very much in the 'here and now' – a present reality which they can neither understand nor accurately describe. There is a danger that attempts to communicate these present day needs will be overlooked, or interpreted as being material from the past.

Another neo-Freudian element which has attracted criticism, not to say some derision, is the account Feil gives of the way disorientated people use objects to symbolise people or objects from their past, claiming that 'after 35 years of working with maloriented and disoriented people around the world, I have found the following typical symbols ... :

Jewellery, clothing – Worth, identity
Shoe   – Container, womb, male or female sex symbol
Purse   – Female sex symbol, vagina, identity
Cane or fist   – Penis, potency, power' (Feil 1992a, p. 47).

Feil's list goes on and is followed by the claim that the symbols are 'universal, regardless of race, religion, culture or sex'. I have yet to meet anyone who works with people with dementia who will ascribe any validity to this claim, and many fear that it is dangerous to promote such an idea without the most rigorous research to support it. One dreads to think what interpretations are being made of behaviours around the world based on this 'code' of the way people with dementia use certain objects. Feil and her supporters may protest that a false interpretation, a mistaken guess, will meet with a negative response – yet how can they know that this is so? To interpret the behaviour of those who no longer possess the communication abilities to correct us if we are mistaken is a dangerous, and unnecessary, approach which is completely out of tune with the person-centred approach. It is encouraging to note that in the most recent publication little mention is made of the use of symbols (Feil 1993).

Feil's theory of dementia

The neo-Freudian account of disorientation had a direct impact on Feil's theory of dementia and this, in turn, had implications for her definition of the group of people for whom validation was useful.

Her belief that disorientation was primarily the result of a psychodynamic process seemed to indicate that she was either denying the existence of a physical disease which caused disorientation or, alternatively, that she had identified a distinct group of disorientated people who were not suffering from dementia. Feil's earlier writings appeared to give support to both of these viewpoints, in that she wrote of the 'disoriented old-old' (who benefit from validation) as showing 'permanent damage to ... brain [and] ... recent memory' Feil (1982, p. 2) whilst at the same time they 'choose on a subliminal level of awareness to retreat from painful present reality' (Feil 1982, p. 2).

The idea that choice is involved in a disorientation that results from damage to the brain is a difficult one. By the time of the second edition in 1992, Feil's thoughts on the subject appear to have become more orthodox and the disorientated old-old are described as very old people who 'have significant cognitive deterioration and can no longer function intellectually to achieve insight' and who 'withdraw from present day reality to survive' (Feil 1992a, p. 26).

Other more recent writings (Feil 1992b, 1993) refer to those with 'late-onset dementia' and 'Alzheimer-type dementia' as forming the target group for validation, although de Klerk-Rubin still suggests that there remains a distinction between, 'an Alzheimer's patient and disoriented elderly person' (de Klerk-Rubin 1994, pp. 14–15).

She supports this claim with the strangely circular argument that whilst the neurofibrillary plaques and tangles might be held to cause the disorientation in younger sufferers (because the deterioration does not fit with the life stage), the fact that those same plaques and tangles are present in a larger number of very old people (some of whom do not become disorientated) means that they do not cause the disorientation (because the disorientation does, according to Feil, fit with the life stage).

Although adopting a less controversial definition of the group held to benefit from validation may reduce the impact of one line of criticism, it creates other problems as it shifts the focus of attention to the four-stage model of disorientation – or the 'four stages of resolution' (Feil 1993) as it has now become known.

The four stages of resolution

The four stages are open to at least three criticisms. The first is that they are simply too tightly defined, and that any individual may display characteristics from at least three of the stages at any one time. Paradoxically, Feil is, on the one hand, at pains to emphasise the uniqueness of each individual with dementia and, on the other hand, lumps them together under one of her four stages, each of which is a description so tight that Feil can role-play each stage.

The stages do not have the backing of credible research and appear to represent generalisations from the people that Feil has worked with over her career. The claim of the four-stage model to represent universal characteristics is unfounded.

Secondly, there is the question of how compatible the four stages are with the notion of a progressive organic disease such as Alzheimer's disease. Feil claims that sufficient validation will prevent an individual from reaching the fourth stage of vegetation.

Is this the same as halting the disease itself? If it is, then presumably the claim is for a 'talking cure' for Alzheimer's disease. If it is not, we are entitled to ask what exactly these four stages are stages of. To complicate matters further, Feil (1993) now talks of individuals who 'wander from stage to stage' during the course of a single day.

Viewed retrospectively, we should note that the four stages were introduced before Feil accepted the idea of a disease process behind disorientation. She has not acknowledged that the notion of a disease process stands in clear opposition to her idea that disorientation is a key component of a developmental task or life stage. Again, her refusal to come to terms with the devastating nature of dementia, at whatever age it begins, is understandable given the way in which sufferers were habitually 'written off' in the past. What better way to remotivate staff and carers than to redefine the illness as a positive 'life task' which, if successful, would prevent deterioration towards 'vegetation'? What better way, on the other hand, of instilling a sense of guilt and failure in the carers of those who have progressed to the final stage? If we accept that 'those who are validated need not progress to vegetation' (Feil 1993), then we cannot escape the conclusion that those who did progress to vegetation did so as a result of insufficient validation.

Erikson's model

A final observation frequently made of Feil's ideas is that she did not need to add a final stage to Erikson's model of life stages as his own final stage of 'integrity versus despair' includes the struggle of resolving of past crises. To accept this idea, and to abandon the four-stage model, might well point the way out of the theoretical morass in which validation finds itself. It would also deal with the awkward point that Feil's description of the 'resolution versus vegetation' stage carries an implication that it is actually necessary to become disorientated in order to achieve resolution. It is unclear whether only disorientated old-old people need to confront this final life task. If not, then it is equally unclear how orientated older people can hope to achieve it, as they do not have the 'ability' to travel to the past to deal with, and resolve, unfinished conflicts.

To ask that supporters of validation abandon the psychodynamic emphasis: the theory of symbols, the four stages model of disorientation, and the 'resolution versus vegetation' life task, is to ask them to abandon many of the defining features of their approach. What would remain would be an approach which fits firmly within the Rogerian tradition, one that was not obliged to deny the presence of a disease in dementia yet remained able to acknowledge the psychosocial factors which contribute to the dementing process. They could, perhaps, learn from some more recently developed therapeutic approaches to dementing people, in particular from Tom Kitwood's more coherent account of the relationship and interplay between the physical (neurological) and the psychosocial in the dementing process (Kitwood 1990). It is to a consideration of Kitwood's work and other therapeutic approaches to dementia that we now turn.

RESOLUTION THERAPY

Like VT, resolution therapy, developed by British clinical psychologists Fiona Goudie and Graham Stokes (Goudie & Stokes 1989), has as its focus the emotional distress which accompanies dementia. There are significant differences between the two approaches, however, and the use of the term 'resolution' should not be confused with Feil's use of the term in the context of the 'resolution versus vegetation' stage of life (a confusion which led Feil to consider legal action against Goudie and Stokes in defence of the copyright of her phrase).

Resolution therapy rests upon a model of communication in which dementia is seen as an ever increasing impediment, or barrier, to meaningful communication. The particular cruelty of dementia is that it robs the sufferer of the communication skills required to attract emotional support just at the time such support is most needed.

The key task of the carer/therapist is to overcome the communication barrier by looking beyond the superficial level of confused speech and behaviour. This involves a tentative interpretation of the failed communication attempt to identify the concealed meaning behind it and the accompanying underlying feelings or needs. When the carer/therapist is given confidence that their interpretation is sound, they can make a response which reflects the underlying feelings and, when appropriate, offer to assist to meet the needs. Person-centred counselling techniques from the Rogerian tradition are employed.

Resolution, then, shares with validation a concern to improve the affective state of the dementia sufferer by establishing contact, and empathy, through the search for meanings and messages behind apparently confused speech and behaviour. It differs from validation, however, in some key respects. As mentioned earlier, Goudie & Stokes (1989) criticise Feil's tendency to make psychodynamic interpretations of incoherent speech; they reject the idea that it is more likely to represent unfinished conflicts from childhood and earlier life than to be failed expressions of current feelings and needs. It should also be noted that Goudie and Stokes neither share Feil's optimistic view of the nature of the dementing process nor make similar claims for the potential of their approach to delay, halt or reverse it. They view the role of the carer, or therapist, as one of helping the dementia sufferer come to terms with the emotional and psychological effects of the disease, rather than addressing the disease itself. Indeed, they accept that there comes a point when the barriers to communication (which result from the

neurological damage) become insurmountable and resolution ceases to be of use. We may find that at this point in the development of dysphasia the use of 'pre-therapy', described later, becomes appropriate.

It makes some sense to describe resolution as the therapy that validation would have been had Feil not attempted to graft the ideas of Freud and Erikson onto her initial Rogerian theory. This gives it the dual advantage over validation of neither being plagued with theoretical inconsistency nor involving an implicit rejection of the idea of dementia as a disease.

It might also be argued, however, that resolution does not really represent a therapy in its own right at all, but is rather an attempt to apply Rogerian therapy to a new group of clients – people with dementia.

This would only represent a partial truth, as Goudie and Stokes are silent on the matter of the relationship between the person with dementia and the carer/therapist. For Rogers, this relationship constitutes the central therapeutic factor and to fail to emphasise it as such is to portray Rogerian counselling as a set of techniques or skills – something he and his followers would vigorously deny. If there is a criticism of resolution therapy it is precisely this, that they do not address the issue of how people with dementia are able to form and maintain relationships, and what we can do to assist in this process.

Having made that point, it must noted that this a criticism of completeness rather than content. Resolution has provided a framework for many who reject validation yet still wish to introduce a person-centred approach to their work in dementia care.

KITWOOD AND THE BRADFORD DEMENTIA RESEARCH GROUP

The work of Kitwood and the Bradford Dementia Research Group (Kitwood 1990, 1993, Kitwood & Bredin 1992a, 1992b) draws upon the traditions of social psychology in its analysis of the types of processes we see in dementia, whilst relying heavily on person-centred approaches to deal with the problems that these processes produce.

Kitwood's starting point is a rejection of the traditional 'medical model' account of dementia (Kitwood 1990). According to this model, the process we understand as dementia can be explained in terms of the neurological damage that is being inflicted upon the brain. In other words, there is a straightforward causal relationship between the disease process and the changes we see in the person with dementia. Kitwood argues convincingly that this account is too simplistic, that in reality there exist a multiplicity of other factors which have a significant bearing upon the course and development of the dementia of any one individual. The most influential of these other factors can be grouped together and described as the individual's 'social psychology' – the total interpersonal and group relationships in which we are involved, a kind of psychological 'environment' or milieu that surrounds us all and through which we all must swim during our waking hours.

The malignant social psychology

Kitwood's account of dementia involves a dialectical interplay between the neurological factors of the medical model and the social psychology which surrounds the dementia sufferer and becomes increasingly 'malignant' as the disease progresses.

The ten aspects of the malignant social psychology (MSP) and the examples with which Kitwood illustrates them have a powerful, even uncomfortable, familiarity for those who have been closely involved with dementia sufferers. They describe how professionals, carers and others unwittingly combine to rob sufferers of their confidence, self-esteem, skills, sense of agency, social status and, ultimately, their 'personhood'. This psychosocial aspect of the dementing process does not involve any malicious intent, it is merely the routine, everyday, typical reaction of others in being over-helpful, thoughtless, 'over-professional', and dealing with dementia in the sanitised and patronising way that we have been conditioned to respond. This in turn results from the fact that our society leaves the majority of people 'extremely lacking in inter-subjective insight' (Kitwood 1990, pp. 181–184) and therefore ill-equipped to meet dementia sufferers with an empathic response. Other factors combine with this tendency to contribute to the malignancy: carers are stressed and under-resourced; a prevalent myth stereotypes dementia as something which destroys 'the person', so dementia sufferers are not accorded the status of persons; and carers tend to defend against their own (usually subconscious) anxiety that the dementia sufferer may represent their own future – a defence which lessens both their ability and their desire to build close relationships.

Kitwood's accounts of the typical social and interpersonal reactions which meet people with dementia (Kitwood 1990) are convincing through their familiarity: we feel he is describing, with accuracy, situations we have been involved in – perhaps even felt uncomfortable and guilty about without being able to articulate why. However, these descriptions do not have much explanatory power. Indeed, his description of the malignant social psychology could be accurately applied – in varying degrees – to the social psychology of an enormous range of people: those with virtually any mental health problem, members of ethnic minorities, women, children, lesbians and gay men, and older people in general. His ten aspects, and four reasons for, the malignant social psychology are in fact vivid depictions of social relationships in which there is a significant imbalance of power and, as such, they do not really explain with any specificity the way in which the social psychology around someone with dementia develops.

A parallel can be drawn here with a search to explain the plight of a large group of soldiers lying injured and dying on a battlefield, in terms of their social psychology with specific reference to the military hierarchy of which they form the bottom rung. On observation, the generals and officers would be found to be lacking in inter-subjective insight, spending little or no time empathising with the experience of their soldiers as they lay dying. Perhaps these military leaders are too busy and stressed to provide an empathic response; maybe the officer corps holds a stereotypical view of the lower ranks as being brutish rabble – not really persons as such; we might even suggest that the officers defend themselves against anxiety at their own possible fate in battle by distancing themselves emotionally from the suffering of those under their command.

This account of the officers' relationships to the soldiers may well be accurate in itself, but it hardly offers an explanation of the predicament of the soldiers – it does not explain how they got into that position. A convincing explanation would have to begin with a description of the power relations between the different ranks and of the mechanisms whereby authority is vested in certain people to command groups of others to take certain actions. It would be an explanation of power, not a description of the effects of that power on the social psychology of the hierarchy in which it was exercised.

This point is important because the way in which the problem is defined has a crucial significance for the possible solutions that will be sought. Kitwood (1990) argues that there is a real causal agent, the malignant social psychology (MSP), which combines with another causal agent, neurological impairment (NI), to bring about senile dementia (SD). He expresses this in the form of an equation: 'SD = NI + MSP'. In treating MSP as a causal agent in this way, Kitwood is guilty of reification – i.e. of treating an abstract idea, or concept, as if it were a real, or concrete, thing.

Improving the malignant social psychology therefore becomes the key task of dementia care, yet we have seen that MSP is itself a product of a wider set of social/power relations and to improve 'it' would necessitate changing those relations – an enormous task!

Properly considered, MSP is, in fact, a general term that can be rephrased as 'the way that people with dementia are treated by others'. If this is acknowledged, we arrive at the simple, if somewhat more obvious, truth that the key task of dementia care is to improve 'the way that people with dementia are treated by others'. This is hardly a conceptual breakthrough and does not lead us to conclude that the work of Kitwood and the Bradford group is qualitatively different or more advanced than other attempts to bring person-centred principles and values to the work of dementia care. The aspect of their work which derives from social psychology may be viewed as their most distinctive, if their most theoretically vulnerable, feature.

When it comes to proposing guidance for improving the quality of dementia care, the Bradford group fall squarely into the approach of those attempting to bring the insights of the Rogerian tradition to bear on the world of dementia care.

Evaluating dementia care

Whilst their work on the social psychology, and 'personhood' may be described as interesting if, ultimately, unhelpful, the Bradford group have developed a person-centred method of assessing the quality of psychological care which is proving to be of great practical value.

Dementia Care Mapping (DCM), is based on extensive observation of the things that happen to a dementia sufferer over a 4–6 hour period. The coding system is devised to 'take the point of view of the person with dementia' and produces a 'dementia care quotient' which assists care staff by highlighting areas where improvement is required (Kitwood 1992). Users of the DCM method report that, when used sensitively, the evaluation it offers is perceived positively by staff and provides them with new insights into the way that care is experienced by those on the receiving end (e.g. Barnet 1993). Whilst necessarily both 'labour intensive' and time consuming, DCM appears to be the only quality assurance tool available that provides a person-centred picture of care, one that is able to enhance the insight of staff and bring about positive change in itself. This immediate benefit should more than compensate for the resources invested.

Communication

The other area of Kitwood's work which has important implications for practice is his account of the communication process (Kitwood 1993, p. 55). He rejects the 'morse code' model of communication which consists of a message that is encoded by a sender and conveyed via a signal which is then decoded by the person receiving the message. This model 'fails to do justice to the subtlety and fragility of the communicative act' and is rejected in favour of a detailed model of a reflexive triad which is illustrated below:

Person X
– (a) an individual with a given temperament, constitution, etc
– (b) carrying his or her unique legacy from past experience
– (c) in a particular sentient state (referring here to mood, emotion, feeling, etc.)
– (d) defines the situation in a certain way and
– (e) having various assumptions (about others' expectations, states, etc.)
– (f) and with certain desires, intentions, expectations etc., makes an action
Person Y
– (a, b, c, d, e)
Interprets Person X's action and (f) responds
Person X
Interprets Person Y's response and reflects, checking in various ways whether the acts he or she is trying to bring off with Person Y is likely to be successful.
(Kitwood 1993, p. 56)

When applied to dementia care, this model provides a useful guide to staff as to their role in the communicative process. At the very least they should recognise actions, utterances and gestures as attempts at communication which deserve a response, learning to treat people with dementia as having a communication disability. As with any other disability, the most helpful response of others is to offer compensatory behaviour which assists disabled people to achieve their goals. In this instance, the person with dementia is attempting a communicative action and the care worker, respecting (a) and (b), provides specific assistance by:

– (c) empathising with mood, emotion and feeling
– (d) defining the situation in a collaborative way and moving with X when that definition changes
– (f) assisting with the conversion of the desire or need into an intention
– sustaining X's action, by compensating for the memory deficit which is needed to carry it through.
(Kitwood 1993, p. 58)

The value of this analytic approach to interactions with dementia sufferers is that it provides a framework for others that is not over-prescriptive. Kitwood uses the analogy of a tennis coach whose task is to keep a rally going with a 'deeply discouraged older person'. As he points out, the attitude and skills of such a coach would bear little resemblance to those required by an average tennis coach.

Kitwood and other approaches

Kitwood's chief criticism of other therapies – reality orientation, reminiscence, validation, resolution and others – is that they define the 'problem' of dementia as residing with the dementing person and do not acknowledge that 'we', the therapist or carer, come to the situation as part of the problem. Rather 'we' are seen as part of the potential solution to 'their' problem (Kitwood & Bredin 1992a).

Unlike psychotherapy and counselling, where it is acknowledged that we are, at least, a potential part of the problem (and thus require therapy ourselves to be able to function effectively as therapists), in dementia care there has been little acknowledgement of the fact that our own personality, behaviour and attitudes contribute to the 'problem' of dementia.

It can be argued that Kitwood is being somewhat unfair, certainly towards validation and resolution, in his classification of their approach, and that his own practical suggestions are no less 'us and them' than the approaches he criticises. More seriously, he is again confusing the wider, societal issue with the specifics of dementia care theory. It is not about the theorists of validation and resolution who problematise people with dementia; it is the way our society structures health care (or rather confuses health care with medical treatment), categorising patients as people with problems who seek out professionals with solutions. This is not a problem that is created by, nor can it be solved by, therapeutic approaches; it is rather a reflection of a social reality – the organisation of health care which is itself a construct of the wider society of which it is part. To posit an alternative theory will do nothing to alter this reality, the true causes of which extend far beyond the boundaries of that with which the theory is concerned.

This helps to explain the tendency of the Bradford group to describe abstract aspects, or characteristics, of good quality dementia care without having anything substantially new to recommend in terms of practice. There is much talk of attitude and little description of skill. When recommendations or illustrations of good practice are made (e.g. Kitwood & Bredin 1992b) they tend to reflect commonly held notions of good practice, communication skills, empathy and social sensitivity. Whilst there is little to disagree with, it is not an approach that is qualitatively different from others described in this chapter.

PRE-THERAPY

Finally we turn to consider the latest arrival on the scene, 'pre-therapy', which owes much to the adoption of ideas and practices developed in the field of learning disabilities by those involved in the dementia care. Wolfensberger's (1983) theory of social role valorisation (formally known as 'normalisation') is echoed in Kitwood's analysis of the social psychology of dementia sufferers, leading to the helpful conclusion that dementia should be categorised as a disability – with all the implications that carries for the struggle to establish and assert people's rights.

The use of sensory stimulation environments, especially for clients with profound communication difficulties, has also crossed into dementia care along with a range of 'complementary' therapies (aromatherapy, massage, drama and music therapy). The latest to cross the divide is pre-therapy, an approach which had earlier migrated to the field of learning disabilities – via the field of chronic psychosis – from the world of person-centred counselling. Unlike the approaches discussed earlier, in which person-centred principles were imported by people already concerned with dementia, pre-therapy represents an expedition which set off from the Rogerian tradition of person-centred counselling to chart new areas previously thought to be beyond the boundaries of its applicability. Initially used with 'psychotic retardates' and 'catatonic schizophrenics' as well as people with learning disabilities, its potential for use with people with dementia is, as yet, largely unexplored.

Pre-therapy was pioneered by Garry Prouty (1990) in the USA, who originally conceived it as being appropriate for those whose communication skills have potential for improvement – hence 'pre-therapy'. Prouty was motivated by a desire to make person-centred counselling available to those who appeared to lack the verbal skills and capacity for insight, without which it would not be possible to establish the 'psychological contact' that Rogers (1959) had identified as an essential condition of a therapeutic relationship. Rogers did not himself define what psychological contact is, or suggest how it may be created or repaired. Prouty suggests that psychological contact is made up of three elements ('contact functions'), which are enhanced by the therapist employing a set of five techniques ('contact reflections') (Prouty & Kubiak 1988, Lambers 1993). If successful, these techniques increase the frequency of 'contact behaviours'.

Levels of psychological contact

According to Prouty (1990), there are three levels of psychological contact: contact with the world, with self and with others.

Contact with the world. This is 'reality contact', awareness of facts, situations, people, environment and events. Contact with the world is enhanced by situational reflections which describe the present situation and environment. For example: 'It is very cool down here'; 'I can hear the children playing'; 'We've been quite a long time in this little room'. Contact behaviour involves the 'verbalisation of people, places, things and events'.

Contact with self. This is 'affective contact', awareness of own mood, feelings and emotions. Contact with self is enhanced by facial reflections in which the therapist states the emotion apparent in the client's facial expressions. For example: 'Your face looks scared'; 'Your eyes are big'; 'Little smile on your face'. Contact behaviour involves 'the expression of emotion', either verbally or non-verbally.

Contact with others. This is 'communicative contact' in which affective awareness and reality are communicated to others. Contact with others is enhanced by word-for-word reflections which pick out and repeat coherent phrases in confused or disordered speech. Contact behaviour involves 'the use of social language'.

The remaining two contact reflections are 'body reflections' and 'reiterative reflections'. Body reflections, either physically or verbally, reflect body movement, posture or state. They enhance all three contact functions. For example:

Client: (sits rubbing legs)

Therapist: 'You rub your legs.'

Client: (continues rubbing legs)

Therapist: (rubs own legs) 'You rub, I rub.' (Prouty 1990, p. 651).

Reiterative reflections re-use reflections which have previously been successful. For example: 'Before you pointed over there and said ... '.

Whilst none of Prouty's published work relates specifically to people with dementia, pre-therapy clearly has the potential to be adapted for use in this area. We might hope that the traditional identification of the client group of person-centred counselling as being verbally articulate and capable of 'insight' is largely a reflection of those who have had the social and financial resources necessary to access it. If this is so, adaptation of the principles of the therapeutic process to those who are experiencing increasing difficulties with communication may well be achievable.

CONCLUSION – WHICH WAY FORWARD?

Whatever the future of validation itself, its historical impact should not be underestimated. For 2 decades, reality orientation dominated the world of dementia care and, in the absence of any viable alternatives, came to be used regardless of the degree of cognitive deterioration. Validation therapy, along with reminiscence, became the most important additions to this paucity of approaches.

Above all, Feil's insistence that we listen to what the person with dementia is saying with the same respect we would give to anyone else has found a great resonance with the more progressive elements working in the field. She turned our attention to the experience of the dementia sufferer, and taught us to respect their viewpoint. Whatever our reservations about her work as a theoretician, her skills as a practitioner and communicator have added greatly to the repertoire of those who care for people with dementia.

Validation therapy and the other three approaches to dementia care outlined in this chapter are part of a wind of change which has grown in force over the past decade. Undoubtedly the demographic reality of an enormous increase in the numbers of people with dementia has added urgency to the creation of what Kitwood has described as the 'new culture of dementia care'. Kitwood's vision is of people with dementia being cared for by staff who have high levels of motivation, respect and empathic understanding.

The key question is how we enable that new culture to spread out to the army of carers – family, friends, volunteers and paid workers in the NHS, social services departments, and in the private sector. It is one thing for a new culture to spread amongst the conference-attending, journal-reading professionals and quite another for it to move into the places, and the cultures, in which people with dementia actually spend their time.

This is ultimately a practical problem, as is the other problem which prevents the person-centred ideals described here from having a real and demonstrable impact on the quality of life of significant numbers of people with dementia. By this I mean the problem of identifying and developing, through rigorous research, the most effective communication methods to combat the multiplicity of different barriers which dementia produces. Naomi Feil's attempt to describe the different communication techniques appropriate to the different 'stages' of disorientation may have been unsuccessful but she, at least, addressed the real problem. If we are to begin to create a therapeutic relationship with anyone who has dementia, we must first be able to identify and assess the particular obstacles to communication and then be sure that we are aware of the most effective methods available to overcome them. This will require extensive high quality research which, hitherto, has been noticeably lacking.

Needless to say, it will take more than improvements in the interpersonal and social milieu to raise the quality of care of people with dementia to an acceptable level. There is, for example, great scope for the further creation of prosthetic environments which could offset many of the disabilities which increase the need for psychological support. There is also the question of resources, human and financial, the absence of which will kill off any new culture before it has taken root.

In the final analysis, we have to acknowledge the extent to which we all need those personal relationships which sustain our sense of being part of a truly human world. When we develop dementia, we need them more than ever.

REFERENCES

Barnet E 1993 Observing care in detail – the DCM method. Alzheimer's Disease Society Newsletter July: 5
Bleathman C 1994 Personal communication
Butler R 1963 The life review: an intepretation of reminiscence in the aged. Psychiatry 26: 65–75
Collins English Dictionary 1986
Erikson E 1964 Insight and responsibility. Norton, New York
Feil N 1967 Group therapy in a home for the aged. The Gerontologist 7: 192–195
Feil N 1972 A new approach to group therapy. Unpublished paper presented to the 25th annual meeting of the Gerontological Society
Feil N 1978a Looking for yesterday (video). Feil Productions, Cleveland
Feil N 1978b Looking for yesterday (video): study guide. Feil Productions, Cleveland
Feil N 1982 V/F validation: the Feil method. Feil Productions, Cleveland
Feil N 1992a V/F validation: the Feil method, 2nd edn. Feil Productions, Cleveland
Feil N 1992b Validation therapy with late onset dementia populations. In: Jones G, Miesen B M L (eds) Care-giving in dementia. Routledge, London
Feil N 1993 The validation breakthrough. Health Professions Press, Baltimore
Goudie F, Stokes G 1989 Understanding confusion. Nursing Times 39: 35–37
Jung C G 1964 Man and his symbols. Doubleday, New York
Kitwood T 1990 The dialectics of dementia: with particular reference to Alzheimer's disease. Ageing and Society 10: 177–196
Kitwood T 1992 Quality assurance in dementia care. Geriatric Medicine September: 34–38
Kitwood T 1993 Towards a theory of dementia care: the interpersonal process. Ageing and Society 13: 51–67
Kitwood T, Bredin K 1992a Towards a theory of dementia care: personhood and well-being. Ageing and Society 12: 269–287
Kitwood T, Bredin K 1992b Person to person: a guide to the care of those with failing mental powers. Gale Centre Publications, Loughton
de Klerk-Rubin 1994 How validation is misunderstood. Journal of Dementia Care 2: 14–16
Lacey A R 1976 A dictionary of philosophy. Routledge and Kegan Paul, London
Lambers E 1993 Pre-therapy. Unpublished workshop handout. Jordanhill Counselling Unit, University of Strathclyde, Glasgow
Mearns D, Thorne B 1988 Person-centred counselling in action. Sage Publications, London
Morton I, Bleathman C 1991 The effectiveness of validation therapy in dementia – a pilot study. International Journal of Geriatric Psychiatry 6: 327–330
Prouty G 1990 Pre-therapy: a theoretical evolution in the person-centered/experiential psychotherapy of schizophrenia and retardation. In: Lietaer G, Rombauts R, Van Balen R Client-centered and experiential pychotherapy in the nineties. Leuvan University Press
Prouty G, Kubiak H 1988 The development of communicative contact with a catatonic schizophrenic. Journal of Communication Therapy 1: 13–20
Rogers C 1959 A theory of therapy, personality and interpersonal relationships as developed in the client-centered framework. In: Koch S (ed) Psychology: a study of a science. McGraw Hill, New York
Wolfensberger W 1983 Social role valorisation: a proposed new term for the principle of normalization. Mental Retardation 21: 234–239

RECOMMENDED READING

Bleathman C, Morton I 1992 Validation therapy: extracts from twenty groups with dementia sufferers. Journal of Advanced Nursing 17: 658–666. *This article describes in some detail the extent to which people with a significant degree of impairment resulting from dementia can be helped to become involved, animated, articulate and even orientated when brought together in validation groups. Group members' enjoyment becomes manifest from the extended verbatim extracts from the transcript of recorded conversation.*

Feil N 1967 Group therapy in a home for the aged. The Gerontologist 7: 192–195. *One of Feil's earliest articles highlights the extent to which her development of validation therapy grew out of her rejection of reality orientation and its replacement with a person-centred approach to people who suffer from dementia.*

Feil N 1992a V/F validation: the Feil method, 2nd edn. Feil Productions, Cleveland. *This book contains the most thorough account of the theory and practice behind validation therapy. Feil's four stages of disorientation model is explained along with helpful techniques for working with people at each stage.*

Feil N 1992b Validation therapy with late onset dementia populations. In: Jones G, Miesen B M L (eds) Care-giving in dementia. Routledge, London. *In this article Feil attempts to harmonise her own four-stage model of disorientation with a more orthodox diagnostic classification of the dementing process.*

Feil N 1993 The validation breakthrough. Health Professions Press, Baltimore. *In addition to restating the principles of validation therapy, this book contains a wealth of anecdotal examples of its use with people at each of the four stages of disorientation. These highlight Feil's status as a great practitioner and as an innovator in developing communication with people with dementia.*

Goudie F, Stokes G 1989 Understanding confusion. Nursing Times 39: 35–37. *The authors argue for an application of Rogerian counselling techniques when working with people with dementia. Examples are given to illustrate how apparently confused speech and behaviour might contain concealed meanings and attempts to make known emotional needs.*

Kitwood T 1990 The dialectics of dementia: with particular reference to Alzheimer's disease. Ageing and Society 10: 177–196. *This excellent article argues convincingly in favour of a theory of dementia which moves beyond the traditional 'medical model' account and demonstrates how the reactions of those around the person with dementia can play a part in the dementing process. The author gives an acutely observed account of the 'malignant social psychology' which we create around people with dementia and which provides the theoretical starting point for Kitwood's person-centred approach to dementia care.*

Kitwood T, Bredin K 1992 Person to person: a guide to the care of those with failing mental powers. Gale Centre Publications, Loughton. *This book is a practical and clearly written guide to the application of Kitwood's principles to everyday care practice. It is targeted at care assistants, family carers and others who are closely involved with people with dementia.*

Kitwood T 1993 Towards a theory of dementia care: the interpersonal process. Ageing and Society 13: 15–67. *This article contains a model of the communicative process which moves beyond simplistic 'morse code' analogies and emphasises the subtlety, complexity and fragility of everyday communication. The author then applies this model to people whose communication abilities are impaired by dementia and demonstrates the most helpful position that carers can adopt in facilitating successful communication.*

Prouty G 1990 Pre-therapy: a theoretical evolution in the person-centred/experiential psychotherapy of schizophrenia and retardation. In: Lietaer G, Rombauts R, Van Balen R Client-centered and experiential psychotherapy in the nineties. Leuvan University Press. *The theoretical basis of pre-therapy and its links with the main body of Rogerian thought are outlined. Pre-therapy techniques are described and illustrated by examples. There is discussion of the results of 2 years of pre-therapy with a single client.*

22

Approaches to reminiscence

Joanna Bornat

This chapter begins with a quotation from Dobroff (1984), who is remembering the impact of a particular piece of writing – *The Life Review: An Interpretation of Reminiscence in the Aged*, by Butler (1963), a US psychogeriatrician. I quote from Dobroff's article at some length because of its importance on a number of counts. Though it was written in the mid 1980s and describes experiences on the other side of the Atlantic, it neatly and dramatically illustrates some key themes relating to reminiscence work in Britain which I will be developing in this chapter:

Perhaps tape recorders and word-processing machines are to the spoken word what the phonograph is to music: they make it possible for us to preserve the voices of our mothers and fathers telling us the history of their times. Technology expands the possibilities, and interest rises with the dawning recognition of the possibilities. In the field of aging, interest began with the publication in 1963 of a seminal paper by Dr Robert Butler ... It is not often that one paper has so important and immediate an effect. I was then a very junior social worker on the staff of a home for the aged. I remember well being taught by our consulting psychiatrists and the senior social work staff about the tendency of our residents to talk about childhood in the shtetls of East Europe or arrival at Ellis Island or early years on the Lower East Side of New York. At best, this tendency was seen as an understandable, although not entirely healthy preoccupation with happier times, understandable because these old and infirm people walked daily in the shadow of death. At worst 'living in the past' was viewed as pathology – regression to the dependency of the child, denial of the passage of time and the reality of the present, or evidence of organic impairment of the intellect.

It was even said that remembrance of things past could cause or deepen depression among our residents, and God forgive us, we were to divert the old from reminiscing through activities like bingo and arts and crafts.

And then the Butler paper came out and was read and talked about and our world changed. The Life Review became not only a normal activity; it was seen as a therapeutic tool ... In a profound sense, Butler's writings liberated both the old and the nurses, doctors and social workers; the old were free to remember, to regret, to look reflectively at the past and try to understand it. And we were free to listen and to treat rememberers and remembrances with the respect they deserved, instead of trivializing them by diversion to a bingo game.

(Dobroff 1984, pp. xvii–xviii)

Talking to long-experienced staff members in health and social care it is often possible to hear a similar watershed experience being described. There was a time, 15 or 20 years or more ago now, when reminiscence or reminiscence work as it has commonly come to be known was not regarded as an acceptable activity. Older staff will remember, like Rose Dobroff, that they were expected to discourage or distract the older people in their care from talking about the past. Some found it very difficult to stick to this prohibition. They knew that many older people, like people from any age group, enjoy talking about the past. They also knew that they themselves enjoyed listening to stories and accounts of past times which were irretrievably lost. One such person was Susan Hale, a psychiatric social worker who, in 1960, wrote how she had become 'quick to spy out possible openings, a give away testimonial or framed photograph on the wall, a presentation clock, a pair of clogs or a case of tropical butterflies, and one sits on tenterhooks manoeuvring to get the conversation round to them.' (Hale 1960, p. 153).

Of course those older workers also remember people whose memories were painful and upsetting. Looking back now it seems cruel to expect that pain and guilt should have to be silently endured in isolation. Again Rose Dobroff recalls how sharing those feelings could help to relieve painful memories. Speaking of a man who blamed himself for the deaths of his wife and daughter in the Holocaust because however hard he worked in the 1920s, he had not been able to save enough money to pay for their fares from Poland to New York, she observes: 'How could anyone understand his pain and try to find an anodyne for it if his story remained private, isolated from the history of the pogroms of the late 1800s and the immigrants' experiences, including their failures, in the New World?' (Dobroff 1984, p. xix).

The memories of older workers are witness to a profound change in thinking about the part which the past plays in the lives of older people. Elsewhere I have called this a 'social transformation' (Bornat 1989, p. 16) because the changes in attitude and in practice were sweeping and dramatic and involved a broad swathe of people caring and working with older people.

Rose Dobroff's (1984) memories of the changes she witnessed provide us with our first focus in this chapter, the emergence of a distinct set of practices which are described as reminiscence work. In the first section we trace the emergence of the idea of reminiscence with older people and its subsequent development; in particular we look at research findings. Mention of a 'therapeutic tool' takes us into the second section where we weigh up the issues in the debate about reminiscence as therapy. The quotation given at the beginning of the chapter (Dobroff 1984, pp. xvii–xviii) also provides us with a key to the next section: identifying contexts for reminiscence work with older people.

Susan Hale's (1960) account provides us with a lead into the fourth section: a review of methodologies. She recalls some of the objects which the older people she met kept by them and how these could evoke memories. In this section we review the different types of stimuli and themes which may be used to encourage reminiscence: not only objects, but sounds, smells and images. In the fifth section we look at different ways of working with reminiscence: in one-to-one and in group settings. Again, Rose Dobroff's (1984) account provides us with a lead when she mentions the need to share painful memories. In this section we evaluate some varied approaches to group work.

The final sections take us further than these quotations, mainly because they relate to issues which have emerged more recently. In the penultimate section we look at specialised work which has developed with older people with special needs. In this section we focus on people with a dementing illness and who have learning difficulties. In the last section we look at ways to improve and support good practice in reminiscence work through training, and discuss the contribution of reminiscence to a number of practice areas in health and social care.

THE RECOGNITION AND DEVELOPMENT OF IDEAS ABOUT REMINISCENCE

I have laid much emphasis on the impact of one person's contribution to a change in thinking about reminiscence. It is certainly the case that Butler's paper in 1963, with its focus on life review as a ' ... naturally occurring, universal mental process characterised by the progressive return to consciousness of past experiences, and, particularly, the resurgence of unresolved conflicts ...' (Butler 1963, p. 66) did much to assert a key role for remembering in a re-evaluation of relationships between psychological processes and old age. Butler's suggestion that life review is a normal part of human mental activity, but with particular significance at later stages in life, helped to initiate debates and research which increasingly looked at old age in more positive and sympathetic terms. The idea that older people faced a certain inescapable existential issue – death, loss, finitude – was increasingly seen by some psychologists as generating particular mental strategies.

Erik Erikson's theory that individuals pass through a series of developmental stages of psychosocial development was particularly important in debates which highlighted the contribution of life review to later life: 'Part of the old-age process of reviewing the sense of oneself across the life-cycle involves a coming to terms with perceived mistakes, failures and omissions – with chances missed and opportunities not taken.' (Erikson et al 1986, p. 141).

Many of the early studies in the 1960s and 1970s sought to validate Butler's theory that life review is a necessary part of successful ageing. McMahon and Rhudick's (1964) study of veterans of the Spanish–American war, for example, found a group of men who were well-adjusted psychologically and who were actively engaged in reminiscence. Lewis (1971), again studying a group of older men, found that reminiscence provided a possible support against threats to present views of self. Kiernat (1979) studied a group of nursing home residents who were mainly women and found that behaviour changed favourably during an opportunity to engage in life review. Lewis and Butler (1974), reporting on life review work with individuals and groups, suggested that life review helps older people to establish meaning in their lives.

Haight, in reviews of the literature (1991, 1992, 1995), suggests that nurses were amongst the first to report on positive research findings in relation to life review in clinical settings. In some cases, nurses pointed to the way in which life review enhanced group processes (Burnside 1978), while Ebersole (1976) and Safier (1976) suggested that life review offered itself as a means to promote self-understanding, to reinforce coping mechanisms and to organise thoughts, feelings and experience more meaningfully.

Early enthusiasm and conviction was informed by two important developments: evaluation and classification. While some of the early and subsequent studies, often experimental in design and using volunteer subjects, showed positive outcomes from exposure to reminiscence stimuli or to encouragement to reminisce, others were more ambiguous. For example Fallot (1980), in an experiment which compared two groups of women over and under 65, found no evidence that reminiscence had an especially

adaptive function for older people. Perrotta & Meacham (1981) assessed the value of reminiscing as a therapeutic intervention amongst older people in a New York day centre. They found no evidence that reminiscing, as a short-term intervention, had an effect on either depression or self-esteem. Brennan & Steinberg (1984), looking for a way to link reminiscence positively to morale and social activity levels, found no correlation amongst the 40 older women they studied at a 'senior centre'. In conflict with disengagement theory they conclude that there was no evidence that 'the elderly substitute reminiscence for reduced opportunities or desire for social interaction' (Brennan & Steinberg 1984, p. 108).

The fact that studies might conflict or be inconclusive has been noted by a number of observers. Thornton & Brotchie (1987), in an often-quoted critical evaluation of the empirical literature, drew three rather damning conclusions: that the role of reminiscence cannot be seen, contrary to Butler's proposition, as specifically functional to the lives of older people, that reminiscence cannot be shown to have any therapeutic value beyond use as a diversionary activity and that there is no clear evidence as to the function of reminiscence in terms of personal or social adjustment.

Despite or because of such criticism, researchers interested in reminiscence have responded by acknowledging conflicting and unclear concepts and findings. For example, Merriam (1989) argues:

Inconclusive findings across approximately two dozen data-based studies of reminiscence may in part be due to different conceptualizations of the phenomenon. Some studies specifically focus on an evaluative reminiscence (the life review), while others do not differentiate life review from other forms. Other areas of confusion have to do with whether reminiscence prompted by the researcher is the same as spontaneous reminiscence, and whether oral or silent, interpersonal or intrapersonal ... forms make a difference.   (Merriam 1989, p. 762)

Partly in response to an awareness of conflicting and, in some cases, negative findings, some researchers have sought clarification through classifications of reminiscence activity. In an early paper, Coleman (1974) put forward the suggestion that there might be three different types:

- simple reminiscence, in which recall of the past provides a source of strength and esteem in the present
- informative reminiscence, where recall of the past is used as a way to pass on knowledge
- life review, which involves 'analysing memories of one's life to integrate a proper image of oneself in the face of death' (Coleman 1974, p. 283).

Watt & Wong (1991) argue that discrepancies in findings stem from researchers having 'treated reminiscence as a unidimensional construct ... [assuming] ... a simple and linear relationship between reminiscence and wellbeing'. They suggest the need for greater realism and to 'conceptualise reminiscence as a multi-dimensional construct, with each dimension serving a unique psychological function and bearing a different relationship with wellbeing' (Watt & Wong 1991, p. 40). They propose a taxonomy of six major types (see Box 22.1).

Watt & Wong argue that their classification has value in both research and therapeutic terms. We come back to the question of reminiscence as therapy in the second section, meanwhile we conclude this section by looking at research which has helped to further refine our ideas about the part played by reminiscence and recall in later life.

One of the main problems which researchers have faced is the observation and measurement of reminiscence as an activity. Most researchers have kept to a strictly experimental design in which a group of people, usually captive as residents in a home or visitors to a day centre, or volunteers invited to a laboratory setting, are subjected to some kind of stimulus to reminiscence. Measurements of, for example, mood, depression, cognition, self-esteem, ego integrity, have then been made before and after the introduction of the stimulus. The problem with this type of research is that it cannot match the natural surroundings in which people live their lives, nor can it allow for changes over time.

Some researchers have divided groups of subjects into age groups to see if the role played by reminiscence changes as people age. Here again there are difficulties. There is the effect of cohort. Elder (1982) in his study of people who lived through the Depression in Oakland, California, suggested that particular historical events and experiences stay with an age group, giving it particular characteristics. In England, Victor (1987) suggests, in a study of take up of welfare benefits, that older people's evaluation of their standard of living tends to be related to their experience early in life, rather than prevailing standards today. And of course, between the ages of 60 and 90 there may be more than one cohort experience.

Another problem arises from the fact that before and after studies, and even observation studies in naturalistic settings, tend only to cover a short period of time. Few studies have been able to show what part reminiscence plays over a number of years.

Finally there is the issue of subjectivity and experience. Most of the experimentally designed projects have tended to focus on older people as objects of research, few have been drawn into the process or have been invited to reflect on their own feelings as part of the research.

All these limitations suggested a need for a longitudinal study which might provide insights into the part played by reminiscence as people age. Coleman's (1986) study of 27 women and 23 men living in sheltered accommodation in the London borough of Camden, whom he visited and talked to over a period of 15 years, more than met this need. His account is richly illustrated by the reminiscences of the people he talked to; however, its greatest strength lies in the theory which he developed from the accounts he heard. While earlier researchers had focused on the process, he focused on the people, drawing the conclusion that reminiscence was not, as Butler and Erikson had claimed, always an acceptable or welcome experience. Analysing his data enabled him to draw up a typology (Table 22.1).

Coleman's work was important for its recognition that reminiscence can be a painful and unwelcome mental activity. Nurses, community workers, social care staff and others are aware of this and, in training sessions, frequently seek guidance. Acknowledging the

---

Box 22.1 Watt and Wong's taxonomy of six major types of reminiscence (Adapted from Watt and Wong 1991)

Integrative, where the main function is 'to achieve a sense of meaning, coherence and reconciliation with regard to one's past'.

Instrumental, which involves 'drawing on past experiences to help solve a present problem, and recalling past efforts in coping with difficult situations'.

Transmissive, where 'the reminiscer passes on to a younger generation some enduring values and wisdoms which s/he has acquired, growing up in a different era'.

Narrative, defined as 'descriptive or factual accounts of the past for the purpose of providing biographical information ... for the pleasure of the audience or the narrator'.

Escapist, where 'reminiscence takes on the tone of fantasy/daydreaming as the reminiscer dwells on the good old days as a means of escaping from a gloomy present'.

Obsessive, which may be 'indicative of the individual's failure to integrate certain problematic past experiences'.

Table 22.1   Coleman's types of attitudes to reminiscence and related morale

Reminiscers	Value memories of past (n = 21)	High morale
	Troubled by memories of past (n = 8)	Low morale
Non-reminiscers:	See no point in reminiscing (n = 15)	High morale
	Have to avoid because of contrast between past and present (n = 6)	Low morale

(Coleman 1986, p. 37)

existence of painful memories and of avoidance of the past has become a focal point for preparation for reminiscence work. However, his work is also important for the emphasis it places on the present. And here we come back again to disengagement theory. 15 of the people Coleman studied saw no point in reminiscing. As he put it 'not reminiscing can be purposeful because there are better things to do' (Coleman 1986, p. 37).

As we have seen, apart from Coleman's longitudinal study, much of the evaluation of reminiscence as a normal human activity has tended to be restricted to experimentally designed interventions. Recently, social gerontologists and some psychologists have begun to focus on the relevance of the context in which reminiscing takes place and to look at the particular role which reminiscing plays in social relationships in particular settings. An early study by Lieberman and Falk (1971) compared reminiscence amongst three separate groups: people living in their own homes, people who were about to be moved into residential care and a third group who were already established as residents in a home for older people. They found that the group which spent most time reminiscing were the middle group who were about to face changes in their lives. Lieberman and Falk's focus was not so much the different effect of the settings so much as the use which people made of reminiscence in their different circumstances. In fact they were unable to show that there was any relationship between the stress of moving and later adaptation to change.

More recently, researchers have begun to explore issues raised by differences in settings and older people's use of reminiscence and references to the past in managing their daily social interactions and relationships. Analysing the verbal interactions of older people, both in reminiscence-based conversation and in unstructured conversation, researchers such as Boden and Bielby (1983) and Buchanan and Middleton (1995) suggest that the past plays a key role for older people both in relation to conversation management and the presentation of identity.

Understanding the importance of setting and context was a motivation in a research project which I carried out with nursing colleagues in traditionally designed continuing care wards in an East Midlands hospital. By interviewing a number of frail older women, patients in the wards, and then by talking to them about what details of their lives they would like to have included in a life story book, it quickly became obvious that each woman had more than one narrative to relate, a public and a private narrative. Moreover, as researchers we became aware that certain women we spoke to were keen to recall particular types of experience; evidence we argue that what is remembered is affected very much by context (Bornat & Middleton 1994).

Issues of context are raised critically by Wallace (1992) in a review of Butler's theories of the life review. Wallace argues that since older people may sense their inequality in relation to money, education and physical abilities, 'it is understandable that personal experiences of the past might become an essential part of their contribution to present social interactions'. Reminiscing, he argues, should therefore be viewed not as a 'psychodevelopmental explanation' but in terms of 'social processes' (Wallace 1992, p. 124).

Gubrium and Wallace (1990) suggest the possibility that exhortations to reminisce may lead to older people seeking to meet the needs of younger people or researchers by looking for cues as to how to tell their stories. In analysing life history interviews they noted that older people often seemed uncertain where to begin and what they should include. This led to different accounts being provided depending on the cues supplied by the interviewer. Biggs' (1993) concern is that this might mean that older people are less able to 'define their own experience' and more likely to comply with nostalgia or a younger generation's perception of the past (Biggs 1993, p. 64).

I introduce these debates and discussions at this stage as part of the scene setting for reminiscence work. Enthusiastic reminiscence work has brought about many positive experiences for older people and those involved in their support and care. However, we need to be aware of the fact that the processes we engage in may be complex, and may bring about results which we may not have anticipated. An awareness of the interaction of the many factors which lead to the generation of recall and memory is a necessary accompaniment of sensitive and appropriate approaches to reminiscence work.

Summary

In this first section we have traced the emergence of thinking about reminiscence amongst psychologists and social gerontologists. We have looked at the way reminiscence has been researched and at some of the findings in relation to discussions about the function of reminiscence in later life. We then looked at the ways in which researchers have begun to organise and distinguish types of reminiscence. Finally we looked at some recent critiques of more psychological approaches to reminiscence and the development of research into the social meanings and uses of the ways people recall the past in old age.

IS REMINISCENCE THERAPY?

As reminiscence-type activities developed their own typical formats and following there was a growing tendency to describe these as constituting a 'therapy'. In this section we look at this claim and review the position which most practitioners have more recently developed.

As we have already seen, claims for the proven ability of reminiscence-based interventions to bring about positive change have not been sustained by research evidence. Thornton and Brotchie's (1987) severe judgement is that 'while reminiscence is undoubtedly a useful and enjoyable activity for elderly persons and care staff in clinical and residential settings, claims for its therapeutic value, except in the most general sense, are largely unsubstantiated' (Thornton & Brotchie 1987, p. 102).

Where does this leave the enthusiastic practitioner who is keen to develop skills and to take part in what is understood to be an established practice and even a 'social transformation'? (Bornat 1989, p. 16).

A possible answer is to distinguish the work that a psychologist does from the work of a reminiscence facilitator or group leader by identifying the former as life review therapy and the latter as reminiscence work. Garland, a psychologist who specialises in work with older people and who uses life review therapy, defines it as, 'a pervasive theme in psychotherapies which work towards a client achieving 'insight' in developing

a more varied and useful set of models for the interpretation and understanding of experience' (Garland 1993, p. 22).

Another psychologist, Norris (1989), well known for his writing on reminiscence themes drawn from clinical experience, suggests that a reminiscence-based approach can combine well with what he describes as 'insight based psychotherapy'. He suggests that older people may find it helpful too if they are encouraged to identify ways in which they were able to deal with stressful situations earlier in life. However, he stresses that, 'It is important ... to ensure that some account is taken not just of the historical chronicle of events but also of how these events are perceived by the individual at the time and in retrospect'. Another helpful combination, he points out, is in bereavement counselling when, for example, someone is unable to express their feelings for reasons of denial or depression. He suggests: 'Reviewing events surrounding the loss of a significant person with a focus on the feelings associated with those events may be helpful in providing the necessary release from the delayed grief process'. He also suggests that combining a reminiscence-based approach with cognitive therapeutic treatment of depression may help to 'challenge the chain of automatic thoughts which result in the person viewing themselves with low self-esteem'. Even with more behaviourist approaches to psychotherapy he argues for a role for reminiscence. For example, a more holistic understanding of an individual generated through an account of their lifestyle, values and background may help to manage behaviours which may appear disruptive to staff but which are rooted in a long-term pattern of life. Norris gives the example of a baker who 'wakes everyone on his ward at three in the morning' (1989, pp. 27–28).

Burnside (1990), a US nurse researcher, has devised a useful table which distinguishes life review from reminiscence work (see Table 22.2).

Psychologists working with older people seem to have few concerns as to the therapeutic value of a life review approach. Garland (1993), in a review of clinical approaches, focuses on what he feels should be the outcomes from successful life review therapy. These are, for the client, the enhancement of 'a sense of being in control of one's own life; understanding self in relation to others; and enjoyment of life' (Garland 1993, p. 31).

What we have been describing so far are strategies which a qualified professional such as a clinical psychologist might adopt when working psycho-therapeutically with people who have been designated as 'clients', and where outcomes are defined in terms

Table 22.2 Burnside's table of reminiscence versus life review (From Issues in Mental Health Nursing 1980, 11: 37, Burnside I, Hemisphere Publishing, Washington. Reproduced with permission. All rights reserved.)

	Characteristics	Qualities of therapist
Reminiscence (supportive)	Do not increase anxiety Reinforce life decision	Psychosocial Astute clinical skills
	Reinforce lifestyle	Sound judgement
	Do not dwell on losses Strategies of leader are ego-supportive	Understand short-term and long-term memory
Life review (uncovering)	Insight Reworking Working through Tolerate anxiety Transference Counter transference	Psychoanalytic Specific education Understand defence mechanism Understand human developmental stages

of personal change and growth in response to specific need.

This chapter is not directed at the reader who is already qualified as a professional clinical psychologist. It starts from a position that the reader has an interest in reminiscence work with older people and has a general sympathy with and understanding of the lives of older people. It is written with the conviction, however, that reminiscence and life review need to be undertaken with an awareness of the possible outcomes for individuals who take part, either in one-to-one sessions, or more commonly, in group settings. A conscious awareness of negative outcomes for some people, or of the possibility that unresolved grief and pain may be stirred up by quite unpredictable cues or stimuli, is an essential part of the range of sensitive strategies which workers should have ready. In answer to the question, 'Can reminiscence groups be run by untrained staff?' Bender responds 'Yes'. However, he qualifies this by insisting on six preconditions for successful group work, including the need for 'a competent supervisor' and 'sufficient time for supervision' (Bender 1993, p. 43).

Bender lays great stress on the need for groups to work to declared outcomes and with leaders who have an awareness of group dynamics. He argues that anyone who does not feel competent to handle all the possible outcomes of group reminiscence or who has had no training in psychotherapeutic techniques should, of necessity, have access to supervision or support from someone who is so skilled or trained. Painful memories of the past may stir up emotions which someone may feel unable to deal with and which neither the group members or the group leader can help with. In such a situation, it is important to know who to ask for help with professional skills, or to whom to refer for advice.

Of course it is also true that expressing unhappy feelings may be helpful to someone who has been dealing with feelings of grief or guilt on their own for years, as Rose Dobroff experienced. The case example below (Box 22.2) is an interesting and moving example of how unexpected emotions may be provoked and, in this case, it seems offered a sympathetic response.

Box 22.2 Responding to an older man's feelings of bitterness and abandonment (From Bornat 1989, p. 23)

Freda Millett is an oral historian who was researching the history of children's homes in Oldham by interviewing older people who had lived there as children or who had worked there during the early decades of the 20th century. In common with other oral historians in interview situations, she found herself confronting bitterness and resentment when she interviewed one elderly man. Freda was struck by the degree of control which Boards of Guardians held over the lives of children and parents. The man she spoke to was in his eighties and had lived in one of these homes. He had only the memory of a young woman who visited him until he was 3. He had one postcard from Australia signed 'mother' and quite late in life heard that his mother had left him a bungalow in Australia in her will. He was bitter and felt all his life that he had been abandoned. Freda's work with the records of the Board of Guardians and her interviews with staff and children helped her to be able to convince this man that his mother had quite probably been unable to go against the powers of the Guardians. Her apparent abandonment was an unwilling act. It was Freda Millett's sensitive work which helped him, late in life, to finally overcome some of his bitter feelings towards his mother.

What is interesting about the case example in Box 22.2 is the way it illustrates a number of issues. It serves as a reminder, should this be necessary, that older people like anyone else may experience powerful and varied emotions and that although some may have been repressed, others may be constantly experienced. It also shows that the resources that a reminiscence worker or facilitator may need to have at hand, or be aware of, may be more than those commonly associated with the roles of health or social care workers. In this case, familiarity with the local history archive proved the key to a helpful approach.

Summary

In this section we have reviewed the reasons for and claims about reminiscence as therapy. While clinical psychologists appear to be clear about the therapeutic contribution of reminiscence, it is important that unskilled practitioners are aware of outcomes which may be unwelcome, or painful to participants in reminiscence group work or one-to-one work. At the same time, amongst the skills which a group leader needs, is an awareness of who to ask for support, should problems arise and a recognition that amongst the people they will be working with there will be a wide variety of different experience.

CONTEXTS FOR REMINISCENCE WORK

So far we have looked at some of the debates about the contribution which reminiscence work can make to the lives of older people. We now want to move on to look at some of the different contexts in which reminiscence activities, one-to-one and group work, may be organised. Evidence from the field and the literature suggests that reminiscence activities may be organised wherever older people happen to be! Examples are cited of work in day centres, residential homes, in wards, in both acute and continuing care settings, at home in the community, in clubs and groups and in sheltered accommodation. Within such different settings reminiscence work can clearly play a variety of roles, contributing to a sense of social solidarity, to assessment of need, to care planning and to the development of an awareness of individual worth and value. In what follows we look at four different types of context for reminiscence work, outlining possible objectives and outcomes for each setting. We look at nursing settings, residential care, clubs and people's own homes.

Nursing settings

Although much of the documented reminiscence work in nursing settings has taken place on hospital wards, usually in what is known as continuing care or rehabilitation, this section has been broadened to include other settings. The closure of continuing care wards in many UK National Health Service hospitals and trusts means that much of the nursing care of frail older people is now taking place in private or voluntary aided nursing homes. Research published in 1993 showed that the proportion of NHS-funded residents as a proportion of all people in long-term settings had declined from 28% in 1970 to 12% in 1992 (Laing 1993).

Despite the variety in the types of setting in which nurses may be working these days, there are still likely to be certain characteristics both in terms of objectives and the older people they will be caring for. Many nurses, and observers of nursing practice (Evers 1981, Adams 1988, Thompson 1989, McKenzie 1991), argue that recall of the past is a normal part of communication with older patients. However, there is also evidence that this will tend to be spasmodic and possibly directed mainly to those people who are considered most likely to respond (Evers 1981).

Reminiscence work in nursing settings may be amongst the most challenging to be tackled. Traditionally these are areas with low skill levels and low morale amongst nursing staff, who frequently operate with outdated and traditional nursing routines which have changed little over the last four decades (Nolan & Grant 1993). Moreover, older people living in continuing care nursing settings are more likely to be characterised by high levels of physical and mental frailty (Age Concern England 1990, Wade et al 1983).

What then might reminiscence activities seek to achieve in a nursing setting? Writing about the work of the Reminiscence Project in Manchester, Sim (1991) suggests that it may be a question of changing practices which focus more on nursing routines than on opportunities for choice and social interaction amongst patients. Nurses who have become part of the project, working in the wards, have sometimes been criticised for spending too much time talking to patients. He explains: 'We've also had hostility from the "old school" who believe that hospitals are meant to be functional and not places where you have fun' (Sim 1991, p. 8). Nurses who have taken part in the Reminiscence Project have found ways to challenge the physical environment of the ward. One nurse who became a link worker at Ladywell Hospital in Manchester described some of the outcomes which they had achieved:

Our ward was a typical Nightingale Ward: drab walls, drab curtains and old lockers by the bed. But we've transformed it. Now we've got pictures on the wall, and a stained glass window in the day room. The patients helped us make table clothes for the tables and we replaced the plastic cups with china ones. The whole feeling of the place has changed ... Before, the patients used to sit and stare at the walls for most of the day. But thanks to all the activities we've been arranging they know each other's first names and they talk to each other. The Reminiscence Project has changed my whole view of the job – I see the patients as my friends now.

(Sim 1991, p. 8)

This example illustrates a whole range of possible outcomes: environmental, social and work-related. Seeking ways to improve levels of esteem, motivation and commitment in an area of health care which possibly has a low value professionally amongst nurses, is a particularly important outcome for reminiscence work.

Nightingale-style wards and traditionally hierarchical approaches to nursing may be less common these days, however the problem of how to individualise care is one which is shared across settings. Some approaches focus on a checklist of items which relate to current preferences and biographical details; for example, 'Have you ever done this activity: art appreciation, politics, arts and crafts activities, music, gardening' and 'name, maiden name, birth date, birth place, languages spoken', etc. (Jones 1992, pp. 107–109, p. 155, O'Donovan 1993). However, such listings, though clearly a useful resource, may do little on their own to change patterns of social interaction, attitudes and motivation. Nor does it facilitate patient control over, or ownership of, what has been generated. The case study in Box 22.3 illustrates an alternative approach.

It is interesting to note how nurses draw on the life story books as a resource for communication. Potentially this should provide a base for semi-formal integration of the patients' biographies into their care planning and management. Certainly this might be an advance on current systems which have been developed in relation to the more medicalised and reductionist approach to delivering and recording care via the nursing process (Adams et al 1996).

Box 22.3 Creating life story books for continuing care

In research carried out in an East Midlands hospital one of our objectives was to find ways in which biographical information might contribute to care planning and management. From participant observation and interviews with members of the nursing staff it was clear that although some of the nurses were familiar with the life stories of patients who were most able to communicate verbally, this knowledge did not easily translate into choices and options for the patients living on the wards. We looked for ways to make the patients' biographies more visible and more easily communicated to all the nurses who worked on these wards. We used a mixture of reminiscence sessions in groups with one-to-one interviews. From these we produced text and pictures. The words were the patients' own and the images were a collection of photocopied family photographs and pictures selected because they related to particular patients' backgrounds and experiences. For example, one patient was fond of animals, another had grown up in the West Country. Their life story books included pictures of dogs and cats and cuttings from tourist brochures describing Somerset and Avon. Our aim was to develop a method which was acceptable to patients and their relatives and which could easily be copied and developed by members of the nursing staff.

The life story books were assembled into attractive scrapbooks and patients were asked where they would like to keep them. Here a problem arose since patients had so little personal space. Most chose to hang them on the end of their beds or to keep them on the top of their bedside cabinets. The nurses were asked to evaluate the contribution of the life story books.

Nurses responded to questions, saying for example: 'I think the patients benefit from this because they are able to talk and reminisce about what went on in their lives and also the staff understand what the patients are talking about' and, 'Knowing what they have been through in the past helps in caring for them'. Asked if they thought the life stories might cause potential problems some responded: 'Looking back on the past may make them sentimental' and, '"Muriel" was very very upset, it brought back that she was here and wanted to go home. For some it may remind them they no longer have homes, their bit of independence, their own world, furniture, ornaments, sadly we haven't got the room to keep'.

Nurses were also asked if they could think of an example from their own experience where knowing about the patient's life story helped to care for her. One nurse responded, 'Yes, lots of times gives a lot of insight into how you approach a patient, areas in conversation to talk or not to talk about; insight into "spiritual needs". Knowledge of family background is always important re Holistic base'.

(Contributed by Joanna Bornat, John Adams, Mary Prickett)

Day centres, classes and clubs

Older people living in the community, in their own homes, may often make their own way to clubs, or be offered places in day centres. For whatever reason they may well be mixing with other people for short periods of time and for a variety of reasons. They may attend a luncheon club purely for social reasons or they may be offered a day centre place as a way to provide respite for carers who are family members or neighbours. Reminiscence activities may provide opportunities for socialising, a means of identifying individual needs and preferences and ways to draw on skills and knowledge.

Centres and clubs may have their own raison d'être, objectives and programmes. Reminiscence may be planned into the life of such forms of provision or it may emerge as groups coalesce or seek a purpose or project to engage in. At a lunch club in West London, older people from the Afro-Caribbean community were involved in reminiscence sessions which ultimately resulted in a publication, *Nice Tastin': Life and Food in the Caribbean* (Bartlett 1991). Choosing the topic 'food' led to discussions about rearing animals, growing and marketing crops and preparing food for occasions like weddings and funerals. Members of the group visited a local school where, as Bartlett, the group's coordinator explains, they took part in a 'carefully organised programme of activities which included art, craft, storytelling, cooking, songs, games and dances [and] they passed on some of their knowledge of the culture of the Caribbean' (Bartlett 1993, p. 7).

A group of men and women retired from the retail drapery trade and living together in the Linen and Woollen Drapers' Cottage Home estate came together with Mace as coordinator to recall their shared experiences as workers in many of the country's largest department stores with a view to 'precipitating new confidence in participants and in creating new knowledge for others' (Mace 1994, p. 68). For this group, the primary objective was the shared recollection of a changed trade; however, the ultimate outcomes were much broader in scope.

Books as an outcome are clearly not always likely to be within the resources or budgets of all centres and clubs and they may not always be an appropriate outcome. What we are more interested in highlighting here are the processes at work in different settings. In all the cases briefly described the objectives were to encourage social interaction and autonomy as groups. These groups, one Afro-Caribbean, the other two mainly white European, shared common disadvan-tages as older people in inner city areas whose personal histories had become eclipsed by more recent social and environmental change. The Afro-Caribbean group undoubtedly experienced the added factor of everyday racism which lent a particular immediacy to their group's goal of identifying their potential as cultural and educational contributors to the wider community. However, while they experienced the disadvantageous status of being members of older, poorer and marginalised groups within the wider community, these groups had certain advantages. They could call on common experiences of place, time and generation to create a sense of solidarity and shared purpose. The actual processes involved, talking, listening, sometimes arguing and supporting one another through different emotional experiences, led on to other activities and interests. Jane Mace's group told her how 'developing pieces of work for our publication and exhibition revived old intentions of making scrapbooks, writing more, maybe even forming a poetry group on the estate' (Mace 1994, p. 68).

Such reminiscence activities demonstrate processes which affirm identity, learning potential, shared interests and links beyond the group. Though the basis for group membership may be ethnicity, housing tenure or occupation, there will undoubtedly be opportunities to highlight diversity and hidden experiences. The differing experiences of men and women, of single and married people, of divorced and gay or lesbian or disabled people and of people from a range of cultural or religious backgrounds can all help to challenge any tendency towards complicity in constructing a past which is without conflict or experience of discrimination. Reminiscence work can then play its own part in developing anti-discriminatory practice (Bornat 1993, Harris & Hopkins 1993).

Clearly the role and responsibilities of the group leader are of great significance in all these processes and we will be looking at issues of group facilitation and dynamics in a later section.

At home in the community

Current 'Care in the Community' policies, with their emphasis on older people 'staying put' in their own homes, clearly pose a challenge to reminiscence work, given its basis in group work and social interactions. As research has shown, life at home in the community can often replicate many of the worst aspects of institutional care (Gavilan 1992).

Given such an environment, how might reminiscence work contribute to the lives of older people without further increasing feelings of institutionalisation at home or interference within a private domain?

Biographical information elicited through interviews and reminiscence enabled workers from the Gloucester Care for Elderly People at Home Project (Dant et al 1989) to find out which long-standing attachments and individual preferences might help to sustain a network of personal care and support which was acceptable to older people living in the community. This biographical assessment draws on the ideas of Malcolm Johnson (1976), who argued that knowledge of an older person's whole life, as described by them, enables a more accurate understanding of what their needs are now. The Gloucester project used care coordinators to assess, plan and operate care packages with older people seen as being 'at risk' in the community. The project's key assumption was that health and social needs are interrelated and that the term 'social' requires an interpretation which includes the life history of a person as well as their current living situation. Using a biographical interview schedule and a lifetime chart amongst other assessment tools, the care coordinators developed an approach which helped them to build care packages which were both individual and arguably more workable than those devised through traditional service-led assessment practices (Dant et al 1989).

Reminiscence may play a part in assessment; it can also help to maintain contacts with the outside world through developing activities tailored to suit the needs of housebound older people. In Bradford, a project run by the Social Services Department matched volunteers with housebound older people. With backup from a local oral history project, they recorded or wrote down reminiscences and copied photographs making life story books. The result in one case was 100 000 words of testimony from a post-war refugee, though others were happy with briefer accounts of their lives (Abendstern 1988). On a South London housing estate, a social worker and a social welfare officer deliberately focused a local history project on the needs of older people who were physically disabled. Their aim was to 'enhance the quality of life of some elderly people who currently have little outside social contact' and they therefore prepared themselves for activities which could be carried out in people's own homes (Wright 1986, pp. 62–63) (Box 22.4).

Box 22.4 Home-based reminiscence work in a South London housing estate (Wright 1986, pp. 62–63)

Our initial task involved contacting colleagues within our work place about our proposed group and requesting referrals of elderly isolated and/or physically handicapped people who were interested in sharing their reminiscences of the area. We received a good response from social work and home care staff. We visited about 20 elderly people who gave a varied response to our initial discussions. Whilst some were interested in only one or two meetings and then said that they had 'told us all they knew', others were interested in us visiting them over a longer period of time and were keen on being involved with the project. The 'group' became established with 10 members and we had a flexible approach to allow new members to be introduced. We discussed reminiscences of the 1920s and 1930s in the area. This included the 'rural feel' of Bellingham, gardening competitions, Second World War, local film studio, local trades services and so on.

Although our aims included discovering information about the Bellingham area, the house visits proved to be important as social contact points for members. We were able to feed back what each had recalled about the early days of the area and distributed a newsletter which helped members identify more as a group, even though they had not all met. Photos and objects were also used and helped to encourage individual and group discussions. Our first newsletter included short pieces of historical information from all the members and reproductions of an old local photograph and an advert. We also included an invitation to a social meeting at our office. The second stage of the group was our first social meeting. Eight members attended, others being too frail or too ill to come. We discussed local history, showed photographs and objects and shared anecdotes and stories. Some members had not been out of their homes for weeks.

The Bellingham History group has been consolidated by ... holding a local exhibition, 'A view of Bellingham'. At this local display we had a special guest, ex-boxer George Cooper, twin brother of European heavyweight Henry Cooper, both Bellingham ex-residents. We also invited local school children, church and community organisations as well as local residents. The display of photos, maps, old adverts, posters, objects, like a flat iron, curling tongs and a rolls razor helped to engage members and visitors in lively discussion. More importantly it seemed to do a lot for the self-esteem of the group who for much of the time have little social contact.

Residential care

Many of the objectives which I have described as appropriate to the three previous settings are also relevant to the lives of older people living in residential care. Issues of autonomy, independence, choice, social interaction, development and participation are clearly implicit when considering the quality of care available in residential settings.

The development of reminiscence work skills has largely taken place in relation to the constraints and opportunities of life in residential care homes. The fact that 'the world of residential care for older people is truly a woman's world' (Pence 1993, p. 139) is a key to a particular aspect of the development of reminiscence work and activities. In addition, those coming into residential care are likely to be widowed or never-married women, in their late eighties. Most are likely to have lived alone before admission and to have had to accept a place in residential care either because of their own, or a carer's, ill health. These demographic issues are worth emphasising since they have, to a large extent, determined the content of much reminiscence activity and the parts the approach tends to play in people's lives. Residential care, unlike continuing or nursing care, is generally an option invoked in response to a variety of factors. These might be inappropriate housing, increased disability and a breakdown in care and support in the community (Peace 1993, p. 139). Coupled with the public nature of life in residential care settings (Willcocks et al 1987) this tends to mean that the goals of care staff are likely to be those which enhance group solidarity and shared perspectives in a heterogeneous group.

Such pressure towards conformity and homo-geneity clearly poses a problem for residents who prize opportunities for privacy and independence. It is here that the best quality reminiscence work can play a part. Opportunities to stress individuality through life experience, while at the same time contributing to a group perspective of the past, are made possible through sensitive recall.

The fact that the boundaries between private and public are so finely divided in residential care provides another pressure towards conformity. Jennifer Hockey suggests that everyday reminiscence is one way in which residents maintain a stable identity in a context in which unexpected and unwelcome change is ever present in the form of increasing disability and eventual death (Hockey 1989, p. 216).

There are clearly a number of tasks which sensitive reminiscence work needs to engage with if it is to succeed in residential care, both in supporting individuality and in maintaining a sense of community. In subsequent sections we shall go on to look at the skills required as well as the form and content of appropriate approaches.

Summary

In this section we have looked at four different contexts for reminiscence work. Each has its own particular environmental constraints, yet each has a similar set of objectives and roles for reminiscence and recall. Though distinctions were drawn between nursing settings, day centres and clubs, at home in the community and residential care, there are also similarities, as much dictated by the existential issues faced by older people as they become more frail and dependent on others as by the social and cultural factors which help to marginalise and devalue older people in society. Each context provides its own challenges for sensitive reminiscence work. In the next section we look at some of the approaches which reminiscence workers have adopted in encouraging older people to recall the past with enjoyment and commitment.

METHODS AND STIMULI

Reminiscence activities in the UK were given a kick-start with *Recall*, a tape/slide programme published by Help the Aged (1981). The importance of *Recall* lay in its apparent simplicity. A cassette player, slide projector and white wall were within the means of most institutions and community settings. The six sequences of sounds and images matched the personal and public history of someone born at the turn of the 20th century, with images of bath night in front of the fire, Prince Edward and Mrs Simpson, the trenches in the First World War and unemployment between the wars. Sounds were edited from films, radio, popular music and older people talking about their childhood and younger years. Showing the sequences led to an instant response as people identified with the images, joined in with some of the music and songs, or, sometimes, questioned what they saw. *Recall* played an important part in popularising reminiscence-based activities. Staff who were keen to encourage older people to share memories found that they had instant proof that this was an enjoyable activity and one in which almost everyone could join. With these outcomes it became a form of instant legitimation of reminiscence as an activity.

Recall is important partly because of its early role in confirming the appropriateness of interest in the past, but it is also important for the legacy it left to later practitioners, a legacy of form and content.

Recall began life as the Reminiscence Aids Project, funded as an experiment by the then Department of Health and Social Security during the late 1970s. The inspiration of an architect with responsibility for advising on the design of residential settings for older people, it employed a team of artists and drew on the expertise of geriatricians, nurses, occupational therapists, psychologists and journalists, BBC sound and television archivists as well as older people.

This particular combination of professional skills has typified much reminiscence work since then. At its best it is multidisciplinary, making use of a wide variety of types of trigger and stimuli to memory and combining these with the skills and personal experience of facilitators and group members. When planning a reminiscence-based activity, there are two aspects which need to be considered:

- The type of activity – is it group based? Will it be focused around audio, visual or other sensory stimuli?
- The content of the activity – are there themes which can be relied upon to include rather than to exclude group members.

Types of activity

This section draws substantially on the handbook of reminiscence work by Osborn (1993). In it she lists 18 types of activity for groups and individuals (Osborn 1993, p. 13) compiled from long experience of working with groups of older people and with reminiscence group leaders in a wide variety of contexts and settings. It draws on what may seem like familiar group work techniques each focusing on the past. We will look briefly at each in turn to see what they entail. This list is not exhaustive and you may well find that it suggests ideas and brings back memories to you too. As you read through you might find it useful to note down any ideas of your own that come to mind, suggested by the activities listed.

Asking around the group. Here the idea is to get everyone to join in who wants to – less confident as well as more confident group members. The group leader begins with a question on, for example, schooldays, or first jobs and asks everyone to say just one thing, perhaps only a word, to start off a longer discussion. As Osborn points out, this may be a useful way to start a session off and to get initial information from everyone.

Display making. Groups like to be able to look at what they have worked on together and a display is a way of keeping a visual record which everyone can share. A display could be a map showing all the places people have mentioned, or it could include objects or craftwork with any writing or drawing which members may have contributed.

Drama ideas. The Age Exchange Reminiscence Centre has for years provided training in reminiscence drama techniques for group leaders. Osborn has worked with drama at the Centre and suggests that drama may be more acceptable to group members than leaders may imagine: 'Sometimes people will hardly realise that they are taking part in a drama activity' (Osborn 1993, p. 14). She gives examples of drama work taking the theme of schooldays and parent–children relationships, such as the following:

Leader, setting the scene,
I am a cross mother because my sixteen-year-old daughter has come home late.
What would the mother say to the daughter?
Contribution from the reminiscence group,
I told you to be back at 10:30, why are you late?
Leader repeating,
I told you to be back at 10:30, why are you late?
Leader going on,
What answer would the daughter give?
Someone in the reminiscence group suggests,
The bus didn't come.
Leader repeats this and asks what the mother might have said next and so on (Osborn 1993, p. 15).

As Osborn points out, this exercise can be extended by asking group members to say what they think the mother and daughter were thinking, but not perhaps saying, what did each really think about it.

Drawing, painting and collage. Some people feel happier painting or representing their memories through drawing or by making a collage from a variety of different materials such as cloth, wool, raffia and different textures and colours. For the group leader this may be a test of skills and ingenuity in terms of creative presentation. It is also an activity which needs to be clearly developed in such a way that it is neither childish nor demeaning. Osborn suggests that people who are unable to draw may prefer to describe and allow someone else to make the drawing for them, but under their instruction.

Handling objects. Here reminiscence work is sometimes seen at its best. Contributors to group sessions may come from any part of an establishment as particular interests contribute to collections of objects. People who enjoy car boot sales, jumble sales or visiting junk shops are the key to a successful session focusing on objects. Coin collections, particularly those which include pre-decimal denominations, different types of tools from the kitchen or garden shed, badges, labels, buttons, medals, souvenirs, ornaments, wrappings, pieces of material or lacework, almost any object may provoke discussion. People enjoy the opportunity to feel the weight of an old penny, to stroke material or to try again the action of a kitchen gadget.

It is in object handling sessions that contributors can often be most inventive with their enthusiasms. For example, a nurse working on a rehabilitation ward combined an enthusiasm for car boot sales with her love of ornaments and her knowledge of beneficial therapeutic movement and made a collection of small brass facsimile objects such as spinning wheels, anvils, cars. Each object was interesting in itself, provoking discussion and polishing the collection became an enjoyable and therapeutic part of the reminiscence session.

In some homes and day centres, object collections have become so large that the items have been distributed amongst different boxes focusing on particular themes, such as the kitchen, babies and children, holidays, cinema. Group sessions can then be planned around a particular theme or collection from a box.

Making a list. Osborn suggests this as a particularly easy way to engage members of a group. By taking a particular theme and then writing down on a large sheet of paper anything anyone says which is related to the topic, whole lists of ideas may emerge. She suggests children's games, household tasks and things sold in different kinds of shops.

Maps. A map of an area known to everyone, or a map of the world can lead to memories of journeys and countries of origin. Some people enjoy drawing their own maps, showing where they were born and what the important landmarks were.

Music and sounds. Music provides a particularly strong way to evoke the past. Songs and tunes heard in the years between ages 10 and 19 seem to be particularly important when it comes to recall. Music provides powerful ways to include even the most disabled people. It is not uncommon for people who have lost virtually all their powers to communicate through speech and conversation to be able to sing verse after verse of songs from their younger days.

Haunting second-hand record and tape shops and keeping an eye open for new collections of old favourites helps group leaders to put together themed sessions around different times, types of music and well-known singers.

Outings. Trips out to places people have mentioned like pubs, fish and chip shops, markets and the seaside, to museums which welcome groups and provide their own handling sessions and to places from people's own past, their schools, streets and parks and places of worship always provoke memories. Staff in museums often value the contributions which older people make, particularly in identifying objects and how they were used.

Practical activities. People enjoy taking part in activities which they used to do as a child, or younger adult, such as cooking, making bread, gardening, carpentry, sewing or looking after animals. Sometimes it may be a question of giving instructions while someone else does the actual work, or of showing how, so that others, younger people, can copy the actions.

Read a quotation. Reading aloud from something that has been published, like an official document, a magazine from years ago or a school text book may provoke discussion and may lead to debates and even argument.

Showing around. Osborn suggests an activity where people are encouraged to describe a place they remember well as if they are showing others around it. This could be the kitchen in the house they grew up in, their parents' farm, a walk to school, or their school playground.

Story telling. This is a well known group activity. Someone starts off a story and others are encouraged to take turns, adding the next section as they go. If they contribute things which they remember happening, then this can help to make the story lively or evocative. Mere describes what she calls a 'collective story' provoked from 'one simple question': 'Do you remember the gypsies?' (Mere 1993, pp. 133–134). Some group leaders write the story down and then read it out at the end. Peter Coleman argues that storytelling is at the root of reminiscing. He explains, 'The most valuable reminiscence ... is that which is related to the lives of others and helps illuminate their experience too' (Coleman 1993, p. 20).

Then and now. A still common criticism of reminiscence is that it distracts from present concerns and provides escapism into the past. Osborn suggests ways to link past and present by inviting people to contrast the modern and the old version of an object, for example a flat iron and an electric iron. Photographs of modern scenes such as school classrooms, workplaces and streets can lead to interesting comparisons and contrasts.

Things learned by heart. Poems, proverbs, sayings, monologues, rhymes, slogans, prayers, hymns and catch phrases are part of most people's verbal repertoire. As Osborn points out, 'The memory of things learned by heart lasts longer than the ability to generate speech' (Osborn 1993, p. 22). Without much encouragement people will enjoy repeating familiar words and perhaps joining in with what others remember.

Taste, touch and smell. Some reminiscence workers have built up ingenious collections of bottled smells: spices, scents, smelling salts, mothballs, cleaning materials. These are powerfully evocative of different aspects of home life and lead to ready discussion. Tastes too can be recalled with old-fashioned sweets and fizzy drinks. Finally, touching objects, particularly from nature when people have become used to a more indoor, institutional life, can bring back memories of country life and outdoor activities.

Prompted reminiscence

Here a leader develops skills in asking questions which draw people out comfortably so that they are able to talk about what they remember. Phrasing questions such as 'How did it feel ...?' or 'Where did you grow up ...?' or 'What was it like ...?' tend to be less challenging or threatening than questions which ask for exact information even about family size or dates of weddings.

Using pictures. This last example brings us back to *Recall* with its emphasis on the visual. Showing slides and encouraging people to notice details in street scenes, interiors or in aspects of people's clothing is a sure way to encourage discussion and talk of the past. Passing round photographs is not always so successful since the act of passing immediately creates a distraction and tends to break up the group. Some people may not be able to see all the detail, or at all. They will still enjoy being brought into the discussion with descriptions of what is included. One reminiscence worker with an interest in photography found that by enlarging people's own photographs, particularly family photographs, people were able to see again faces and images which their eyesight had found too small to distinguish easily anymore.

Having read through this section, did you find that you were recalling any memories of your own, or thinking of particular objects, places, words, or tunes? You might find it helpful to keep any list you make. It could become part of your own reminiscence resource material, useful when planning group or individual reminiscence sessions.

Themes

Gibson, who, like Osborn, has long experience of involvement in reminiscence groups and activities has worked on themes which groups and individuals can use to focus their reminiscence activities. In planning a programme, or even structuring a single session, the choice of a theme is of key importance. Group members will want to be involved in choosing the theme and deciding how long they spend discussing it. The theme gives the group facilitator and the members useful boundaries within which to think creatively and develop ideas and connections between each other's memories.

Gibson suggests a number of themes. These are: 'home life, clothing, childhood, washday and other housework, school, work, wartime, leisure' (Gibson 1994, p. 60).

She goes on to elaborate each theme and to suggest appropriate triggers for each. Taking the theme 'home life' we might suggest the following topics for discussion: the place where you lived, the house you grew up in, bath night and hairwashing, neighbours and friends, courtship, marriage, childbirth, deaths at home, illnesses, home cures and remedies, celebrations and festivals, cooking and shopping, etc. In order to evoke such memories, certain types of trigger are appropriate, for example: photographs, maps, kitchen utensils, lamps, cookery books, a safety razor, ornaments, sewing kits, buttons, etc.

You might like to try working out your own topics and triggers for the eight themes she suggests and you could also add your own themes – holidays, journeys, pets and animals are other possibilities.

Summary

In this section we have had a glimpse of just some of the ideas which help to focus a reminiscence session. This is the content, the material which provides the stimuli, often the enjoyment and sometimes the pain of remembering in groups or in one-to-one sessions. As you read it through you almost certainly found yourself remembering experiences from your own life. This is an important part of becoming a sympathetic and successful reminiscence worker. Being able to relate to other people's memories, even if they come from quite different backgrounds and generations, is the key to organising sessions which meet a wide range of needs. Next we come to look at the ways of structuring and running sessions and address some of the issues raised by working together and managing social interactions amongst staff and group members.

WORKING TOGETHER

In this section we consider reminiscence as a form of social interaction, between individuals and in groups.

We look at ways of working together towards successful outcomes and consider some of the problems which both older people and reminiscence workers may face. First we look at one-to-one work.

Working on a one-to-one basis

Occasions when possibilities for one-to-one work arise range from opportunistic moments, or 'spontaneous recall' (Gibson 1994, p. 67) when talk and conversation turns to memories of the past, to more planned reminiscence sessions.

Nurses and residential care workers often suggest that their daily life caring for older people naturally leads them into reminiscence, particularly at points when physical care needs such as bathing, toileting and dressing are being carried out. The research evidence does not wholly back this up. Evidence from observation suggests that such care is seen principally as work and that interactions are fairly restricted and in any case largely task-oriented (Wells 1980, Evers 1981, Brocklehurst & Andrews 1987, Salmon 1993, Lee-Treweek 1994).

How then to find ways to integrate reminiscence into daily work and to respond to spontaneous reminiscence? We might like to consider the following principles:

- talk to the older person you are working with, not across them to colleagues
- make the task a focus for discussion, about bathing, choosing clothes, dressing, hair brushing, shaving, nail cutting, etc.
- listen out for any stray or chance remarks which you can respond to with a question or showing interest
- if you really haven't got time to listen to a long story, let the person know that you'll be back to hear more later on
- pay attention to times when talking about the past while you work or sit with someone may be comforting or reassuring, for example if someone is new to an establishment, has to move their bed or room or has been bereaved
- staff under pressure sometimes need reassurance that time spent talking and listening is worthwhile; you may be in a position as a manager to influence attitudes positively amongst staff

Some workers find that reminiscence fits quite naturally into the work they do. Wright (1984) cites his own experience:

My initial reminiscence-work consisted of talking to older people about their past ... whilst delivering bath aids, seats, mats and rails. I found elderly people more than willing to be engaged in recall when I asked, 'How long have you lived here?' 'What work did you do?' 'I suspect that you have seen a lot of changes?' Although these were fairly basic and unimaginative questions they always led to an enjoyable discussion about the past and, sadly, often much bitterness over the present. (Wright 1984, p. 60)

Planned one-to-one sessions present quite different challenges and may be organised for quite specific reasons. Reminiscence should be a natural accompaniment to assessment, though time may not always permit prolonged and detailed discussion. Gibson (1994) explains:

In some care homes, reminiscence with a key worker may be an established way of assisting assessment, helping newcomers settle, establishing a relationship with a staff member and developing a care plan. Life stories reveal how different people think about their own lives, and the process of gathering a life story helps the carer to grasp the essence of the other person. (Gibson 1994, p. 66)

Adams (1993), working as a nurse on a continuing care ward, became aware that although some people were happy to take part in group sessions, others preferred to remember on an individual basis. He cites interesting examples of how insights into previous experience helped staff to understand current behaviour: ' ... the discovery that one woman who seemed to be obsessed with the standard of the cleaning achieved by the domestic staff on the ward had spent her working life as a cleaner in a wide range of government buildings, including Number 10 Downing Street, helped to transform resentment into a lively interest' (Adams 1993, p. 84).

The tape recordings which he made with individual patients helped him, he argues, to hear 'the patient's own perspectives expressed in her own words' (Adams 1993, p. 95).

Group work

Group approaches to reminiscence are perhaps the most common and most popular amongst both care workers and older people. So popular have they become that the question inevitably arises, 'Has the reminiscence group become the easy equivalent to bingo?' Evidence from the field is that in some cases this may be precisely the case. Reminiscing becomes an unfocused activity with little personal meaning or awareness of sensitivities. What follows is a brief attempt to prepare reminiscence group facilitators for more appropriate and thought-through group work.

Group reminiscence offers particular opportunities, including:

- social interaction
- changed relationships
- an opportunity for people to meet as equals
- collaborative project work
- shared understanding and empathy.

Naturally such outcomes require careful planning and organisation if they are to be achieved. Gibson (1994) identifies a number of key aspects which facilitators need to prepare for:

- the responsibilities of the group leader
- the responsibilities of senior staff
- the responsibilities of group members
- awareness of group dynamics
- setting of objectives and outcomes
- ensuring that there is an agreed and acceptable ending to the life of the group.

We will look at each briefly in turn.

The group leader. As Gibson explains, the leader, to be effective, must act as 'an enabler, a facilitator, not an authority'. The leader's aim should be to create a 'safe environment' (Gibson 1994, p. 28) and, as Bender also points out, be able to 'communicate respect and interest' (Bender 1993, p. 43) in what group members are saying. One obvious way in which this can happen is if the group leader shows a preparedness to learn from the group members. This is a welcome opportunity for role reversal, when the members become the experts about the past and the facilitator and helpers learn about the history of their community or society from those who lived it.

It is the group leader's responsibility to identify the different stages that the group goes through, from preparation and planning, through beginnings, middles and endings in group life. This means being able to identify and resolve such issues as where and when to hold the group, how big it should be, whether it should be open or closed, how people should be invited and whether they should be interviewed beforehand about their interests and backgrounds.

Senior staff. It is the senior staff who can make sure that a reminiscence group is valued by the whole staff group and the older people too. Issues like staff rotas, routines, timing of staff meetings and handovers and the support of staff initiatives in reminiscence work all need to be treated seriously if good quality reminiscence work is to be achieved. Thus, for example, the timing and journey of the daily tea trolley round which interrupts rather than supports the reminiscence group in the lounge needs to be reviewed. The tendency to take time out rather than support or join in the reminiscence group needs to be discussed rather than allowed to develop into established practice.

Burnside (1990) gives an example of problems she encountered when trying to start a reminiscence group in a nursing home. She kept weekly logs:

Entree difficult; got run-around for a week ... staff not knowledgeable about gerontological nursing ... staff hold negative views about residents ... there is great emphasis on pills and great emphasis on charting and chart maintenance ... group members are unsure, tentative, almost bewildered ... only three members know one another ... group members are severely depressed; one has attempted suicide three times ... energy levels noticeably low in two of members, especially the 90-year-old ... 'excessive disability' seems to be the norm ... all have multiple diagnoses ... food and beverage important to the members ... staff not at all interested in the group meetings ... help with ambulation needed ... am expected to teach the principles of reminiscence group therapy to a 19-year-old activities director who is getting married in a few weeks and shows little interest in continuing the group when I leave.

(Burnside 1990, pp. 40–41)

Her scenario may include aspects which are familiar. Clearly, such situations make heavy demands on the skills of senior staff if reminiscence group work is to succeed. Often such group work is introduced as a means of bringing about institutional change, without discussion with junior staff or with residents or patients. It is important to identify what is positive in such situations, to make sure that staff with enthusiasm for reminiscence are enabled to take part. It is also important to find ways to draw as many people into the process as possible, some may have objects to lend, others may have useful contacts with local community groups such as photography societies, or sports clubs, others may simply need to be encouraged to realise that this is a legitimate part of their work and role as carers.

The responsibilities of group members. Some groups demonstrate a tendency to assume that older people will enjoy their membership without being considered and without having their own sense of purpose or outcomes. This is clearly to underestimate the strengths and contributions which people bring to reminiscence groups. One way to make sure that people have a sense of their own responsibility and commitment is to make the processes which lead to the setting up and running of the group as open as possible. This means:

- inviting rather than taking people to the group
- discussing with group members how often and how long the group should meet
- choosing topics for discussing with group members
- agreeing group rules as to confidentiality
- agreeing what the outcomes are to be with the group.

Each of these aspects requires open and thorough-going discussion. Some may need time to be explained, particularly if people are not used to group work. However, it would be wrong to underestimate people's interest and willingness to build up group norms and practices. The clearer these are to everyone then the more likely it will be that the group itself will find that it is able to deal with potentially 'difficult' issues and moments, rather than the leader or facilitator taking action on their behalf. For example, older people who have experienced loss and bereavement, maybe several times over, may have skills which enable them to support a group member who feels unable to contain emotions. They should be permitted and encouraged to do so.

Bender describes the way a successful group feels to a leader:

... there is that lovely moment, a few sessions into the life of a group, when you notice that you're not saying much and that you feel relaxed and you know that the group no longer needs you as the provider of the energy. They can now sort out their own problems, they can set their own agendas. To add to the wealth of experience that is their lives, they now have confidence and trust. The wisdom is in the group.
(Bender 1993, p. 4)

Group dynamics. We have already touched on the possibility that a successful group may develop ways to deal with situations which are upsetting. However, there are issues which a skilled group leader and facilitator needs to be prepared for. These include:

- being aware of impairment and disability amongst group members and making sure that they are able to take part on an equal basis
- not allowing certain people to dominate discussions
- creating space and time for quiet people to speak and be heard
- not allowing a consensus to develop which excludes or marginalises a particular experience, for example the woman who never married, the wartime experiences of black or Asian older people, the person whose first language is not English, the war widow and the person who spent significant periods of their life abroad.

Setting of objectives and outcomes. Some reminiscence groups set up on a casual diversionary basis have no sense of beginning and ending, nor of why they are meeting at all beyond the immediate fact of encouraging older people to talk about the past. It is likely that such groups will achieve very little for their members, beyond a degree of socialising. Given the potential of reminiscence-based activities to change

and develop understandings on both an individual and group basis, it is worthwhile putting some effort into thinking about why the group is needed in the first place and what it could aim to achieve.

Some reminiscence groups are set up with specific purposes, for example, to change patterns of social interaction in settings where people seem unable or unwilling to communicate. Fielden's (1990) work in a sheltered living complex and Bender's (1993) example of working with residents singled out as 'difficult' provide interesting insights into how such people are identified and then a group formed. Other groups are set up as part of a programme of developmental work, more in the nature of education, with the aim of learning about the past and sharing this with an outside audience often of younger people. Somewhere in between are most reminiscence groups, meeting on a weekly basis and with fairly modest objectives of involving members, learning about individual life stories and building more supportive structures within the group and its setting.

Even the most modestly conceived group needs to have a sense of achievement and outcome even if this changes during the lifetime of the group. For example, one group set up to take part in a local oral history competition with a tape and display, later found itself publishing a small book based on members' memories. Another group began with a focus on writing history but found that taping and transcribing memories was a more feasible outcome (Duffin 1993). Lawrence and Mace (1992) describe this process as 'planning for surprise' and see this need for flexibility as extending right through the lifetime of a group's work, whether the chosen outcome is an exhibition, a play, film or writing (Lawrence & Mace 1992, p. 22).

Endings. An agreed outcome – such as an exhibition, publication or open day – is a way of reaching a point which says, 'We've done something'. However, there may be groups which are not aiming for such ambitious ways to mark an achievement. Even groups which are not time-limited need opportunities to stop and review what they have been doing. This means that endings come in different forms. Some are there to create a time for reflection and change, a pause for perhaps a few weeks, while changes are taken on and plans for a new phase are made. It may be necessary to change the meeting place, choose new themes, introduce new members or simply stop for a rest! Members need to be aware of this planned pattern and the reasons why it has been devised.

Other groups are time-limited. For these, the ending phase will be more dramatic as members have to prepare themselves for a time when they cease to meet.

As Gibson (1994) points out, this may come as a relief for some! She insists on the need for the facilitator to be able to deal with what may be strong feelings as the group comes to an end and not to be tempted into making promises about the future when there is no realistic possibility of continuing.

Summary

In this section we have looked at some of the dynamics of leading and supporting reminiscence work in one-to-one and in group situations. In both cases there are responsibilities for the initiator or the facilitator, but in both cases there is also a need to recognise the contribution which the older person will be making to the social relations generated in reminiscing. This may be a contribution in terms of knowledge, adding to our knowledge of the past, but it may also be a contribution based on experience of life in all the richness of its emotion.

In the next section we look at two groups of people for whom, because of their special needs, reminiscence may play a particularly significant role.

PEOPLE WHO HAVE SPECIAL NEEDS

The researchers attached to the Reminiscence Aids project which led to Help the Aged's programme, *Recall*, hoped that the triggers and prompts devised would 'increase reminiscence in the elderly with mental infirmity' (Help the Aged 1981). Success in achieving this objective was evaluated when reactions among people in the early stages of dementia were tested during exposure to reminiscence materials. The findings were inconclusive; no effect on the ability to reminisce was observed (Department of Health and Social Security 1979). The result was that, in the early years at least, many organisers of reminiscence-based activities tended to exclude those seen as more 'difficult' or unmanageable. A purely medical model of their illness supported the maintenance of such boundaries (Kitwood & Bredin 1992).

More recently, sensitive work with people with dementing illnesses such as Alzheimer's disease has shown that although the early aim to improve or change the course of such conditions is likely to remain unachievable, reminiscence does have a role to play in relation to providing appropriate care.

The tendency to select the natural reminiscers and people who manage well in groups led to the exclusion of others. Amongst those who tended to be selected out were older people with learning difficulties, particularly those who had spent a large part of their lives in long-term care institutions such as mental handicap hospitals. Care in the community policies resulting in the closure of some of these larger institutions, together with a more enlightened set of attitudes amongst some reminiscence workers, has shown the importance of attending to the stories and memories of older people with learning difficulties.

People with dementing illnesses and those who have learning difficulties have special needs when it comes to organising reminiscence work. In this section we will look at these two groups of people in turn.

People with dementing illnesses

In Chapter 11 of this book, Trevor Adams discusses the nature of dementing illnesses, including Alzheimer's disease. In relation to memory, what we know is that memory for recent things is first affected and that the ability to recall the more distant past stays least affected far into the illness. The example of the person who cannot remember what time it is, or when her relative is coming to pick her up from the day centre, but who can give a rich account of her early years in the East End of London together with details of the wages she earned, her social life and where she met her husband is probably familiar to anyone who has worked with people with dementing illnesses.

Gibson and others who have used reminiscence-based activities with people with dementia refers to this long-term recall as a 'memory bank'. She argues that reminiscence can be used to 'encourage conversation and increase sociability' (Gibson 1994, p. 89).

Adams (1989), writing as a nurse, argues for the need to 'take the dry bones' of someone's memories and to 'add flesh to them'. He describes an approach to anamnesis – that is, the construction of a patient's personal and medical history before illness – with people who have dementia. He considers the situation of people who are unable to give coherent accounts of themselves and who have no relatives who can fill in the story. Without evidence of personal biography such patients will tend to be neglected at worst, or stereotyped at best. He describes researching with the help of scraps of conversation and the local history archives to build up a picture of a patient's childhood in South London.

Gibson and Adams make a strong case for reminiscence work with people who have dementing illnesses. Both suggest that there are gains to be made from listening, responding and building a picture of the life of the person and that this can lead to more sensitive and appropriate care management. Gibson argues for a selective approach which targets those whose behaviour may be challenging. She gives two reasons for this:

First, the troubling individual is worthy of help in his or her own right. Individualisation is now readily accepted as a major principle in child care practice but is still all too rare in gerontological care. Second, if the behaviour of the troubled and troubling people could be improved, then the quality of life for everyone else around them – residents, families and staff – could also be improved. By making things better for them, things could be improved for others.

(Gibson 1993, p. 55)

She gives the example of 'Mary' (Box 22.5).

Box 22.5 Mary

Mary was selected for 'specific' reminiscence work. She was a most unhappy, isolated, aggressive, underweight woman who pushed, hit, spat or shouted at anyone who came near. The key worker collected a detailed life history from Mary's niece and discovered that, when younger, Mary had always liked nice things such as fine china, good linen and small delicate flowers.

So the key worker decided to try to tempt her to eat by setting a breakfast tray with a linen tray cloth, special china and a posy of flowers. Mary started to eat better and some days she asked for a second piece of toast. Her aggression decreased and her isolation lessened.

On the days when the key worker was off duty the special arrangements were ignored because the cook refused to set the tray, so opposed was she to the idea of one resident being singled out for special attention.

It took the officer in charge several weeks to confront the cook and instruct her not to undermine the care plan and to set the tray.

(From Gibson 1994, p. 93)

Working with individuals will mean spending time constructing a life history from a number of different sources as well as the person with the dementing illness. Gibson recommends that workers should:

Start reminiscing with the older person themselves. Learn to listen very attentively. Often their conversation needs to be decoded, translated. If you begin by assuming truth rather than falsity, belief not disbelief, much valuable information can be gathered. You have to learn to decipher symbolic and partial information. You must learn to recognise and respond to people's underlying emotion connected to what they are struggling to tell you instead of being preoccupied with establishing facts. (Gibson 1994, p. 95)

Working with groups, she recommends a similar approach, one which involves careful observation and attention to behaviour patterns. Group facilitators will have to take a lead and provide the necessary stimuli.

Sessions should be short and held more than once each week, but in the same place and at the same time, following a pre-set pattern. She quotes a day centre worker in Northern Ireland:

People with dementia come to our day centre for 2 days a week. It's in an area of the town where a lot of people live who once worked in the local mill so we have gathered up a lot of old bobbins, spools, wool and different types of cloth. We also have old newspapers with pictures of mills and mill workers, and our local museum gave us a recording of a mill hooter ... We use all these things with two or three women together, or sometimes with just one person to get them talking. (Gibson 1994, p. 91)

Gibson provides a detailed account of ways of communicating with people with dementia and makes a strong argument for taking a life history approach. She concludes with five key points:

- Reminiscence work requires adaptation for people with dementia; it is more effective in very small groups or with individuals.
- It provides a constructive role for professional staff and family carers.
- It appears not to improve short-term memory but does improve quality of life.
- It increases job satisfaction.
- Gains will be small, but important none the less.

Reminiscence work with people with learning disabilities

Margaret:

When I was a little girl I was put away. I was 14 and a half. I went to Cell Barnes to live because they said I was backward. My dad refused to sign the papers for me to go, but the police came and said he would go to prison if he didn't. I cried when I had to go with the Welfare Officer.

(Atkinson 1993a, p. 43)

The quotation above is from *Past Times*, a book which is the outcome of a project which involved a group of older people with learning difficulties recording their memories. Atkinson points out in the book's introduction why such publications and experiences are important. The memories shared by the group are not exceptional or unusual in many aspects. They are memories of rural childhoods and the descriptions of domestic routines, games, toys, shopping fit in with a familiar pattern, typical of their age and generation. This sense of a common, shared, past helps to refocus understandings about people who have for most of their lives been made to feel different and apart. The memories are also important for the light they shed on institutional life. As Atkinson points out: 'The view from the inside, of life in the long-stay hospital makes this a rare and valuable document. The oral historians do not emerge in their accounts as victims, but as people who survived, and often defied the worst aspects of the system.' (Atkinson 1993a, p. iv).

This particular project met over a period of 2 years on a weekly basis at first. The group of seven men and two women were encouraged to talk in response to particular themes. Staff who were present joined in, adding their memories, prompting more reminiscence. After a while various aids to memory were introduced, Help the Aged's tape/slide sequences *Recall* and objects such as cigarette cards. People were helped to talk by breaking the group up into pairs and small groups. This gave quieter members an opportunity to talk without interruption.

A first draft of the book, compiled from the transcribed tapes, led to additions and amendments which were also tape recorded and added in. Eventually, after a third period of drafting, a final version appeared. In its final form the book has become an object of pride for members of the group who have been pleased to share it with members of their families as well as friends.

Tracking the process of production here and in other accounts (Potts and Fido 1991, Bender 1993) helps to emphasise aspects of reminiscence work with older people with learning difficulties which are worth identifying:

- The importance of having a tangible outcome, in this case a written history even though most of the group were unable to read their book (Gibson 1994).
- Taking part in the project brought increased self-esteem – this was an 'intrinsically enjoyable' (Atkinson 1993b, p. 103) experience for the group members.
- The revealing of a 'hidden history' is an important contribution to the 'reclaiming of a shared or collective past' (Atkinson 1993b, p. 103).
- At the same time, it is a means to rescuing the personal and the individual for people who for a large part of their lives have had few opportunities for individual self-expression or recognition.
- For people who are moving from long-stay hospitals into the community, reminiscing provides a means to re-establish links and to identify personal choices and preferences (Potts & Fido 1991, p. 136).

Working with groups of people with learning difficulties, Bender (1993) has found ways to include people exhibiting challenging behaviour and suggests

a need to group people according to verbal ability in order to be able to find the right pace for everyone as far as possible. One outcome was the growth of group cohesion. The reminiscence group grew into a house committee for the members who were all users of a day centre for people with learning difficulties.

Summary

In this section we have looked at two groups of people who traditionally tended to be excluded from opportunities to reminisce. The examples and case studies show that while work with people who have dementing illnesses or who have learning difficulties may have special features, there are many common aspects, such as selection of themes, stimuli, group management and awareness of outcomes.

ACHIEVING QUALITY IN PRACTICE

This chapter has presented a brief overview of the achievements of reminiscence work with older people, its evaluation as well as suggestions as to encouragement and support with individuals and groups. We end with some indicators which we feel should underpin reminiscence work and which, if adhered to, should provide a guarantee of quality in practice.

These are:

Embedding evaluation

As group leaders or facilitators, or in one-to-one situations we should constantly be on the look-out for opportunities to evaluate our practice. Evaluation in the case of reminiscence work means monitoring the work we do by involving all the participants: older people, staff and relatives. It means finding ways to discuss what we do with other practitioners and asking others with more experience for comments and supervision. It also means sharing what we do with others, exposing both our successes and failures to their scrutiny.

Identifying wider outcomes

Evidence that reminiscence work has brought about changes amongst the older people we work with should be followed up and reinforced with positive action. We know that on its own, reminiscence as an individual or group activity can only do so much. Our practice needs to focus on those wider outcomes which can make all the difference to the quality of life of older people. Through reminiscence work we may identify views and experiences which enable us to highlight the isolated lives of some older people living in residential and nursing home settings or in the community. We may be able to blow the whistle on poor care delivery and management. We may even find that we can contribute to the ending of practices which are rooted in racism and discrimination.

Valuing difference

One of the key contributions of reminiscence work has been the opportunity to dispense with the stereotypes which deny individuality. We need to make sure that we value the differences which we learn about and incorporate this knowledge into our practice. This means allowing modest and mundane lives to be celebrated as well as those which challenge convention

and tradition. Younger people need to take care that they are not imposing their own views of the past, and the present, on older people's understanding. One way to guarantee this is to allow for, and value our different experiences.

Support for self determination

Right from the start, reminiscence workers pointed out the way knowledge of the past undermines established relationships between younger and older people, carers and cared for. Reversing roles by acknowledging past expertise, knowledge and skills is at the heart of good reminiscence practice. Taking this further, reminiscence work should act as a basis for advocacy and promote ways to change status and unequal access to resources. If we listen for the things that people identify as important in their past lives, then we can support them in determining how they live their lives in the present.

REFERENCES

Abendstern M 1988 Me and you – them and us: conferences and workshops. Oral History 16(2): 3–7
Adams J 1988 Ghosts of christmas past. Nursing Times 84(50):62–64
Adams J 1989 Anamnesis in dementia: restoring a personal history. Oral History 17(2): 62–63
Adams J 1993 A fair hearing: life review in a hospital setting. In: Bornat J (ed) Reminiscence reviewed: perspectives, evaluations, achievements. The Open University Press, Buckingham
Adams J, Bornat J, Prickett M 1996 'You wouldn't be interested in my life, I've done nothing': care planning and life history work with frail older women. In: Penhale B, Philips J (eds) Reviewing care management for older people. Jessica Kingsley, London
Age Concern England 1990 Left behind? Continuing care for elderly people in NHS hospitals. Age Concern England, London
Atkinson D (ed) 1993a Past times. The Open University Press, Buckingham
Atkinson D 1993b 'I got put away': group-based reminiscence with people with learning difficulties. In: Bornat J (ed) Reminiscence reviewed: perspectives, evaluations, achievements. The Open University Press, Buckingham
Bartlett L (ed) 1991 Nice tastin': life and food in the Caribbean. Kensington and Chelsea Oral History Group, London
Bartlett L 1993 Between life and death: a space for memory. Reminiscence 6: 6–8
Bender M 1993 An interesting confusion: what can we do with reminiscence groupwork? In: Bornat J (ed) Reminiscence reviewed: perspectives, evaluations, achievements. Open University Press, Buckingham

Biggs S 1993 Understanding ageing: images, attitudes and professional practice. Open University Press, Buckingham
Boden D, Bielby D D V 1983 The past as resource: a conversational analysis of elderly talk. Human Development 26: 308–319
Bornat J 1989 Oral history as a social movement: reminiscence and older people. Oral History 17(2): 16–24
Bornat J 1993 Representations of community. In: Bornat J, Pereira C, Pilgrim D, Williams F (eds) Community care: a reader. Macmillan, Basingstoke
Bornat J, Middleton D 1994 Context and interpretation in accounting for experience. Paper presented at Biographical Methods for Comparative Social Policy Seminar, London
Brennan P L, Steinberg L D 1984 Is reminiscence adaptive? Relations among social activity level, reminiscence and morale. International Journal of Aging and Human Development 18(2): 99–110
Brocklehurst J, Andrews K 1987 Nurse staffing in geriatric wards. Nursing Times Occasional Papers 83.1
Buchanan K, Middleton D 1995 Voices of experience: talk, identity and membership in reminiscence groups. Ageing and Society 15(4): 457–491
Burnside I 1978 Working with the elderly: group processes and techniques. Belmont, California
Burnside I 1990 Reminiscence: an independent nursing intervention for the elderly. Issues in Mental Health Nursing 11: 33–48
Butler R N 1963 The life review: an interpretation of reminiscence in the aged. Psychiatry 26: 65–76
Coleman P G 1974 Measuring reminiscence characteristics from conversation as adaptive features of old age. International Journal of Aging and Human Development 5: 281–294

Coleman P G 1986 Ageing and reminiscence processes: social and clinical implications. Wiley, Chichester

Coleman P G 1993 Reminiscence within the study of ageing. In: Bornat J (ed) Reminiscence reviewed: perspectives, evaluations, achievements. The Open University Press, Buckingham

Dant T, Carley M, Gearing B, Johnson M L 1989 Co-ordinating care: the final report of the care of elderly people at home project, Gloucester. The Open University School of Health and Social Welfare, Milton Keynes

Department of Health and Social Security 1979 Reminiscence aids: the use of audio-visual presentations to stimulate memories in old people with mental infirmity. Unpublished report

Dobroff R 1984 Introduction: a time for reclaiming the past. Journal of Gerontological Social Work 7(1/2): xvii–xviii

Duffin M 1993 Turning talking into writing. In: Bornat J (ed) Reminiscence reviewed: perspectives, evaluations, achievements. The Open University Press, Buckingham

Ebersole P 1976 Problems of group reminiscing with the institutionalized aged. Journal of Gerontological Nursing 2(6): 23–27

Elder G H 1982 Historical experience in the later years. In: Hareven T K, Adams K J (eds) Ageing and life course transitions: an interdisciplinary perspective. Tavistock, London

Erikson E H, Erikson J M, Kivnick H Q 1986 Vital involvement in old age: the experience of old age in our time. Norton, New York

Evers H 1981 Care or custody? The experience of women patients in long-stay geriatric wards. In: Hutter B, Williams G (eds) Controlling women: the normal and the deviant. Croom Helm, London

Fallot R D 1980 The impact on mood of verbal reminiscing in later adulthood. International Journal of Aging and Human Development 10(4): 385–400

Fielden M A 1990 Reminiscence as a therapeutic intervention with sheltered housing residents: a comparative study. British Journal of Social Work 20: 21–44

Garland J 1993 What splendour it all coheres: life review therapy with older people. In: Bornat J (ed) Reminiscence reviewed: perspectives, evaluations, achievements. Open University Press, Buckingham

Gavilan H 1992 Care in the community: issues of dependency and control. Generations Review 2(4): 9–11

Gibson F 1993 What can reminiscence contribute to people with dementia? In: Bornat J (ed) Reminiscence reviewed: perspectives, evaluations, achievements. The Open University Press, Buckingham

Gibson F 1994 Reminiscence and recall: a guide to good practice. Age Concern England, London

Gubrium J F, Wallace J B 1990 Who theorises age? Ageing and Society 10: 131–149

Haight B K 1991 Reminiscing: the state of the art as a basis for practice. International Journal of Aging and Human Development 33(1): 1–32

Haight B K 1992 The structured life-review process: a community approach to the aging client. In: Jones G M M, Miesen B M L (eds) Care-giving in dementia: research and applications. Tavistock, London

Haight B K, Hendrix S 1995 An integrated review of reminiscence. In: Haight B K, Webster J D The art and science of reminiscing: theory, research, methods and applications. Taylor & Francis, Washington

Hale S 1960 The horse buses stopped north of the Rye. Case Conference 7(6): 153–155

Harris J, Hopkins T 1993 Beyond anti-ageism: reminiscence groups and the development of anti-discriminatory social work education and practice. In: Bornat J (ed) Reminiscence reviewed: perspectives, evaluations, achievements. Open University Press, Buckingham

Help the Aged Education Department 1981 Recall: a handbook. Help the Aged, London

Hockey J 1989 Residential care and the maintenance of social identity: negotiating the transition to institutional life. In: Jefferys M (ed) Growing old in the twentieth century. Routledge, London

Johnson M L 1976 That was your life: a biographical approach to later life. In: Munnichs J M A, van den Heuvel W J A (eds) Dependency and interdependency in old age. Martinus Nijhoff, The Hague

Jones G 1992 A nursing model for the care of the elderly. In: Jones G M M, Miesen B M L (eds) Care-giving in dementia: research and applications. Tavistock, London

Kiernat J M 1979 The use of life review activity with confused nursing home residents. American Journal of Occupational Therapy 33: 306–310

Kitwood T, Bredin K 1992 Towards a theory of dementia care: personhood and wellbeing. Ageing and Society 12(3): 269–287

Laing W 1993 (ed) Laing's review of private health care. Laing and Buisson, London

Lawrence J, Mace J 1992 Remembering in groups: ideas from reminiscence and literacy work. Oral History Society, London

Lee-Treweek G 1994 Bedroom abuse: the hidden work in a nursing home. Generations Review 4(1): 2–4

Lewis C N 1971 Reminiscing and self-concept in old age. Journal of Gerontology 26: 240–243

Lewis M I, Butler R N 1974 Life review therapy: putting memories to work in individual and group psychotherapy. Geriatrics 29: 165–169

Lieberman M A, Falk J M 1971 The remembered past as a source of data for research on the life cycle. Human Development 14: 132–141

Mace J 1994 Reminiscence, retailing and change. Oral History 22(1): 66–68

McKenzie S 1991 A positive force. Nursing the Elderly May/June: 22–24

McMahon A W, Rhudick P J 1964 Reminiscing: adaptational significance in the aged. Archives of General Psychiatry 10: 292–298

Mere R 1993 Arthos Wales: working in hospitals. In: Bornat J (ed) Reminiscence reviewed: perspectives, evaluations, achievements. The Open University Press, Buckingham

Merriam S B 1989 The structure of simple reminiscence. The Gerontologist 29(6): 761–767

Nolan M, Grant G 1993 Action research and quality of care: a mechanism for agreeing basic values as a precursor to change. Journal of Advanced Nursing 18: 305–311

Norris A 1989 Clinic or client? A psychologist's case for reminiscence. Oral History 17(2): 26–30

O'Donovan S 1993 The memory lingers on. Elderly Care 5(1): 27–31

Osborn C 1993 The reminiscence handbook: ideas for creative activities with older people. Age Exchange, London

Peace S 1993 The living environment of older women. In: Bernard M, Meade K 1993 (eds) Women come of age: perspectives on the lives of older women. Edward Arnold, London

Perrotta P, Meacham J A 1981 Can a reminiscing intervention alter depression and self-esteem? International Journal of Aging and Human Development 14(1): 23–30

Potts M, Fido R 1991 'A fit person to be removed': personal accounts of life in a mental deficiency institution. Northcote House, Plymouth

Safier G 1976 Oral life history with the elderly. Journal of Gerontological Nursing 2(5): 17–23

Salmon P 1993 Interactions of nurses with elderly patients: relationship to nurses' attitudes and to formal activity periods. Journal of Advanced Nursing 18: 14–19

Sim R 1991 Reviving memories. Reminiscence 2: 7–9

Thompson A 1989 Times past. Nursing Times 85(6): 31–32

Thornton S, Brotchie J 1987 Reminiscence: a critical review of the empirical literature. British Journal of Clinical Psychology 26: 93–111

Victor C 1987 Old Age in a modern society. Croom Helm, London

Wade B, Sawyer L, Bell J 1983 Dependency with dignity. Paper 68. Bedford Square Press, London

Wallace J B 1992 Reconsidering the life review: the social construction of talk about the past. The Gerontologist 32: 120–125

Watt L M, Wong P T P 1991 A taxonomy of reminiscence and therapeutic implications. Journal of Gerontological Social Work 16(1/2): 37–57

Wells T 1980 Problems in geriatric nursing care: a study of nurses' problems in care of old people in hospitals. Churchill Livingstone, Edinburgh

Willcocks D, Peace S, Kellaher L 1987 Private lives in public places: a research-based critique of residential life in local authority old people's homes. Tavistock, London

Wright M 1984 Using the past to help the present. Community Care 533: 20–22

Wright M 1986 Priming the past. Oral History 14(1): 60–65

RECOMMENDED READING

Bornat J 1993 (ed) Reminiscence reviewed: perspectives, evaluations, achievements. The Open University Press, Buckingham. *This edited collection brings together leading practitioners in the field of reminiscence work. Psychologists, social workers, educationalists, community workers, a nurse and academics review what had been achieved in reminiscence in the UK. The book provides critical and evaluative insights into the work in a range of contexts including hospital wards, the community, residential care, social work training and clinical settings.*

Butler R N 1963 The life review: an interpretation of reminiscence in the aged. Psychiatry 26: 65–76. *This is the article which arguably set the whole issue of reminiscence and life review for older people going. Butler makes a case for viewing reminiscence as a normal, rather than a pathological, activity in old age. The article should be read in the light of its later impact on memory work with older people.*

Coleman P G 1986 Ageing and reminiscence processes: social and clinical implications. Wiley, Chichester. *This is a classic study and the best known example of UK research by the leading exponent of reminiscence and life review in the UK. Taking a longitudinal view of reminiscence, the research findings suggest the need to take a discriminating view of the role of reminiscence in different people's lives. The book includes accounts from older people, unusually for much reminiscence literature, and is an accessible and well-argued account of research and of key issues in reminiscence and life review work.*

Haight B K 1991 Reminiscing: the state of the art as a basis for practice. International Journal of Aging and Human Development 33(1): 1–32. *This extremely helpful article provides an overview of almost the entire literature on reminiscence published between 1960 and 1990, though drawn mainly from the USA. In a tabular form it records the study variables and findings of 97 articles describing reminiscence. Of the 97 only 7 report negative findings, the rest are positive or provide no definite evaluation.*

Haight B K, Webster J D 1995 The art and science of reminiscing: theory, research, methods and applications. Taylor & Francis, Washington, USA. *This edited collection brings together many of the main US proponents of reminiscence and life review approaches to working with older people. Contributors include Butler, Fry, Merriam, Burnside, Meacham, Wong and of course Haight and Webster themselves. British contributors add their own reviews of research and recent findings as well as ways of working with reminiscence with people suffering from depression and dementia.*

Fielden M A 1990 Reminiscence as a therapeutic intervention with sheltered housing residents: a comparative study. British Journal of Social Work 20: 21–44. *This is one of the few published UK studies evaluating reminiscence through an intervention. The study produced positive findings in relation to organised reminiscence activities. However, the article is most valuable for its description of the research process and should therefore be helpful to students interested in developing research methodologies for their own project work.*

Gibson F 1994 Reminiscence and recall: a guide to good practice. Age Concern, London. *This thoughtfully argued book provides the ground for sensitive individual and group reminiscence work. Key chapters focus on work with people with dementing illnesses. A particular strength of the book is the way it carefully outlines the necessary steps and protocols in preparing and running reminiscence groups which seek to meet the needs of individual members.*

Jones G M M, Miesen B M L 1992 (eds) Care-giving in dementia: research and applications. Tavistock, London. *Several chapters in this comprehensive book (Chs 3, 4, 6–9 and 16) discuss aspects of reminiscence in later life and review work with people suffering from dementing illnesses. Chapters 3, 4 and 6 provide useful overviews of aspects of memory change, learning, attachment theory and communication with dementing patients. Chapter 8 includes a critical review of reality orientation, while Chapter 9 outlines an evaluation of reminiscence intervention in a group setting. Chapters 7 and 16 propose life review based approaches to nursing care in hospital and community settings respectively.*

Osborn C 1993 The reminiscence handbook: ideas for creative activities with older people. Age Exchange,

London. *This is a lively compendium of ideas and activities for reminiscence work in a wide variety of settings. The book is laid out clearly and is well illustrated with ideas for group activities including drama, writing, craftwork and talk. Drawn from the experience of 10 years of practice and training, this is a resource book for workers and carers working in community and clinical settings.*

Thornton S, Brotchie J 1987 Reminiscence: a critical review of the empirical literature. British Journal of Clinical Psychology 26: 93–111. *This article is the most quoted critical review of approaches to reminiscence. The authors compare definitions of reminiscence in the literature, consider evidence for reminiscence and life review amongst older people, evaluate evidence for the functional role of reminiscence and arrive at a controversially negative set of conclusions.*

Wallace J B 1992 Reconsidering the life review: the social construction of talk about the past. The Gerontologist 32: 120–125. *This is a good example of a 'second wave' approach in reminiscence debates. Theorising is beginning to encompass the social meanings of reminiscence. This article argues against Butler and his followers, suggesting that reminiscence should be viewed as being appropriate only to the particular coping strategies required by older living in residential care.*

Watt L M, Wong P T P 1991 A taxonomy of reminiscence and therapeutic implications. Journal of Gerontological Social Work 16(1/2): 37–57. *This article is interesting for the way it approaches the organisation of evidence about types of reminiscence. Students involved in project work should find the typology adopted a helpful approach to theorising and to interpretative work. By identifying six types of reminiscence the authors draw readers' attention to the meaning and context of what is recalled. The article usefully describes the methodology adopted, providing a helpful insight for students interested in teaching and evaluating reminiscence data.*

23

Pharmacological treatments and electroconvulsive therapy (ECT)

Dinah Gould

This chapter discusses the role of pharmacological and physical treatments in the care of elderly people with mental health problems.[1] The distressing symptoms associated with anxiety, depression and lack of sleep can often be alleviated with the help of drugs used in conjunction with appropriate non-pharmacological interventions. Electroconvulsive therapy (ECT) can be of benefit in the treatment of depression in carefully selected patients.

DRUGS AND THE ELDERLY

Prescription of anxiolytics, hypnotics, antidepressants and antipsychotic drugs is the responsibility of the medical practitioner, but other members of the caring professions often have closer and more regular contact with their elderly clients, often visiting or providing physical care for years. Regular contact and familiarity with the habits and behaviour of the individual place them in an ideal position to help with drug administration. They can observe side-effects, monitor progress, provide information and supervise when necessary. The task is considerable. Elderly people account for approximately one-third of all National Health Service drugs expenditure, with those over 75 receiving three-quarters of all prescribed drugs (Burns & Phillipson 1986). In recent years prescriptions for hypnotics and anxiolytics have declined, but there has been substantial increase in the number of prescriptions overall, particularly for the elderly (Cartwright &

---

[1] I have made every effort to ensure that the information and drug dosages in this chapter are correct at the time of publication but mistakes may have been made and therapeutic regimes may have been altered. Where there is any doubt, dosage should be checked against the manufacturer's data sheet or other authoritative source.

Smith 1988). This increases the opportunity for mistakes when medicines are taken and for drug interactions. Both are very common in this age group, accounting for hospital admissions which might otherwise have been unnecessary (Bliss 1981). Sometimes problems arise through over-prescription, especially in nursing homes where old people may receive psychotropic drugs unnecessarily (Wade et al 1983). It is particularly important for professionals involved in the care of elderly people to understand the goals of drug therapy and to be familiar with the therapeutic regime of each of their patients, not only because drug-related problems are so common in this age group, but because they are also potentially very dangerous. Burns & Phillipson (1986) present evidence that suggests that the elderly suffer twice as many dose-related and hypersensitivity reactions as younger people. Knowledge of drugs and their properties is essential for the professional carer because elderly people are often required to take several different types of drug (polypharmacy) and their absorption and metabolism may be altered in elderly subjects (Fielo & Rizzolo 1985).

Changes in response to drug therapy with age

The best way of taking any drug is the most simple and straightforward – by mouth. This is possible when the individual is cooperative and the drug is absorbed readily from the gastrointestinal tract. However, oral administration is not always the most efficient. The amount of drug given via this route does not automatically coincide with that entering the circulation and eventually the tissues (bioavailability). A drug administered by intravenous injection has 100% bioavailability, but in the case of orally administered medicines, bioavailability may be considerably less – 0% if the medication is forgotten or omitted for some other reason. Sometimes people experience difficulty swallowing tablets. This can be overcome by giving preparations in liquid form. Depot injections may be used for psychotic patients who fail to take oral medication. The issue of compliance is discussed below.

Absorption

Absorption is affected by the physical properties of the substance, including those modified by the manufacturer during formulation (slow release tablets, etc.) and by factors relating to the patient. These include the rate at which the stomach empties, interactions with other drugs and the effects of gastrointestinal disease. There is little evidence to suggest that absorption is affected by age per se but the older patient may be receiving a cocktail of drugs and is more likely to have coexisting disease which may influence drug metabolism. For example, drugs belonging to the atropine group delay gastric emptying. They are sometimes used to treat diverticular disease which is common in the elderly. Metoclopramide, often given to help reduce nausea, speeds gastric emptying. The effects on drug action and absorption can be subtle and unpredictable.

Drugs administered by injection enter the systemic circulation via capillaries in the subcutaneous or muscular tissues. Reduced muscle tone through lack of activity may result in the fluid remaining as a depot at the site of entry for longer than usual, so action is delayed. People in this age group have delicate skin, especially if taking steroids, and bruise easily, so remembering to rotate the site of injection is an important point when individuals receive injections frequently. Patients responsible for their own injections may welcome someone else who can use a site which they find inaccessible.

Metabolism

Drugs absorbed from the gastrointestinal tract are carried via the portal vein to the liver before gaining access to the systemic circulation (Figure 23.1)

This is of clinical significance as many drugs are metabolised in the liver, explaining why only a proportion of the amount absorbed enters the systemic circulation. Destruction of a drug by the liver before it gains access to the general circulation (and target

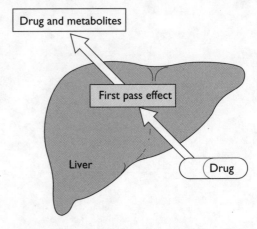

Figure 23.1 First pass effect in drug metabolism. (Adapted from Trounce & Gold 1994 with permission)

tissues) is known as the first pass effect. The first pass effect tends to be increased in older people for two reasons: reduction in hepatic blood supply and reduced activity of hepatic enzymes. The net result is a lower rate of metabolism, accumulation of the drug and the possibility of overdose if the signs and symptoms are not recognised and reported. Reporting often falls to a relative or to a member of the caring professions who must be taught what to look out for.

Carriage

Drugs are poorly soluble in plasma, so like most naturally occurring metabolites carried in the blood, they are transported attached to plasma proteins, chiefly albumin. This is the most abundant plasma protein in the body. In elderly people the amount of circulating albumin is reduced, so more of the drug is carried freely in the plasma (Montamat et al 1989). From Figure 23.2 you will see that it is the amount of free drug in the circulation which determines rate of diffusion into the tissue fluid and ultimately its pharmacological action, which thus tends to be greater in older people.

Excretion

Drugs and their breakdown products are mainly excreted via the kidney. The speed of elimination is clinically important as it is the chief factor to determine the duration of action. The length of time that active drug remains in circulation is known as its plasma half-life. Chronic conditions affecting the renal system are more common in the elderly, but even in the physically well older person there is marked decline in renal function. Glomerular filtration rate and tubular absorption fall so that by 80 years of age renal function is only half that at 40 (Montamat et al 1989). The use of diuretics requires particular care in the elderly for whom they are often prescribed (Lamy 1985).

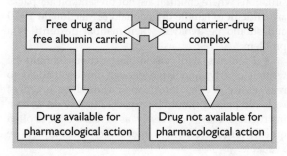

Figure 23.2 Plasma carriage of pharmacologically active substances.

Relative proportions of muscle and fat

The proportion of fat increases with age, producing a larger depot for lipid-soluble drugs such as the benzodiazepines and barbiturates. These are taken up readily by adipose tissue and released slowly for metabolism and excretion. As a result elderly people recover from the effects of treatment slowly. Problems are exacerbated if they have to undergo general anaesthesia because the agents normally used are also fat soluble. The patient becomes confused and may remain disoriented for several days (Platzer 1989). This is distressing for friends and relatives and a major difficulty for staff working in acute hospital settings: if an old person is admitted in an emergency, typically after falling, staff meeting them for the first time will have no yardstick against which to measure usual behaviour.

Tolerance

With repeated use some drugs are metabolised more effectively by the liver – the phenomenon of tolerance. Increasingly larger doses become necessary to produce therapeutic effect. This may occur with narcotic analgesia such as morphine.

Organ sensitivity

There is evidence that some systems become increasingly sensitive to certain drugs as the individual ages. In particular, functions of the brain tend to become disturbed in older people with the result that hypnotic drugs readily produce confusion during the night and excessive drowsiness or hangover effects the next day.

Individual idiosyncrasies

These may be the result of lifestyle, especially diet, or response to the drug itself. This is an area which has so far attracted little research. However, genetic differences in the hepatic enzymes responsible for metabolising drugs are known to exist, resulting in individual variations in plasma concentration. If the individual has never taken the drug before their reaction will not be known.

Effects of drugs on general health

Drugs may affect individuals' general health. Specific side-effects are discussed in conjunction with each of the main groups below. However, it is important to remember that taking large numbers of tablets may reduce the appetite, especially in hospital where they are usually presented immediately before a meal, or if taking them makes the mouth sore (Lamy & Lamy 1985). Nutritional deficiency can result from prolonged use of drugs which suppress appetite or reduce absorption. Amphetamines and anticonvulsants may behave in this way. It is not unknown for the responsibility of managing a complex regime of drugs to generate marked anxiety, either in the individual taking them or a lay carer supervising medication at home. In other cases, side-effects from the drugs themselves may lead to problems, or the apparent mental disorder may prove to be the result of physiological disturbance.

Drug interactions

These are particularly common among older people for the following reasons:

- They are more likely to be prescribed several drugs, often to treat a number of different complaints. There is an established relationship between the number of different drugs taken and the number of adverse reactions reported (Montamat et al 1989). Many people take over the counter medicines which may interact with those that have been prescribed (Conn 1991). For example, many proprietary cough mixtures contain mild sedatives. This effect is then added to that of hypnotics they are already taking.
- Deterioration in renal function alters the plasma half-life of drugs. Elimination is impaired, exposing elderly people to higher concentrations for reaction if dosages are not adjusted.
- Concurrent illness may interfere with drug metabolism. For example, many old people suffer some degree of congestive cardiac failure. This reduces hepatic blood supply, so metabolism in the liver is reduced over and above any normal age-related effects, contributing to build up and overdose.
- Hypnotics which have well established side-effects on cerebral function are often prescribed for old people, especially old people with mental health problems.
- Compliance. This is an important topic, particularly in relation to this client group and is considered in detail below.

Compliance

There is no doubt that people who receive information about their drugs comply better with their regimes of medication (Weibert & Dee 1980). Patients in hospital can be encouraged to take responsibility for looking after their tablets and taking them at the appropriate times. They are then less likely to make mistakes when they go home because they have been involved in their own care and are not suddenly overwhelmed with too much information shortly before discharge (Webb et al 1990). Whether or not older people can realistically be expected to participate in these schemes will depend on a number of factors including mental capability, willingness to learn and issues such as manual dexterity. A recent study by Cargill (1992), conducted with 70 elderly people in the community, indicated that after assessment to indicate specific areas of difficulty, a group receiving a tailored teaching intervention geared to individual need and followed up by telephone were more likely to remember instructions, stick to regimes and avoid over the counter medication. Cargill (1992) points out that contrary to popular belief, there is no documented evidence that older people wilfully fail to take their medicines more often than those in any other age group. However, there are numerous barriers to compliance to which the elderly are especially prone. Some may be resolved quite easily providing that time is spent with individuals observing practical difficulties and listening to their worries. Problems include:

- Difficulty or dislike of swallowing tablets or problems handling them, especially if they are very large or small. Most medications can be supplied as elixirs or syrups. Advice should be sought from the pharmacist before tablets are crushed because the presentation of medicines is closely related to the special properties required of them. For example, slow release tablets will not work as they are intended if fragmented.
- Difficulty opening medicine bottles with arthritic hands. Child-proof containers are no advantage in situations where children are not present. Blister packs are difficult to handle (Macdonald & Macdonald 1982) and should be avoided when manual dexterity is a problem.
- Problems with vision. Instructions should be written clearly, and large enough for the patient to read easily. Verbal information should be given as well. No patient should be expected to rely on written instructions only. Conversely, as verbal advice is often quickly forgotten, written information must always be available.
- There has long been a feeling that elderly people receive too much medication and a call to simplify

regimes to avoid confusion and the likelihood of drug-induced reactions (Wade & Bowling 1986). Problems may arise if drugs are prescribed by repeat prescription over long periods without the patient seeing the doctor, as the regime is not reviewed. Those in close contact with elderly people in the community play an important role monitoring the number and range of medications the individual is expected to take.

• Cognitive functioning is related to ability to understand and comply with medication and can be used as an indicator of likely non-compliance (Macdonald & Macdonald 1982), especially when regimes are complicated (Parkin et al 1976). An important factor to bear in mind is that over time the health and cognitive level of the individual may deteriorate. Someone who was once independent may not remain so. Assessment is important periodically to determine capability.

• Non-compliance may occur because the drugs have side-effects which the individual is not prepared to tolerate. Of course in some cases the medication may not be responsible for the symptoms that have been noticed, but when related to drug non-compliance this is a logical conclusion. Unfortunately many of the drugs which older people have to take have acknowledged side-effects which are known to be unpleasant. Diuretics are a nuisance, especially for those with problems of mobility, because of the frequent need to empty the bladder. Hypotensives may cause dizziness. Some of the tranquillisers and antidepressants are difficult to tolerate, as discussed below, but taking medication as instructed is vital.

Errors with medication may involve: omission; mistiming; and extra doses. The research evidence indicates that omission and mistiming are the most common (Parkin et al 1976), probably because most people feel that they have to take too many medicines (Morrow et al 1988). Anyone prescribed medication should be given all the information shown in Box 23.1. It should also be made clear that swapping drugs with other people or 'trying out' someone else's medication is extremely dangerous.

Those with mental health problems present particular challenges when compliance with drug regimes is sought. People suffering severe depression may have little motivation to help themselves. Even taking responsibility to obtain their medicine may initially lie beyond them. For some people paranoid ideas may extend to medication and there may be refusal to comply for reasons which are not rational to anybody else. Individuals with suicidal ideas pose a special risk because some psychotropic drugs are

---

Box 23.1   Information essential for anyone receiving prescribed medication

• Name of the drug
• Strength
• Appearance (pink pills, red capsules, etc.)
• Purpose
• Dose
• Frequency that it must be taken
• Storage (safety, how to dispose of unused medication if discontinued)
• The importance of expiry dates
• Common side-effects
• Common adverse reactions and early signs that they are occurring
• Common interactions and the need to mention existing medication when seeing a doctor
• Avoidance of over the counter prescriptions when this is relevant
• Special instructions – may be related to the route of administration or foods to avoid.

---

dangerous, even in small quantities. The following points are of a practical nature and may go some way to help avoid obvious problems:

• If at all possible, a responsible friend or member of the family should be included in discussions concerning treatment and they should be supplied with a telephone number for contact in case they become worried or particular problems arise.

• The amount of medication which the individual possesses should be continually monitored. Nobody should be given more medicines than they need for a specific amount of time to reduce the risks of overdose or hoarding by individuals who are forgetful and confused. Drugs are expensive. Once dispensed they cannot be used for anyone else and will have to be destroyed if they are no longer needed.

• In some cases, especially for patients with schizophrenia, drugs may be administered by injection as depot preparations. Fluphenazine and flupenthixol may be given by deep intramuscular injection into the upper, outer quadrant of the buttock or the lateral aspect of the thigh. However, there are numerous disadvantages including inflexible dosage, inability to discontinue medication quickly if adverse effects occur and patients' dislike of injections which may be painful.

DRUGS AND MENTAL DISORDER IN ELDERLY PEOPLE

In many cases the cause of mental health problems is undoubtedly related at least in part to social factors such as loneliness or bereavement, for example. However, chemical abnormalities in the brain are also thought to contribute to the development of some disorders because studies have shown that their levels tend to be altered in people suffering from specific mental health problems. It now appears that Alzheimer's disease, some depressions, anxiety and schizophrenia involve alterations in the amount of neurotransmitter substances in the brain (Figure 23.3).

The distribution and normal functions of the main neurotransmitters thought to play a role in the genesis of mental health problems are shown in Table 23.1.

Most of the drugs presently given to alleviate the symptoms of mental health disorders influence the cerebral cortex, the limbic system and the reticular formation (Fig. 23.4). These areas are concerned with maintaining the state of consciousness and arousal. Additionally the limbic system appears to play a role in the control of mood and the emotions entering consciousness. Amine oxidase inhibitors operate as

Table 23.1 Neurotransmitters: distribution and function in the brain

	Distribution	Function
Acetylcholine	Basal nuclei Cerebral cortex Limbic system	Not clear. Depressed levels in Alzheimer's disease.
Adrenaline	Hypothalamus	Control of mood.
Noradrenaline	Hypothalamus Cerebellum Cerebral cortex Spinal cord	Maintaining arousal, dreaming, regulation of mood.
Dopamine	Midbrain Cerebral cortex	Emotional response. Control of movement.
5-hydroxy-tryptamine (5-HT)	Brainstem	Induces sleep. Sensory perception. Control of mood.
Gamma-amino-butyric acid (GABA)	Hypothalamus Thalamus Cerebrum	Control of mood.

stimulators by retarding the breakdown of adrenaline and noradrenaline, while drugs belonging to the tricyclic antidepressant group produce a similar effect by interfering with their reabsorption. Reserpine appears to exert its depressant effect by reducing the levels of adrenaline and noradrenaline. Gamma-aminobutyric acid (GABA) has a sedative effect.

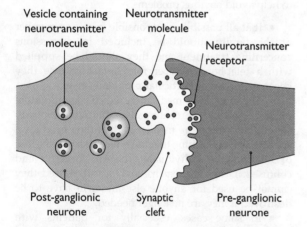

Figure 23.3 Neurotransmitters. Neurotransmitters are chemicals which carry the nervous impulse across the synaptic cleft between adjacent neurones or between a neurone and a muscle. About 50 chemicals are known to operate as neurotransmitters, but some have additional functions outside the nervous system. For example, noradrenaline operates as a neurotransmitter in the brain and as a hormone when released into the blood by the adrenal medulla during stress (sympathetic 'flight and fight' reaction). Some chemicals operating as neurotransmitters are found within the central and peripheral nervous systems. Acetylcholine falls into this category. Others such as gamma-aminobutyric acid (GABA) seem to be found exclusively within the brain. Some neurotransmitters operate quickly to open or close ion channels within the cell membrane, altering permeability. Others operate more slowly and their main influence appears to be to alter enzyme reactions taking place within the cell.

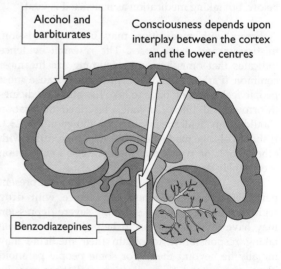

Figure 23.4 The mode of action of hypnotics and tranquillisers. Source: Adapted from Trounce J, Gould D J 1994 Clinical pharmacology for nurses, 14th edn. Churchill Livingstone, Edinburgh with permission.

These represent only a few of the many drugs which have been used with varying success to treat mental health problems over the last 30 years. A problem common to all is the difficulty of testing them adequately on animal models as it is impossible to reproduce the symptoms of mental illness in non-human subjects. Trials with animals intended to assess therapeutic usefulness are therefore difficult to conduct and the results' hard to interpret. Trials with human volunteers seldom involve elderly people and evaluative studies tend to include outcome measures geared to younger populations (Katona 1993).

The main groups of drugs used in the treatment of elderly with mental health problems are discussed below.

Drugs and the elderly person with anxiety or agitation

Major tranquillisers

The purpose of these drugs is to induce a state of calm in the patient while avoiding unwanted drowsiness. They do not have any influence on the disease itself and are not prescribed with a view to 'cure'. Instead they help alleviate symptoms so the individual feels more comfortable and is in a better condition to benefit from non-pharmacological treatments such as psychotherapy.

Neuroleptics exert their effects directly on the central nervous system. They are valued for their effectiveness in treating psychotic symptoms and controlling the agitation associated with schizophrenia, mania and delirium. Although the precise mode of action is unknown they are believed to block the action of dopamine, an effect which not only produces their antipsychotic and sedative functions but also their well-documented side-effects, including disorders of posture and movement (Culshaw 1994). The main groups of narcoleptics are discussed below.

Phenothiazines. These drugs modify behaviour by blocking receptors for dopamine and acetylcholine, chiefly in the reticular formation and basal ganglia. They reduce restlessness, agitation, delusions and hallucinations and have thus been widely used in the treatment of schizophrenia. These drugs purport to produce a feeling of detachment from external worries which leaves the patient in a better position to cope with day-to-day problems without becoming overwhelmed. However, they also have some sedative effect which is often a cause of complaint from users. The phenothiazines exert a number of peripheral effects by blocking adrenergic and anticholinergic receptors outside the CNS. This causes fall in blood pressure and faintness, which can lead to falls.

Most phenothiazines are absorbed readily when given by mouth and are metabolised in the liver. Table 23.2 shows those most commonly prescribed with their usual doses. However, the table is meant to be an indication only, as the amounts actually prescribed for individuals are subject to wide variation according to the disorder treated and the response of the person receiving them. For older people lower doses may be required. Professionals have an important role monitoring response to treatment and documenting side-effects, which are quite common with the phenothiazines, especially when older people are treated (Gomez & Gomez 1990).

The incidence of side-effects varies between individual drugs in this group. Symptoms to watch for include:

- Jaundice. The cause has not been fully established but it is thought to be an allergic response in which the canaliculi of the liver become blocked due to local swelling. This effect is most common with

Table 23.2 The phenothiazines

Drug	Trade name	Use	Dose/24 hour
Promazine	Sparine	As for chlorpromazine but less potent	25 mg
Thioridazide	Melleril	Agitated elderly	30–100 mg
Trifluoperazine	Stelazine	Schizophrenia	10 mg
Fluphenazine	Modecate	Schizophrenia	6.25 mg depot injection, repeated at intervals of 14–35 days, depending on response.
Chlorpromazine	Largactil	Sedative for the confused patient. No longer much used for the elderly because of the risk of hypotension and falling.	Orally: 50–800 mg IM injection: mg

chlorpromazine. Patients can be reassured that the effect is reversed when treatment stops.

• Depression of the leucocyte count. Susceptibility to infection increases.

• Skin rashes, particularly light sensitivity and contact dermatitis when the drug is handled. This can be avoided by wearing gloves when injections are prepared.

  • Hypothermia in elderly people.
  • Dry mouth.
  • Weight gain.
  • Gynaecomastia in men.

• Hypotension and faintness due to the alpha blocking effect on the sympathetic nervous system, as noted above.

• Disordered body movement caused directly or indirectly by blocking dopamine receptors in the brain. These include:

— Parkinsonian syndrome
— akathisia (a sensation of restlessness with inability to stand still)
— dystonia (uncontrolled body movements)
— tardive dyskinesia (abnormal movements of the lips, tongue and occasionally the upper limbs).

Tardive dyskinesia develops in approximately 20% of all people receiving neuroleptic drugs long term. This is an unfortunate side-effect of treatment as psychotic patients may need this type of medication for a very long time, sometimes in high doses. The onset is not usually immediate but control is difficult even if treatment ceases. The other side-effects may develop soon after treatment begins, but it is possible to reduce them by adjusting the dose. In some cases additional treatment with a benzodiazepine helps. The antimuscarinic drug, procyclidine, is helpful in cases of acute dystonia. It can be given orally, 2.5 mg three times daily, by intramuscular injection (5–10 mg) or by intravenous injection (5 mg). If symptoms are severe this may have implications for the individual living alone as independence is threatened.

Thioridazine is particularly useful with elderly people because of its side-effect profile, having few extrapyramidal side-effects and being moderately sedative. The latter can be helpful in relieving agitation and restlessness in dementia sufferers, starting with a low dose of, say, 10 mg twice daily. Its antipsychotic action is important in treating schizophrenia, again with careful adjustment of dose according to response. Hypotension is always a possibility so needs to be monitored, particularly in an elderly person living alone. The case of Mrs Atkinson (Box 23.2) illustrates the value of thioridazine for an elderly person suffering from schizophrenia.

Box 23.2 The value of thioridazine for Mrs Atkinson, an elderly person suffering from schizophrenia

Mrs Atkinson, aged 75, suffered from schizophrenia. She was especially disturbed at night when she experienced auditory hallucinations, hearing music and dancing in the flat above. She believed that the people upstairs were involved in drug dealing and that the noise was aimed at getting her to move from the flats, these being delusions. Consequently she slept little at night and might spend hours in night vigils on the corridor outside her flat, trying to identify any of the drug dealers. She agreed to take a tablet 'to help her sleep'. Thioridazine 25 mg taken half an hour before bedtime made little difference but when the dose had been gradually increased to 75 mg the auditory hallucinations ceased and she slept well. The combined antipsychotic and sedative action of the thioridazine was probably responsible for this. Consequently her quality of life was much improved.

An uncommon but serious complication of neuroleptics is neuroleptic malignant syndrome. This is characterised by muscle rigidity, high temperature, fluctuating level of consciousness and autonomic dysfunction including pallor, sweating and labile blood pressure. Patients with dementia of Lewy body type may be particularly prone to this.

Thioxanthines. Drugs belonging to this group are similar to the phenothiazines. They are antipsychotic and can be used to treat schizophrenia. The advantage is that they are less sedative than phenothiazines but akathisia is a common side-effect. The most commonly prescribed is flupenthixol. This can be given orally or as a depot injection every 2 weeks. The dose is 20–40 mg.

When more sedation is required, for disturbed behaviour in mania or schizophrenia for example, zuclopenthixol is useful.

Butyrophenones. Again, these drugs are similar to the phenothiazines but less sedative. The two used most widely are haloperidol and droperidol. Haloperidol can be taken orally by cooperative patients. The dose is 0.5–2 mg three times daily. In the case of confusion or mania it may be given by intramuscular injection in doses of 2–10 mg every 6 hours. High doses are avoided because they result in the development of Parkinsonism. Droperidol is similar, but acts more rapidly within the same dose range.

Other neuroleptic drugs. A number of other neuroleptic drugs are available. These include:

• Pimozide, a drug which causes side-effects less often than the phenothiazines. The dose is 2–16 mg by tablet.

• Sulpiride, which specifically blocks the action of dopamine. It is given twice daily at a dose of 200–400 mg and is responsible for the same disorders of posture and movement.

• Clozapide. This has little influence on posture and movement and is thus a useful drug for schizophrenic patients who require long-term therapy. The lowest effective dose is 25 mg daily, but this can be increased to as much as 300 mg daily. Unfortunately clozapide is associated with serious side-effects. Approximately 3% of patients receiving it for a year or longer develop neutropenia. Regular blood tests to monitor white cell count are therefore essential. Other undesirable effects include seizures, hypotension, excess salivation and sedation.

Benzodiazepines

The benzodiazepines are widely used as hypnotics but they are also prescribed as minor tranquillisers for anxious patients. They are thought to act on the reticular formation where specific receptors able to bind to the drugs have been detected. They enhance the action of gamma-aminobutyric acid (GABA), a neurotransmitter which is known to depress brain function, thus exerting a sedative effect.

Individually the benzodiazepines vary in duration of action although all have similar tranquillising and sedative effects. The variation in the duration of effect is due to the rate at which the body metabolises different members of the group. The products of breakdown themselves have sedative action in some cases, prolonging the length of time that they exert action. For example, diazepam is partially converted to a compound called desmethyldiazepam which continues to exert sedative effects.

The benzodiazepines are usually effective in relieving anxiety symptoms but there are a number of disadvantages:

• They are less effective if use continues over an extended period.

• If patients stop taking the drug, even after 2 or 3 weeks, they may develop withdrawal symptoms, including renewed anxiety and sleeplessness.

Withdrawal symptoms are troublesome but generally short-lived unless benzodiazepines are taken in large doses or over a long period of time. In this case the patient may also experience seizures, psychotic symptoms, muscular twitching and pain, all indications that dependence has developed. Recovery usually occurs in a week or so, but may take longer in

patients who are badly affected. The problem may be avoided or reduced by cautious prescription of benzodiazepines and careful withdrawal over several weeks. During this time the dose should be gradually reduced (Potter et al 1991). Help may be required even for individuals usually responsible for their own drug regime, as written instructions may be complicated and confusing.

Misuse of benzodiazepines is now extremely common. A study by the National Addiction Centre in London has revealed that large numbers of young people are acquiring the drugs for intravenous use, especially temazepam (Strang et al 1994). Drugs are frequently obtained by theft from dispensaries. The extent of misuse of benzodiazepines amongst elderly people is less clear. However, health care professionals employed in institutional settings should adhere to their local policies for the safe handling and custody of drugs with care, while those working in the community should remind clients about safe storage, involving informal carers if necessary.

Providing that the benzodiazepines are prescribed with care, avoiding large doses and prolonged use with gradual withdrawal, this group of drugs is safe. Overdose results in sedation, lack of coordination and loss of memory. A more serious problem is respiratory depression. This is not common, but is most likely to be a problem in the older patient with coexisting respiratory disease. For the patient who has taken an overdose, treatment is possible with flumazil, which is a benzodiazepine antagonist. Given intravenously it will reverse sedation within a few minutes, but the effects last for only a short time (about 1 hour) so treatment must be repeated. Those taking benzodiazepines should be aware that the sedative effect is increased with alcohol. The most commonly prescribed benzodiazepines with their usual doses are shown in Table 23.3.

Table 23.3 The benzodiazepines

Drug	Daily dose	Duration	Comment
Diazepam	4–30 mg	24 hours	Control of status epilepticus
Chlordiazepoxide	30–60 mg	24 hours	
Oxazepam	45–120 mg	12 hours	
Lorazepam	1–4 mg	12 hours	Used as pre-medication
Medazepam	15–30 mg	12 hours	
Clonazepam	4–8 mg	24 hours	Epilepsy

Because the benzodiazepines, although safe, are associated with so many undesirable side-effects, there have been attempts to find alternative drugs (Potter et al 1991). The most recent is buspirone. It appears to be anxiolytic without sedative effects or risk of addiction. Side-effects include occasional nausea and headaches. Other disadvantages are the slowness with which it begins to exert its therapeutic effects and its apparent ineffectiveness if the patient has already taken benzodiazepines. Essential information for people taking benzodiazepines is given in Box 23.3.

Box 23.3 Essential information for people taking benzodiazepines

- You will be given tablets for a short time only to help relieve your anxiety/tension.
- This medication must be taken exactly as prescribed because excessive use long-term can result in side-effects when it is discontinued.
- The tablets may cause drowsiness or dizziness and impair judgement or coordination. You must not drive or operate machinery when you are taking them.
- You must avoid alcohol because the drug will react with it.
- You must consult your doctor before taking any other medicines.

Drugs and the depressed elderly person

When clinical levels of depression occur there is accompanying reduction in the amines, particularly 5-hydroxytryptamine (5-HT, serotonin) and noradrenaline at neurosynaptic junctions in the brain. Many of the drugs used to treat depression increase the amount of these chemicals. This supports the hypothesis that amines are associated with the control of mood. The most frequently used groups of antidepressant drugs include: tricyclic antidepressants, tricyclic anxiolytics, 5-HT re-uptake inhibitors, monoamine oxidase (MAO) inhibitors, lithium, and other miscellaneous antidepressants

These are powerful drugs with well-known side-effects. Their use should be carefully monitored with any patient, but especially when they are given to elderly people (Glassman & Roose 1994).

Tricyclic antidepressants

These drugs are convenient for patients because they are readily absorbed in tablet form. Both imipramine

and amitriptyline have a long duration of action and need to be taken only once a day. Amitriptyline is best given at night because its sedative action will promote sleep. Metabolism in the liver results in the formation of therapeutically-active breakdown products. Therapeutic effect probably results because the drugs prevent re-uptake of amines at neurosynaptic junctions within the brain (Figure 23.5).

Some tricyclic antidepressants have a greater effect on noradrenaline (nortriptyline, amitriptyline), others on 5-HT (imipramine, amitvirtyline). Those in common use are shown in Table 23.4. Patients and their families need to be warned that although most tricyclic anti-

Before treatment

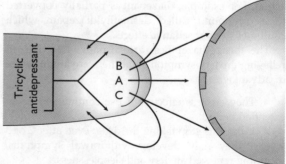

Catecholamines are released and stimulate receptor. Some only re-enter the nerve endings

After antidepressant

Antidepressant on nerve ending prevents re-entry of catecholemines – thus nerve receptors are stimulated leading to relief of depression

Figure 23.5 How tricyclic antidepressant drugs work. Source: Adapted from Trounce J, Gould D J 1994 Clinical pharmacology for nurses, 14th edn. Churchill Livingstone, Edinburgh with permission.

Table 23.4 The tricyclic antidepressants

Drug	Dose	Comments
Desipramine	75–150 mg	
Nortriptyline	20–50 mg	
Protriptyline	15–60 mg	Least sedative
Clomipramine	30–100 mg	Used for patients with obsessive disorder
Lofepramine	140–210 mg	Few side-effects. Minimal sedation

depressants relieve the sleeplessness so often associated with depression quite rapidly, it may take longer, sometimes several weeks, for other symptoms of depression to be relieved. They should be encouraged to persevere with treatment for at least 6 weeks, otherwise it will be impossible to determine whether the drug is of any value. Treatment is successful for about 80% of patients.

Side-effects are troublesome and include: fall in blood pressure sometimes accompanied by light-headedness and fainting, weight gain, and anticholinergic effects: dry mouth, urinary retention, dilation of the pupil and constipation.

Adverse effects associated with the tricyclic antidepressants occur in particular groups of patients:

• Patients with glaucoma because the pupil dilates in response to anticholinergic drugs.

• Epileptics. Fits may become more frequent. If there is no alternative the dose of anti-epileptic drugs may have to be increased.

• Patients known to be suffering from heart disease. Tricyclic drugs depress the conduction system in cardiac muscle and a number of sudden deaths have been reported in people with cardiac conditions who have taken these drugs.

• Treatment may have to be suspended for patients likely to receive drugs with a stimulating effect on the sympathetic nervous system (sympathomimetic drugs) such as adrenaline and noradrenaline. These are included in many local anaesthetics. Dangerous reactions occur because of the conflicting effects of the two groups of drugs on blood pressure: the tricyclic antidepressants are hypotensive, while adrenaline and noradrenaline cause a rapid increase in blood pressure.

• Tricyclic antidepressants are extremely dangerous in overdose. They cause cardiovascular disturbance, coma and seizures.

Anxiolytic tricyclic antidepressants

Drugs in this category share many similarities with the tricyclic antidepressants. However, their antidepressant action is weaker so they are considered particularly useful in the treatment of anxiety in people who are mildly depressed. Other advantages are their more rapid action and side-effects which though similar to the tricyclics, are less marked. Two commonly prescribed drugs are: doxepin taken as 50–100 mg tablets at night and dothiepin taken as 75–150 mg tablets at night.

5-HT re-uptake inhibitors

Deficiency of 5-hydroxytryptamine (5-HT) is thought to be linked with depression owing to its role in the control of mood. In consequence, a number of drugs have been developed to inhibit the re-uptake of 5-HT at neural synapses in the brain so that its concentration is raised. Examples are shown in Table 23.5. These drugs are not regarded as any more effective than the tricyclic antidepressants, but they have a number of distinct advantages. They are neither cardiotoxic nor anticholinergic and do not cause any increase in weight. Side-effects documented so far include occasional nausea and dyspepsia. Unfortunately, they reduce the effectiveness of anticoagulant drugs such as warfarin and interact with alcohol (Song et al 1993).

The benefits of fluoxetine are illustrated by the case of Mrs Benbow (Box 23.4).

Lithium

The body handles lithium in a manner very similar to sodium because the two chemicals are closely related. Lithium is thought to enter neurones in the brain and decrease their excitability. It can be used in the acute phase of mania and for prevention in bipolar disorder. It can also be used to prevent relapse in recurrent depression and may add to the action of antidepressants. Treatment must be planned carefully, especially for older people with reduced renal function

Table 23.5 5-HT re-uptake inhibitors

Drug	Dose
Fluvoxamine	100–200 mg
Fluoxetine	20 mg ⟶
Setraline	50 mg
Paroxetine	20 mg ⟶

Mrs Benbow, aged 80, was severely depressed. She lived alone, with poor eyesight, and an unsteady gait and tended to get muddled with medication. She was seen at home by a psychiatrist who arranged attendance at a day hospital twice a week and prescribed fluoxetine 20 mg one tablet daily. The simple once daily regime, together with the fluoxetine being dispensed in a clearly labelled drug drawer/dosette box helped to ensure good compliance considering the problems described. The prescription of fluoxetine also avoided the risk of postural hypotension, a problem of many tricyclic antidepressants, thus minimising the possibility of falls. The combination of antidepressant and day hospital ensured a full recovery from the depression.

---

because lithium will be retained if the kidneys are not working properly. Renal function tests are essential before the first dose is given. The usual daily dose is 0.5–1.2 g adjusted to produce a plasma level of 0.4–0.9 mmol/litre in blood withdrawn 12 hours after medication. Health professionals should be aware of the following and advise their patients accordingly:

- Lithium is lost slowly from the body so several days may pass before a steady plasma level is achieved. Monthly blood tests are necessary beginning a week after treatment starts.

- Lithium excretion is reduced and toxicity may develop if therapy coincides with taking loop diuretics. These are often prescribed for older people, probably by a different doctor. The dose of lithium will have to be reduced and more frequent blood monitoring may be necessary.

- Adverse effects fall into two categories, those associated with the dose and those which are not dose-related. Overdosage with lithium may result in weakness, drowsiness, confusion and ultimately coma. Other side-effects not related to dose include thyroid deficiency, increased urine output and weight increase.

Other antidepressant drugs

Members of this group exert their effects by modifying the amount of amines in the brain, but the mechanisms appear to be different from the drugs discussed above.

Mianserin. Mianserin does not inhibit re-uptake of catecholamines. Instead it is thought to operate by increasing the release of noradrenaline, although this

is not certain. The usual daily dose is 30–60 mg for younger adults and 30–40 mg for elderly people. The most troublesome side-effect is sedation. Older people may also develop serious haematological disorders; leucopenia, agranulocytosis and aplastic anaemia. Regular blood tests are essential.

Monoamine oxidase (MAO) inhibitors. These drugs result in accumulation of adrenaline, noradrenaline and 5-HT in the brain by interfering with degradation. The MAO inhibitors were first developed in the 1950s and until recently had been superseded by newer products such as the tricyclics because of their marked and potentially very serious side-effects and the dietary restrictions which have to be imposed when they are taken. However, some authorities believe they have a place in the treatment of atypical depression resistant to other forms of therapy (Potter et al 1991). Nevertheless it is felt that patients should only receive this type of medication if they can be monitored by health professionals experienced in their use. The least toxic and most commonly prescribed is phenelzine. It is given in doses of 15–60 mg orally.

Side-effects include: insomnia, nervousness, urinary retention, and (rarely) jaundice.

Interactions occur with other centrally-acting drugs and with many common types of food. MAO inhibitors dangerously exaggerate the effects of barbiturates, alcohol, morphine, pethidine and cocaine. They interact with adrenaline, amphetamines and vasoconstrictor substances including proprietary cold cures taken to reduce symptoms of congestion. The result is likely to be restlessness, severe headache, hypertension and possibly coma. Similar effects occur if the patient eats many types of food. The list is long: cheese, meat and meat extracts, yeast extracts, game, broad beans, pickled herrings, many red wines and beers. The reactions occur because these items contain vasopressor chemicals which are usually metabolised by amine oxidase acting in its normal fashion as an enzyme. If breakdown is inhibited the vasopressors build up to produce toxic effects. People taking MAO inhibitor drugs are often given cards to carry in case of emergency and need to be given the information shown in Box 23.5.

Any patient scheduled to undergo surgery should be warned to stop taking the tablets at least 2 weeks before the operation is planned, to avoid the possibility of interaction with pethidine or morphine. It is particularly important for patients to hand in or destroy all their old drugs because interaction with tricyclic antidepressants is exceptionally dangerous. If people living at home are taking these drugs it is helpful if they are visited regularly by a health

---

Box 23.5   Essential information for people taking monoamine oxidase inhibitor drugs

This treatment card must be carried at all times while you are taking your drugs and for 2 weeks afterwards. If you go to the doctor or receive any other medical or dental treatment you must show this card first.

You must not:

- Eat cheese, pickled herrings or broad beans.
- Drink Bovril®, Oxo®, Marmite® or any similar meat or meat extract or yeast extract.
- Take any other medicines. You must not use any other tablets, nose drops, sprays, suppositories or powders. You must not take any cures for coughs or colds.

You should:

- Report any side-effects at once.
- Report any food which disagrees with you at once.
- Avoid alcohol.
- Eat only fresh food, especially fresh meat, offal, poultry and fish. Avoid game.

---

professional who is able to monitor them for side-effects. Complaints of headache should never be ignored because this is an indication of increased blood pressure. Arrangements for the blood pressure to be taken should be made as soon as possible. Moclobemide is a newly introduced member of this group, prescribed only for people with major depression. It is reported to cause fewer problems with food. The dose is 300 mg daily, usually given in divided doses after meals. Side-effects include sleep disturbance, dizziness, nausea, headache and restlessness. Disturbance in liver function is a rare side-effect, but for this reason the drug may be unsuitable for some elderly people.

Drugs and elderly patients who cannot sleep

Elderly people often have problems sleeping, particularly if they are anxious or depressed. Insomnia itself may generate anxiety, difficulty concentrating and debility, especially if the problem is long-standing. However, sleep requirement varies between individuals and tends to diminish with age. Whereas the typical adolescent requires about 10 hours sleep a night and the typical adult about 8 hours, by old age sleep requirement has fallen. It is believed that elderly people need approximately 6 hours sleep and that insomnia may be exaggerated (Prinz 1990). This is

understandable as time passes slowly at night, especially for the person who feels worried or distressed. Some people doze during the day and in consequence sleep less well at night, not realising how long they are regularly spending nodding over the television or a book. The best action is to explore reasons for lack of sleep and recommend simple, natural remedies. Worries can be discussed and practical solutions suggested. Treatment for depression will usually resolve any associated insomnia. Patients may benefit from taking more physical exercise so that they are more tired at the end of the day. Warm drinks may help providing that they do not contain caffeine: some people do not realise that it is in tea as well as coffee. Gradual 'winding down' at the end of the day with a long, dull book is helpful too. Pain interferes with sleep and must be controlled.

Hypnotics, the drugs which induce sleep, should be used with caution because tolerance develops rapidly, sometimes within as little as 2–3 weeks and patients can soon become dependent (Perry and Wu 1984). Withdrawal at this stage results in increasing wakefulness at night which may take some time to settle down. Hypnotics operate on the cerebral cortex, but in most cases the sleep that they induce is not natural. They suppress the REM sleep associated with rapid eye movements and dreaming. People deprived of REM sleep display psychological changes during waking hours. It is now believed that although hypnotics have a place in alleviating insomnia for short periods during times of excessive stress or worry, their use should be discouraged. The number of prescriptions has fallen in recent years but they are still used widely in hospital and it is here that a lifetime of dependence may begin. A recent study indicates that this situation is unnecessary and need not occur if other therapeutic interventions are encouraged. This study showed that nurses working in hospital wards with a team approach to care gave out almost three times as much night sedation as those on wards where primary nursing had been implemented. Their attitudes correlated more closely with a 'medical model' of care delivery than attitudes of nurses in the primary nursing ward where a more client-centred approach was apparent (Duxbury 1994).

Unfortunately there is evidence that sleeping problems are not taken seriously in hospitals and other institutions (Wilkie 1990). Staff may contribute to the problem through lack of care about noise (Hodgson 1991). However, the individual responsible for providing care is usually the one to notice lack of sleep or to receive complaints of sleeplessness and it is this same person who will decide whether or not to give hypnotics if they are prescribed. If the use of a hypnotic is considered to be justified, the nature of insomnia must be considered carefully before a suitable drug is selected, so observation of the patient is important. There are three categories of insomnia:

- Transient insomnia occurring in people who do not generally have a problem sleeping. This is usually caused by some upset in the normal routine: hospital admission, being away from home. A short-acting benzodiazepine is the most appropriate drug. Temazepam is widely prescribed in these circumstances.
- Short-term insomnia is caused by anxiety, illness or other worries. Again, short acting benzodiazepines may be given, but if anxiety is marked diazepam may be more appropriate because its effects will persist into the next day. Treatment should cease as soon as possible because of the risks of tolerance and dependence with this drug.
- Chronic insomnia is a symptom of moderate or severe mental disorder, especially depression (Dample 1989). However, simple explanations may exist such as excessive use of tea or coffee. Discussion of bedtime habits is always worthwhile. The drug of choice in the case of genuine chronic insomnia is diazepam. This can be given intermittently for about a month. If this is not successful antidepressants may be indicated, but management of chronic insomnia is likely to be difficult and ongoing. The main hypnotic drugs used with elderly people are examined below.

Benzodiazepines

These have already been discussed in conjunction with the management of anxiety. Their main advantage with older people is their safety. The three most commonly prescribed are:

- Nitrazepam, the first benzodiazepine to be recommended for use as a hypnotic. Originally it was welcomed in response to claims that it would not produce confusion in elderly people. Such optimism was unfounded. Another disadvantage is that the sedative effect may be evident the next day.
- Diazepam is used chiefly as a minor tranquilliser, but is also an effective hypnotic in cases when a person is anxious. Its persistent sedative effect is desirable in these circumstances.
- Temazepam has a shorter half-life and duration of action than most other benzodiazepine drugs because metabolism does not produce other metabolites with sedative action. These are valuable

properties because they reduce residual drowsiness the following day.

Zopiclone

This drug is not related to the benzodiazepines chemically but its action is probably similar. It is thought to exert its effects via gamma-aminobutyric acid (GABA). Zopiclone is rapidly absorbed. It produces sleep lasting for several hours without inducing hangover, but tolerance and dependence may still be problems. It is unsuitable for some people because it can cause hallucinations. The usual dose is 7.5 mg before retiring.

Chlormethiazole

This drug is related chemically to vitamin B_1. It is used orally or intravenously as a sedative and a hypnotic. Its effects are of short duration. Chlormethiazole is particularly valuable for elderly people, especially if they become agitated or confused. This may occur in response to withdrawal of alcohol. For people who cannot sleep the usual dose is two 192 mg capsules. For agitated patients requiring sedation three capsules of chlormethiazole are given four times a day. Intravenous chlormethiazole is used to control severe epilepsy (status epilepticus) and delirium tremens. The patient must be observed carefully because intravenous use is associated with risks of respiratory depression and low blood pressure. Oral use is very safe. A few patients report nasal congestion after taking their capsules, but no other side-effects have been reported.

Paraldehyde

The most striking characteristic of this drug is its distinctive odour which lingers hours after it has been taken, and its equally unpleasant taste. Not surprisingly, paraldehyde has never been a popular medicine. Paraldehyde takes the form of an oily liquid soluble in water. It can be given orally, rectally or as an intramuscular injection administered with a glass syringe (it undergoes chemical interaction to destroy plastic). The dose is 5 ml for adults, repeated 2 hours later if required. Care is necessary because paraldehyde injections are painful and may result in the formation of an abscess at the site of administration. Although once used widely for the management of disturbed behaviour, paraldehyde has been superseded by newer drugs, and is now mainly of historic interest.

Chloral hydrate

This a drug that can be used safely with older people who cannot sleep, although a benzodiazepine is more likely to be prescribed if the individual is confused. The usual dose is 500 mg–2 g at bedtime but this will be reduced when it is intended for a frail elderly person because it may depress respiration. Chloral is dispensed either as 500 mg capsules or as an elixir and is rapidly absorbed to produce hypnotic effect within approximately 30 minutes. Its effects wear off after about 4 hours. It is not suitable for anybody who suffers from symptoms of indigestion because it is a gastric irritant.

Barbiturates

These drugs operate directly on the cerebral cortex. They were once used in the treatment of severe, intractable insomnia. Occasionally they still have to be prescribed for people who have become dependent on them, but they have no other place in the treatment of sleeping problems because dependence and tolerance develop so easily. They are dangerous drugs which have a cumulative effect with repeated use, leading to excessive sedation. This may have tragic consequences. Withdrawal is also problematic, resulting in rebound insomnia, anxiety, tremor, dizziness, fits and delirium. Most barbiturates are now controlled drugs, used therapeutically for the treatment of severe epilepsy. Patients who do have to use barbiturates must be monitored with great care and warned that interactions with other drugs are common, especially alcohol.

Alcohol (ethanol, ethyl alcohol)

Some people think that alcohol is a good sedative. In sufficient amounts, varying with build, tolerance and other factors related to the make-up of the individual, it will certainly induce sleep, but this is not really a desirable use of alcoholic beverages. Like most hypnotics it depresses REM sleep and many people wake up later in the night with rebound insomnia. The diuretic action of alcohol interferes with sleep. Small amounts may be comforting to older people. They should not be denied a regular drink when they come into hospital or sheltered accommodation if it has formed part of their usual routine. Individuals may become restless and agitated if they are denied alcohol to which they have become accustomed. However, the dangers of accidents in relation to the use of alcohol should never be forgotten, especially if it is combined with other drugs or if the individual is in unfamiliar surroundings. Many accidents among elderly people, especially the frail elderly, are related to the use of alcohol or to sedatives, especially benzodiazepines (Askham et al 1990).

Special points to remember when hypnotic drugs are used with older people are:

- Minimum doses used for the minimum length of time are essential.
- Careful observation for giddiness, instability and tendency to fall is essential.
- Individuals should be aware that the effects may be potentiated by the use of alcohol or other drugs.
- Distressing dreams or hallucinations may occur. These are frightening for elderly clients.
- Observation for symptoms of disorientation or confusion is important.
- Tablets should never be stored on a bedside table. Individuals may forget that they have taken night sedation and repeat the dose or wake up and think that it has not worked properly and take some more.

Information which should be given to the patient or carers when hypnotics have been prescribed is shown in Box 23.6.

Box 23.6 Special information for people taking sedatives and hypnotics

- Take your tablets with a full glass of water. If they upset your stomach you may take them with a snack, e.g. a biscuit.
- You will not fall asleep immediately. You will probably begin to feel drowsy within 15–30 minutes.
- Do not keep the bottle at your bedside. Keep all tablets in a safe place, out of sight.
- Do not smoke in bed after taking your tablets.
- Be careful if you have to get up during the night. You may feel unsteady.
- Do not take any other medicines without consulting your doctor.

Drugs and the management of confused elderly people

Confusion may be the result of physical or mental health problems or a combination of the two. In older people the cause is likely to be multifactorial and treatment is not easy. In the above discussion mention has been made of a number of drugs which can be given to help calm individuals who become agitated and disruptive. Compliance by patients themselves is not often a problem because confused people are usually reliant on other people for administering their medicines. However, the person giving them needs guidance on their proper use. Two scenarios are possible:

- Over-use by exhausted relatives who depend on the action of the drug to achieve peace for themselves, or in institutions for the sake of other residents who would otherwise endure disruption and loss of sleep.
- Under-use because relatives or staff feel guilty about sedating someone who will not be the foremost beneficiary of treatment.

There is no easy solution to either of these situations. Relatives entrusted with the care of someone who is severely disoriented deserve sympathy and practical support. The option of respite or night hospital care should be offered if at all possible. Time should be spent to allow relatives to voice their worries, including any that relate to medication. Frequent recourse to the maximum prescribed dose of a sedative may indicate that the carer needs more help to cope. At the same time, they should be left in no doubt that all medicines, but particularly the major tranquillisers, antidepressants and hypnotics discussed above are potent drugs with marked and undesirable side-effects if misused. Those inclined to under-medicate should be aware that confusion and delusions are frightening experiences for the person suffering from them and that it is not kind to deny them medication designed to help, providing that adverse reactions have not arisen.

In some cases, however, the cause of confusion and agitation may be related to a particular circumstance and can be alleviated without heavy reliance on drugs. Unfamiliar surroundings may be a contributory factor. Elderly people who function well in their own homes may suddenly become disoriented when they are removed to another environment, especially towards the end of the day when they become tired. A tranquilliser may be helpful short term, but the best solution is return to the comforting familiarity of their own home. In these circumstances hospital admission to assess and treat acute symptoms is most effective if of short duration. If long-term institutional care is essential treasured possessions from home will help. In other cases the drugs themselves may be the cause of the problem. Over-medication with hypotensives may cause low blood pressure associated with nausea, dizziness, light-headedness and risk of falls. Over-use of major and minor tranquillisers and hypnotics, especially benzodiazepines, will result in side-effects

which initially increase rather than decrease as the individual is weaned off them. There are many ethical dilemmas in deciding which care and treatments are in the best interests of elderly people, especially those with mental health problems, and deciding when to have recourse to sedating and tranquillising drugs features prominently among them.

Cerebral vasodilators

These drugs are claimed to improve mental function by enhancing cerebral blood supply. This may become diminished in old age due to arteriosclerosis, with symptoms of confusion further exacerbated by poor oxygenation through low haemoglobin or coexisting respiratory disease. In trials individuals may perform better with psychological tests after they have received cerebral vasodilators, but clinical benefit seems slender. Drugs in this group include:

- Cyclandelate which is sometimes given during the acute phase of cerebrovascular accident (CVA). The normal daily dose is 1.2–1.6 mg. It is available as capsules or in suspension.
- Naftidrofuryl given parenterally in cases of atrioventricular block. The normal dose is 200 mg infused over 90 minutes twice a day.
- Co-dergocrine mesylate. This is sometimes prescribed for elderly patients with dementia. It can cause postural hypotension in hypertensive patients. The usual dose is 1.5 mg three times a day.

ELECTROCONVULSIVE THERAPY (ECT)

Recently there has been a resurgence of interest in the use of electroconvulsive therapy (ECT) especially for older people who do not respond well to drug therapy (Wilkinson 1993). Many of these patients respond slowly to treatment with antidepressants or have a medical condition which contraindicates treatment with any of the currently available medications (Katona 1993). For this group ECT provides a valuable and effective alternative. Its chief advantage is speed of action, especially for elderly people who are so seriously depressed that suicide or decline in health through self-neglect pose real dangers.

The procedure and what it involves

ECT has had a bad press. Members of the public and many health professionals have exaggerated ideas of what this treatment involves and the effects that it may have on the recipient. Possibly this is because their fears have been fuelled by films featuring the treatment of aggressive mentally disturbed patients. In the past ECT was indeed a source of dread, not surprisingly; it was administered to conscious patients without safeguarding them against physical injury (Mawson 1985). This situation is unfortunate because ECT can be very effective in the treatment of people with delusional depression, although controversy reigns concerning its use for other conditions (Potter et al 1991). Fears can be allayed by giving careful explanations to patients and their families. It has proved helpful if they are allowed to see the ECT equipment before treatment is planned and this is routine in some units (Wilkinson 1993). It is recommended for individuals who have not responded to tricyclic antidepressant drugs or those who are so severely depressed that rapid treatment is essential because they have suicidal tendencies or cannot eat. This may include frail elderly people. Their depression may have been overlooked or its severity not recognised. They may not be able to take tricyclic antidepressants because of poor compliance or side-effects.

ECT involves passing an electric current through the brain. There are two types (see Figure 23.6):

- Unilateral, where the route is longitudinal through the dominant hemisphere. In right-handed people

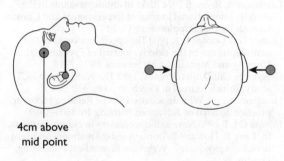

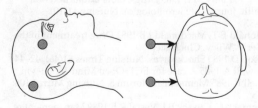

Figure 23.6 Bilateral and unilateral electroconvulsive therapy.

this is the left hemisphere. In left-handed people the right hemisphere tends to be dominant. Short-term cognitive impairment, one of the adverse effects of ECT, is reported to be reduced with this method (Weeks et al 1980).

- Bilateral, where the current follows a transverse route through the brain. This is said to be the most rapidly effective (Gregory et al 1985).

Passage of the current induces a grand mal type seizure which with modern equipment with a properly prepared and sedated patient may be detectable only through the use of a sophisticated monitoring device. It is quite safe for use with the elderly. Broken limbs and bitten tongues have long ceased to be side-effects of ECT. Nowadays safety is further promoted by the following safeguards:

- The ECT machine must conform to British Standards.
- A very small current (a few mA) is used for any patient, but especially older people.
- The patient is given a short-acting general anaesthetic combined with a muscle relaxant.

The nurse is involved in the patient's preparation for general anaesthesia and recovery. Careful assessment is particularly important with older people as they may have arthritic limbs making positioning difficult or sensory defects (impaired hearing, vision) which may impair communication and reduce their understanding of events. Care is the same as that for any unconscious patient and recovery occurs in about 10 minutes. Older people may feel a little dizzy or unsteady after lying down and should if possible be accompanied home. The most common side-effects associated with ECT include confusion in the immediate recovery period and longer-term memory disturbance. Immediate confusion is reported to last between 15 minutes and several hours, but can be reduced if unilateral ECT is given. This is generally the treatment of choice for elderly people, especially those receiving ECT as out-patients. Longer-term effects on the memory of elderly people are difficult to assess, especially when other variables such as depression may affect cognitive function.

The action of ECT

The development of ECT dates from the 1930s. At this time it was believed that epilepsy and schizophrenia could not coexist within the same individual (Mitchell 1985). The origin of both treatment and the theory to support it are attributed to a physician called Von

Meduna. The hypothesis was rapidly disproved (Whyte 1983), but by this time ECT had become an established treatment and has been used ever since. There have been numerous controlled trials to examine its efficacy. The results suggest that ECT must have some therapeutic effectiveness because patients who have undergone treatment show better short-term improvement than those acting as controls (Brandon 1984). However, the manner in which treatment exerts its effects remains to be established and there are a number of acknowledged side-effects including loss of memory, although this is probably short-term only and may be more related to cognitive function than the treatment itself (West 1981).

Ethics

Despite evidence that ECT can benefit severely depressed patients, many nurses, social workers and other members of the caring professions feel concerned about its use on ethical grounds, because its mode of action remains unclear. It has even been argued that persistent use of ECT operates as a barrier to the development of newer, better approaches (McDowall 1985). But, at present, for some people with such severe and intractable depression that all the activities associated with normal life are suspended, there is no alternative. It could thus be argued that to withhold ECT under these circumstances would not be morally defensible. After all, very little is known about the action of many centrally-acting drugs used every day with mentally ill patients. At present it appears that ECT will remain a treatment option for several years to come. In the meantime, members of the health professions have an important role dispelling alarmist stories and explaining the simple procedure involved.

ACKNOWLEDGEMENT

I thank Colin Hughes for his comments on an earlier draft of this chapter and for providing the case examples.

REFERENCES

Askham J, Gucksman E, Owens P, Swift C, Tinker A, Yu G 1990 Home and leisure accident research: a review of falls among elderly people. Age Concern Institute of Gerontology, King's College, London

Bliss M 1981 Prescribing for the elderly. British Medical Journal 283: 203–206

Brandon S 1984 Electroconvulsive therapy: results in depressive illness. British Medical Journal 288: 22–25

Burns B, Phillipson C 1986 Drugs, aging and society: social and pharmacological perspectives. Croom Helm, London

Cargill J M 1992 Medication compliance in elderly people: influencing variables and interventions. Journal of Advanced Nursing 17: 422–426

Cartwright A, Smith C 1988 Elderly people: their medicines and their doctors. Routledge, London

Conn V 1991 Older adults: factors that predict the use of over the counter medication. Journal of Advanced Nursing 16: 1190–1196

Culshaw F 1994 Composition and effects of commonly used neuroleptics. Nursing Times 90(38): 38–40

Dample A 1989 Psychiatric aspects of sleep disorders. Geriatric Medicine 10(2): 67–70

Duxbury J 1994 An investigation into primary nursing and its effect upon the nursing attitudes about and administration of PRN night sedation. Journal of Advanced Nursing 19: 923–931

Fielo S, Rizzolo M A 1985 The effects of age on pharmacokinetics. Geriatric Nursing 6(6): 328–331

Glassman A, Roose S 1994 Risks of antidepressants in the elderly. International Journal of Experimental and Clinical Gerontology 40(Supplement): 15–20

Gomez G E, Gomez E A 1990 The special concerns of neuroleptic use in the elderly. Journal of Psychosocial Nursing and Mental Health Services 28(1): 7–14

Gregory S, Gill D, Shawcross C 1985 The Nottingham ECT study. British Journal of Psychiatry 146: 520–524

Hodgson A 1991 Why do we need sleep? Relating theory to practice. Journal of Advanced Nursing 16: 1503–1510

Katona C L E 1993 New anti-depressants in elderly patients. In: Levy R, Howard R, Burns A (eds) Treatment and care in old age psychiatry. Wrighton Biomedical Publishing, London

Lamy P P 1985 Side effects of diuretics; a danger for the aged. Journal of Gerontological Nursing 11(6): 44–45

Lamy P P, Lamy M L 1985 Drugs, older adults and oral health. Journal of Gerontological Nursing 11(10): 36–37

Macdonald E T, Macdonald J B 1982 Drug treatment in the elderly. Wiley, Chichester

Mawson D 1985 Shockwaves. Nursing Times 81(46): 42–44

McDowall A 1985 A case for ECT. Open Mind 16: vii–viii

Mitchell R 1985 Mental heath forum 5. Nursing Mirror 106: iii–v

Montamat S C, Cusack B J, Vestal R E 1989 Management of drug therapy in the elderly. New England Journal of Medicine 321: 303–309

Morrow D, Leirer V, Sheik J 1988 Adherence and medication instructions: review and recommendations. Journal of the American Geriatrics Society 36: 1147–1159

Parkin D M, Henney C R, Quirk J, Crooks S J 1976 Deviation from prescribed treatment after discharge from hospital. British Medical Journal 200: 686–688

Perry S W, Wu A 1984 Rationale for the use of hypnotic drugs in a general hospital. Annals of Internal Medicine 3: 441–446

Platzer H 1989 Post-operative confusion in the elderly. Nursing Times 85(14): 66–67

Potter W Z, Rudorfer M V, Manji H 1991 The pharmacological treatment of depression. New England Journal of Medicine 325: 633–641

Prinz P N 1990 Sleep disorders and aging. New England Journal of Medicine 323: 520–521

Song F, Freemantle N, Sheldon T A, House A, Watson P, Long A 1993 Selective serotonin uptake inhibitors: meta-analysis of efficacy and acceptability. British Medical Journal 306: 683–686

Strang J, Griffiths P, Abbey J 1994 Survey of injected benzodiazepines among drug users in Britain. British Medical Journal 308: 1082–1083

Wade B, Bowling A 1986 Appropriate use of drugs by elderly people. Journal of Advanced Nursing 11: 47–55

Wade B E, Sawyer L, Bell J 1983 Dependency with dignity. Occasional Papers on Social Administration No. 68. Bedford Square Press, London

Webb C, Addison C, Holman H, Saklaki B, Wagner A 1990 Self-medication for elderly patients. Nursing Times 86(16): 46–49

Weeks D, Freeman C P, Kendall R 1980 ECT: enduring cognitive defects. British Journal of Psychiatry 137: 26–37

Weibert R T, Dee D A 1980 Improving patient medication compliance. The Medical Economics Company, New Jersey

West E 1981 Electric convulsion therapy in depression: a double blind controlled trial. British Medical Journal 282: 355–357

Wilkie K 1990 Golden slumbers. Nursing Times 86(51): 36–38

Wilkinson D G 1993 ECT in the elderly. In: Levy R, Howard R, Burns A (eds) Treatment and care in old age psychiatry. Wrighton Biomedical Publishing, London

Whyte L 1983 In our right senses? Nursing Mirror 156(42): 20–21

RECOMMENDED READING

Ballinger B R 1990 Hypnotics and anxiolytics. British Medical Journal 300: 456–457. *The history of the development and use of benzodiazepine and other hypnotic drugs is discussed, especially in relation to dependence and side-effects. The need for careful monitoring and evaluation of treatment is emphasised. This is a medical report, but clearly written without medical jargon.*

Bateman D N, Chaplin 1988 Centrally acting drugs. British Medical Journal 296: 417–419. *A succinct short article debating the advantages of the newer tricyclic drugs and speculating on possible modes of action.*

Bergen A, Labute L 1993 Promoting effective drug taking by elderly people in the community. In: Dines A, Cribb A (ed) Health promotion concepts and practice. Blackwell Scientific Publications, Oxford. *Issues surrounding compliance with drug regimes among elderly people in the community are clearly discussed in this well-referenced chapter and there is useful debate concerning 'intelligent non-compliance' when the individual is justifiably worried about the side-effects of medicines. A number of case studies are presented. Teachers would find these particularly useful to initiate discussions with students on pre- and post-registration programmes.*

Bird C, Hassall J 1993 Self-administration of drugs: a guide to implementation. Scutari Press, London. *This slim little volume provides a general introduction to the topic of patient self-administration. There are numerous practical tips which would be of immense value for practitioners keen to involve clients more closely in their own care whether in hospital or the community, although the book does not provide much in the way of theoretical discussion.*

Crossfield T 1988 Curse or cure? Nursing Times 84(5): 66–67. *An informative short article examining the different forms of ECT in current use and presenting differing perspectives on the ethics of participating or refusing to participate in the application of this controversial treatment.*

Koller W C, Huber S J 1989 Tremor disorders of aging: diagnosis and management. Geriatrics 44(5): 33–41. *A helpful account of the main causes of Parkinsonism among elderly people and approaches to treatment.*

Quilligan S 1990 Tablets to take away: why some elderly people fail to comply with their medication. Professional Nurse 5(11): 566–568. *A good review of the literature specifically related to compliance. Easily readable and suitable for those with little prior knowledge of the subject.*

The organisation of care for elderly people with mental health problems

SECTION CONTENTS

24

The development of service provision

Anthea Tinker

INTRODUCTION AND SCOPE OF THE CHAPTER

This chapter is concerned with the development of services for elderly people with mental health problems. Many of the developments and issues are common to people of all ages. However, in this chapter there is a particular focus on older people. It should also be noted that some of the issues and developments, such as community care, are applicable to elderly people with both physical and mental disabilities. For a more detailed discussion of this see Tinker (1992).

A number of useful historical accounts of service provision do already exist. Two of the best are Kathleen Jones's *Asylums and After* (Jones 1993b) and Elaine Murphy's *After the Asylums: Community Care for People with Mental Illness* (Murphy 1991). Both of these are very readable. They differ, however, from this chapter in two main ways. First, both of them are historical accounts and second, they are not specifically about elderly people. Both do, of course, analyse policy changes and do look at elderly people but this is not their focus.

The purpose of this chapter is to look at the development of services and also to consider certain themes and in these to make some assessment of the changes.

This chapter is divided into six sections which deal in turn with:

- major policy changes and why they have taken place
- the development of services
- how services are organised and who provides them
- the responsiveness of the providers
- financial and economic aspects of provision
- the importance of links between services and integrated provision.

441

The focus is on the UK, where it can be seen that there is much to learn from what has happened over recent years. The Appendix gives a summary of recent key events, policies, reports and legislation in the UK.

It must always be remembered that there are a number of different kinds of elderly people involved and that generalisations may be dangerous. Elderly people with learning disabilities may have different needs from those with dementia. For those with mental illness, the 1972 Department of Health and Social Security (DHSS 1972) circular, *Services for Mental Illness Related to Old Age*, distinguished between three main groups among people with mental illness symptoms to whom the term 'psychogeriatric' is often loosely applied. These are:

- patients who entered hospital before modern methods of treatment were available and have grown old in them
- elderly patients with functional mental illness
- elderly people with dementia.

MAJOR POLICY CHANGES AND WHY THEY HAVE TAKEN PLACE

The majority of elderly people with mental health problems have always remained in their own homes with care given in the main by relatives. In a few cases some special provision was made available. For example the Bethlem Hospital in London, originally a priory, started caring for 'mad' people around 1350. For some, institutional care has been available but the nature of this has changed. In some cases it had been of a reasonable standard but in many cases people with mental health problems were kept apart, as much out of fear as for any other reason. Incarcerated in buildings which were often far from other people, they lived out their lives with little in the way of treatment. Living alongside mentally ill people would often be others who had been institutionalised for other reasons, but who had subsequently aged there. These would sometimes include women who had had illegitimate children.

There are many reasons why policies have changed so that institutional care is less acceptable. Some of these reasons are negative and some are positive. Many of the negative ones are to do with the problems of institutions. Foremost among these has been research on the unsatisfactory conditions in institutions. Unsuitable buildings, sometimes badly maintained, often had their origins in accommodation designed for people who had to be provided for under the Poor Law Amendment Act 1834. This was supposed to provide a lower standard of living than that enjoyed by the population outside. Poor food and clothing was often the norm. Added to this was, in many cases, an institutional atmosphere with rigid rules and time-tables. What was even more damning was the often low standard of medical care. Many old people presently alive in the UK remember these conditions and fear being sent away from home in case the hospital or home resembles the dreaded 'workhouses' of earlier days. Indeed, many buildings which were used for this purpose do still exist.

Studies such as Robb's *Sans Everything* (Robb 1967) and Meacher's *Taken for a Ride* (Meacher 1972) painted a bleak picture of conditions in institutions for elderly people. Official reports on psychiatric hospitals have also been damning, for example those in the early 1970s on Ely Hospital, Cardiff, Farleigh Hospital and Whittingham Hospital.

In some cases the way the patients acted was blamed on 'institutionalisation'. As Murphy (1991) puts it:

Apathy, passivity, social withdrawal, egocentric behaviour and helpless dependence on staff for daily care were regarded as an inevitable consequence of remaining for years under the control of an institutionalised, repressive regime where social conformity and acquiescence to the rules were rigidly imposed. Although it was clear that bad institutions did have many detrimental effects, and research had demonstrated that less restrictive regimes promoted improvements in patients' social behaviour, many of the disabilities observed in long-term patients were later shown to be symptoms of mental disorder itself, not a consequence of the institution.   (Murphy 1991, pp. 10–11)

And, she tellingly added: 'These symptoms are not miraculously prevented by keeping people out of institutions' (Murphy 1991, p. 11).

The second negative reason against institutions is the cost. Although costings of all kinds of provision are still in their infancy, there is no doubt that institutional care is not cheap. (This is further developed in the section dealing with financial and economic aspects of provision later in this chapter.) A further reason is the problem of getting and keeping staff. In part this is practical, in that many institutions are outside or on the outskirts of towns, with consequent problems of transport. But it is also likely to be due in part to the stigma which is attached to institutions. Apart from acute hospitals, others such as long-term and psychiatric hospitals are less likely to be favoured by doctors and nurses.

There is also a range of positive reasons why the emphasis has changed from institutional to community care. The development of drugs and other forms of treatment have meant that many previously very disturbed people can remain in their own communities without causing disruption and problems. Another reason has been the development of a range of services to enable elderly people to remain in their own homes. These include day care, special housing, respite care, lunch clubs and holidays. Some of them are primarily designed for the elderly person and some for their carers.

Added to these reasons is the growing awareness of patients' rights underlined in the Mental Health Act 1983, and greater policy stress on the importance of choice for service users.

The focus of policies has, therefore, been twofold. The first has been on closing institutions. Some would argue that this policy has gone too far and that institutions still have a real role, including the provision of asylum for the person and to enable their carer to live a more normal life. It is worth looking carefully at the traditional role of the old psychiatric institutions. The House of Commons Health Committee (1994), in its report *Better Off in the Community? The Care Of People Who Are Seriously Mentally Ill*, described the institution as intending 'to provide a "total" environment for their patients so that the full range of their needs would be met' (House of Commons Health Committee 1994, p. viii). It listed the functions of the old psychiatric hospitals as:

- assessment and treatment (both physical and mental)
- long-term care for people with learning disabilities or those who contravened 'normal' behaviour (e.g. illegitimate pregnancy)
- food
- clothing
- a basic income
- some occupational and vocational rehabilitation
- respite care
- out-patient care
- protection of patients from the public
- protection of the public from patients
- asylum (peace and quiet)
- shelter
- recreation
- a social world
- some care for forensic patients.

Although the Committee went on to make critical comments, some of the advantages were also evident. They stated:

The benefits of centralisation in an institution give the 'illusion' of comprehensive care and real economies of scale. These are considered to be offset by the lack of independence, choice and individualised care for patients. While the hospital provides an element of safety and protection from exploitation, this is at the expense of allowing individuals the responsibility for their own affairs.
(House of Commons Health Committee 1994, p. viii)

An earlier House of Commons Social Services Committee (1990) in their report, *Community Care: Services for People with a Mental Handicap and People with a Mental Illness*, had also said that there were some advantages in some kind of 'asylum' provision. However, they discussed at length other possible names including sanctuary, haven and refuge. They suggested that the Government give further and detailed consideration to what is meant by the term 'asylum', who this type of service is for, and how it can best be provided and financed. The Government tacitly accepted the need for some institutional care when they identified the need for continuing and terminal care beds for people with dementia (Department of Health 1993b, p. 36).

Arie (1986) argues that there are some patients, including some with dementia, for whom institutional care is the only humane and right solution. Others have also argued that dementia in old age is the most likely mental illness to require institutional care (Blessed 1988).

The second focus of policies has been on the provision of services at home – or community care as it is usually (and sometimes misleadingly) called. The philosophy behind this policy, which has been adopted for all groups who need help and not just elderly people or people with mental health problems, was summed up in the White Paper *Caring for People: Community Care in the Next Decade and Beyond* (Department of Health 1989b) which preceded the National Health Service and Community Care Act 1990. The objectives were to:

- 'enable people to live as normal a life as possible in their own homes or in a homely environment in the local community'
- 'provide the right amount of care and support to help people achieve maximum possible independence and, by acquiring or re-acquiring basic living skills, help them to achieve their full potential'
- 'give people a greater individual say in how they live their lives and the services they need to help them to do so'.
(Department of Health 1989b, p. 4)

These were the policy aims underlying the Act. More specific policy objectives for people with mental health problems were given in *The Health of the Nation: A Consultative Document for Health in England* (Department of Health 1991). This stated that, 'There is a clear and urgent need to realign the resources tied up in the old hospitals into more appropriate services' (Department of Health 1991, p. 87).

Despite these broad policy aims there has not been a great deal of official guidance in terms of objectives and standards. There is even less which is specific to elderly people. For example, *The Health of the Nation Key Area Handbook: Mental Illness*, which had as its targets improving the health and social functioning of mentally ill people and reducing the suicide rate, only says that: 'Particular issues for people who are elderly will include the need for:

- continuing and terminal care beds for people with dementia
- respite care
- practical advice and support for carers in dealing with, for example, behavioural problems, incontinence or immobility' (Department of Health 1993b, p. 36).

However, the objective of the Mental Health Task Force, which was set up in 1992 by the Department of Health, was to ensure the substantial completion of transfer of mental health services away from obsolete hospitals to a balanced range of locally based services (Audit Commission 1994, p. 105).

What then have been the consequences of the policies?

Looking first at closures of the large psychiatric institutions, there were 130 open in 1960, but by March 1993 only 89 remained (House of Commons Health Committee 1994). The Department of Health estimates that only 22 will remain by the end of the century. The policy director of MIND has argued that another 'bone of contention is whether psychiatric hospital closures should be speeded up, slowed down or halted altogether' (Sayce 1994, p. 10).

The number of beds for mentally ill people declined from a peak of 149 000 in 1955 to 50 278 in 1991/1992 in England (House of Commons Health Committee 1994). This marked decline is well illustrated by the Audit Commission in Figure 24.1. There is some evidence that the rate and extent of bed closures has not happened on the same scale in other continental countries except possibly Italy (Hirsch, quoted in Jones 1993b, p. 244).

It is not always easy to obtain statistics to estimate the effect of policies. Jones points out that 'when mental hospitals were separately designated, and most patients stayed in hospital for comparatively long periods, admissions, discharges and average length of stay could be calculated with some confidence. Now that many acute patients stay for very short periods of time (see Fig. 24.2), accurate compilation even of hospital data has become much more difficult' (Jones 1993b, p. 244). She gives figures for the decline in the

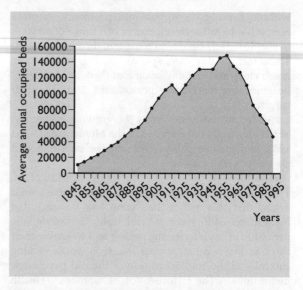

Figure 24.1 The number of hospital beds. The number has declined markedly since the 1950s. Source: Audit Commission 1994 (p. 6) Finding a place: a review of mental health services for adults. HMSO, London.

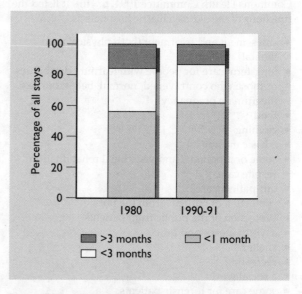

Figure 24.2 Length of stay in hospital. Shorter stays have become more common. Source: Audit Commission 1994 (p. 6) Finding a place: a review of mental health services for adults. HMSO, London.

number of beds available for mental illness and shows that this has been balanced by an equally marked and continued rise in admissions (see Table 24.1). The latter is borne out by figures given by the Department of

Table 24.1 Beds available for mental illness, admissions and bed turnover, England 1976–1991

Year	I Beds available (000s)	II Admissions (000s)	III Annual turnover
1976	97	179	1.8
1977	93	175	1.9
1978	91	171	1.9
1979	89	165	1.9
1980	87	174	2.0
1981	85	176	2.1
1982	84	186	2.2
1983	82	192	2.3
1984	79	197	2.5
1985	76	204	2.7
1986	72	204	2.8
1987/8	67	304	4.5
1988/9	63	212	3.4
1989/90	59	215	3.6
1990/1	55	219	4.0

Source: Jones K 1993 After the Asylums, p. 244.

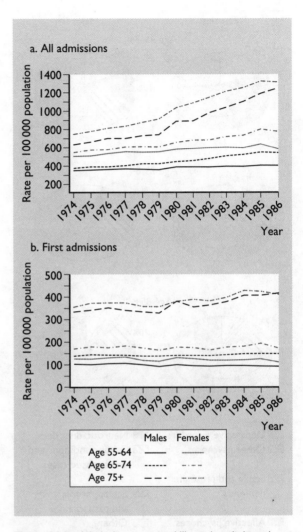

Figure 24.3 Admissions to mental illness hospitals and units by sex and age, England 1974–1986. Source: DOH 1992 (Fig. 37, p. 57) The health of elderly people: an epidemiological overview. HMSO, London.

Health (1992a) in *The Health of Elderly People: An Epidemiological Overview* (see Figs 24.3 and 24.4).

A more encouraging picture is presented by the decline in numbers of residents with a stay of over 5 years for mental handicap and mental illness hospitals and units. Figure 24.5 shows that numbers in England and Scotland fell from 67 000 to just 22 000 in 1993. Murphy (1991) presents a useful diagram showing the rise and fall of residents in lunatic asylums/mental hospitals (see Fig. 24.6). She points out that numbers of people resident in mental hospitals in England and Wales reached a peak in 1954 at 148 000 but have fallen steadily since then. In 1990 it was approximately 59 000.

Some figures on occupancy are available and show the drop in percentages of people occupying hospital beds. At the end of the 1950s, about 40% of National Health Service (NHS) hospital beds were occupied by people suffering from mental illness. In 1986 the figure was 20% (Taylor & Taylor 1989). On the other hand, mental illness outpatient attendances have risen by 50% in the last decade and the number of short-stay admissions has also gone up (Taylor & Taylor 1989).

THE DEVELOPMENT OF SERVICES

Potential growth in numbers of patients

One of the main reasons why the development of services is of such crucial importance in all countries

of the world is the effect of an ageing population. As the proportion of the population which is old (of whom a larger proportion will be very old) grows, the more likely it is that more will have dementia and possibly more mental illness. In the UK a constant theme of government advice has been to point to this. For example, *The Rising Tide* (HAS 1982), by the NHS Health Advisory Service (HAS), suggested that rising numbers and increased expectations would mean that 'the flood is likely to overwhelm the entire health system' (HAS 1982, p. 1).

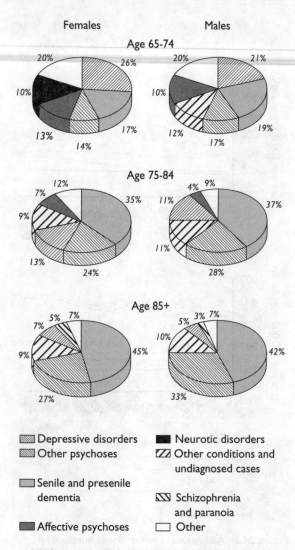

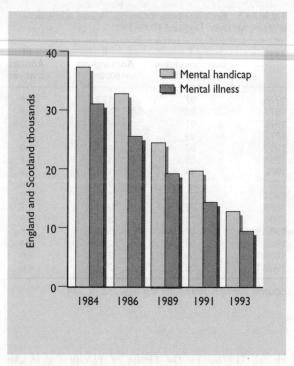

Figure 24.5 Residents with a stay of over 5 years for mental handicap and mental illness in NHS hospitals and units. Source: Statistical Office 1995 Social Trends No. 25. HMSO, London.

Depressive disorders

Other psychoses

Senile and presenile dementia

Affective psychoses

Neurotic disorders

Other conditions and undiagnosed cases

Schizophrenia and paranoia

Other

Percentages may not add to 100 due to rounding

Figure 24.4 First admissions to mental illness hospitals and units by diagnostic group, sex and age, England 1986. Source: DOH 1992 (Fig. 38, p. 58) The health of elderly people: an epidemiological overview. HMSO, London.

The influence of the medical profession and the development of specialisms among staff

The medical profession has had a great influence on all aspects of the National Health Service, from the organisation to the methods of payment of doctors. Perhaps inevitably, they have also chosen to 'focus on providing a service for those who were the most rewarding to treat, that is those with reversible, short-

term illnesses which responded best to the new drugs' (Murphy 1991, p. 10). As a consequence doctors and nurses working in long-stay care became very much the 'cinderellas' of the professions.

The medical profession has not always been united in its approach to mental illness. For example, following the Ministry of Health's goal in 1961 and 1962 to close many long-stay institutions some, mainly right wing, were in favour and thought that this was the most progressive policy. Others, more to the left, were pessimistic and thought that community services were unlikely to cope and that the influence of drugs was limited (Jones 1993b).

The development of psychogeriatrics has been a welcome one. Similarly, nurses and social workers increasingly undertook additional training in mental health. Social workers now all undergo basic training and many then go on to specialise. However, the demise of the specialist mental health social worker is regretted by many. Approved social workers have taken their place. They have undertaken specialist training in mental health and been approved by the local authority. They have statutory responsibilities when people are compulsorily admitted to hospital

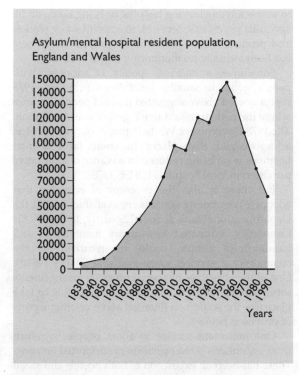

Asylum/mental hospital resident population, England and Wales

Figure 24.6 The rise and fall in residents of lunatic asylums/mental hospitals 1930–1990. Source: Murphy E 1991 (Fig. 1, p. 9) After the asylums.

and have a duty to examine alternatives to hospitalisation.

This is not the place to argue the case for and against a specialist geriatric or an integrated service. However, as Twining (1993) has argued, 'The interface between the specialities of geriatric medicine and old age psychiatry is clearly an important one. Any experienced clinician will recognise that many mentally ill older people have serious physical pathology and, likewise, many of those with physical illness have accompanying mental frailty' (Twining 1993, p. 28). The Department of Health has maintained that, 'In assessing need, age-determined cut-off should be sensitively applied. For example, an existing patient with schizophrenia who reaches the age of 65 might have their needs better met by remaining within existing service provision' (Department of Health 1993b, p. 36).

The themes of policy change

The development of services has focused on the four main themes of policy change:

- preventing people going into institutions
- returning people from institutions to the community
- improving conditions in institutions
- building up community care.

Preventing people going into institutions

A major thrust of policy has been that of preventing people going into institutions. In 1961 the Minister of Health, Enoch Powell, announced that in 15 years there would probably only be half the number of places for mental illness in hospitals. He said that he hoped that most patients would, in the future, be placed in wards or wings of general hospitals and not in large institutions. The 1962 Hospital Plan called for the closure of the old mental hospitals and their replacement by psychiatric units based in district general hospitals. Later documents (e.g. the 1972 DHSS circular *Services for Mental Illness Related to Old Age*) envisaged the eventual closure of hospitals for mentally ill people and, as has been seen, this is what has happened to many.

It is easy to prevent people going into institutions, especially if the number of hospital beds is declining. But to what extent are people already in the community remaining there successfully? The real question is how they and their carers are coping. What evidence is there that this is a 'successful' policy? In order to answer this question one has to look for evidence of elderly people living in the community. Although there is not a great deal of research specifically on elderly people with mental health problems that has focused on keeping them out of institutions, there are some studies which have looked at this. For example, the Kent Community Care Project showed that 50% of a group of elderly dementia sufferers who were at risk of going into institutional care were still at home at the end of a year compared with only 23% of a matched control group (Challis & Davies 1986, Challis 1989). The former group received a well planned and designed package of care whereas the control group received only conventional services. A replication of this study in Gateshead showed similar findings (Luckett 1989). Other research has also confirmed these findings.

Returning people from institutions to the community

There is evidence that there are a disproportionate number of elderly people who are left in institutions. 'Research and evidence has also shown that those still resident in long-stay hospitals are the more elderly, the more physically and mentally disabled, and are generally the ones who will require the most support and input of services to enable them to live as full and normal a life as possible in the community. Thus their needs are almost certain to be greater than those already discharged' (House of Commons Social Services Committee 1990, p. 13, para 29).

Other researchers have found that the majority of long-stay patients currently in hospital are seriously disabled but could manage to live in the community with support (Clifford et al 1991).

Allowing people to return from institutions is not an easy policy. Some of the people may have been there for a long time and are, therefore, likely to be old. For example, the DHSS National Development Group for the Mentally Handicapped, in their 1978 report, said:

Most elderly residents are only mildly intellectually handicapped. Many of them were admitted over 20 years ago, and some have even lived in hospital since early childhood, having been admitted under Poor Laws and similar legislation at a time when society relied on mental handicap hospitals to provide care and shelter for people who would under no circumstances be admitted today. For this group more than any other the mental handicap hospital is their home.

(DHSS National Development Group for the Mentally Handicapped 1978, p. 67)

The House of Commons Health Committee (1994) distinguished between those patients who were long-stay in-patients in psychiatric hospitals and those who were admitted to these hospitals for shorter periods of treatment (House of Commons Health Committee 1994). In their view, 'In some instances reprovision has been more successful for the former than for the latter group. The functions served by old hospitals have not always been picked up by the new community developments to meet the needs of those with long-term mental illnesses, with many acute episodes and resulting social disabilities' (House of Commons Health Committee 1994, para 12).

When people do move out of institutions there needs to be some assurance that some kind of provision is available. In 1985 the House of Commons Social Services Committee in their report, *Community Care with Special Reference to Adult Mentally Ill and Mentally Handicapped People*, maintained that no-one should be discharged from an institution without an individual care plan. Under the NHS and Community Care Act, 1990, there is a requirement for there to be a plan for everyone who is assessed as being in need of care. In 1991 the Government introduced the Care Programme Approach. This requires health authorities

to assess anyone leaving hospital or being taken on by specialist psychiatric services, to appoint a key worker and produce a care plan with other agencies. There has been virtually no monitoring of this system.

Sometimes a half-way policy is adopted, with people going to smaller institutions first. The 1978 report quoted above suggested that old people's homes where the patients could live together was one option. The 1978 Government White Paper, *A Happier Old Age*, acknowledged that places in some large mental hospitals were being reduced in advance of alternative provision in local hospitals (DHSS 1978).

But there is also the problem of ensuring that adequate community services are available. In 1981 the Department of Health & Social Security, in *Care in the Community*, estimated how many mentally ill and handicapped people could be returned to the community if services were available (DHSS 1981d). One of the objectives of special financial arrangements set up under Joint Finance was to enable this to take place (see the section on financial and economic aspects of provision below).

One important service to allow people to return from institutions is the provision of supported housing. There has been an expansion of both hostels and small houses in the community where a number of ex-residents can live together.

The primary health care team should also play a crucial role in people returning from hospital. The Audit Commission (1994) argues that hospital care should be reserved for those with the most serious problems. It has recommended that:

• Most mental health problems – the least severe ones – should be treated in the primary care setting. GPs and primary health care teams need to be better trained and resourced to carry out appropriate interventions.
• Provided the advice and assistance is available at times of vulnerability, GPs should be encouraged to take responsibility for the people on their list with long-term needs for mental health care. They should participate in care programme arrangements (Audit Commission 1994, p. 51).

What indications are there of the success or otherwise of returning people (especially elderly people) to the community? Research in London by the Institute of Psychiatry on the run down of Friern Hospital and St Bernard's Southall (previously called Hanwell Asylum) shows that on the whole these closures did bring about improvements in living conditions for the patients (Jones 1993b quoting Leff). For example, only six out of 500 patients who moved into staffed group homes became vagrant (House of Commons Health Committee 1994). However, there are sometimes consequences for the areas into which the patients move, such as increased pressure on acute beds. Other research on the closure of Friern and Claybury Hospitals showed that costs for community care were lower than those in hospital and users generally preferred living in the community (Knapp et al 1990). Further research evidence is available on other hospital closures (House of Commons Social Services Committee 1990). Although caution is urged over the findings, because a period has to elapse before there can be certainty about what has happened, the results are reasonably encouraging.

The results of a demonstration programme in 1983 to move 900 people from long-stay hospitals to the community has been what the House of Commons Social Services Committee called a 'measured success' (House of Commons Social Services Committee 1990, p. 31, para 75). 28 projects were funded. Eight were for people with mental health problems, 12 for people with a learning disability, four for elderly people with mental impairment, three for physically frail elderly people, and one for people with physical disability. The evaluation by The Personal Social Services Research Unit (PSSRU), University of Kent, found that community living was preferred to hospital life by the majority of people in the programme, that coordinated individual care planning worked better than the fragmented responsibilities it replaced and that the costs of community care were not prohibitively expensive. A useful summary of the Care in the Community demonstration programme can be found in Higgins & Richardson (1994).

The House of Commons Committee summed up the problems:

The problems that emerged tended to be that some projects were slower to start than others, especially those for day care; getting the right kind of accommodation in the right location, at the right time and within the budget was more difficult than was anticipated; social security and local joint finance funds did not always meet the total costs required to establish and continue the operation of new forms of service provision; some of the joint working aims foundered at an early stage and some projects ran into staff difficulties.

(House of Commons Social Services Committee 1990, p. 32, para 76)

Another indicator, and this is one often used by lay people, is to look at homeless people and to suggest that they are the ones who have been turned out of institutions. There have not been many studies specifically of elderly homeless people. One is *Elderly Homeless People Sleeping on the Streets in Inner London: An Exploratory Study* (Crane 1993). This was a study of 75 homeless elderly people. It found that 84% of the sample appeared to have mental health problems and one in five had had psychiatric treatment in the past. However, only 14% said that they had been in a psychiatric hospital and only one of the 75 respondents had that as their last home. The largest number (20) had rented. However, 17 were unable to say where they had been. There is now a Government Central London Homeless Mentally Ill Initiative.

Crane's findings about the small number of homeless people who had come from institutions has been borne out by the House of Commons Health Committee report (1994). This states: 'We establish that the closure of the old institutions is not the principal cause of the numbers of homeless people who are mentally ill, and that the majority of mentally ill people who are homeless are those who have lost touch with services or have never properly engaged them' (House of Commons Health Committee 1994, p. vi, para 6). They found that, for adults, the main reasons for becoming homeless were inability to meet rent payments or difficulties with families or landlords. However, an earlier report stated: 'We have become convinced that the numbers of homeless people with a mental illness is increasing' (House of Commons Social Services Committee 1990, p. 49).

Another indicator is the extent to which problems are caused by the person discharged. The most dramatic cases have nearly all involved the discharge of someone who has then gone on to murder or severely injure someone. Few, if any, of the most publicised cases have involved an elderly person. A systematic study would be needed to look at the profile of people released and what has happened to them.

To summarise – returning people to the community may involve:

- half-way provision (perhaps a smaller hospital or hostel)
- special financial help either to other providers or to the individual.

But it certainly *must* include:

- an individual care plan
- adequate support services which include medical, social and housing elements.

Improving conditions in institutions

As previously indicated, there has been great criticism of conditions in institutions for people with mental health problems of all ages. In general the Health Advisory Service has found that conditions have improved (for more details see Chapter 27).

Building up community care

There is little point in allowing people to remain in the community or returning them there from institutions if support and services are not available or are insufficient. As is well known, most community care is provided by families, but support services from statutory and independent sources are essential. It is also vital for those who do not have relatives or whose relatives are not able to help. From the 1970s there has been an acknowledgement by succeeding governments that community services are not adequate. In 1975, the White Paper *Better Services for the Mentally Ill* admitted that, because of limited resources and competing demands, adequate support services in the community were not available.

The influential House of Commons Social Services Committee chaired by Renee Short in 1985 reported in *Community Care: With Special Reference to Adult Mentally Ill and Mentally Handicapped People*. They called for a wide variety of services in the community. A subsequent House of Commons Social Services Committee in 1990 called for adequate financial provision for community care to be transferred to local authorities from the social security budget. The NHS and Community Care Act, 1990 did introduce a specific grant to local authorities for the development of social care services for people with a mental illness (see the finance section below).

A series of critical reports on community care came out in the 1980s (see Tinker 1992). One of the most influential was the Audit Commission's report, *Making a Reality of Community Care* (Audit Commission 1986). Its main criticisms were about the slow and uneven progress towards community care. Following advice from Sir Roy Griffiths (Griffiths Report 1988) the Government issued a White paper in 1989 entitled *Caring for People: Community Care in the Next Decade and Beyond* (Department of Health 1989b). Its main recommendations formed the basis of the NHS and Community Care Act, 1990.

The Government stated its position in 1991: 'There is also a firm commitment that Ministers will not approve any hospital closure until they are satisfied that adequate alternatives have been developed' (Department of Health 1991, p. 86). This was emphasised in 1993 when the Mental Health Task Force was set up to help ensure the substantial completion of the transfer of services away from large hospitals to a balanced range of locally based services, including community-based beds.

Not to be forgotten is the role of housing in community care policies. Supported housing such as hostels can provide help for elderly people both with mental illness and learning disabilities. For those with dementia very sheltered housing (i.e. sheltered housing with additional elements such as meals and 24-hour care) have proved very successful (Tinker 1989). (See also section above on returning people from institutions to the community.)

HOW SERVICES ARE ORGANISED AND WHO PROVIDES THEM

Increasing attention is being paid, at least in theory, to the recipients of services. Not only is there concern for the person with the problems but also for the carer. In the UK, services for elderly people with mental health problems and their carers are split between a number of different authorities. The main statutory ones are illustrated in Figure 24.7.

In health the authorities come under appointed Boards, whereas social services and housing are part of elected local authorities. In some areas the local authority is a unitary one and provides both social services and housing, whereas in others they are separate, with the County Council providing social services and the District Council responsible for housing. From the point of view of the elderly person it would seem that a service might be better provided

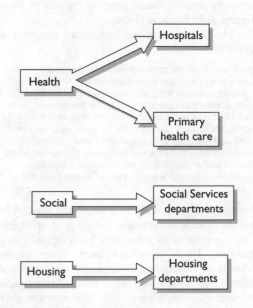

Figure 24.7 Authorities responsible for services for elderly people. Source: the author.

by one authority so that there was more possibility of coordination. In Northern Ireland for example, health, social services and housing all come under one Board.

One of the main changes brought about by the NHS and Community Care Act, 1990 was the distinction between purchaser and provider of services. This followed recommendations about health services in the Government's White Paper, *Working for Patients* (Department of Health 1989a). The district health authority as purchaser can enter into contracts or agreements with hospitals and community health units. Service providers include the district's directly managed hospitals and units, those from other districts, NHS trusts or the independent sector. General practitioners who are fundholders can also purchase services. Those who seek to emulate the British system need to be aware that there may be problems.

Criticisms and comments about the performance of purchasers and providers have been made by the Audit Commission (1994). These include the need for purchasers to review the balance of expenditure on hospital and community resources as well as making more use of information. The need for the two to work together was also stated: 'Purchasers and provider managers together, bearing in mind the wishes of users and carers, should develop clear guidance on the appropriate balance of hospital and community services in the local area with a definite timetable for its achievement' (Audit Commission 1994, p. 25). Concerns have also been expressed about good purchasing practice and measures by which to judge services (Jones 1993a).

The purchaser/provider split also operates in social services. In some cases the majority of providers are in the independent sector. On mental health services it has been held that local authorities are not experienced in purchasing nursing home beds and would be well advised to learn from their health service colleagues (Walker 1993).

A separate point is the need for joint commissioning between health and social care providers not only of services but to obtain an adequate and integrated database of mental health services (Audit Commission 1994). Joint commissioning of residential and nursing home facilities seems a sensible approach.

As indicated, some services are provided by the independent sector. This means private (for profit) and voluntary (not for profit) organisations. Private provision can mean:

- separate provision alongside statutory (e.g. public and private hospitals)

- services contracted out by the statutory sector (e.g. cleaning or catering in hospitals)
- services transferred or sold by the statutory sector (e.g. the transfer or sale of council housing).

The situation is even more complicated than this; for example, services may be publicly provided and privately funded (e.g. private pay beds in NHS hospitals), publicly provided and part funded privately and part publicly (e.g. local authority residential homes which take people who are funded from different sources) and other permutations (see Glennerster 1992 for a fuller discussion).

In many countries health care is mainly provided by the private sector but in the UK the National Health Service has been the main provider. Even though the private sector has expanded, this has been mainly in the provision of acute medical care. Neither old people nor mental health provision have been targeted as profitable by firms. The main expansion has been in private residential and nursing home care. For social care again most provision has been by the state via local authorities. Private domiciliary care has been slow to be taken up by the private sector.

Voluntary organisations have a long history of providing for elderly people with mental health problems. Residential homes and day care are two areas. Advice and support for carers is another. They are increasingly taking on more services as these are contracted out. For example, Age Concern is providing a growing amount of day care.

In some cases these voluntary bodies both provide services and act as other functions. For example, MIND has carried out demonstration projects to help mentally ill people as well as publicising good practice and supporting the involvement of patients ('consumers') who receive care. They have also pressed for national standards (Sayce 1994).

Under the 1990 NHS and Community Care Act and subsequent regulations and advice from the Department of Health, it was planned that the independent sector would take on more provision for all people who need support. A special transitional community care grant was given and 85% of this had to be spent in the independent sector.

The variety of providers ensures that there is not a monopoly. It may also mean that innovations take place (though these are not the exclusive prerogative of the independent sector), but the very tight contracts offered by statutory bodies may give little scope for innovation. In addition, the profit element may mean that services are not of a high standard in order to maximise the amount made. There is also the problem of standards. Who is to enforce these and how is quality to be measured? Chapter 27 throws some light on measurement.

THE RESPONSIVENESS OF THE PROVIDERS

In order to provide a good service, providers need to ensure that they are both responsive to the needs of an area and also to individuals. Where a statutory body is given responsibility, they are obliged to take into account everyone in that area, for example social services have a duty to plan for the needs of their whole area; an independent provider will inevitably take a narrower perspective.

An important aspect of services is that they should be appropriate for the person receiving them. For this to take place there has to be a clear assessment of needs. As early as 1972 the DHSS stressed this in the circular *Services for Mental Illness Related to Old Age.* They advised that those needing hospital treatment were best treated in the psychiatric departments of district general hospitals. For the rest, the emphasis was on rehabilitation with the use of day hospitals and, where necessary, residential care.

An NHS view of standards for elderly mentally ill people lists some clear criteria (Jones 1993a). These features of high quality services are shown in Boxes 24.1 and 24.2.

Box 24.1 Features of high quality services – 1
Ease of referral

Encouragement for primary care involvement
Responsiveness – speedy opinions offered
Comprehensiveness – any old person in the community
Specialist involvement
Home assessment
Further assessment available in:
- outpatient clinics
- day hospital
- multidisciplinary team
- district general hospital
Services offer care to a reasonable sized locality
Carer involvement in:
- care planning
- support groups
Communication with primary care services.

(Source: NHS Health Advisory Service 1993
Comprehensive Health Services for Elderly People.
NHS/HAS, p. 44)

Box 24.2 Features of high quality services – 2

Liaison with social services/voluntary sector
Collaboration with geriatric medicine
Specialised manpower in specialist teams
Appropriate resources and facilities
Respite care system
Community nursing team and other community workers
Long-term care in health provision
Follow-up review and monitoring practice
Education (and prevention)
Training and audit
Exploring advocacy.

(Source: NHS Health Advisory Service 1993
Comprehensive Health Services for Elderly People.
NHS/HAS, p. 44)

There has been growing stress on the rights of patients to have a say both in their own treatment and in more general issues of policy. Their rights have also increasingly been recognised. Some of this has been enshrined in legislation. In 1983 the Mental Health Act expanded the range and degree of safeguards for patients and set up the Mental Health Commission as a watchdog on the new legislation.

Those with or who have had mental health problems are becoming more willing to speak out on their own behalf. There is not a great deal of evidence that older people are becoming more willing to do so. The evidence is also scant about the special needs of older women and of people from ethnic minority groups and how providers are responding (see Chapter 13).

Complaints are a different issue. Largely as a result of the hospital inquiries in the 1960s, the Hospital Advisory Service was set up in 1969. This later became the Health Advisory Service. Teams of staff from different disciplines visit hospitals and advise on practice and where improvements could be made. Since 1991 the Health Advisory Service has kept its previous role of giving advice on improving standards of management and clinical care and focusing on mental health services, on services for substance misusers and on services for elderly people. But it has also taken on new roles of advising purchasing and providing authorities in relation to services on:

- the strategic and practical aspects of needs assessment for the service specification for, and the monitoring of, quality standards
- achieving *Health of the Nation* targets.

The first Health Service Commissioner (Ombudsman) was appointed in 1972. Although the terms of the Commissioner are limited and patients have to have gone through other channels first, the office has proved to have value (see also Chapter 28).

Some of the most interesting innovations have been for elderly people with dementia and their carers. Many stress the importance of treating people as individuals with rights to dignity, choice, respect, participation and high quality professional services. Some services are particularly aimed at the carers (e.g. Askham & Thompson 1990). (More details are given in Chapter 25.)

FINANCIAL AND ECONOMIC ASPECTS OF PROVISION

As has already been seen, a major impetus for a change from institutional to community care was because of the cost of the former. Recent costings show this still to be the case. In 1991 about three-quarters of the NHS mental health budget went on hospital and medication costs, and only a quarter on community services (Sayce 1994). In some cases it is likely that costs will rise (Robins & Wittenberg 1992). The Short Report in 1985 stressed that none of the services they were calling for would be cheap.

Costings of services are still in their infancy but have developed greatly in the last 10 years. One costings exercise of elderly people with cognitive impairment showed that large-scale improvements in the provision of care for people living in private households and local authority homes required significant increases in funding (Kavanagh et al 1993). But they also found that reductions in the provision of long-stay hospital beds can significantly reduce the cost burden to the public purse. Their analyses suggest that, 'widespread improvements in provision can be achieved with comparatively modest injections of additional resources, and might even be accommodated largely within existing resources if long-stay hospital provision was reduced' (Kavanagh et al 1993, p. 78).

To enable changes of policy to take place it is often necessary to offer some kind of financial inducement. One of these in the UK was the introduction of Joint Finance in 1976. This enables health authorities to give grants to social services, and subsequently, housing and voluntary bodies, to help with the costs of community care so that health authorities would not have to spend so much. The thrust of this was then changed. The 1981 DHSS report *Care in the Community* was concerned with how patients 'together with resources for their care' could be transferred from the NHS to the personal social services in addition to existing joint finance arrangements (DHSS 1981d). The subsequent advice (DHSS 1983b), *Explanatory Notes on Care in the Community*, said:

The joint finance arrangements have assisted the development of community care and in doing so have contributed to the important objective of enabling people to remain in the community instead of having to be taken into hospital. But the Care in the Community initiative has a different and quite specific aim: to help long-stay hospital patients unnecessarily kept in hospital to return to the community where this will be best for them and is what they and their families would prefer.   (DHSS 1983b, p. 1)

Among the suggestions put forward were transferring funds centrally and transferring hospital buildings. Another idea was a lump sum or annual payment. The latter was one of the options which was subsequently tried and, from 1983, district health authorities were empowered to offer both lump sums and annual payments to local authorities or voluntary bodies who would take people from hospital and provide community care. This system, which does not seem to be very well known, is sometimes called the 'dowry' system. It was only used to a limited extent and primarily for people with learning disabilities. Joint financing was also extended and could run for 13 instead of 7 years. After that the provider had to pay the amount. From 1983 a series of pilot projects were started. They were subsequently evaluated. How successful were they and how far did they help elderly people with mental health problems?

Research on joint finance shows mixed findings. It has led to many innovatory and worthwhile projects such as hospital at home schemes but the money has not always been spent on community care services. In fact the National Audit Office in Community Care Developments has demonstrated that a growing proportion has been going to the NHS (National Audit Office 1987). This may be due in part to the reluctance of local authorities to venture into schemes where they have, ultimately, to pick up the full costs.

A rare example of a specific grant which is targeted to people with mental health problems is the Mental Illness Specific Grant. This was part of the NHS and Community Care Act 1990. It goes to local authorities to enable the development of social care services. Over 500 projects were funded in the first year of the grant's operation. The grant is monitored by the Social Services Inspectorate (SSI) who have reported that these projects have had a 'very significant impact on the lives of users and carers, and represented good value for money' (Department of Health and Social Services Inspectorate 1993, p. ix, para 20).

What of the long-term prospects for financing and providing services for people with mental health problems? There appears to be an acceptance by both the left and right in politics that some degree of self-insurance in old age is going to be a serious option for the future in most countries. But will people be able to insure for a sufficient sum to be able to cover costs of medication and treatment which may be very high? And what of the costs for people with dementia if they have to receive 24-hour care? It seems that premiums are high and conditions requiring long-term care are often excluded from coverage (Robins & Wittenberg 1992).

THE IMPORTANCE OF LINKS BETWEEN SERVICES AND FOR INTEGRATED PROVISION

The first need is for a clear strategy to be adopted which is agreed by all the parties. Detailed advice to central government, purchasers, providers and other agencies has been given by the Audit Commission (1994).

The ideal service must be one which allows comprehensive assessment and treatment. The DHSS publication, *Better Services for the Mentally Ill* (DHSS 1975), visualised both a hospital-based 'specialist therapeutic team' and a primary care team consisting of a general practitioner, health visitor, district nurse and social worker. The Royal Colleges of Physicians and Psychiatrists (1989) have argued for a comprehensive psychogeriatric service aimed at both elderly people and their carers.

The Care Programme Approach (CPA), introduced in 1991, has been commended as helping links. A single plan is worked out for the individual which all the relevant services agree on. The District Health Authority has to collaborate with the social services department in the plan. One worker makes sure that all the elements of care are delivered. The care programme is to provide for the effective treatment in the community of all in-patients considered for discharge and all new patients accepted by the specialist psychiatric services. Any mental health worker can be the key worker but would usually be a community psychiatric nurse or a social worker. Care Management is a similar system, with one key worker but operated by social services for all vulnerable people and not just those with mental health problems. A monitoring exercise of mental health services by the Department of Health Social Services Inspectorate (SSI)

showed that there were still some problems to iron out (DH/SSI 1993).

As far as the CPA was concerned, the difficulties were found 'to concentrate on four issues: who receives CPA, who is the key worker, how CPA relates to care management and how information systems can be set up' (DH/SSI 1993, p. 52).

The boundaries between community and institutional care are blurring. Some argue that institutions, especially small ones, are part of the community. For example, Bergmann & Jacoby (1983) suggest that, for elderly people with dementia, home-like institutions in the community are appropriate in the absence of the family or when it collapses.

Close links between services are essential if people are not to slip through the net of provision. The importance of coordination and joint planning was, for example, stressed in the 1972 DHSS circular *Services for Mental Illness Related to Old Age*. Hospital discharge is a classic case where coordination is needed.

CONCLUSIONS

For the growing number of elderly people across the world with mental health problems the experience of the UK holds some lessons. Obviously different circumstances, including varied patterns of family care, will prevail. Developments which will have a major impact are:

* changes in treatment methods
* changes in treatment settings, e.g. the move from institutions to local services
* changes in working patterns, e.g. the development of multidisciplinary teams and the greater involvement of users and carers (Department of Health 1993b).

What does seem apparent is that there:

* is need for both institutional and community care
* are advantages and disadvantages for all sectors but it is likely that the statutory sector will predominate
* may be advantages in giving financial incentives to providers though this may bring problems in the long term over who will then pay
* should be a multidisciplinary approach by staff
* is need for flexible services to meet gender specific and multi-cultural services
* must be involvement by clients in the assessment of services.

ACKNOWLEDGEMENT

The author is grateful to Hannah Zeilig, previously research associate and now research student, Age Concern Institute of Gerontology, King's College London, for a preliminary literature search.

REFERENCES

Arie T 1986 Recent advances in psychogeriatrics. Churchill Livingstone, London

Askham J, Thompson C 1990 Dementia and home care. Age Concern England, London

Bergman K, Jacoby R 1983 The limitation and possibilities of community care for the elderly demented. In: DHSS Elderly people in the community: their service needs. HMSO, London

Blessed G 1988 Long stay beds for the elderly severely mentally ill. Psychiatric Bulletin of the Royal College of Psychiatrists 12: 250–252

Central Statistical Office 1995 Social trends no. 25. HMSO, London

Challis D 1989 Elderly dementia sufferers in the community: the needs, service and policy background. In: Morton J (ed) Enabling elderly people with dementia to live in the community. Age Concern Institute of Gerontology, King's College London

Challis D, Davies B 1986 Case management in community care. Gower, London

Clifford P, Charman A, Webb Y et al 1991 Planning of community care: long stay populations of hospitals scheduled for rundown or closure. British Journal of Psychiatry 158: 190–196

Crane M 1993 Elderly homeless people sleeping on the streets in Inner London: an exploratory study. Age Concern Institute of Gerontology, King's College London

Department of Health Central Health Monitoring Unit 1992a The health of elderly people: an epidemiological overview. HMSO, London

Department of Health Central Health Monitoring Unit 1992b The health of elderly people: an epidemiological overview: companion papers. HMSO, London

Department of Health and Social Security 1972 Services for mental illness related to old age. DHSS Circular (72) 71, HMSO, London

Department of Health and Social Services Inspectorate 1993 Inspection of projects funded by the mental illness specific grant. HMSO, London

Glennerster H 1992 Paying for welfare the 1990s. Harvester Wheatsheaf, Hemel Hempstead

Health Advisory Service (HAS) 1982 The rising tide. HMSO, London

Higgins R, Richardson A 1994 Into the community: a comparison of care management and traditional approaches to resettlement. Social Policy and Administration 328(3): 221–235

House of Commons Health Committee 1994 Better off in the community? the care of people who are seriously mentally ill. 28.3.94 HMSO, London

House of Commons Social Services Committee 1990 Community care: services for people with a mental handicap and people with a mental illness. HMSO, London

Jones B 1993a Contemporary demands on services for elderly mentally ill people – a view from the national health service. In: NHS Health Advisory Service Comprehensive health services for elderly people. NHS/HAS, London

Jones K 1993b Asylums and after. Athlone Press, London

Kavanagh S, Schneider J, Knapp M, Beechman J, Netten A 1993 Elderly people with cognitive impairment: costing possible changes in the balance of care. Health and Social Care 1(2): 69–79

Knapp M, Beecham J, Andersen J et al 1990 The TAPS Project 3: predicting the community costs of closing psychiatric hospitals. British Journal of Psychiatry 157: 661–670

Luckett R 1989 The Gateshead community care scheme. In: Morton J (ed) Enabling elderly people with dementia to live in the community. Age Concern Institute of Gerontology, King's College London

Meacher M 1972 Taken for a ride. Longman, London

Morton J (ed) 1989 Enabling elderly people with dementia to live in the community, proceedings of an ageing update conference. Age Concern Institute of Gerontology, King's College London

Murphy E 1991 After the asylums: community care for people with mental illness. Faber and Faber, London

NHS Health Advisory Service 1993 Comprehensive health services for elderly people. NHS/HAS, London

Robb B 1967 Sans everything. Nelson, London

Robins A, Wittenberg R 1992 The health of elderly people: economic aspects. In: Department of Health, Central Health Monitoring Unit The health of elderly people: an epidemiological overview: companion papers. HMSO, London

Royal College of Physicians and Royal College of Psychiatrists 1989 Care of elderly people with mental illness: specialist services and medical training. Royal College of Physicians and Royal College of Psychiatrists, London

Sayce L 1994 An alternative view. In: Care in the Community, Community Care Supplement 26 May–1 June 1994: 9–11

Taylor J, Taylor D 1989 Mental health in the 1990s: from custody to care? Office of Health Economics, London

Tinker A 1989 An evaluation of very sheltered housing. HMSO, London

Tinker A 1992 Elderly people in modern society, 3rd edn. Longman, London

Twining C 1993 The interface between geriatric medicine and old age psychiatric services. In: NHS Health Advisory Service Comprehensive health services for elderly people. NHS/HAS, London

Walker M 1993 Contemporary demands on services for elderly mentally ill people – a view from the personal social services. In: NHS Health Advisory Service Comprehensive health services for elderly people. NHS/HAS, London

RECOMMENDED READING

Audit Commission 1994 Finding a place: a review of mental health services for adults. HMSO, London. *Although this excludes services for older people with dementia it is a stringent critical look at services.*

Department of Health 1993 The health of the nation: key area handbook: mental illness. *Detailed policy advice and practical guidance intended to be used to develop local strategies.*

House of Commons Health Committee 1994 Better off in the community: the care of people who are seriously mentally ill. HMSO, London. *Another critical account of policies and possible ways forward.*

House of Commons Social Services Committee 1985 Community care: with special reference to adult mentally ill and mentally handicapped people. HMSO, London. *This report of a Committee chaired by Renee Short (usually referred to as the Short report) is a powerful account of problems for people with mental health problems and some solutions.*

House of Commons Social Services Committee 1990 Community care: services for people with a mental handicap and people with mental illness. HMSO, London.

Another House of Commons report which both reinforces and updates that of 1985 (the Short report – see above).

Jones K 1993 Asylums and after. Athlone Press, London. *A comprehensive historical account of mental health services in the UK from the early 18th century to the 1990s.*

Morton J (ed) 1989 Enabling elderly people with dementia to live in the community. Proceedings of an Ageing Update Conference, Age Concern Institute of Gerontology, King's College London. *Papers from a conference which discussed innovations and policies for elderly people with dementia.*

Murphy E 1991 After the asylums: community care for people with mental illness. Faber and Faber, London. *Another comprehensive historical account of mental health services in the UK which complements that by Kathleen Jones.*

Tinker A 1992 Elderly people in modern society. Longman, London. *A critical account of policies, practice and research on all aspects of social policy to do with elderly people. It includes chapters on health, social services, care by families, etc. It also contains excerpts from key documents such as reports from the Audit Commission.*

APPENDIX: Recent key events, policies, reports and legislation in the UK

All of the following are published by HMSO except where indicated.

Note: The term mental handicap has been used instead of learning disabilities when the former term was used in the literature.

1948: In the new NHS, psychiatric hospitals were placed under the same management as general hospitals.

1950s: Drugs revolution (e.g. antidepressants, tranquillisers, sedatives, etc.).

1957: Report of the Royal Commission, *The Law Relating to Mental Illness and Deficiency*, HMSO, London.

1959: Mental Health Act.

1960s: Policies (e.g .1962 Hospital Plan) to run down large psychiatric hospitals and put patients in small local hospitals or community care.

1963: DHSS, *Health and welfare: the development of community care*. Local authority plans.

1969: Hospital Advisory Service set up.

1969: Local Authority Social Services Act.

There was then a series of four DHSS documents all stressing the need for priority to be given to people with mental health problems:

1971: DHSS, *Memo on hospital services for the mentally ill*.

1971: DHSS, *Better services for the mentally handicapped*.

1972: DHSS Circular (72) 71, *Services for mental illness related to old age*.

1975: DHSS, *Better services for the mentally ill*.

1976: DHSS, *Priorities for health and personal social services in England*.

1976: Start of Joint Finance.

1978: DHSS, *A happier old age*.

1978: DHSS, The National Development Group for the Mentally Handicapped, *Helping mentally handicapped people in hospital*.

1978: Review of Mental Health Act.

1979: Jay Report, *Report of the committee of enquiry into mental health, nursing and care*.

1981a: DHSS, *Mental handicap: progress, problems and priorities*.

1981b: DHSS, *Care in action: a handbook of policies and priorities for the health and personal social services in England*.

1981c: DHSS, *Growing older* (White Paper).

1981d: DHSS, *Care in the community*.

1982: NHS Health Advisory Service, *The rising tide*, called for extra resources for expected growing numbers.

1983: Mental Health Act.

1983a: DHSS Health Service Development Circular HC(83)6 LAC(83)5, *Care in the community and joint finance*.

1983b: DHSS, *Explanatory notes on care in the community*.

1985: House of Commons, Social Services Committee, *Community care: with special reference to adult mentally ill and mentally handicapped people*. (Short report.)

1986: Audit Commission, *Making a reality of community care*. Very critical of all aspects of community care.

1987: National Audit Office, *Community care developments*.

1988: Department of Health, The Firth Report, *The funding of residential care*.

1988: Griffiths Report, *Community care: agenda for action*.

1988: House of Commons Public Accounts Committee, *Community care developments*.

1988: Wagner Report, *Residential care: a positive choice*.

1989a: Department of Health, *Working for patients* (White Paper).

1989b: Department of Health, *Caring for people: community care in the next decade and beyond* (White Paper).

1990: House of Commons Social Services Committee, *Community care: services for people with a mental handicap and people with mental illness*.

1990: NHS and Community Care Act brought in new community care arrangements and introduced a specific grant to local authorities for the development of social care services for people with mental illness.

1990: Department of Health Joint Health/Social Services Circular, *The care programme approach*, HC(90)23/LASS(90)11, September 1990.

1991: Department of Health, *The health of the nation: a consultative document for health in England.*

1992: Department of Health, *The health of the nation: a strategy for health in England.*

1993a: Department of Health, *The health of the nation one year on.* (Published by Department of Health.)

1993b: Department of Health, *The health of the nation: key area handbook – mental illness.*

1994: House of Commons Health Committee, *Better off in the community: the care of people who are seriously mentally ill.* 28.3.94.

1994: Audit Commission, *Finding a place: a review of mental health services for adults.* (Although this excluded older people with dementia.)

25

Supporting elderly people and informal carers at home

Janet Askham

THE ISSUES AND PROBLEMS IN SUPPORTING ELDERLY PEOPLE AT HOME

Most people want to live in their own homes rather than elsewhere, whether that alternative be an hotel, the street or an institution providing care. Everyone needs help of some sort to do this, but those with mental health problems often need more support. Supporting elderly people and their caregivers at home means:

1. Helping the older persons to carry on living at home, and helping to improve or maintain the quality of their lives at home.
2. Helping caregivers to carry on supporting the older person, and to do it at less cost, or at no increased cost, to themselves or to the person for whom they are caring.

By cost, of course, we mean not merely financial or employment cost but also costs in relation to their physical and mental health and wellbeing, their social lives and relationships (and maybe also their spiritual and intellectual lives, though such factors are rarely mentioned in research about caring). For example, a study of the caregivers of confused elderly people (Levin et al 1989) found that of those who said they had difficulty supporting their relative two-thirds said this was because of behavioural or interpersonal problems with him, half said they had difficulty in providing practical help, and two-fifths said they had difficulty because of the social restrictions on them. Support may also refer to helping people to know when the time has come for the elderly person to cease living at home or for the carer to end her caregiving role.

This sounds straightforward, but of course it is not. One type of support may conflict with another, and the interests of the older people and of their family caregivers may also be at odds; for example, it may be possible to give someone enough extra help so that they can carry on at home, but with serious long-term effects on their physical and mental health; or the interests of an older person may best be advanced by trying to keep them at home, while the interests of their carer may be quite the reverse. It may be that support which helps with one aspect of the older person's or the caregiver's life causes greater problems in another. For example, respite care may help a caregiver by giving her a break but add to practical problems of care if the older person comes home disorientated and less able to do things for himself than before. Or if a dementia sufferer's physical health is improved by one kind of support he may become more of a problem to a caregiver if, for instance, improved mobility leads to more behavioural problems.

The topic of this chapter therefore is complex. It is also broad in that its aim is to include organic and functional mental illness among older people as well as learning difficulties. Unfortunately, however, the discussion will concentrate more on supporting the carers than the care recipients, and more upon dementia than other forms of mental illness, because that is where most interest has lain.

In the main this chapter will not be concerned with health services, but with social care services (though some of these may be provided by the health services). The chapter does not cover preventive services, health assessment and diagnosis services, or treatment, therapy and monitoring services (though they may all be *involved* in support services).

Support needs of caregivers and care recipients

The first question to be asked is, what are the support requirements and needs of people affected personally or as a carer by mental health problems in later life? One can classify these by drawing out the implications of what has been said above, and by other researchers elsewhere. For example, in their study of 150 caregivers in the London area, five initial items were identified by Levin and her colleagues (Levin et al 1989, p. 130) as comprising the kinds of help which the supporters of confused elderly people required: 'recognition, explanation, advice, practical help, and time off'. From sources such as this one can see that the main things with which older people, and those who help to care for them at home, need or want support are:

Improving or maintaining their physical health and fitness

This makes personal and household care easier, and has been shown to be related to psychological health and wellbeing, though as stated above it can make a person – whether carer or care recipient – more demanding and therefore in some ways perhaps less easy to be with. The kinds of support likely to help with physical health and fitness will include anything which helps them to endure less direct physical strain (e.g. in lifting someone), or enables them to get a better diet, more fresh air and exercise, warmth, rest or sleep.

Improving or maintaining psychological wellbeing

This may make people more content with their lives and may make their relationships with others easier and happier. It may result in carers becoming more capable of carrying on caring, or, conversely, acknowledging their inability to do so. Support likely to help people's psychological wellbeing would include relief from the more stressful aspects of their lives, training in how to manage stress more effectively, counselling, sympathy and companionship.

Maintaining or improving knowledge and skill

Improved understanding of a mental health problem often makes it easier to know the most effective course of action to take, and improved skills mean that these actions are carried out more effectively. The former, however, is not necessarily an unmixed blessing; sometimes people cope better with their own lay knowledge (e.g. of a prognosis – see Askham 1995). Support to improve knowledge and skills might include specific information and advice facilities or services, also courses of training run by the education or other services, and the information or teaching of skills which might be given by a professional treatment or care worker concerned with elderly mentally ill people.

Maintaining or improving social life or relationships

A social or family life seen as satisfactory improves people's general life satisfaction and psychological wellbeing. It may involve a recognition that someone cannot go on living at home, or, conversely, it may help to maintain them at home. Support to help maintain or improve social life and relationships most obviously for caregivers means time and opportunity to devote to these other relationships, and an environment which is congenial to them. For those with the mental health problem, it may involve a befriending service at home, or services which take them out of the home and into the company of others, counselling to help them relate better to others, and so on.

Maintaining or improving leisure, spiritual or intellectual life

Again, if such wants are satisfied, people's general life satisfaction and psychological wellbeing has been found to improve. It may help carers to go on caregiving or it may have to be recognised that it can only be improved if they do not. Again, it may be relief from care for carers, opportunities for the desired activities or facilities, information or advice about achieving them which provides the support needed.

Maintaining or improving financial wellbeing

Such support may be vital to help people stay or care at home in a way that they or others see as satisfactory. The support needed may include advice about how to manage finances better, as well as about what financial assistance is available; also advocacy to help people achieve that financial assistance; or help which relieves people to enhance their income through greater opportunity for paid employment (see Laczko & Noden 1993).

Seen in terms of actual services, it is not difficult to identify the kinds of service which may address each of these support needs; and one can see immediately the prime importance of respite care, home care, home nursing, etc. For example, Levin et al (1989) found in their study of the caregivers of confused elderly people that those who said they had no difficulties in supporting their relative attributed it to 'assistance given by day care, nursing and home help services'.

Next in this section we will discuss some of the key factors, first in the mental illnesses themselves, and secondly in the caring role, which have implications for support.

SOME KEY THEMES FROM THE ILLNESSES THEMSELVES RELEVANT TO THE KIND OF SUPPORT WHICH PEOPLE NEED AT HOME

Reversibility versus inexorable decline

Can older people and carers expect or hope for improvement? If they can, then support during the possible stress and anxiety of waiting for such

improvement may be what is needed, or short-term support of various kinds. If there is no hope of improvement, then what is needed in the way of support may be quite different: a long-term career as a carer or sufferer in which needs may change as time progresses; support in helping people to adjust and adapt to a permanent change in relationships and roles; helping people come to terms with grief and sense of bereavement.

Independence versus dependence

Support services, etc., will have to determine to what extent independence can be maintained and/or encouraged (even a perceived need for support services at all), and to what extent they must assume dependence. For example, a study which looked at spouses caring for dementia sufferers (Pollitt et al 1991) found that there was one group of husbands and wives who did not see the dementia as a problem at all. They were mainly diagnosed clinically as having mild dementia, but tended to be seen by their spouses as merely forgetful or 'suffering from old age', and were in receipt of very few support services, and that was what the spouse preferred (out of 11 couples, 7 received no support services at all, 4 had a home help, 3 a community nurse, 2 meals-on-wheels).

Services for specific symptoms versus whole person care

Depending on the nature of the illness the support services will have to take into account whether what is needed is general support for the person (carer or ill older person) in looking after self and household, or the combatting of some specific problems such as eyes, feet, bathing. It is not necessarily the case that what people want or need is care rather than services (see Askham 1991). Many people may prefer to take the care themselves, and just want specific services which will fit in with their own care package.

Place of care

The nature and severity of the illness is implicated in the choice of place of care. Can people be better taken care of or treated outside or in the home? Leaving aside questions of cost and of the necessary location for effective treatment, most people prefer to be at home, but, equally, most would accept temporary care outside the home if it helped them or their carers. But not everyone under all circumstances prefers to live outside an institution. For example, people who have spent much of their lives in institutions are likely to see them as home; and a person with very poor short-term memory who cannot remember that people come to visit her every day, and is therefore always lonely, would be likely to feel happier in residential care because of the almost 24-hour a day face-to-face contacts. However, most elderly people with mental health problems do not of course live in institutions; even those with advanced cognitive impairment mainly live at home. Thus a survey giving a representative sample of older people with advanced cognitive impairment in England (Schneider et al 1993, using the OPCS Disability Surveys of 1985/1986) found that 63% were in private households, 22% in nursing care establishments, and 15% in residential care establishments.

The place of care may also be an institution but on a daily basis. Here too it has to be borne in mind that getting out of the house for a few hours a day may be very disorientating for some, but for others a welcome and stimulating change of environment.

Supporting the individual versus supporting the group/family

Should services see as their 'client' the person who has the mental health problem, or the family or other group to which that person is seen as belonging? There may be a need to tread a fine dividing line between taking into account the fact that the illness and support services affect others as well as the ill person, and assaulting that individual's right to be treated as an autonomous individual and not being seen to 'go behind his back' in dealing with other family members.

SOME KEY THEMES IN THE CARING ROLE RELEVANT TO SUPPORT AT HOME

The extent to which someone sees her or himself as a 'carer'

'Carer' is an identity or role which has become much more specific in recent years; through its gradual evolution it has achieved a public and professional recognition involving certain kinds of expectation and image. In general such recognition must be beneficial to caregivers but in individual cases it may constrain and direct behaviour and relationships which would otherwise have taken a different course. 'Are you the carer?' may be a daunting question to, for example, a nephew who drops in to share a meal once a week with a dementing aunt living on her own, and he may

find himself involved in decisions and responsibilities of which he had no expectations. Even for those who readily see themselves as 'the carer' it has to be remembered that this role will affect their self-image and will fit more or less easily with their other identities. For example, studies show that there are both positive and negative perceptions of the effects of caregiving on identity: people may see themselves as becoming more responsible, dutiful, morally worthy people, tolerant and understanding (see for instance Clifford 1990); but more frequently they see themselves as becoming more irritable, less relaxed, inadequate, resentful, and a more passive and resigned person (Anderson 1986, Brody et al 1989, Lewis & Meredith 1988, Nissel & Bonnerjea 1982, Qureshi & Walker 1989). For many people being a 'carer' will not be their prime identity, their caring tasks not the only or even the main things they have to do, nor their relationship with the elderly mentally ill person their prime relationship. The carers' own conceptions of what being a carer means (Taraborrelli 1994) may also be different from professional conceptions. And as Twigg (1989) has suggested, the role of 'carer' can be conceptualised by service-providing agencies in different ways (carers as 'resources', 'co-workers' or 'co-clients'), and this will affect the kinds of support seen as necessary.

The extent to which the caring role is shared or not

Research shows that one family member, etc., usually assumes – or is encouraged to adopt – the main role, with other family members either not involved at all, involved to a much lesser extent, or involved only on a substitute basis (Martin et al 1989). But just because they appear to fulfil a secondary role, other carers should not necessarily be ignored by support services; family conflict or conversely family cooperation may be a very important factor in an elderly person's care at home.

Attributes of the carer

The attributes of the carer and her relationship with the elderly person with mental health problems (including whether or not the person cared for lives with the caregiver) are all key issues. The gender, cultural background and attitudes of the caregiver, the way in which she is related to the care recipient, the quality of the relationship in the past as well as present, and whether or not they are co-resident are all relevant to the way in which they go about home care and how they react to it (Twigg & Atkin 1995).

The kind of tasks carers have to carry out

The variety of aspects of caregiving have already been mentioned; they are not all likely to be involved at all times for all mentally ill older people, nor for all caregivers. Support will therefore need to be sufficiently flexible to allow for diversity and for change; in one case companionship and sympathy may be required, in another help with incontinence and bathing.

The fact that caring has been shown to be very stressful

The stress of caregiving may be so great that it has been shown occasionally to have serious consequences such as severe psychological morbidity or risks of elder abuse (see Cooney & Howard 1995, Cooper et al 1995, Coyne et al 1993).

Studies show that in any general sample of caregivers the vast majority express a willingness to continue caring, even under considerable strain. For example, in the study by Levin et al (1989) only 13% said at first interview that they would definitely accept permanent residential care if offered. Indeed, findings show that most people who help to care for elderly mentally frail people find something satisfying about doing so. However, they also report problems, and these are related to levels of strain. As far as reported problems are concerned, a study of a community sample of dementia sufferers and their carers in Cambridge (O'Connor et al 1990) found that the problematic symptoms most frequently mentioned were mainly to do with the sufferer's physical dependency or his inertia or forgetfulness (things like sitting doing nothing, needing help dressing, being unsteady on his feet, needing help getting in or out of a chair). Much less frequently mentioned, though less easily tolerated, were disturbed behaviours such as temper outbursts, demands for attention and disruption to the carer's life. All types of problem area were 'significantly and positively associated with measures of strain' (though other researchers have placed most emphasis on 'demanding behaviour' (Twigg 1992)). O'Connor et al go on to say that their findings underline the importance of support services such as community nurses, occupational therapists and physiotherapists (to help with the physical dependency problems), but that the other kinds of problem are much less easily remedied, i.e. those to do with inertia or the disturbed behaviours.

As far as stress is concerned, the study by Levin et al (1989) found that one-third of the caregivers had high GHQ scores (a measure of their psychological health). Scores were higher where there had been an actual diagnosis of dementia and where another psychiatric disorder had been diagnosed in addition to or rather than dementia. This latter finding is particularly interesting since as Levin et al say (p. 136), it: 'draws attention to the strain upon those who look after elderly persons with depressive illnesses, anxiety states, paraphrenia and long-standing personality disorders. The experiences of such supporters have to date received scant attention from researchers'.

Strain as measured by GHQ score varied by health and gender of the caregiver, the number and nature of the caregiving problems, and the quality of their present relationship with the elderly person. What was also particularly striking was that at the 1-year follow-up, the GHQ scores of those who had ceased to provide routine care went down (showing improved psychological health). This study is a key source of evidence because it is one of the few which followed up caregivers over a period of time and can thus show with greater confidence than most the direction of association between factors like the health of caregivers and support.

These then are some of the problems which support services need to address, and some of the issues which they have to take into account as far as the people they support are concerned.

HOW ARE PEOPLE GENERALLY SUPPORTED? THE SUPPORT SERVICES

A number of questions need to be asked about each of the services available as well as about services overall. The prime one must concern how much and what kind of support people receive. If receipt is low, is this to do with lack of availablility, lack of awareness, lack of access or resistance to the service?

We must also ask whether they are appropriate, that is, whether they are meeting people's needs or wants, or addressing the problems? There are some limited indications that individual formal service providers involved in supporting the carers of dementia sufferers think they are doing so adequately (Clarke et al 1993) – but what is the evidence? Are the services effectively meeting their objectives? Are they of sufficiently good quality? Are they coordinated, and does this matter? What are the main gaps in service provision?

Despite the wealth and growth of evidence (discussed below) the answers to these questions remain partial. We still know little about the best way to help older people with mental health problems and their families (Evans 1992). We still do not know when, because of conflicting interests within a family, on balance, one form of support does more harm than good; or the point at which continued home care constitutes neglect rather than maintenance of independence.

A brief preliminary look at the overall picture (through analysis of the national OPCS Disability Surveys of 1985/1986) shows that, as far as older people with advanced cognitive impairment living in private households are concerned (Schneider et al 1993), the most likely services for people to have received in the previous 12 months were (as one would expect) the general practitioner (91%), informal care (56%), community nurse (36%), and home help/care (24%). For people with moderate to severe dementia this looks disturbingly low; nearly one in 10 dementia sufferers had not seen their general practitioner in the past year, nearly half had had no informal care, two-thirds had not had a community nurse, and three-quarters no home help. For people with severe dementia, however, the picture may be somewhat less bleak. For example, O'Connor et al (1989) found in their Cambridge study that among the most severely dementing people, 70% had seen the community nurse in the previous 4 weeks, and two in five a home help and similarly two in five meals-on-wheels in the previous week (though these findings involved a very small sample).

As for functional illnesses in older people, we know comparatively little about their receipt of services in the community. Further analysis of the OPCS Disability Survey (Gerontology Data Service 1996), similar to that mentioned above (Schneider et al 1993), shows for community services that functionally mentally ill older people were less likely than the cognitively impaired to have received the services of a community nurse in the past year (21%) but just as likely to have had a home help/carer (25%); approximately 10% had seen a health visitor, chiropodist or social worker or had meals-on-wheels. These are small proportions, and it appears that functionally mentally ill people may be no more likely (or even perhaps somewhat *less* likely) to use support services than those not psychiatrically distressed. Here, however, findings are inconsistent: Bowling & Farquhar (1991) found that psychiatric morbidity was a poor predictor of health and social services use among elderly and very elderly people living at home in an Inner London borough and a semi-rural area. Studies of adults of all ages show that those with psychiatric illness are more likely to use health and social services, but it looks as though it is different for

elderly people, whose perceived need for services may be lower. The authors draw rather bleak conclusions from this finding, though, as we shall see below, others draw rather more optimistic conclusions from similar findings.

The services potentially available are very varied, and it is possible to categorise them in a variety of ways. One could divide them according to where the support is provided, as follows:

- inside the home
- outside in the neighbourhood
- outside in institutions.

Alternatively, they could be divided according to the kind of support they primarily offer, for example:

- information and advice
- emotional support
- respite or relief from caring
- help with tasks: personal or daily living activities
- financial/benefits aid
- environmental/housing improvements.

The following discussion of each of the services divides them by whether the service is provided inside the person's home or outside because although no classification works very well (there being lots of overlap between categories), the least precise is the most manageable.

Support provided inside the home

The types of support available inside the home are summarised in Box 25.1, and discussed under the relevant headings below.

Assessment for support services

With the implementation of the NHS and Community Care Act in the UK in 1990 the importance of assess-

---

Box 25.1 The main support services at home

Assessment for services
Advocacy
Community nursing/bathing
Home help/care/sitting service
Home aids/adaptations
Laundry service
Meals delivery
Social workers
Wardens/alarms
Packages of care

ment has received greater emphasis through its aim of making services needs-led rather than supply-led. The assessment of needs has long been acknowledged as complex, with the influence of funding constraints, professional ideologies, elderly people's self-images and expectations, caregivers' views, etc., all playing a part (McWalter et al 1994). For older people with mental health problems, assessment is likely to be even more difficult. We still know little about whether all those who want an assessment receive one, or about the best ways of carrying it out, though there have been some innovatory schemes. For example, a project in Gloucester (Dant et al 1992), though not aimed specifically at older people with mental health problems, sensitively tried to take into account the older person's past life experience in assessing the kind of services which he or she required and would find acceptable. Although they found this approach welcomed by older people, it was very time-consuming and had to be used with restraint as the project developed.

Advocacy schemes

As a recent report on advocacy (Wertheimer 1993) states that, 'access to individual advocacy may be particularly important for people suffering from dementia' (p. 27). The same is probably true for older people with other kinds of mental illness who may also be vulnerable to disregard or exploitation. As Wertheimer says: 'a central aim of advocacy is to protect the individual's quality of life and safeguard their rights' (p. 27). Emphasis is not normally on the caregivers; in fact the concern is usually for people without carers or close family, though it is recognised that one of the problem areas for advocacy, but also one where it may be most needed, is where the interests of carers and care recipients appear to conflict (Wertheimer 1993). Although advocacy has long been part of the social worker's stated role, specific advocacy schemes for older people are comparatively new in the UK. There is as yet, therefore, little systematic evidence about their role and effectiveness (Leat 1992), though their importance is acknowledged as well as the difficulty of providing the service for elderly mentally ill people. There may also be some opposition to the schemes, and there is a suggestion that advocacy may be played down by centres offering advice and support in order not to alienate funders or potential funders, who may see advocacy as confrontational (Hills 1991).

Community nursing (including community psychiatric nursing and bathing services)

These services are difficult to evaluate because they perform multiple roles. Depending upon their expertise, agency affiliation, etc., community nurses may give information and advice, emotional support, personal care, medical care and treatment and arrange access to other services. Despite this multiple role, however, studies provide evidence of the under-provision of the community nursing service. For example, in 1986 only a third of those elderly people with advanced cognitive impairment living in the community had received such a service in the previous 12 months, according to the OPCS Disability Survey (Schneider et al 1993). And Levin et al (1989) found that sizeable proportions of people with problems with which community nurses dealt were not receiving any visits from them: 'For example, at least two-fifths of elderly persons with serious physical problems, of those who were incontinent, and of those who had a lot of help with personal care, lacked nursing support ...Moreover, although most supporters found behavioural problems particularly trying, few families had contact with community psychiatric nurses who have skills in managing these problems' (Levin et al 1989, p. 230).

This under-provision is particularly sad in the light of the evidence about the effectiveness of community nursing. Levin et al found that community nursing services had a beneficial effect on the psychological health of supporters coping with incontinence, though they did not appear to affect the likelihood of an elderly person entering permanent residential care.

Home help/care

Increasingly in the UK, home care (the term nowadays usually preferred to 'home help' since it reflects the greater emphasis on personal care as opposed to housework) is provided by private or voluntary agencies and purchased for elderly people by the social services department, though often with a means-tested contribution from the recipient. We could include any voluntary or paid worker who comes into the house to help with domestic or personal care (so, as well as home helps or home carers it could include shoppers, housekeepers, cleaners and sitting services). As such, and in the total number of hours of work provided, home care comprises the main form of community support to older people.

As with other services, home care is generally welcomed and well-received and there is evidence of under-provision. For example, in the case of dementia an examination of a small group of spouse carers in the Cambridge project (Pollitt et al 1991) found that eight out of 13, in a group of spouses who defined physical problems as the major difficulty rather than the dementia, said they could use more home help or district nurse or 'a sitting service, help with transport, laundry, the garden or someone to talk to'. Also some of those in another group (where the major problem was seen as dementia) said they would like more of a service or something they were not getting 'like a housekeeper, someone to take an interest in her, someone to be there in an emergency, a good night's sleep' (p. 456). Some of the spouses complained that private home or gardening care was expensive and hard to find though sometimes services had to be refused because the dementia sufferer would not have them in the house. Refusal of services can be an issue with people suffering from dementia; schemes which use care coordinators or managers can be especially good at allowing the development of confidence and trust which can break through this refusal (see, for example, the Ipswich/Newham Home Support Project, under the section dealing with multidimensional home support packages, below). There has been much debate about whether home care services are well-targeted; that is, whether they are reaching the people who may need them most. For instance, research has suggested that where there is a male caregiver people are more likely to receive a 'home carer' than where the supporter is female (though this has been disputed: see Arber et al 1988); and that those with milder dementia are as likely – or even more likely – to have such help as those with more severe conditions. Indeed Levin et al (1989) found that supporters dealing with more severe symptoms of confusion were considerably less likely to receive home care than those looking after someone with milder confusion. However, such a pattern is not universal; O'Connor et al (1989) found that receipt of home help was positively associated with level of dementia. The most undisputed connection, both in the UK and the USA, is between receipt of home care and whether the sufferer lives alone or not: those living alone are more likely to get such help than those living with a caregiver (O'Connor et al 1989, Webber et al 1994).

How effective are home care services in either maintaining willingness to continue caring or in combatting stress? As far as dementia is concerned, two Scottish studies in the 1980s found that the home help service alone was not significantly associated with willingness to continue caring (Gilhooly 1984) or with carer wellbeing as measured by the GHQ (Gilleard et al 1984). Levin et al (1989), in the London area, did find an association (though not significant on its own): carers receiving a home help were less likely to show an increase in strain (as measured by the GHQ) over a period of 1 year than those not in receipt. They also found evidence of the special importance of the home help service to male carers: 'men with home helps were as likely as women to go on looking after relatives with dementia, but without home helps they were far less likely to do so' (Levin et al 1989, p. 224).

There is limited evidence about the importance of home help/care to depressed older people, and it is hard to interpret. For example, a London study (Evans et al 1991) found that having a home help was 'inversely related to depressive illness, that is, the subject was less likely to be depressed if he/she received this service' and the authors concluded that the lower level of depression among those receiving a home help indicated the service's protective function and suggested 'the value of this service in supporting the emotional as well as the physical needs of its clients' (Evans et al 1991, p. 792). Findings generally suggest higher levels of psychological morbidity among those in receipt of services since it is such people who are more likely to be seen as in need of services. However, Bowling & Farquhar (1991), in a study of elderly and very elderly people living at home in an Inner London borough and a semi-rural area, drew a more sombre conclusion from a similar finding about the low level of home help receipt by older people suffering from depression, seeing it as due to the low priority given to the needs of such people by the home care services.

Home aids/adaptations

Elderly people with mental health problems and those who help to care for them may also be assisted at home by physical aids or adaptations such as bath aids, commodes, safety adaptations to stairs or to coal fires, electrical or gas equipment. For example, the 1985 OPCS Disability Survey showed that for disabled people of 60 years and over, 50% of women and 36% of men had bathing aids, and 16% of women and 6% of men had toileting aids (Jarvis et al forthcoming). These data, however, refer to people with any disability; there is little evidence about the scale of such assistance to those with mental health problems, or about its effect on the elderly person's wellbeing or morale, or on the carer's wellbeing or willingness to continue caring, though anecdotal evidence confirms that it is valued by caregivers and said to allay anxieties.

Laundry services

Incontinence is understandably one of the problems least easy for carers to tolerate. It is particularly likely to afflict those with severe dementia, and for them a laundry service may make all the difference to carers' willingness to continue caring. It is therefore a pity that the service is not more widespread. For instance, Levin et al (1989) found that the laundry service was very thinly spread; only a small minority of their caregivers received it, but for those who did it was of great value in helping them to cope with incontinence.

Meals delivery

If people have lost the ability or the motivation to prepare meals for themselves, as may well be the case with depression or dementia sufferers, then one would expect meals-on-wheels to be an important part of their community support. Levin et al (1989) found – as one would expect – that this service was most relevant to those who lived alone, and was greatly appreciated by their caregiving relatives, and that most of those who said they would find it helpful already got it. It is therefore perhaps surprising that it has not been shown to be an important factor, for example, in delaying institutionalisation or promoting carer wellbeing. Elderly people with mental health problems seem no more likely to receive meals-on-wheels than other elderly people. A London survey of depression among older people (Evans et al 1991) found no significant link between the presence of depression and having meals-on-wheels, and the service does not appear to have a significant effect on the care situation (for example, Gilhooly 1984, in a Scottish study of dementia sufferers, found no association between meals-on-wheels and either carers' psychological wellbeing or their willingness to continue giving care).

Social workers

The role of social workers with elderly people has always been difficult to assess because of the range of their responsibilities, their changing role, and the difficulty older people (who are often the source of research data) may have in recalling the frequency and outcome of their visits. Where social workers are involved at all, their most frequent role is likely to be in mobilising other resources, and it is these which may have an impact on the home care situation rather than the social worker himself. Apart from this activity, they may be involved in giving emotional support, counselling, helping with family conflicts, and assisting with finances/benefits. Since the implementation of the community care reforms in the UK in 1993, case management (or perhaps more likely 'care management' – see Hugman 1994) has become an increasingly important role. Research carried out before that date has limited relevance though it may provide some indications. Thus, for instance, Levin et al (1989) found that three-quarters of the caregivers in their study who had seen social workers said they found them helpful, particularly in 'the provision of information, counselling and practical services including day, relief and permanent residential care' (Levin et al 1989, p. 209).

However, there are indications that social workers in general have not been well-informed about the symptoms of dementia and therefore perhaps not as helpful as they might be (O'Connor et al 1989), though with the increased awareness of dementia this may have changed. Also, there is little evidence of carers coming into contact with trained social workers, and certainly not on an on-going basis (Twigg 1992).

Wardens/alarms

As with the wider population, very small proportions of older people with mental health problems live in warden-assisted housing or have alarms which they can activate in order to obtain help in an emergency. We know very little about the prevalence of confusion or functional mental health problems among those who do live in sheltered housing or with access to alarms, though there is evidence that it is low; for example, a study by Tinker (1989) of older people living in very sheltered housing found that 5% of a sample of just over 1000 were assessed by interviewers as 'very confused'. Studies of dementia sufferers, for example those by Levin et al (1989) and Askham & Thompson (1990), generally make no mention of sheltered housing or alarms; in the case of the latter study – and probably the former also – this was because it applied to such a small proportion of the sample.

The consensus of opinion is that alarms are of only limited value to older people with mental health problems unless their condition is very mild, since they may lack either the ability or the motivation to use them (Tinker 1984). As far as sheltered housing is concerned, it is generally held that other tenants and wardens will tolerate and support those who develop mental health problems while already in the accommodation (Tinker 1989), but that sheltered housing is not suitable for those who already have a mental health problem, unless it is very mild (when limited but regular help is all that is needed), or unless accommodation is provided in small separate units (Tinker et al 1995). Units of this kind have been found to work well, even though they are expensive.

Multidimensional home support packages

The piecemeal nature of social service provision for older people in the UK was increasingly criticised throughout the 1970s and 1980s, and led to a number of innovatory schemes to provide care in a more coordinated way. The pioneering scheme was the Kent Community Care Scheme (KCCS) first established in 1977 (and subsequently mirrored and developed elsewhere, and researched by both the Personal Social Services Research Unit at Kent University and other research bodies). The Kent scheme was very influential in the evolving community care policies eventually culminating in the NHS and Community Care Act of 1990. The scheme was designed to redress some of the major problems of community service delivery to older people: lack of coordination, fragmentation of services, their inflexibility, the limited range of services, the fact that they were service- rather than client-oriented. The key features of the scheme were: to use social workers as case managers with devolved budgets, and allow them to incur expenditure on clients up to a limit of two-thirds of the cost of residential care; they worked solely with people defined as being on the margins of institutional care, and could use existing services or buy in helpers from the community. Researchers evaluated the scheme using a control as well as the experimental sample in order to see whether those with the new system were maintained in the community longer than those with standard services (Challis & Davies 1986). Their findings showed a clear success for the KCCS model. In this original scheme, and as far as elderly people with mental health problems are concerned, the researchers concluded that the KCCS:

- more frequently identified minor psychiatric disorders and got treatment for them
- was more successful in ameliorating depressed mood than standard services
- helped people suffering from alcohol abuse through provision of an adequate diet and support
- helped to counter isolation and loneliness and therefore helped to prevent the onset of depression
- 'Even in the case of the dementing elderly, where particularly great care problems are found', had 'some degree of success in the establishment and maintenance of care and reduction of risk through

a more structured approach' (Challis & Davies 1988, p. 195).

Challis & Davies concluded that there are two groups for whom KCCS is especially cost effective. The first of these is the extremely dependent person with mental and physical frailty who receives a considerable degree of informal support ... The second group is the socially isolated elderly person, with only a moderate degree of dependency, likely to suffer from depression. These are people whose difficulties are frequently undetected in usual circumstances' (Challis & Davies 1988, p. 199).

The same research unit was involved in other later related schemes (e.g. in Gateshead and Darlington). These projects were also evaluated, but the researchers' conclusions remained fundamentally the same: 'These studies all indicate that it is possible, with case management and flexible use of resources, to provide both community care of a higher quality and reduce levels of stress on carers of very frail elderly people at no greater cost than the usual pattern of provision for these people' (Challis et al 1990, p. 88).

However, it is not easy to assess the beneficial effects of the Kent Community Care Scheme model specifically for the carers of elderly people with mental health problems because:

1. the scheme was not specifically directed at those with mental health problems
2. it was not specifically directed at the needs of carers. (For a fuller critique see Parker 1990.)

In the experimental group of the original evaluated Kent Community Care Scheme most of the 92 elderly people did not have informal carers (only 21 carers were in fact interviewed) and by no means all had mental health problems (26% had moderate to severe confusion or disorientation and 48% moderate to severe depressed mood). However, the researchers concluded that in general the scheme was better than standard services at providing support for carers because it could organise relief care specifically to suit the needs of the carer (often in the home rather than outside) and also help them set limits to their involvement. The Kent scheme showed 'evidence of some degree of improvement in the wellbeing of carers, and no evidence of decline' (Challis & Davies 1991, p. 69). One would expect this kind of result, since the scheme's approach explicitly involved aspects which would be welcomed by carers, for example:

- continuity of contact with more experienced staff
- a service designed to respond to the elderly person's and the carer's definition of problems

- involvement in defining solutions
- provision of more appropriate services and filling gaps in service provision.

However, it is not possible to say what particular aspects of this package of support were most beneficial to carers.

Different groups of researchers and development workers have been involved in other multidimensional care schemes. For example, there was the Gloucester Care for Elderly People at Home Project which, while not primarily concerned with supporting caregivers, and not concerned solely with older people with mental health problems, clearly confirmed the importance, both for elderly service recipients and for their family supporters, of a coordinated approach. The use of care coordinators with responsibility for devising and maintaining an apppropriate 'package of care' (Dant & Gearing 1990) was responded to positively by both service recipients and caregivers; 'most (66%) felt that their support had either been better or much better as a result of the Care Co-ordinator's involvement' (Dant et al 1992, p. 193).

Another scheme focused solely on dementing elderly people in order to try and provide clearer indications of the value of such approaches with people suffering from organic mental illnesses. This was the Age Concern/Guy's Hospital (UMDS) Home Support Scheme (Askham & Thompson 1990), which operated in a London borough and a market town in southern England (the London borough of Newham and Ipswich, Suffolk). The main aim of the new service was the construction of flexible packages of care for dementia sufferers living at home, first by liaising with other services to provide or increase where necessary the client's receipt of existing services, and secondly by 'topping up' existing services (where the development worker thought extra care was needed to maintain someone at home) through the employment of local support workers. Unlike the Kent Community Care Scheme, there was no clear indication from the evaluation that extra home support was effective in keeping people with dementia at home longer than those with standard services. Detailed case study analysis suggested, however, that the intensive coordinated approach of the kind offered was particularly beneficial in the support of severely demented people living alone and without wholly involved informal carers, yet not requiring 24-hour-a-day care (Askham & Thompson 1990). For these people the scheme appeared to substitute for the family caregivers they did not have, but for most people the more coordinated approach and the topping up of

services, although warmly praised, were either not really essential to continued home care, were already adequately addressed, or were not adequate to keep people at home who were severely dementing and needed even more than the Home Support Project could offer. As for the scheme's support to carers, again there was no overwhelming evidence that it relieved them of strain sufficiently to prolong their willingness to go on caring. In fact:

The findings would support a conclusion that what helps carers of dementia sufferers most is the temporary removal of the sufferer from the home, either for day care or for temporary institutional care, rather than extra help in the home whilst the dementia sufferer is still there. If this is the case then the Home Support Project was unlikely to have a marked effect on carers' views except when it was instrumental in organising or increasing respite care.

(Askham & Thompson 1990, p. 106)

There is a problem in evaluating these multidimensional care schemes, for by their very nature they involve a huge variety of variables: a diverse population of older people, and a wide variety of service innovations. Even if they can be shown to have made a difference it is not possible, without huge samples, to show precisely what it was that made the difference. However, services outside the home seem to be crucial, especially for dementia sufferers, and it is to these we now turn.

Support outside the home

The main support services are summarised in Box 25.2 and discussed under the relevant headings below.

Box 25.2   The main support services outside the home

Caregivers' support groups
Day hospitals/centres/care
Information and advice services
Institutional respite care/holidays/overnight care
Primary care
Specialist psychiatric community service

Caregivers' support groups

Support groups, often led by a professional worker such as a social worker or community nurse, grew rapidly in the UK and elsewhere in the 1980s. They provided a forum for carers to discuss their problems and circumstances with others in the same position and to obtain advice, confirmation and information both from each other and from professional sources.

There have been many evaluations of such schemes, though mainly in the USA. For example, Toseland and Rossiter (1989) examined 29 American evaluations of the effectiveness of support groups. They found that satisfaction with the groups was high, and people saw them as informative and helpful. Nevertheless, they found no clear link between satisfaction and other important outcome measures, such as carers' coping skills, stress, carers' support systems, or psychological disturbance. The evidence is not consistent; some studies show that self-help groups have resulted in reduced burden (Kahan et al 1985, Glosser & Wexler 1985, Toseland et al 1992). Also, of course, reduction of burden is not the only purpose of support groups; Gubrium (1986) and Gubrium & Lynott (1985) describe in some detail the important educative role of such groups in helping people to make sense of and categorise the illness. Also, support groups may be provided directly for elderly people with functional mental illnesses rather than for their relatives or caregivers. These have been little researched and what evidence we have is largely descriptive (e.g. Procter & Alwar 1995).

Day hospitals/centres/care

Apart from the typical forms of such day provision (funded and/or run by the statutory services and provided in normal working hours), there is also the voluntary sector provision, and variants such as lunch clubs, evening care and travelling day care. Evaluation of some of these more innovatory forms of care is still inadequate, though there are some encouraging signs; for example, an evening club for elderly mentally ill people in West Glamorgan, though still in its infancy, appears to be popular, has developed within existing resources, and is seen by staff as providing 'an improved quality of life for carers in reducing their stress through providing more choice of care for clients' (Sansom et al 1993, p. 374).

Day respite of whatever sort is liked by caregivers of dementia sufferers, many of whom say they would like more (Twigg & Atkin 1993). Levin et al (1989), for example, found it warmly praised by the two in five supporters of elderly confused people who received day care, though it was less likely to be wanted by spouse carers than some other groups. Other research confirms this; for instance Pollitt et al (1991) found some negative comments about day care from spouse carers of dementia sufferers, who complained about the kind of people with whom their husbands or wives were associating.

Again there is no unanimity about the beneficial effects of day care. Some have found it beneficial to carers, for example Levin et al (1989), who saw the psychological health of those with access to day care deteriorating less over a year than that of those without such access (though the difference was not significant). Gilhooly (1990) found a complex picture from North American studies, where, according to some outcome measures, day care had a positive effect (continued maintenance of the older person in the community, satisfaction with the day care service), and according to others no effect (death rates, carer wellbeing).

Part of the debate about day care is about whether day hospitals are any more beneficial than day centres in supporting the carers of elderly people with mental health problems. Among this group of older people, their main client group is dementia sufferers, and there is little doubt that as a means of giving their carers some respite from care they are useful (see Lennon & Jolley 1991, Levin et al 1994), but not necessarily any more useful (and certainly more expensive) than day centres run by voluntary organisations (Fasey 1994, Murphy 1994). Day hospitals have been shown to have little effect on the need for institutional care (Diesfeldt 1992, Woods and Phanjoo 1991). Some studies have found them to relieve strain on carers; for example, a recent study by Jerrom et al (1993) examined the stress levels of the carers of 63 dementia sufferers attending an assessment day hospital, and found that after 12 weeks at the day hospital the stress levels of the carers had fallen to normal population levels; this was not through any change in the behaviour of the dementia sufferers, so was probably due to the respite from care itself or to carers feeling that their problems were being recognised and that others were sharing their responsibilities (see also Gilleard 1987).

However, this finding is not supported in other studies; for instance Gilhooly (1984, p. 42) found that 'day hospital attendance was not significantly correlated with morale, a measure of carers' mental health or with carers' willingness to continue caring'. One study (Berry et al 1991) from the USA showed that getting the older person ready for the day hospital increased the carer's workload rather than decreased it. It also disrupted familiar routines, and in that sense may cause more of a burden to the carers.

There has been very little evaluative research on the effectiveness of day hospitals or day centres for elderly people with functional as opposed to organic mental illness. Indeed, the authors of a recent review of research on day care for elderly mentally ill people (Warrington & Eagles 1995) concluded that day care for this group of people had in general been poorly evaluated, making it very difficult for any conclusions about its benefits for elderly people and carers to be drawn.

Information/advice/education services

There is little evaluation of schemes to provide advice (Leat 1992), written or verbal information, though what there is tends to support the view that it reduces stress among carers by reducing uncertainty (see Toner 1987, Brodaty & Gresham 1989). The latter study involved the evaluation of an Australian training programme including education, therapy, skills training, and support group discussions for dementia sufferers and their carers, in which participants were placed in experimental and control groups. A much lower rate of institutionalisation was found for patients in the experimental group, and lowered psychological morbidity amongst carers. Numbers were small, however, and the authors, though optimistic, were cautious in their conclusions.

Institutional respite care

Relief care for short periods is provided in hospitals, nursing homes or residential care establishments. Its aim is generally to give some respite to caregivers, but Nolan & Grant (1992) have shown that it may also serve other functions, such as providing skills training and emotional support. In addition, some agencies may arrange holiday breaks for people with dementia (sometimes in conjunction with their carers) but these are very rare (Micklewood 1991).

Pollitt et al (1991) found some complaints about respite care (dislike of the diet, loss of the patient's clothes, etc.), and there is some evidence from other studies of deterioration in the condition of the person admitted on his or her return home (Hirsch et al 1993, Wright 1986). But studies show mixed reactions; for instance Melzer (1990), in a small-scale study of one respite care unit for dementia sufferers, found in a semi-structured interview study of 19 carers that while those who went on using the unit spoke very highly of it, many had stopped using it for various reasons (these included the sufferer becoming more confused when moved from home, physical illness, or the carer being able to obtain preferred respite via other family members, etc.). He also found that 'the belief in a preventive role for respite care in avoiding admission to hospital was both unsupported by the available evidence, and also obscured the unit's main role as one of many forms of social help to carers' (p. 66).

Moriarty and Levin (1993) say that research on the effectiveness of respite care provides 'a tentatively optimistic picture' of its contribution to delaying institutional care. Research from the USA (e.g. Lawton et al 1989) showed that, among carers who were offered institutional or in-home respite, day care, or a combination of services, over a period of a year, families with respite care maintained their relative at home for a significantly longer period. Similarly, Montgomery and Borgatta (1989) found that respite care delayed the use of nursing home placements (see also Donaldson et al 1988). But it is not possible to demonstrate conclusively an association between levels and types of respite care and continued stay in the community; and as Nolan (1994) says, even against limited criteria, such as effects on carers' stress or willingness to go on caring, research to date suggests that the positive outcomes of respite services are by no means certain.

In Levin et al's own earlier study (1989) it was found that one in four elderly confused people had had a short stay in hospital or residential home, and two in five of the carers who had not been offered it said they would accept it if offered. If received it was particularly strongly praised by the caregivers and thought to be extremely helpful. A minority criticised it for having negative effects upon the elderly person. On the question of effectiveness, the striking finding was that it appeared to be associated with an *increased* likelihood of the elderly person being in residential care at follow-up interview. This was because it was targeted at those on the margins of institutional care, and was often a precursor to it. Relief care appeared to have beneficial effects on carers' psychological health (though on its own not significantly so).

There are few evaluative studies of night care (when elderly people go to a centre just during the night-time hours), though there are indications of its increasing use. A study of one scheme shows a familiar pattern of findings (Watkins 1994): carers were likely to see a night centre as valuable, but there was no suggestion that it was effective in delaying institutional admission or in controlling psychological morbidity in carers or service users.

The primary care service

The support which GPs can give to elderly people and their carers will of course depend (apart from occasions like the 75 plus assessment) on whether people contact the GP in the first place. There is some evidence that people are reluctant to go to their GP about a mental health problem. As one of Pollitt's interviewees (the wife of a dementia sufferer) said: 'Our GP is a dear, but I wouldn't want to bother him about that' (Pollitt et al 1991, p. 461).

The same study also found that although GPs were well-informed about the nature of dementia, 'they rarely intervened, partly because families failed to inform them that they were in difficulty, but also because the doctors felt that they had little to offer' (O'Connor et al 1989, p. 343).

GPs can be useful for support not only in what they give directly but also, of course, in referring people on to other services. But the study by Levin et al (1989) identified some of the weaknesses of GPs as links in the referral system. These were:

- unawareness of many of their patients' medical and social problems
- great variation between them in whether patients find them easy to talk to
- variation between them in the extent to which they are willing to consider the social consequences of disease.

These findings are supported by recent evaluation of an open access community psychiatric service in London (Macdonald et al 1994) which found that only 45.3% of the psychiatric service users came via GPs, and 36% from non-medical services.

Specialist psychiatric community services

The move towards community mental health teams appears to bring some additional support to older people with mental health problems and their carers. One example from London is in North Southwark and Lewisham, where a change was introduced in the mid 1980s, from the traditional consultant service to a multidisciplinary team of doctors, community psychiatric nurses, occupational therapists and clinical psychologists. Referrals became more open (not just taken through general practitioners) and clients were dealt with by a team but with one member acting as the key worker for each client. The key worker would make an assessment, formulate a list of problems and a treatment plan. Researchers found that this system enabled the service to pick up more referrals, more time was spent with clients and their families, and it was better at identifying carers' problems (though it was of course more labour intensive and therefore expensive; however, its long-term cost-effectiveness was not studied) (Coles et al 1991). A later study of the same area (Macdonald et al 1994) showed that over the first 58 months of a new team service, GPs referred less than half the cases seen and researchers concluded

that if the service had been confined to patients referred from traditional (i.e. medical) sources, 463 patients with a psychiatric diagnosis 'would have had to await referral via these sources' (Macdonald et al 1994, p. 711).

The coordination and setting up of services may also be done through the psychogeriatric team. For example, Tym (1991, p. 317) says, in discussing a rural service in East Anglia, that the burden of caring for a dementing patient can be 'shared and lightened by appropriate supporting measures such as counselling, respite care arrangements, day care, relative support groups, and assistance with home care. If these are not available in the community, the psychogeriatric team needs to be innovative and to set about trying to arrange networks of provision' (Tym 1991, p. 317).

Such services have still to prove their worth, though early findings look promising for carers. However, developments in the organisation of health care services may well threaten their existence.

THE STATE OF CURRENT PROVISION AND THE WAY FORWARD

Neither all older people with mental health problems nor their carers have a need for formal service support. Although we do not know what proportion might be managing satisfactorily with what they see as normal family help, we do know that people with milder conditions are less likely to say they need extra outside support.

Service support is, however, very important to huge numbers of people. Because of the enormously varied support needs and difficulties mental health problems bring to older people and those who help to care for them at home, facilities and services must inevitably be varied, and available in different combinations to different kinds of people. It is very difficult to research them adequately, and impossible to draw together the threads of widely different research projects and knowledge on such a diverse subject to give an overall picture of the situation in the UK today. This difficulty is compounded by the fact that there are no adequate national data on the receipt of support services by older people with mental health problems; the most recent and appropriate survey was the OPCS Disability Survey carried out in 1985/1986, but a great deal has happened to the organisation of services since then. However, one can tentatively make some general points:

1. Support services, of whatever kind, are almost always warmly praised when recipients are asked

for their views; people particularly praise those services which give them most relief or relieve them from especially burdensome tasks (e.g. day relief or incontinence laundry services). It is clear, also, that the kind of support services wanted or welcomed are conditional upon the characteristics and circumstances of caregiver and dependant. For example, spouse carers have different preferences from adult children, male carers from female, and those in paid employment from those who are not. Equally, preferred support for someone with mild dementia is likely to be different from that desired for someone with depression or severe dementia.

On their feelings about the volume of support, most people appear satisfied with what they get (see Gilhooly 1990, Pollitt et al 1991). The danger here is that if people express satisfaction then, because resources are limited, their views are likely to be taken at face value when perhaps in some cases they should not be. As Pollitt et al (1991, p. 463) say, 'sometimes it seemed to us that it suited the professionals to turn a blind eye'. In today's quasi-market situation such findings are a reminder that carers and older people themselves are not able to act like 'real' consumers, and therefore of the huge responsibility towards their clients held by the statutory purchasers and the providers.

2. It is easy to conclude that people are not receiving as much support as they would find beneficial. This service deficit may be partly to do with uptake, which some research suggests is lower than availability (see for example Pollitt et al 1991), but it is much more to do with limited availability and the lack of resources. Clear exceptions are the general practitioner service (lack of receipt of this service must be due to lack of access, awareness, perceived need or to resistance), and information and advice (where, because there is a great deal in existence, lack of receipt must be due to lack of access, lack of awareness or the information not being in the required form). Underprovision seems to be evident in most of the common types of support service: community nursing, home care, day care, institutional respite care. There is some evidence that people with the severest problems are most likely to be receiving the services, that is, that the services are being targeted appropriately; but even this is not uncontested. For example, there is no clear evidence about how well targeted the home care service is. It is clear that many factors influence the scale and nature of the services a person receives (Twigg & Atkin 1995).

It is also true that very little seems to be provided specifically for the support of older people and their caregivers when the mental health problem is a functional mental illness rather than dementia. For example, there is no consistency of findings about whether depressed people are more or less likely to have good social support in general than non-depressed. And it is a difficult area to research. For instance, one New Zealand study (Walton et al 1990) found that elderly people with psychiatric morbidity (depression or phobias) were no less likely to have social support and to be socially integrated, yet they were more likely to perceive them as inadequate.

3. There is no evidence to support any further fundamental change in the mixture of support services (e.g. a change in the balance of services or the introduction of major new kinds of services). Research generally concludes with the not very surprising finding that the gaps in support are to do with the inadequacy of existing services rather than with the need for something completely different (Levin et al 1989).

Lack of coordination and fragmentation of services have been recognised, particularly in the period leading up to the implementation of the NHS and Community Care Act, and, to some extent, have been addressed.

4. Beyond questions of satisfaction or scale of provision are the even more important questions of the effectiveness or value of support services. First there is the issue of whether support services are beneficial to mental health, that is, whether they can allay further psychological problems or improve psychological health. As far as carer stress is concerned, unfortunately, there is no simple answer to the question about the extent of the contribution of formal services to its alleviation. The main problem is that most studies only show associations between receipt of services and stress, and not the direction of the link. There is agreement also that other factors are important influences on a caregiver's psychological wellbeing. For example, there is the closeness of the relationship between the carer and cared-for (the closer the kinship tie the greater the stress), the quality of the previous relationship (the better it was the lower the stress), informal support to carers (found to reduce carer stress; see Morris et al 1989), caregiver style and coping strategies, and the extent to which the carer can continue to find rewards in the relationship with the sufferer (Morris et al 1988).

There are very few longitudinal studies of any magnitude. One of the few is the study by Levin et al (1989) of the caregivers of confused elderly people, which because of its longitudinal design was able to answer the question about the contribution of support services fairly clearly: as far as the carers of confused elderly people are concerned, those receiving more support services do better than those with fewer. Levin and her colleagues found that supporters receiving a relatively high number of community services showed less deterioration in their psychological health over a period of time than those receiving fewer or none. However, this study needs replication with other populations, particularly amongst people with other mental health problems.

5. The second important question about effectiveness of support services is whether they can help people who would otherwise be in institutions to remain living at home longer. The most realistic answer is that they can do so to a limited extent. Below a certain level of disability it is unlikely that institutional care would even be suggested (and very unlikely to be wanted). Above a certain level of disability there would be perhaps very little question: it would not be cost-effective for someone to remain in the community with very high levels of formal support, and family caregivers would find the volume of support needed unmanageable. But somewhere in between there are people for whom support services are the crucial factor in helping them to remain at home longer. But it is by no means clear what are the characteristics of this group nor at what point they cross the line between community and institution.

It is important to emphasise that evidence about the contribution of support services to continued home domicile is about delaying rather than preventing institutionalisation altogether. Gilhooly (1990), in a review of community services for dementia sufferers, found no evidence, either in the UK or in the USA, that services (i.e. information and counselling, home care, respite care, dementia therapies and financial help services) prevent institutionalisation altogether (and very unclear evidence about whether they delay it).

For the future we can still only make very broad recommendations. Of course, ideally we need more support services for older people and their caregivers, but no piecemeal, across-the-board increase would be sensible; nor is it at all likely to happen. To set priorities, and to give people what will help them most when they are faced with the diverse difficulties of mental illness, we need to know more about the varying benefits of different types of support to different kinds of people in different circumstances.

REFERENCES

Anderson D 1986 The experiences and needs of the carers of the elderly mentally infirm. Social Services Research 15(2): 95–127

Arber S, Gilbert N, Evandrou M 1988 Gender, household composition and receipt of domiciliary services by elderly disabled people. Journal of Social Policy 17(2): 153–175

Askham J 1991 The problem of generalizing about community care of dementia sufferers. Journal of Aging Studies 5(2): 137–146

Askham J 1995 Making sense of dementia: carers' perceptions. Ageing and Society 15: 103–114

Askham J, Thompson C 1990 Dementia and home care. ACIOG Research Report 4. ACE Books, London

Berry G, Zarit S, Rabatin V 1991 Caregiver activity on respite and non-respite days: a comparison of two service approaches. The Gerontologist 31(6): 830–835

Bowling A, Farquhar M 1991 Psychiatric morbidity and service use among elderly people. Ageing and Society 11: 275–297

Brodaty H, Gresham M 1989 Effect of a training programme to reduce stress in carers of patients with dementia. British Medical Journal 299: 1375–1379

Brody E, Hoffman C, Kleban M, Schoonover C 1989 Caregiving daughters and their local siblings: perceptions, strains and interactions. The Gerontologist 29(4): 529–538

Challis D, Davies B 1986 Case management in community care. Gower, Aldershot

Challis D, Davies B 1988 The community care approach: an innovation in home care by social services departments. In: Wells N, Freer C (eds) The ageing population: burden or challenge. Macmillan, Stockton Press

Challis D, Davies B 1991 Improving support to carers: a considered response to Parker's critical review. Ageing and Society 11(1): 69–73

Challis D, Chessum R, Chesterman J, Luckett R, Traske K 1990 Case management in social and health care: the Gateshead community care scheme. PSSRU, University of Kent, Canterbury

Clarke C, Heyman R, Pearson P, Watson D 1993 Formal carers: attitudes to working with the dementing elderly and their informal carers. Health and Social Care in the Community 1(4): 227–238

Clifford D 1990 The social costs and rewards of caring. Avebury, Aldershot

Coles R, von Abendorff R, Herzberg J 1991 The impact of a new community mental health team on an inner city psychogeriatric service. International Journal of Geriatric Psychiatry 6: 31–39

Cooney C, Howard R 1995 Abuse of patients with dementia by carers: out of sight but not out of mind. International Journal of Geriatric Psychiatry 10: 735–741

Cooper B, Ballard C, Saad K, Patel A et al 1995 The prevalence of depression in the carers of dementia sufferers. International Journal of Geriatric Psychiatry 10(3): 237–242

Coyne A, Reichman W, Berbig L 1993 The relationship between dementia and elder abuse. American Journal of Psychiatry 150: 643–646

Dant T, Gearing B 1990 Keyworkers for elderly people in the community: case managers and care coordinators. Journal of Social Policy 19(3): 331–360

Dant T, Gearing B, Johnson M, Carley M 1992 Care for elderly people at home: the Gloucester study. In: Morgan K (ed) Responding to an ageing society. Jessica Kingsley, London

Diesfeldt H 1992 Psychogeriatric day care outcome: a five-year follow-up. International Journal of Geriatric Psychiatry 7: 673–679

Donaldson C, Clark K, Gregson B et al 1988 Evaluation of a training support unit for elderly mentally infirm people and their carers. Health Care Research Unit Report 34, Newcastle

Evans J G 1992 From plaque to placement: a model for Alzheimer's disease. Age and Ageing 21: 77–80

Evans M, Copeland J, Dewey M 1991 Depression in the elderly in the community: effect of physical illness and selected social factors. International Journal of Geriatric Psychiatry 6: 787–795

Fasey C 1994 The day hospital in old age psychiatry: the case against. International Journal of Geriatric Psychiatry 9: 519–523

Gerontology Data Service 1996 Further analysis of OPCS Disability Survey, carried out by Gerontology Data Service, Age Concern Institute of Gerontology, King's College, London

Gilhooly M 1984 The impact of caregiving on caregivers: factors associated with the psychological wellbeing of people supporting a dementing relative in the community. British Journal of Medical Psychology 57: 34–44

Gilhooly M 1986 Senile dementia: factors associated with caregivers preference for institutional care. British Journal of Medical Psychology 59: 165–171

Gilhooly M 1990 Do services delay or prevent institutionalization of people with dementia? Research Report 4, Dementia Services Development Centre, Stirling University

Gilleard C 1987 Influence of emotional distress among supporters on the outcome of psychogeriatric day care. British Journal of Psychiatry 150: 219–223

Gilleard C, Bedford H, Gilleard E, Whittick J, Gledhill K 1984 Emotional distress among supporters of the elderly mentally infirm. British Journal of Psychiatry 145: 172–177

Glosser G, Wexler D 1985 Participants' evaluation of educational/support groups for families of patients with Alzheimer's disease and other dementias. The Gerontologist 25: 232–236

Gubrium J 1986 Old timers and Alzheimer's: the descriptive organisation of senility. Jai Press, Greenwich, Connecticut

Gubrium J, Lynott R 1985 Alzheimer's disease as biographical work. In: Peterson W, Quadagno J (eds) Social bonds in later life. Sage, Beverley Hills

Hills D 1991 Carer support in the community: evaluation of the department of health initiative, demonstration districts for informal carers 1986–1989. HMSO, London

Hirsch C, Davies H, Boatwright F, Ochango G 1993 Effects of a nursing home respite admission on veterans with advanced dementia. The Gerontologist 33(4): 523–528

Hugman R 1994 Social work and case management in the UK: models of professionalism and elderly people. Ageing and Society 14(2): 237–253

Jarvis C, Hancock R, Askham J, Tinker A (forthcoming) Getting around after sixty. HMSO, London

Jerrom B, Mian I, Rukanyake N, Prothero D 1993 Stress on relative caregivers of dementia sufferers and predictors of the breakdown of community care. International Journal of Geriatric Psychiatry 8(4): 331–337

Kahan J, Kemp B, Staples F, Brummel-Smith K 1985 Decreasing the burden in families caring for a relative with a dementing illness. Journal of the American Geriatrics Society 33: 664–670

Laczko F, Noden S 1993 Combining paid work with eldercare. Health and Social Care in the Community 1(2): 81–89

Lawton M Powell, Brody E, Juperstein A 1989 A controlled study of respite services for care givers of Alzheimer's patients. The Gerontologist 29(9): 8–16

Leat D 1992 Innovations and special schemes. In: Twigg J (ed) Carers: research and practice. HMSO, London

Lennon S, Jolley D 1991 An urban service in South Manchester. In: Jacoby R, Oppenheimer C (eds) Psychiatry in the elderly. Oxford University Press, Oxford

Levin E, Sinclair I, Gorbach P 1989 Families, services and confusion in old age. Avebury, Aldershot

Levin E, Moriarty J, Gorbach P 1994 Better for the break. HMSO, London

Lewis J, Meredith B 1988 Daughters who care: daughters caring for mothers at home. Routledge, London

Macdonald A, Goddard C, Poynton A 1994 Impact of open access to specialist services – the case of community psychogeriatrics. International Journal of Geriatric Psychiatry 9: 709–714

McWalter G, Toner H, Corser A, Eastwood J, Marshall M, Turvey T 1994 Needs and needs assessment: their components and definitions with reference to dementia. Health and Social Care in the Community 2(4): 213–219

Martin J, White A, Melzer H 1989 Disabled adults: services, transport and employment. OPCS Surveys of Disability in Great Britain, Report 4. HMSO, London

Melzer D 1990 An evaluation of a respite care unit for elderly people with dementia: framework and some results. Health Trends 22(2): 64–67

Micklewood P 1991 Caring for confusion. Scutari Press, London

Montgomery R, Borgatta E 1989 The effects of alternative support strategies on family caregiving. The Gerontologist 29: 457–464

Moriarty J, Levin E 1993 Services to people with dementia and their carers. In: Burns A (ed) Ageing and dementia: a methodological approach. Edward Arnold, London

Morris L, Morris R, Britton P 1989 Social support networks and formal support as factors influencing the psychological adjustment of spouse caregivers of dementia sufferers. International Journal of Geriatric Psychiatry 4: 47–51

Morris R, Morris L, Britton P 1988 Factors affecting the emotional well-being of the caregivers of dementia sufferers. British Journal of Psychiatry 153: 147–156

Murphy E 1994 Editorial: the day hospital debate. International Journal of Geriatric Psychiatry 9: 517–518

Nissel M, Bonnerjea L 1982 Family care of the handicapped elderly: who pays? Policy Studies Institute, London

Nolan M 1994 Developing the potential of respite care: a carer's perspective. In: Moriarty J, Nolan M Research on breaks. Dementia Services Development Centre, University of Stirling

Nolan M, Grant C 1992 Regular respite: an evaluation of a hospital rota-bed scheme for elderly people. ACIOG Research Paper 6. ACE Books, London

O'Connor D, Pollitt P, Hyde J, Brook C, Reiss P, Roth M 1988 Do general practitioners miss dementia in elderly patients? British Medical Journal 297: 1107–1110

O'Connor D, Pollitt P, Brook C, Reiss B 1989 The distribution of services to demented elderly people living in the community. International Journal of Geriatric Psychiatry 4: 339–344

O'Connor D, Pollitt P, Roth M, Brook C, Reiss B 1990 Problems reported by relatives in a community study of dementia. British Journal of Psychiatry 156: 835–841

Parker G 1990 Whose care, whose costs, whose benefits? A critical review of research on case management and informal care. Ageing and Society 10: 459–467

Pollitt P, Anderson I, O'Connor D 1991 For better or for worse: the experience of caring for an elderly dementing spouse. Ageing and Society 11: 443–469

Procter E, Alwar L 1995 A therapeutic group in the community for the elderly with functional psychiatric illnesses. International Journal of Geriatric Psychiatry 10(1): 33–36

Qureshi H, Walker A 1989 The caring relationship: elderly people and their families. Macmillan, London

Sansom G, Thomas W, Wilkinson M 1993 Alternative community evening care to elderly mentally ill people. Health and Social Care in the Community 1(6): 372–375

Schneider J, Kavanagh S, Knapp M, Beecham J, Netten A 1993 Elderly people with advanced cognitive impairment in England: resource use and costs. Ageing and Society 13: 27–50

Taraborrelli P 1994 Innocents, converts and old hands: the experiences of Alzheimer's disease caregivers. In: Bloor M, Taraborrelli P (eds) Qualitative studies in health and medicine. Cardiff paper in qualitative research. Aldershot, Surrey

Tinker A 1984 Staying at home: helping elderly people. HMSO, London

Tinker A 1989 An evaluation of very sheltered housing. Department of the Environment/HMSO, London

Tinker A, Wright F, Zeilig H 1995 Difficult to let sheltered housing. HMSO, London

Toner H 1987 Effectiveness of a written guide for carers of dementia sufferers. British Journal of Clinical and Social Psychology 5(1): 24–26

Toseland R, Rossiter C 1989 Group interventions to support family caregivers: a review and analysis. The Gerontologist 29(4): 438–449

Toseland R, Labrecque B, Goebel S, Whithey M 1992 An evaluation of a group program for spouses of frail elderly veterans. The Gerontologist 32(3): 382–390

Twigg J 1989 Models of carers: how do social care agencies conceptualize their relationship with informal carers? Journal of Social Policy 18(1): 53–66

Twigg J (ed) 1992 Carers: research and practice. HMSO, London

Twigg J, Atkin K 1993 Carers perceived: policy and practice in informal care. Open University Press, Milton Keynes

Twigg J, Atkin K 1995 Carers and services: factors mediating service provision. Journal of Social Policy 24(1): 5–30

Tym E 1991 A rural service in East Anglia. In: Jacoby R, Oppenheimer C (eds) Psychiatry in the elderly. Oxford University Press, Oxford

Walton V, Romans-Clarkson S, Multen P, Herbison P 1990 The mental health of elderly women in the community. International Journal of Geriatric Psychiatry 5: 257–263

Warrington J, Eagles J 1995 Day care for the elderly mentally ill: diurnal confusion? Health Bulletin 53(2): 99–104

Watkins M 1994 An evaluation of 'Crest', a night hospital for elderly people suffering from dementia. PhD Thesis, Department of Nursing Studies, King's College London, London University

Webber P, Fox P, Burnette D 1994 Living alone with Alzheimer's disease: effects on health and social service utilisation patterns. The Gerontologist 34(1): 8–14

Wertheimer A 1993 Speaking out: citizen advocacy and older people. Centre for Policy on Ageing, London

Woods J, Phanjoo A 1991 A follow up study of psychogeriatric day hospital patients with dementia. International Journal of Geriatric Psychiatry 6: 183–188

Wright F 1986 Left to care alone. Gower, Aldershot

RECOMMENDED READING

Askham J, Thompson C 1990 Dementia and home care. ACIOG Research Report 4. ACE Books, London. *A report on an innovative scheme for the home support of dementia sufferers in London and Suffolk, and its evaluation. The difficulty of assessing the effectiveness of such schemes is demonstrated and the study draws a cautious conclusion that enhanced home support can help some groups of people with dementia to remain in the community.*

Challis D, Davies B 1988 The community care approach: an innovation in home care by social services departments. In: Wells N, Freer C (eds) The ageing population: burden or challenge. Macmillan/Stockton Press, London. *A description in summary form of the evaluation of the highly influential Kent Community Care Scheme and subsequent schemes elsewhere. For full details of the evidence about the effectiveness of the Kent scheme see also* Challis D, Davies B 1986 Case management in community care. Gower, Aldershot.

Dant T, Gearing B, Johnson M, Carley M 1992 Care for elderly people at home: the Gloucester study. In: Morgan K (ed) Responding to an ageing society. Jessica Kingsley, London. *A chapter describing an actio-research project using care coordinators, designed to help elderly people at risk of institutional care to remain at home. The elderly people included, though were not confined to, those with dementia. The project showed that a keyworker scheme had benefits for older people.*

Gilhooly M 1990 Do services delay or prevent institutionalisation of people with dementia? Research Report 4, Dementia Services Development Centre, Stirling University. *A thought-provoking review of research on the effectiveness of community care services in helping people with dementia to stay at home, concluding from the available evidence that they are not effective in this respect.*

Gubrium J 1986 Old timers and Alzheimer's: the descriptive organisation of senility. Jai Press, Greenwich, Connecticut. *A US study which describes the way in which Alzheimer's disease is socially constructed as a pathology rather than part of normal ageing, how it is defined and explained at the level of public culture and at an individual level through, for example, interaction at caregivers' support groups.*

Levin E, Moriarty J, Gorbach P 1994 Better for the break. HMSO, London. *A study of respite services for the carers of confused elderly people in Britain, examining the effects of respite on carers' psychological health, on the elderly people themselves, and on their admission to permanent residential care.*

Moriarty J, Levin E 1993 Services to people with dementia and their carers. In: Burns A (ed) Ageing and dementia: a methodological approach. Edward Arnold, London. *A useful chapter which summarises the range and effectiveness of services available in Britain to people with dementia and their caregivers.*

Twigg J (ed) 1992 Carers: research and practice. HMSO, London. *Whilst not focused on people with a mental health problem, this article has general applicability to the analysis of the caregiving situation. Drawn from a qualitative study of 90 carers and 60 service providers, it describes the kinds of factors – such as the attitudes of carers, the assumptions made by the service providers – which influence whether or not informal carers receive services.*

26

Supporting paid carers

Ian J Norman

There are at least three reasons why we should be concerned with the wellbeing of paid carers of elderly mentally disordered people which go beyond a concern for the workers' welfare alone. First, there is an expectation that paid carers, particularly those who are professionally qualified, demonstrate and promote a healthy lifestyle (Clarke 1991). Second, occupational stress has economic costs which take the form of sickness absence and high levels of staff turnover which disrupt organisational performance (Firth & Britton 1989, Gray-Toft & Anderson 1981). Third, and most important in the context of this chapter, is the contention that occupational stress can lead to deterioriation in work performance, personal relationships and the ability to care for others; thus to poor quality patient care.

The focus of this chapter is the day-to-day paid carers of elderly mentally disordered people, in particular, nurses, health care assistants, residential social workers and home care workers. We look at the nature and sources of stress for these people, at their characteristic coping responses, and at how they can be supported and their performance at work enhanced.

STRESS AND COPING: THEORETICAL AND METHODOLOGICAL CONSIDERATIONS

First we consider the central concepts of stress, burnout and coping and highlight some of the methodological issues involved.

Within the literature on stress in the health care professions there are two distinct, but overlapping, research traditions (Wynne et al 1993). The first is the study of burnout, a term which refers to a particular set of psychological responses to stress associated with working in close contact with other people. Burnout refers to negative changes in work-related attitudes and behaviour (Cherniss 1980). Burnt out care workers are emotionally exhausted, they depersonalise patients (treat patients as objects) and they have difficulty in accomplishing their own personal goals (Maslach & Jackson 1981). Research into burnout emphasises it as an outcome and searches for predictors. For example, Firth and Britton (1989), in a study on care of nurses in long-stay care settings for elderly mentally frail people, found that perceived lack of support and emotional exhaustion were reliable predictors of frequency of sickness absence, reported feelings of depersonalisation and resignation within 2 years.

The second tradition in occupational stress research, which is older than the burnout research, emphasises sources of stress and its multiple outcomes. Here stress has different meanings. It can refer to an *input* variable or agent such as work demands (difficulty, time pressure), environmental factors (sleep loss, noise), or events outside work which impinge on the ability to work. Or it refers to an *output* or effect: the behavioural, subjective and physiological responses produced under strain. These responses are understood as adaptive attempts to cope with the demands of aversive inputs, some of which are temporary pathological alterations (e.g. shock, anxiety) and others are permanent changes (e.g. cardiovascular disease, recurrent depressive episodes).

Both types of meaning present difficulties of definition and measurement, as Dunn and Ritter (1995) explain. A central problem of stress as an input is that factors or events which are accepted as aversive (e.g. loss of a loved one, experience of a road traffic accident) do not affect people in the same way, whether assessed by self-report measures or observation of psychological state. Even events which are seen as agreeable, like winning the National Lottery or job promotion, may be distressing. With stress as an output, accurate physiological measurement may require invasive – and therefore, unacceptable – methods. Furthermore, self-report measures of emotional state, such as depression scales, enable inferences, but not causal links, to be drawn. For example, it is widely held that depression is a consequence of altered physiology but the converse could also be true.

Current theories prefer to perceive stress as a *process* involving a *transaction* between individuals and their environment. Central to transactional theories are the concepts of cognitive appraisal and coping. Dewe et al (1993) identify three main elements in transactional definitions of stress as: a cognitive and dynamic state, an imbalance in normal functioning (homeostasis) and the need for resolution of this imbalance. Thus, stress does not reside in either the individual or the environment but in the perceived interaction between the two. Through cognitive appraisal, individuals represent to themselves:

- an account of the demands which impinge on them and challenge them to adapt or cope
- the incentives for dealing with that demand
- the likely results of dealing with it
- a prediction of what dealing with it is likely to feel like.

Appraisal may change the individual's definition of threats and challenges, possibly through activation of neuroendocrine systems (Dunn & Ritter 1995). Although conceptually researchers now accept the benefits of defining stress as a transaction, this has yet to be translated into empirical measurement (Cox & Ferguson 1991).

The concept of coping usually refers to any response to external life strains (stresses) that prevents, avoids or controls emotional distress (Aldwin & Revenson 1987). So coping serves to solve problems or regulate emotions; the former deals directly with threatening demands and the latter alters the distress that accompanies the threat (Lazarus & Folkman 1984). Coping therefore covers overt and covert actions to reduce psychological distress, is dynamic and specific to the stage and circumstance of the stressful encounter and incorporates failed as well as successful coping efforts; those which lead to physical and psychological disorders following bereavement, for example.

Transactional theories of stress, in which coping is a central factor, tend to see coping as both relational, in that it reflects the relationship between people and their environment, and as a process rather than as an enduring trait or characteristic of individuals (Dewe et al 1993). This conception of coping is criticised by Ritter et al (1995) for ignoring specific information which could be used to make decisions about coping strategies. In transactional theories of stress behavioural, psychological and physiological responses are interdependent and covary. The effect, according to Ritter and her colleagues, is for advice to be given to health care professionals (notably mental health nurses) based on commonsense but simplistic interpretations of the literature; for example, the suggestion by Wright et al (1992) that active coping – readiness to undertake difficult tasks or meet a challenge, for instance – occurs in response to moderately difficult challenges, whereas more difficult challenges do not evoke active coping behaviour.

It is often assumed that coping is an individual

responsibility, but this can lead to 'victim blaming'. There is much evidence to suggest that leaving people to cope with their work stress is not effective in reducing their stress levels nor in managing stress in the workplace (Pearlin & Schooler 1978). What is important is the level of control people perceive themselves to have over the stresses they confront. When control is high individual coping tends to be successful (for example in coping with marital problems), but when control is low (as in many work situations) individual coping strategies are more likely to fail. The implication is that in helping professional carers with their stress organisational support is important, for without it individual coping is unlikely to be successful. We look at coping strategies later in this chapter. The issues outlined above convey the complex dynamics of the stress and coping processes and the danger of making simplistic inferences to guide clinical practice.

STRESS AND SERVICE QUALITY IN ELDERLY CARE SETTINGS

We turn now to consider the relationship between occupational stress and service quality in elderly care settings, a relationship few studies – an exception is Cronin-Stubbs and Brophy (1985) – have investigated directly. However, the effects of occupational stress of staff on patient care can be inferred from research on continuing and long-stay care settings for elderly people carried out since the early 1960s. Virtually all of these describe environments, activities and patterns of care which are undesirable (Norton et al 1962, Clark & Bowling 1989, Tomlin 1989, Age Concern 1990). The concern in most of this research is less with standards of basic physical care, which are often considered satisfactory (RCN 1987), than with aspects of psychosocial care provision. These aspects include lack of attention to individual needs of elderly people and to promoting principles of choice, privacy and dignity (Norman 1987), low levels of patient activity, and staff-patient interaction that is minimal and confined to instrumental needs during direct care provision. Gallagher's (1986) conclusion is that, in spite of 40 years of research in the long-stay care field, standards have not improved.

Elderly patients who are perceived by staff as confused or demented fare even worse than those regarded as lucid. For example, Armstrong-Esther & Browne (1986) found that nurses spent only 10.7% of their time on average interacting with patients and much less time with confused/demented (5.6%) than with lucid patients (15.6%). Patients spent 88.5% of the time sitting and only 9.1% standing or walking. Again the level of inactivity was most pronounced with demented and confused patients. Whereas lucid patients spent 30.5% of the time in purposeful activity (e.g. self care, eating, drinking, craft work, reading), the equivalent figure for confused patients was 18%. This and other hospital studies support Galliard's (1978) conclusion reached over 15 years ago that elderly patients, especially those who are confused, are likely to spend their time sitting doing nothing, and uninterrupted by staff, unless they are active or sufficiently motivated to seek assistance.

Although some studies reveal hospital care staff with high morale and a positive orientation to patients, the dominant picture to emerge from research into continuing and long-stay hospital settings for elderly people is of depressed and demoralised staff whose emotionally challenging work is undervalued by the public and other health care professionals. Moreover, this picture is also found in the literature on residential homes. The low morale of residential social care staff emerged as an important theme in evidence given to the Wagner review (Wagner 1988), and the Howe Report made particular mention of the poor image and status of residential care as a service (Howe 1992, cited in Youll & McCourt-Perring 1993).

Staff behaviours described in this research reflect the syndrome of burnout as described in the occupational stress literature. These findings are also consistent with those described by Menzies in her classic studies of nurses in general hospital wards in the 1950s (Menzies 1960). Her work revealed that close physical care of patients generates complex feelings in carers such as revulsion, problems of coping with intimacy and dependency, fear of failure and lack of competence. Nurses defend themselves from the stress of patient encounters by developing practices and structures to protect them from conflicts and anxieties related to the demands of the job. These practices are manifested in rigid routines, authoritarian staff attitudes, and batch processing rather than individualised treatment regimes.

Menzies' work demonstrates the tendency for all human service systems to develop practices and structures which serve to protect staff. In mental health care settings, in which fear of madness and loss of control are fundamental, the temptation to adopt institutional modes of care delivery that perform a defensive function for staff is particularly seductive. As Clifford et al (1989) point out, institutional modes of care delivery are not confined to hospital and other residential care settings; they also pose a major threat to the quality of the new community-based services.

The implication is that care staff need to be supported in new ways of managing the emotional impact of the work if the aspirations of the community care movement are to be realised.

A recent study of long-stay continuing care wards for elderly mentally disordered people in Scotland (Gilloran et al 1995) has investigated the link between quality of patient care and levels of work satisfaction among staff, a variable often associated with occupational stress. They observed the care activities of feeding, toileting and bathing and took choice, information, conversation, privacy and personal attention as indicators of high quality care. The quality of care was better in wards with more satisfied staff. A key difference between the high and low satisfaction wards was the level of staff-patient interaction during these care activities; in particular, conversing and giving information whilst bathing and toileting were more frequently practised by nurses in the high satisfaction wards. The nurses also respected the patients' privacy more. The authors emphasise conversation between staff and elderly patients as an integral and important part of care in high satisfaction wards. They note that staff looked more comfortable when sitting with patients and talking with them in the high satisfaction than in the low satisfaction wards. Given their conclusion that work satisfaction is associated with high quality care, improving satisfaction of the workforce will benefit patients. Although correlation does not imply causation, this conclusion seems reasonable. Given the negative association between work satisfaction and occupational stress, reducing work stress is likely to impact positively on the quality of patient care.

Burnout or rustout?

Most studies of occupational stress in nursing and other paid care work assume that it takes the form of quantitative or qualitative overload. As applied to care work in long-stay elderly care settings, quantitative overload refers to too much to do, time pressures (even if created by the nurses themselves) and a repetitive daily grind of routine activities. Qualitative overload refers to concern about not doing a job well and the emotional impact of the work, in particular the anxiety generated by close relationships and intimate contact with patients and attempts to respond to their emotional needs.

Our clinical experience suggests that overload in terms of workload and/or emotional demands explains only part of the stress experienced by carers of mentally disordered elderly people. There are, we suggest, similarities between the pressures of low status, unchallenging routinised care work in long-stay elderly care settings and pressures of other types of work, including highly automated work assignments, shift work, routine office work and mass production work. Levi et al (1983) point to the pernicious consequences for workers of these forms of work because they involve quantitative overload, qualitative underload, lack of control and lack of social support. Qualitative underload refers to the unvarying content of work – mainly physical care routines – and little social interaction with patients because of difficulty in communicating and forming relationships with them. This contrasts with other areas of health care, perhaps terminal care or acute psychiatric care, which typically generate qualitative overload in the form of deep emotional involvement with patients over time.

Lack of control is evident in the research on hospital care of elderly people referred to earlier. For example, Evers (1981a, b) found that individualised care of elderly patients who require continuing care depends on whether the ward sister takes account of patients' individuality when organising work, and whether both sister and consultant see 'care work' as being as valid as 'cure work'. Ward sisters who organise care on a patient-centred basis and create individualised long-stay 'careers' for patients, were to be found where doctors specified care work as valid and valuable. Evers attributes low quality long-term care of elderly patients to medical control of care work and the resulting dominance of cure over care work. Nurses can similarly be instrumental in reducing the quality of care work if they leave it to their assistants but give them little support. Nurses who retreat into administrative and office work as a means of coping and leave care assistants, who have no formal qualifications and little training, to do the care work unsupervised and unsupported epitomise this kind of control (see for example, Wells 1980). Lack of support can include non-work pressures and lack of organisational and personal support in the form of social and professional networks as well as negative attitudes of other professionals and of society about the worth, skill and knowledge base of elderly care.

The ideas expressed here resonate with those discussed by Nolan & Grant (1993) who refer to Pennington & Pierce's (1985) concept of 'rustout' in seeking to explain the poor quality of care in long-stay settings for elderly people. Rustout, which affects nurses working in unchallenging environments, is contrasted to the more commonly reported burnout. Burnout results from stress whereas rustout stems from tedium and lack of stimulation (Nolan & Grant

1993). However, the notion of imbalance in normal functioning and the desire to return to homeostasis which are central to transactional theories of stress (Dewe et al 1993), support the view that both burnout and rustout are outcomes of a stress process, although the causes of the stress are different. This view is supported by Pines et al (1981) who propose that burnout symptoms can develop either through emotional involvement with patients over time or through a heavy and tedious workload. Firth et al (1987) support this in suggesting that rustout is similar to 'professional depression', a process identified by Oswin (1978) as affecting nurses in long-stay mental handicap hospitals. So, in burnout, isolation and emotional detachment occur in an attempt to escape the agony of over stimulation and high stress whereas in rustout, or professional depression, isolation and emotional detachment occur to escape the tedium of under stimulation. Thus rustout and burnout have similar features – isolation and emotional detachment – but they have different causes.

In this section we have suggested that the work environment of many long-stay care settings for elderly people may have pernicious consequences for direct care workers because they exhibit Levi et al's (1983) four features of:

- quantitative overload
- qualitative underload
- lack of control
- lack of social support.

Empirical support for this comes from the Scottish study of work satisfaction and quality of care in wards for elderly mentally ill people (Gilloran et al 1994). This study involved a survey of direct care staff drawn from a stratified sample of 121 wards in 39 NHS hospitals. Staff nurses were significantly less satisfied than other nursing grades, mainly because of their experience of the work itself. The staff nurses complained that they were not being stretched to their full potential (qualitative underload) and that they had no control over the pace of work (lack of control). The tedious nature of work in these wards was revealed in the 82% of staff who agreed with the statement that 'each day it's the same old routine' (qualitative underload).

We do not want to imply that the nature of daily caring work with elderly mentally disordered people is intrinsically tedious; it can be quite the reverse. But this work is unlikely to be satisfying for carers unless Levi et al's four features are overcome. These features are reflected in the two other components of work satisfaction, in addition to the experience of the work

itself, found by Gilloran's group: the quality of supervision and of hospital management.

With respect to clinical supervision, staff nurses were more reluctant than other nursing staff to identify their charge nurses as good leaders. They were particularly critical of the charge nurses' capacity to promote innovation and they reported feeling frustrated in their own attempts to introduce change into the ward. In fact many nurses were critical of their supervision. For example, a third of all the staff did not think that their opinions were listened to, over a half thought that the charge nurse showed favouritism, and three-fifths reported that the charge nurse did not give them positive feedback. Staff nurses were also markedly less satisfied with other aspects of hospital management; specifically with laundry and catering facilities and with the practice of 'lending' staff to other wards. Over three-quarters of all the nurses were dissatisfied with this practice.

As the authors point out, staff nurses occupy an important position in wards for elderly mentally frail people, transmitting knowledge and ideas and as role models for junior staff and students. In view of this, they are perhaps more likely to feel frustrated and inhibited at work than other nursing grades, so accounting for their significantly lower level of satisfaction. It is interesting, however, that staff nurses who were satisfied with their job in general were still significantly more negative about the charge nurse and their own ability to introduce change than were satisfied staff in other nursing grades. Thus the charge nurse's leadership ability and nurses' opportunity to introduce changes into practice do not by themselves account for work satisfaction. Perhaps not surprisingly, a significantly greater number of dissatisfied than satisfied staff nurses did not want to be assigned to a ward for the elderly mentally ill and this trend occurred for all nursing grades. Thus commitment to the specialty seems to be important in explaining work satisfaction, although whether working in the specialty promotes commitment in previously uncommitted staff or knocks commitment out of them is not clear.

In sum, the Scottish study indicates that the association between work satisfaction on the one hand and factors such as staff supervision, management policies, experience of work and commitment to caring for elderly mentally frail people on the other is complex. If some nurses say they are satisfied with their work even when stressful features of the working environment persist – quantitative overload, qualitative underload, lack of control and lack of support, for example – then it is clear that individual differences in work experience play a major role. That is to say, one nurse's stress does indeed seem to be another nurse's challenge. The clear implication for supporting professional carers is that a multidimensional approach is required which addresses managerial and organisational factors as well as individual concerns.

LEVELS OF WORK STRESS IN ELDERLY CARE SETTINGS

Macpherson et al (1994) point out that, given the high stress levels in informal carers of elderly people with mental health problems, particularly those with dementia, and the complex relationships between stress and factors such as severity of dementia and levels of problem behaviour (Morris et al 1988), it follows that carers who work in institutions for elderly mentally ill people will also experience high stress levels. It is the care workers in long-stay residential units with the most demanding and disturbed patients who are likely to experience high stress. This line of argument seems reasonable, although it assumes underlying stress as quantitative overload, whereas stress in long-stay settings may more likely be associated with qualitative underload. It is possible that care workers experience high work stress in long-stay settings where docile residents sit comfortably doing nothing, as well as in settings where residents are demanding.

The empirical evidence confirming these assumptions is sparse. A consistent finding in the occupational stress literature is that nurses who look after older people experience low levels of work satisfaction compared to nurses in other specialties. This is often attributed to the low status of the specialty and the fact that they are working with people who usually get worse. This finding is supported by a survey of Irish nurses, by Wynne et al (1993), who found nurses in elderly care wards to be less intrinsically satisfied with their work than nurses in all other specialties surveyed; nurses in wards for the elderly mentally ill were not singled out. Nurses working in accident and emergency departments and medical and surgical wards reported experiencing stress more often than nurses in other specialties. However, this survey, as with Macpherson et al's (1994), drew upon the over stimulation (quantitative overload) model of occupational stress which may be too restrictive for long-stay care settings.

Most studies of stress in care workers have avoided elderly care settings of all types, preferring to focus on acute care environments. Nursing research, in particular, has been mainly concerned with coronary and intensive care units, the hypothesis being that stress is greater in these units because of the 'high-tech' nature of the work. There are few studies which have compared levels of staff stress in elderly care settings with other nursing specialties.

One of these (Hipwell et al 1989) compared stress in an elderly care ward with a coronary care unit, a renal unit and a general medical ward in Birmingham, UK and found the similarities between the specialties more striking than the differences. Dealing with death and dying was most stressful for nurses in the coronary care and renal units, and work overload was reported as a major stressor in the medical and elderly care wards. The fact that the elderly care ward catered for acutely ill rather than long-stay patients, may explain why work (quantitative) overload was identified as a stressor, rather than qualitative underload which may be a more common source of stress in long-stay elderly care settings.

In social work there is a similar assumption that work stress is higher in acute care specialties. This is supported by a national survey of 1196 North American gerontological social workers, using Maslach and Jackson's (1981) Burnout Inventory, which found lower levels of burnout among this group than among social workers in child health, public welfare and mental health. Whether care of mentally ill old people was covered by gerontological or mental health social workers is not clear. However, 26% of the gerontological social workers had high emotional exhaustion scores and 34% had moderate scores, which indicates considerable distress. Other research also demonstrates high stress. Greene (1986) found gerontological social workers experienced higher levels of death anxiety than other social workers, and Carrilio and Eisenberg (1984) found that working with elderly clients constantly reminded social workers that they too may end up alone, sick and vulnerable.

A few studies have sought to establish rates of staff stress in care settings for elderly physically and mentally frail people but many of these suffer from methodological shortcomings which make it difficult to assess the validity of the findings. Benjamin and Spector's (1990) study of stress in nursing staff in three wards for elderly mentally ill people in Hertfordshire, UK demonstrates a high level of stress symptoms although there was an element of selection bias and no clear definition of stress 'caseness' (the likelihood of an emotional disorder being so severe that the worker would be expected to seek psychiatric help).

Another study to report high levels of stress symptoms or outcomes was a survey of 142 nursing staff (nurses and care assistants, both full- and part-time) working in 10 wards for elderly mentally frail people in north east England (Norfolk & Stirton 1987). The staff reported feelings of stress (63%), tension (63%), long periods of tiredness (63%), periods of depression (41%), anxiety (33%) and lack of interest in the work (51%). 23% (all women) reported currently receiving treatment from a doctor and, of those feeling under stress, 73% considered problems at work to be the main contributory factor. This contrasts with the 23% who blamed problems at home principally. These findings give cause for concern but should not be generalised to other similar wards. The authors did not select a random, representative sample of wards (the 10 wards were chosen because they had received the most complaints) and the study was commissioned by the National Union of Public Employees. It seems likely, therefore, that the problems in these wards stemmed from local difficulties rather than from universal characteristics of wards of this kind.

In contrast to the work by Benjamin & Spector (1990) and Norfolk & Stirton (1987), Macpherson et al (1994) report low rates of 'caseness' as assessed with the General Health Questionnaire (Goldberg 1978) using the CGHQ scoring scheme (Goodchild & Duncan-Jones 1985), for nursing staff working in 16 elderly care units in Bristol when compared with a representative UK community sample. The findings of this study are reasonably generalisable because the Bristol units were selected randomly and represented elderly care institutions comprising long-stay wards, private nursing homes, residential homes for the elderly and homes for elderly mentally infirm people. However, the mean response rate, whilst respectable at 67.4%, raises the question of whether a vulnerable group of non-responders was missed. This is acknowledged by the authors who point in particular to the lowest rate of caseness being for staff in one elderly persons' home in which there were also high rates of long-term sickness. It seems possible that the most stressed staff did not respond.

The Macpherson study supports Ritter et al's (1995) observation, made in relation to research on stress in psychiatric nurses, that incomplete data sets resulting from non-response is a consistent feature of the stress and coping literature. Ritter et al's observation is also relevant to more specific elderly care studies and provides one explanation for lower than expected rates of stress amongst direct care workers. A study of stress in staff of elderly care nursing homes by Dunn et al (1994) – in which Ritter was a co-investigator – achieved only a 30% mean response rate and Poulin and Walter's (1993) survey of gerontological social workers reached a mean response rate of 61.5%. The

loss of, at best, over a third of respondents questions whether the most vulnerable workers are missed in the study of occupational stress.

Reluctance to participate in research studies may in itself be evidence of a coping style in which denial and repression are dominant features (Ritter et al 1995). Support for this hypothesis comes from a study of stress amongst paid home carers of elderly people by Bartoldus et al (1989) who investigated self-perceptions of stress and coping of 32 home care workers in New York. Using the Tedium Scale (Pines et al 1981), scores indicated little reported stress but in group interviews the respondents revealed many more stresses in their lives.

In summary, stress seems to be a significant problem for care workers in elderly residential care settings and those who work with elderly people at home. Whether these levels are similar to worker stress in other specialties is uncertain. It seems likely, though, that research studies underestimate rates of stress amongst paid workers who care for elderly people because of the high rates of non-response as a result of which the most vulnerable workers may be missed.

SOURCES OF STRESS IN CARE SETTINGS FOR ELDERLY MENTALLY FRAIL PEOPLE

Most stresses experienced by paid care workers of elderly people are not major events and disasters but take the form of frequently occurring irritations and hassles which Lazarus & de Longis (1983) suggest are the better predictors of psychological symptoms and somatic distress. Major sources of stress in care settings for elderly mentally frail people arise from organisational factors, patient demands and individual characteristics and circumstances (e.g. personality characteristics, responsibilities and home pressures).

Organisational factors

Organisational climate, supervisory style and work group relations have been identified as important psychosocial influences in all health care settings (e.g. Gray-Toft & Anderson 1985). Organisational climate refers here to conditions created by management which influence the work environment. It has been shown to influence job satisfaction and role perceptions (Dewe 1987, Revicki & May 1989) and to be a major source of stress (OPCS 1978, cited in Harris 1989). Dunn and Ritter (1995), in their review of the psychiatric nursing stress literature, point out that nurses' perceptions of their work organisation are almost universally negative. For example, Sullivan's (1993) study of staff in acute psychiatric wards identified poor and minimal communication, lack of consultation and constant organisational change as major stressors for nurses. Dawkins et al (1985) found that all the top 10 stressors identified by their sample of 43 psychiatric nurses referred to administrative and organisational factors.

A number of nursing studies have singled out difficulties in nurse relationships with peers or the head nurse as a major source of stress experienced by staff nurses. Trygstad's (1986) study of 22 registered psychiatric nurses working in nine units found that staff relationships accounted for one-third of all stressors identified and problems between unit staff and head nurses for a further 17% of stressors. Similarly Dawkins et al (1985) found a fifth of job stresses were related to work group conflicts. Particular problems identified by these studies include inadequate or ineffective communication, infighting between individuals and groups, working with poorly motivated staff, working with staff who resist new ideas and having others take credit for their ideas or hard work.

The behaviour of supervisors has been found to exert a particularly significant impact on work group relations, and the satisfaction, motivation and performance of staff. Nursing studies show that work environments in which nursing supervisors enable open expression of views and collaborative problem solving are associated with increased job satisfaction, lower levels of absenteeism and reduced experience of role conflict and ambiguity (Gray-Toft & Anderson 1985, Revicki & May 1989). Participation in decision making and two-way communication between supervisor and supervised is also associated with lower levels of interpersonal conflict and hostility and more cooperative relationships in the staff group (Oaklander & Fleishman 1964). These findings are consistent with the results of the Scottish study of wards for elderly mentally infirm people discussed earlier (Gilloran et al 1994) in which quality of supervision was found to be an important component of work satisfaction.

The research studies discussed above in relation to organisational factors are drawn from nursing and not all are specific to the care of elderly people. However, clinical experience suggests that in long-term elderly care work, in particular the care of elderly mentally infirm people, the impact of negative organisational factors may be exacerbated by the low status of the work and the progressive nature of many conditions. These features can lead to difficulties in recruiting high

calibre staff and establishing a culture to support the provision of high quality care. In care settings in which relationships between carers and patients are distant or are disrupted by communication difficulties, organisational factors have an increasingly important impact on the morale and commitment of care staff. Domus units, which are residential units developed for mentally frail people, have gone a long way to solving these problems (Lindesay et al 1991). These units regard the needs of the staff as being as important as the residents' needs and priority is put on adequate staffing levels, staff training and support (see Ch. 27 for further discussion).

Patient demands

Patients exert demands on care workers in all settings but the nature of these is likely to vary according to client group and care setting. The study of home care workers for elderly people in New York by Bartolus et al (1989), although not specific to clients with mental health problems, highlights the stressful nature of providing services for elderly people living at home. These workers carried out shopping, laundry and housecleaning duties and some also performed personal care tasks such as bathing and hairdressing. However, many reported carrying out affective tasks too; for example, talking with clients about the clients' problems, holding their hands, and massaging their necks.

Of the instrumental tasks performed, shopping was seen as the most difficult. The workers commented on the stressful nature not only of the task itself, but also the associated interactions with clients on issues such as what to buy, how much to pay and money given and change returned. However, affective and relational aspects of the job were considered more stressful than instrumental tasks. Workers described finding it difficult to refuse clients who made inappropriate or excessive requests for services which went well beyond the worker's job description (e.g. washing windows, bathing pets, shampooing large rugs) particularly if they felt they had a good relationship with the old person. These requests made the workers feel that they were treated like servants and were not respected. Workers also described the stress they felt when elderly clients followed them around the house checking on their work and also of being suspected of stealing. One worker described how a client used to check her shopping bag every day before she left the house.

Depressed elderly people were singled out as being

particularly stressful to be with. Workers described how these clients wept about their physical problems, their loneliness and their children and this made the worker feel sad and uncomfortable. Moreover, workers were often the focus of anger and hostility felt towards family members, from clients who were unable to express it directly. Some workers described feeling emotionally drained by these experiences. Others described feeling burdened by family secrets which were revealed to them in confidence and by being asked for financial and medical advice, which they felt ill prepared to give, but to which they felt obliged to respond.

The stresses of dementia care

Dementing patients present particular demands and challenges to care workers and these have been the subject of several research studies, particularly in Sweden. Hallberg and Norberg (1993) examined nurses' views of the characteristics of severely demented patients, the difficulties created by them and the emotional reactions evoked by them in giving daily care. Data collection methods included completion of two instruments developed as part of the study, the Strain in Nursing Care Scale and the Emotional Reactions in Nursing Care Scale by staff who were drawn from two wards in a psychogeriatric clinic in Sweden. Agitated behaviour, being unresponsive and unruly behaviour were identified as the most common characteristics of dementing patients confronting care staff. However, the most difficult problems to handle in providing care were 'emptiness' (including submissive behaviours, leading a meaningless life, being on the verge of death and being unpredictable), 'agony' (including being disorderly, anguished, aggressive and seeming to feel abandoned) and 'wilfulness' (patients demonstrating a will of their own and contradicting the nurse's wishes).

In another Swedish study, Åström et al (1991) looked at the relationship between the experience of burnout (and tedium), empathy and attitudes towards dementing patients of 60 nurses (registered and licensed practical) and aides working in wards for physically and mentally frail elderly people. Data collection methods included semi-structured interviews with the staff and completion of LaMonica's Empathy Construct Scale (LaMonica 1981) and Pines et al's (1981) Burnout Scale. Correlation analysis showed that high burnout was associated with low empathy and less positive attitudes of the staff. This supports other research which has shown that burnout

has a negative effect on attitudes (Maslach 1982) and is related to decreased empathy (Pines et al 1981).

More surprising is that the nurses' aides and licensed practical nurses in the Åström study were at higher risk of burnout and had less positive attitudes towards patients and lower empathy scores than registered nurses. The inverse relationship between risk of burnout and grade of staff member contrasts with most other studies of nurse stress. For example, Wynne et al (1993) note that Guppy and Gutteridge (1990) found that nursing auxiliaries reported far less stress than nurses, and charge nurses and that ward sisters were the most stressed. In their own survey, though, Wynne et al found that students reported the most stress. Åström et al hypothesise that the higher risk of burnout of less qualified nurses in establishments for dementing patients is a result of greater exposure than registered nurses to the patients' behavioural disturbances and communication difficulties. Lengthy daily exposure to these behaviours raises what the authors call ethical conflicts, by which they seem to mean ambivalent feelings staff had towards the patients which left the staff with negative attitudes. This interpretation is supported by another Swedish study which found that vocally disruptive dementing patients present a conflict for care workers in that they want to help yet feel powerless, sometimes hatred towards the old person and that their care is meaningless (Hallberg & Norberg 1990).

Regression analysis of Åström et al's data showed that experience of feedback of performance at work and length of time in the job were the most important predictors of staff burnout. The authors suggest that staff who are empathetic and deeply involved with patients may increase their risk of burnout, particularly if they have worked with demented people for many years. The relationship between empathy and burnout seems, from the Åström study, to be complex. They found that high burnout was associated with low empathy yet they also suggest that staff are at risk of burnout if they have worked with demented people for a long time and are empathetic and committed to them. Disentangling cause and effect is the difficulty with research of this kind and other variables, like job tenure, grade of nurse, involvement in the job and feedback of performance, might moderate the empathy–burnout relationship.

Interestingly, the staff with lowest empathy reported improvement in the patients' condition as the most important stimulating factor at work, whereas those with high empathy scores identified close contact with the patient as the most important factor. This finding supports the two possible burnout pathways described earlier: whereas high empathy staff may be at risk of burnout through close involvement with patients, low empathy staff may be at risk because of lack of positive health outcomes of patients. This hypothesis is supported by Babb's (1994) study of nurses working in elderly care wards which found that caring for dementing patients was stressful for some nurses because it contradicts their image of their professional role. Others, though, had found ways of accepting the challenges posed by dementing patients and had come to enjoy the physical and emotional demands of the work.

The complexity of the relationship between the patients' demands and stress in care workers is illustrated in the UK study by Benjamin and Spector (1990) of three residential facilities for dementing people: a short-stay ward in a general hospital, a long-stay ward in a psychiatric hospital, and a bungalow. A questionnaire, administered as an interview, identified stressful events for the staff which related to one of three categories: resident-related (behaviours of residents which may affect the worker's ability to cope); facility-related (aspects of the work environment); and self-related (personal characteristics which may influence how well a person copes at work). Staff were asked to identify events that they had experienced and to rank them for stressfulness.

Benjamin and Spector found that more staff in the bungalow than the hospital wards reported resident-related behaviours as stressful, in particular residents being unresponsive and incomprehensible in their attempts to communicate. The authors put this down to the underlying value system of the bungalow staff which was to encourage emotional expression by residents. Also to previous research which has found that nursing home staff feel they are better able to alleviate the physical discomfort of residents than to change their affective state (Kane et al 1986). Benjamin and Spector argue that the bungalow staff, who were less well qualified than the hospital staff, were less likely to have much success in improving the affective state of residents. The nurses in the hospital wards were specialists in meeting the physical needs of residents and had the satisfaction of administering drugs that would help the residents' physical condition. The values underpinning the mode of work organisation in the wards was more in line with the nurses' skills than was the case for staff in the bungalow. It is not surprising then, that the impoverished resources (lack of skills and drugs) available to the bungalow staff left them feeling more stressed.

In contrast to staff in the bungalow, those in the short-term ward were much more likely to attribute stress to the organisation rather than to residents' behaviour, even though the cognitive impairment and physical disability of the residents in both facilities were similar. Benjamin and Spector suggest that this may be because the bungalow staff had high expectations of developing long-term relationships with residents which was not so for the short-term ward staff. It seems possible that the sources of stress for staff in the bungalow may be similar to those experienced by informal carers who look after their elderly relatives at home (see Ch. 25 for information on care at home).

The level of functioning of residents in Benjamin and Spector's study may also be an important influence on perceptions of stress by staff. In the long-stay ward, in which residents had lower behavioural and cognitive function and higher levels of physical disability, few staff attributed stress to residents being unresponsive, but many identified attempts by the resident to communicate as stressful. Benjamin and Spector put forward the hypothesis that severe cognitive and physical disabilities in residents decrease the expectations staff have for a meaningful relationship and so reduce the stress attributed to residents' behaviour; the staff do not attempt to develop a relationship because they know it would not succeed. In contrast, lower levels of disability may increase expectations of staff and raise their stress when a meaningful relationship does not emerge. However, these relationships are complex in that elderly residents' level of functioning may be improved by interpersonal stimulation, so highlighting the interplay between cognitive function and type of care.

The bungalow catered for only eight residents whereas the short-term and long-stay wards housed 23 patients (including 15 day patients) and 21 patients respectively. It is probably easier to provide individualised and personalised care in small residential facilities (Norman 1987). Holden and Woods (1982) cite a number of studies which report positive correlations between small living units and residents who are vocal, active, not too disoriented nor incontinent. Benjamin and Spector do not discuss the effects of unit size on staff perceptions of stress although, with just eight residents, it seems possible that the expectations of the bungalow staff of their residents' abilities was higher than might have been the case.

Self-related events were less likely than resident-related and facility-related factors to be identified as sources of stress by the staff in all three settings. This suggests that care staff may not be aware of the possible influence of their personal attributes on their ability to relate to and cope with the demands of dementing people.

Interestingly, the staff in the hospital wards were nurses (qualified) whilst the bungalow was staffed by care workers who had experience but no nursing or social work qualifications; the possible effects of training on the results of this study are not discussed by the authors. But, in a later study, Benjamin (1991) compared ratings of the frequency of stressful events experienced by nursing staff in two traditional long-stay care wards for elderly people and a newly adapted unit with no nurses. No significant differences were found between the three settings. The more senior staff, from staff nurse to manager, experienced the greatest number of stressful events. However, it is uncertain how far a count of stressful events is a valid indicator of the degree of stress experienced. It is the perception of stressful situations that is important (Dewe 1989).

The stressful characteristics of dementing patients found by Benjamin's group are supported by a series of studies of nurses working in wards for elderly physically and mentally frail people which also reveal the stresses of working in poor quality care environments (Wallis 1986, reported in Jones 1987). Nurses working in these wards reported contact with psychotic and dementing patients to be a major source of frustration and saw the problem as intractable. Incontinence was regarded as endemic in these wards and nurses described the stress of having to deal with unpredictable behaviour, ranging from virtual withdrawal to violent outbursts. The long-term nature of care and lack of improvement in patients' abilities were other sources of stress. Many patients had been in the wards for more than a decade and few were expected to leave alive. Thus, unlike most other patients who improve or remain in a stable state, nurses in these wards saw these patients following a relentless path of slow deterioration. The nurses had no option but to cope with inevitable death of their patients and with ethical issues about quality of life as best they could. They also reported working long hours caring for large numbers of patients – up to 30 in each ward – in drab and sparsely equipped surroundings. Any empathy they might have had for the patients disappeared long ago, it seems.

In sum, the studies of stress of staff who look after dementing people demonstrate the complexity of relationships between stress, staff characteristics, client functioning and type of care facility. A number of behaviours and demands of dementing people have been identified as potential stressors. These are influenced by the actions of staff who can, for example, reduce a resident's level of functioning by reinforcing dependent behaviours and ignoring independent behaviours (Bond & Bond 1987). For this reason dementing behaviours are best conceived as the outcomes of interactions between the dementing person and care staff.

The research reviewed here suggests two pathways to worker stress in which quantitative overload, qualitative overload and qualitative underload are implicated. One pathway indicates that stress is generated in workers by interpersonal relationship demands from less cognitively impaired and less physically dependent residents (qualitative overload). The other pathway suggests that boredom, tedium and the absence of rewarding interpersonal relationships with clients (qualitative underload) are the major stresses. It is this second pathway that seems to be the greater problem for staff in continuing care. The evidence is contradictory on which grade of staff is most prone to stress. Some studies have shown staff in positions of responsibility to be under the most stress whereas others have reported higher stress in care assistants who do the direct care work.

Individual characteristics and circumstances

'The only certainty is that different individuals will differ in the precise nature and severity of the symptoms and reactions they produce' (Shouksmith & Wallis 1988, p. 52). That is to say, individuals respond differently to potential stressors because one person's personality characteristics and situational variables are different to another's. These individual differences moderate the effect of a stressor on a person's health and wellbeing. As Shouksmith and Wallis go on to say, ' ... some moderating variables can nullify undesirable effects, others may operate to aggravate what would otherwise be only mild reactions' (p. 52). The major individual differences that affect reactions to job demands fall into the following categories:

- demographic factors
- personality variables
- coping strategies
- work expectations, preferences and commitment
- health-related factors, like smoking, drinking alcohol and exercise
- abilities and skills, including job, organisational and social skills (Parkes 1994).

Personality variables

In this section we are concerned mainly with personality variables. The personality characteristics that can moderate reactions to stress at work are the 'Type A' personality, neuroticism, locus of control, hardiness and optimism. These are the most powerful moderators of the relation between work stress and health outcomes (Parkes 1994).

People with the Type A personality are obsessional, emotionally charged workaholics. As Parkes (1994, p. 115) puts it: 'Type A behaviour is characterised by impatience, hostility, irritability, job involvement, competitiveness and achievement striving'. Type A nurses report higher stress from work overload, time pressures and role conflict, and have a higher blood cholesterol level and systolic blood pressure than nurses with the more easy-going Type B personality (Ivancevich et al 1982, cited by Wynne et al 1993). Another common personality factor that can increase stress is being susceptible to 'cognitive failure', or momentary lapses of concentration and memory (Shouksmith & Wallis 1988) – not to be confused with the true cognitive failure of dementia.

Shouksmith and Wallis describe a study by Walker (1986) of psychiatric nurses and students in a UK hospital which showed how internal personality factors and external situational variables can moderate people's response to stress so that it is difficult to establish how stressful a known stressor is. Walker reported only moderate levels of stress reactions by the nurses – measured by sickness absence from work and General Health Questionnaire scores – even though the amount and type of dissatisfactions, frustrations and weaknesses of managerial practices were considered to be high. Walker argued that moderating variables were masking the full picture and that more detailed analysis would show significant differences in stress levels. This turned out to be so. When the respondents were separated into psychiatric nurse and student subgroups, the stress level amongst the experienced nurses was much lower than for the students, and the range of individual differences was wide. Walker explained this finding by arguing that, rather than being less vulnerable to stress, the experienced nurses were less likely than the students to recognise or admit to psychiatric symptoms in themselves because of their daily exposure to severely disordered patients and their self-image of being psychologically well balanced.

The so-called unstable, or neurotic, personality can increase vulnerability to stress. Research has shown that about 25% of the variance in perceived stress and stress reactions is related to an anxious, i.e. neurotic, personality (Shouksmith & Wallis 1988). This is supported by research that shows that nurses high on trait anxiety experience high stress (Gray-Toft & Anderson 1981). Neuroticism reflects ' ... emotional vulnerability, pessimism and a general tendency to react negatively to life and work stressors' (Parkes 1994, p. 116).

Shouksmith and Wallis wonder whether prolonged exposure to nursing induces a more unstable personality, so making the effect of occupational stressors on nurses more serious than might be the case for other professions. This hypothesis would need to be tested when holding length of experience as a nurse constant. It would also be important to hold perceived control at work constant if, as we have seen, this reduces the stress even in highly demanding jobs. Perceived control is a situational factor that can mitigate high stress. Highly demanding work is not so stressful when workers are able to exercise discretion in how they do the job. That is to say, the job is not tightly controlled, closely supervised and constrained. If responses such as feelings of tension, frustration and powerlessness continue over many years, as Firth-Cozens (1988) found with medical students and junior doctors, then a sense of learned helplessness can result and, perhaps, depression later on. Burnout is the likely unintended consequence. Burnt-out staff in long-stay nursing tend to direct anger inwards and to avoid problems and decision-making (Firth et al 1987).

WHAT CAN BE DONE ABOUT STRESS?

Coping strategies

Parkes' (1994) review of the literature on personality and coping as moderators of work stress reports significant correlations between personality variables and coping strategies. For example, internal locus of control and Type A behaviour are associated with active coping, forward planning and problem-solving strategies. People who are high on extraversion and low on neuroticism use coping strategies judged to be more effective than those used by neurotic introverts. Parkes argues that coping style may be a stronger predictor of health outcomes than personality because coping is integral to stress management.

'Coping' in the occupational stress literature includes adaptive and maladaptive strategies; it does not refer only to positive responses which common-sense understanding of the term would imply. Categories of coping include problem solving, positive reappraisal, seeking emotional or instrumental support, acceptance or resignation, avoidance and expressing emotions (Parkes 1994). The larger the number of strategies in a person's coping repertoire the more effective the coping response is likely to be, although a hugely versatile repertoire might become counterproductive. Research into the association between stressors and personality and coping is complicated by interactive effects of demographic factors (e.g. age, gender, job level) and other psychosocial variables. The moderating effects of the many possible variables on a stress response can form a complex web that requires sophisticated methodological techniques to disentangle. For example, work overload and a Type A personality might interact to predict extreme distress only if social supports at work and at home are low (Parkes 1994).

Stress management programmes

Introducing a stress management programme of some kind is a commonly used active coping strategy. Techniques that can help reduce work stress of psychiatric nurses and other care workers include relaxation, distraction, exercise, changing shift patterns, social support and reduction in smoking, alcohol consumption and illicit drug use (Ritter et al 1995). Ritter and her colleagues reviewed the literature on coping with stress in psychiatric and mental health nursing. They report that relaxation techniques are helpful in the short term but may be more effective if used in conjunction with other coping strategies. Distracting the mind from the stressful incident by concentrating hard for a few minutes on something else can be an effective short-term strategy in that it clears the mind in preparation for other thoughts. Exercise, especially aerobic exercise, is known to reduce certain stress-related health problems and has been introduced in industrial companies to help the workforce. We are not aware of any health and social care settings following suit.

Shiftwork

Ritter et al describe three interventions that can help reduce stress from shiftwork.

1. The first rotates morning, evening and night shifts rapidly to minimise the adjustment required to workers' circadian rhythms.
2. The second allows workers to choose the shifts they prefer so that early rising 'larks' work morning shifts and late night 'owls' work late shifts.

3. The third stabilises eating and sleeping times within irregular shift patterns so that circadian rhythms are disrupted as little as possible.

Shifts in psychiatric hospitals are traditionally long and often exclude paid time off for meal breaks.

Individual and supervisory strategies

Burnout in mental health work settings can be prevented or reduced by implementing individual and supervisory strategies. Effective individual strategies based on reality therapy principles help employees work within the organisation and include problem solving, personal and career development and relaxation. Supervisory strategies include in-service training and staff development, job rotation, morale boosting and seminars on stress and burnout (see Ritter et al's 1995 review). Staff support groups have benefited mental health nurses in that they are successful in helping nurses to improve staff relationships, cope with challenges, increase their sense of control, provide support to each other and encourage teamwork (Ritter et al 1995). What is not explained, however, is the activity within these groups that makes them beneficial. As Ritter et al (1995, p. 169) say: 'Most mental health units tend to put a group of staff into a room once a week and expect them to get on with it'.

Social support intervention

Ritter et al (1995) proceeded to evaluate a social support intervention with 25 psychiatric nurses in a hospital setting. Seven of the nurses were exposed to the intervention and 18 acted as controls. The baseline levels of stress and emotional exhaustion (measured with the General Health Questionnaire and Maslach's Burnout Inventory) were high in the intervention group and decreased after the intervention whereas the scores for the controls remained much the same. Most striking was the reduction in GHQ scores for the nurses whose scores indicated 'caseness'. The intervention consisted of a social support programme which involves six 3-hour sessions run over 3 weeks. The sessions cover:

1. understanding the concept of social support
2. drawing illustrative graphs of participants' life satisfaction
3. rating and ranking their roles in life
4. mapping their support networks
5. understanding social awareness and popularity

6. setting goals for developing their own social networks.

The authors conclude that the social support programme was successful in reducing the nurses' work stress and burnout and increasing their ability to relate to and empathise with patients. The implication is that social support ensures a high standard of care as well as professional survival.

Smoking and alcohol

Smoking continues to be widespread in mental health care settings and nurses also admit to using alcohol and drugs to alleviate stress. But exposure to cigarette smoke and alcohol is thought to contribute to stress and ageing because of the damage they do to body cells (Ritter et al 1995).

Social support, time management and other strategies

Nurses' perceived stress levels are higher than their stress reactions (Shouksmith & Wallis 1988). These authors report different coping strategies by nurses in their response to stress at work. Some keep an emotional distance or aloofness from patients which can harden them in their efforts to protect themselves from the effects of illness and misery around them. Others find humour a good antidote to stress. Most important is the presence of strong support networks among colleagues and family and friends outside work.

The Claybury study of stress and coping compared 323 ward-based psychiatric nurses from seven psychiatric hospitals and psychiatric wards in district general hospitals in the North East Thames Region of England with 250 community psychiatric nurses (CPNs) from the same region (Leary & Brown 1995). The nurses completed the Coping Skills Questionnaire (Cooper et al 1988) which covers six subscales:

- social support from others
- task strategies used to reorganise work
- the use of a logical and rational approach to work
- the interaction between home and work relationships
- time management strategies used
- involvement in and commitment to work.

The coping strategies used on average most often by both groups were reorganising their tasks and committing themselves more deeply to the work. The use of time management strategies was successful in reducing the level of emotional exhaustion (measured with the General Health Questionnaire and the Maslach Burnout Inventory) for the CPNs but was not significant for the ward nurses. Another difference between the groups was the value of task reorganisation strategies in coping with emotional exhaustion. There was no association for the ward nurses but a significant one for the CPNs; reorganising their work tasks was associated with less exhaustion. As the authors explain, efficient use of time and task reorganisation strategies are more important in reducing stress for CPNs who work largely alone and autonomously than for ward nurses who can rely on help from the ward team and benefit from established work practices and structures. The coping strategy that most effectively reduced the ward nurses' level of emotional exhaustion was social support, from professional and personal sources. Discussing work-related problems with colleagues at work to relieve stress was a strategy used by most of the nurses in both groups (89% of the ward nurses and 93% of the CPNs).

A study in Winnipeg, Manitoba, Canada evaluated the effect of social support at work and at home on work stress and burnout of nursing assistants working in long-term residential care homes for senior citizens. 26 homes participated and 10 nursing assistants were randomly selected from each home; 245 were interviewed, 93% of whom were women. The outcome measures used included burden, burnout and job pressure (Chappell & Novak 1992). The findings indicated that the most effective strategy in reducing work-related stress of nursing assistants is for home managers to introduce training in how to work with cognitively impaired old people, to reduce or change the workload and to increase job-related rewards. The provision of social support was not as effective for this group of workers.

A study in southern Sweden found that systematic clinical supervision and individualised planned care decreased tedium and burnout and increased creativity at work for nurses (registered and licensed practical) and care assistants in wards for severely demented patients (Berg et al 1994). The authors argue that support strategies for staff that affect the work itself are most successful in relieving work-related stress.

Training at work

Provision of training at work is an effective strategy for helping workers cope with stress and can be extremely cost effective. A Swedish study, which compared group living for demented elderly people to traditional institutional care, found that a staff training programme led to increased knowledge, more favourable attitudes, greater competence and higher motivation, job satisfaction and quality of work among staff in the group living facilities than the traditional settings (Alfredson & Annerstedt 1994). The staff were head nurses (registered nurses), nursing assistants with 2 years of nursing training and nurses' aides, with a few weeks of training. The training programme for the staff in the group living units consisted of an initial 2-week course on psychodynamic concepts, staff–patient relationships, gerontology, psychopathology of dementia diseases, treatment strategies and the group living ideology. Following this course the staff were supported and supervised at monthly intervals over 12 months by a nurse, a social worker and a geriatrician. The focus of the continuing programme was individual care planning and evaluation of patient outcomes. The staff in the traditional units received the usual training which focused on 'general geriatric topics' rather than on more specific dementia care.

The Training for Care Staff Programme (TCSP)

The need for support and training for all residential care staff is clear: ' ... inadequate support, conflicts or inconsistencies, lack of relevant training or opportunities for staff development and team building can contribute to staff feeling undervalued, of low status and uncertain how to cope with the considerable demands of the work' (Youll & McCourt-Perring 1993, p. 117). The Wagner (Wagner 1988) review recommended that all residential settings should have a staff training plan which would be inspected regularly.

The Caring in Homes Initiative was commissioned by the Department of Health, as a result of the Wagner review, to set up a national programme of developmental research in residential care to promote residents' quality of life (Youll & McCourt-Perring 1993). The brief from the Department of Health linked the status and morale of care staff to good standards and high quality of care. Within this initiative, the National Institute of Social Work set up the Training for Care Staff Programme (TCSP) for basic-level care staff. The Department of Health saw this training as equipping care assistants with competencies compatible with national vocational qualifications (NVQs). NVQ training in social work and nursing was developing at the same time and care workers in social and health care settings are encouraged to acquire NVQs. Alongside this development, the TCSP focused on the contribution care workers can make to the management of residential homes. The NVQ

programme encourages workers to develop their knowledge and practice through externally validated courses and the TCSP, which is based in the workplace, encourages workers to improve the quality of care as individuals and teams.

Up until recently, education and training in social work and nursing have concentrated on professional qualifications and have not done much to help support workers acquire training and qualifications. Both professions were slow to dovetail recruitment, training and development with the changing requirements of the services. Instead the professions assumed that competent workers could be recruited either from professionally qualified people or from mature job seekers. Mature people – usually women – can cope with the tasks associated with caring for people and do not need training, or so it was thought. Although many residential establishments provide orientation courses or induction training for new staff, many do not and the effects have been piecemeal. The development of the NVQ programme and the TCSP are welcome, therefore.

The TCSP specifies seven principles which are summarised in Box 26.1.

Training projects were set up in over 100 residential care homes in a way that ensured that the managers and workers in the homes were closely involved. Imposing change on them was not the objective. The attitudes of the staff were, predictably, a mixture of enthusiasm and doubt about the value of training. Positive reactions included needing specialised

---

Box 26.1 Principles of the Training for Care Staff Programme (TCSP)

The TCSP specifies seven principles which are summarised as follows:

- Training opportunities follow the values, practices and purposes of the home.
- Residents contribute to identifying training needs by helping to formulate the purposes and reviewing standards of the service.
- Staff training and development are an integral part of service provision and quality assurance.
- Managers accept provision of training as their reponsibility.
- Education and training are integral to practice and staff are involved in identifying training needs.
- Training enhances teamworking.
- The climate for learning recognises existing knowledge and skills and values shared learning.

(Youll & McCourt-Perring 1993, p. 122)

knowledge to do the work, meeting others in the same field, having time to reflect on one's practice and the opportunity to develop special skills and, therefore, status. Scepticism included doubts about the worth or necessity of training, fears that it would be intellectually too demanding and concern that they might be expected to make difficult decisions or take on unwanted responsibility afterwards.

The training programme had to be seen to give good value for money and not be too expensive in time and effort. Some costs were inevitable, of course, including:

- allocation of time for staff to plan for and attend training sessions
- cover for staff at training sessions
- manager time to plan and run the programme
- costs of external advice and support
- cost of materials and equipment.

Some homes saw these costs as part of the service. Others, particularly private homes, saw them as extra costs. In-house training that used team-based approaches were regarded as the most effective.

Outcomes of the training programme for the establishment, the residents and the care staff were substantial (Youll & McCourt-Perring 1993). For the establishment, major benefits were clarification of purpose and generation of new ideas for improving care management, many of which became resident focused. At first the staff wanted help with how best to undertake physical care tasks but their concerns gradually turned to requests for help in understanding people with mental illness, dealing with death and bereavement and with managing their own stress at work. The style of communication between staff became freer and more creative than was the case before when their views were sought in management and progress meetings. The level of confidence and morale of the staff increased as they became involved in setting the training agenda, discussing how the home should be run and the details of care strategies.

There were considerable benefits for the residents. They participated in some of the training projects and the outlook of the staff changed when they saw how much the residents benefited. The staff became more sensitive and receptive to residents' needs and interests and relationships became more relaxed. Many small improvements occurred. For example, all the residents in a home for confused elders now have their own door key, to the delight of many. In another home, the staff noticed that the level of disturbed and wandering behaviour had declined; where staff anxiety had decreased so did resident anxiety.

All the training projects demonstrated benefits for the staff. Morale and confidence increased. Attitudes and expectations shifted and the staff showed a greater understanding of dementing residents' experiences and needs. The participative approach to training increased the staff's sense of responsibility to improve the service. The staff began to make contact across boundaries – between day and night staff and with staff from other homes – and they supported each other more than before. They realised that they enjoyed learning from each other through discussion of practice. This gave them a sense of identity and they began to value their own experience. But some staff, who were reluctant to adapt to change, were put under pressure. The move to a climate of openness meant that individual and group difficulties were exposed which increased the anxiety and stress of the less flexible care workers.

Four important conclusions to emerge from the TCSP were drawn by Youll & McCourt-Perring. First, training is not successful if it is 'bolted on' to a care establishment without taking account of the context and circumstances of the home. Second, the attitudes of the staff and climate of the home influence the receptiveness of staff to training. Third, training cannot solve a problem that is the management's responsibility; and audit may be necessary before the content and goals of a training programme can be agreed. Finally, the management must be prepared for greater assertiveness and critique of their policies and practices by staff who complete training. Staff who have learned to change themselves will not tolerate managers who are closed and defensive; the management culture must change too and become open and responsive to staff development

CONCLUSION

In this chapter we have looked at theoretical and methodological issues in occupational stress research with particular emphasis on stress as a transactional process between individuals and their environment, and its concomitant elements of cognitive appraisal and coping. In considering stress in workers who look after elderly people in long-stay settings – particularly those who are mentally frail – we have discussed the concepts of quantitative and qualitative overload (burnout) and qualitative underload (rustout or professional depression). We conclude that burnout and rustout have similar features – isolation and emotional detachment – but the cause of one is work overload and of the other is work underload. Both overload and underload are stressful features of continuing care work and can have pernicious consequences for direct care workers, many of whom are care assistants with little control over their work. Our review of the literature suggests that research has underestimated rates of stress in staff who care for elderly people because the workers most vulnerable to stress probably do not respond to surveys.

Sources of worker stress in care settings for elderly mentally frail people concern organisational factors, patient demands and individual characteristics and circumstances of the staff. The research literature illustrates the complexity of relationships between perceptions of stress, worker characteristics, the functioning level of dementing people and the type of care facility. Individual differences in workers, such as biographical factors, personality variables, coping strategies, work expectations and commitment, skills and abilities, and health-related activities (smoking, drinking alcohol, exercise), all operate to reduce or aggravate undesirable reactions to stress.

Coping strategies that can reduce stress reactions include problem solving, positive reappraisal, seeking support, acceptance or resignation, avoiding the stressor and expressing emotions. Stress management programmes, staff support groups and training in how to work with cognitively impaired elders are effective if they help workers to increase their knowledge and skills, improve staff relationships, cope with challenges, increase their sense of control and support each other through enthusiastic teamwork. Training programmes that involve the residents and are arranged by managers and care staff working closely together benefit the establishment, the residents and the care staff.

Caring for elderly mentally ill people is an important and skilled task which requires able, creative, trained and well motivated staff working in close contact with elderly people themselves. Arguments that favour an all-trained nursing workforce are unrealistic; the bulk of caring will always be done by care assistants. These workers suffer from low esteem and low status. They have little control over their work and their views are rarely sought when decisions about care management are taken. Yet they are the backbone of the caring services for elderly people with mental frailty and enlightened self interest alone should be enough to ensure that their work-related needs are given prominence. Residential care establishments that support their care workers as much as they do their residents reap the rewards of high quality care and a high quality working environment.

REFERENCES

Age Concern 1990 Under sentence: continuing care units for older people within the NHS. Age Concern, London

Aldwin C M, Revenson T A 1987 Does coping help? A re-examination of the relation between coping and mental health. Journal of Personality and Social Psychology 53: 237–248

Alfredson B B, Annerstedt L 1994 Staff attitudes and job satisfaction in the care of demented elderly people: group living compared with long-term care institutions. Journal of Advanced Nursing 20: 964–974

Armstrong-Esther C A, Browne K D 1986 The influence of elderly patients' mental impairment on nurse–patient interaction. Journal of Advanced Nursing 11: 379–387

Åström S, Nilsson M, Norberg A, Sandman P-O, Winblad B 1991 Staff burnout in dementia care – relations to empathy and attitudes. International Journal of Nursing Studies 28(1): 65–75

Babb P J 1994 Dual role stress and coping in nurses. Unpublished PhD thesis, Birkbeck College, University of London

Bartoldus E, Gillery B, Sturges P J 1989 Job related stress and coping among home-care workers with elderly people. Health and Social Work 14(3): 204–210

Benjamin L C 1991 Stress, role and training in carers of the elderly. International Journal of Geriatric Psychiatry 6: 809–813

Benjamin L C, Spector J 1990 The relationship of staff, resident and environmental characteristics to stress experienced by staff caring for the dementing. International Journal of Geriatric Psychiatry 5: 25–31

Berg A, Welander Hansson U, Hallberg I R 1994 Nurses' creativity, tedium and burnout during 1 year of clinical supervision and implementation of individually planned nursing care: comparisons between a ward for severely demented patients and a similar control ward. Journal of Advanced Nursing 20: 742–749

Bond J, Bond S 1987 Developments in the provision and evolution of long term care for dependent old people. In: Fielding P (ed) Research and the nursing care of elderly people. Churchill Livingstone, Wiley, New York

Carrilio T, Eisenberg D 1984 Using peer support to prevent worker burnout. Social Work 65: 307–310

Chappell N L, Novak M 1992 The role of support in alleviating stress among nursing assistants. The Gerontologist 32(3): 351–359

Cherniss C 1980 Professional burnout in human service organisations. Praeger, New York

Clark P, Bowling A 1989 An observational study of quality of life in NHS nursing homes and a long-stay hospital ward for the elderly. Ageing and Society 9: 123–148

Clarke A C 1991 Nurses as role models and health educators. Journal of Advanced Nursing 16: 1178–1184

Clifford P, Leiper R, Pilling S 1989 Assuring quality in mental health services. Research and Development in Psychiatry and Free Association Books, London

Cooper C L, Sloan J M, Williams S 1988 Occupational stress indicator management guide. NFER-Nelson, Windsor

Cox T, Ferguson E 1991 Individual differences, stress and coping. In: Cooper C L, Payne R (eds) Personality and stress: individual differences in the stress process. Wiley, Chichester

Cronin-Stubbs D, Brophy E 1985 Burnout: can social support save the psychiatric nurse? Journal of Psychosocial Nursing and Mental Health Services 23(7): 8–13

Dawkins J E, Depp F, Selzer N 1985 Stress and the psychiatric nurse. Journal of Psychosocial Nursing 23(11): 9–15

Dewe P 1987 Identifying the causes of nurses' stress: a survey of New Zealand nurses. Work & Stress 1(1): 15–24

Dewe P J 1989 Stressor frequency, tension, tiredness and coping: some measurement issues and a comparison across nursing groups. Journal of Advanced Nursing 14: 308–320

Dewe P, Cox T, Ferguson E 1993 Individual strategies for coping with stress at work: a review. Work and Stress 7(1): 5–15

Dunn L A, Ritter S A 1995 Stress in mental health nursing: a review of the literature. In: Carson J, Fagin L, Ritter S (eds) Stress and coping in mental health nursing. Chapman and Hall, London

Dunn L A, Rout U, Carson J, Ritter S A 1994 Occupational stress amongst care staff working in nursing homes: an empirical investigation. Journal of Clinical Nursing 3: 177–183

Evers H 1981a Tender loving care? Patients and nurses in geriatric wards. In: Copp L A (ed) Care of the ageing. Churchill Livingstone, Edinburgh

Evers H 1981b Care or custody? The experiences of women patients in long-stay geriatric wards. In: Williams G, Hutter B (eds) Controlling women: the normal and deviant. Croom Helm, London

Firth H, Britton P 1989 'Burnout', absence and turnover among British nursing staff. Journal of Occupational Psychology 62: 55–59

Firth H, McKeown P, McIntee J, Britton P 1987 Burnout, personality and support in long-stay nursing. Nursing Times 83(32): 55–57

Firth-Cozens J 1988 Stress among medical students. In: Wallis D, de Wolff C J (eds) Stress and organisational problems in hospitals, Croom Helm, London

Gallagher A P 1986 A model for change in long-term care. Journal of Gerontological Nursing 12(5): 19–23

Galliard P 1978 Difficulties encountered in attempting to increase social interaction among geriatric psychiatry patients – clean and sitting quietly. Paper presented to the British Psychological Society Annual Conference, York University

Gilloran A, McKinley A, McGlew T, McKee K, Robertson A 1994 Staff nurses' work satisfaction in psychogeriatric wards. Journal of Advanced Nursing 20: 997–1003

Gilloran A, Robertson A, McGlew T, McKee K 1995 Improving work satisfaction amongst nursing staff and quality of care for elderly patients with dementia: some policy implications. Ageing and Society 15: 375–391

Goldberg D 1978 Manual of the general health questionnaire. NFER-Nelson, Windsor

Goodchild M E, Duncan-Jones P 1985 Chronicity and the general health questionnaire. British Journal of Psychiatry 146: 56–61

Gray-Toft P, Anderson J 1981 Stress among hospital nursing staff: its causes and effects. Social Science and Medicine 15A: 639–547

Gray-Toft P, Anderson J 1985 Organizational stress in the hospital: development of a model for diagnosis and prediction. Health Services Research 19(6) February, part 1: 753–774

Greene R 1986 Countertransference issues in social work with the aged. Journal of Gerontological Social Work 9(3): 79–88

Guppy A, Gutteridge T 1990 Job satisfaction and occupational stress in UK general hospital nursing staff. Work and Stress 5(4): 315–323

Hallberg I R, Norberg A 1990 Staff's interpretation of the experiences behind vocally disruptive behaviour in severely demented patients and their feelings about it: an exploratory study. International Journal of Aging and Human Development 31: 297–307

Hallberg I R, Norberg A 1993 Strain amongst nurses and their emotional reactions during one year of systematic clinical supervision combined with the implementation of individualised care in dementia nursing. Journal of Advanced Nursing 18: 1860–1875

Harris P E 1989 The nurse stress index. Work and Stress 3(4): 335–346

Hipwell A E, Tyler P, Wilson C M 1989 Sources of stress and dissatisfaction among nurses in four hospital environments. British Journal of Medical Psychology 62: 71–79

Holden U P, Woods R T 1982 Reality orientation: psychological approaches to the confused elderly. Churchill Livingstone, London

Howe E 1992 The quality of care: a report of the residential staffs inquiry. Local Government Management Board

Ivancevich J, Matteson M, Preston C 1982 Occupational stress, Type A behavior, and physical well being. Academy of Management Journal 25(2): 373–391

Jones J G 1987 Stress in psychiatric nursing. In: Payne R, Firth-Cozens J (eds) Stress in health professionals. Wiley, Chichester

Kane R L, Bell R M, Riegler S Z 1986 Value preferences for nursing home outcomes. Geront. Soc. Am. 26: 303–308

LaMonica E L 1981 Construct validity of an empathy instrument. Research in Nursing and Health 4: 389–400

Lazarus R S, de Longis A 1983 Psychological stress and coping in aging. American Psychologist 38: 245–254

Lazarus R S, Folkman S 1984 Stress, appraisal and coping. Springer, New York

Leary J, Brown D 1995 Findings from the Claybury study for ward based psychiatric nurses and comparisons with community psychiatric nurses. In: Carson J, Fagin L, Ritter S (eds) Stress and coping in mental health nursing. Chapman and Hall, London

Levi L, Frankenhauser M, Gardell B 1983 Work stress related to social structures and processes. In: Elliott G, Eisdorfer C (eds) Research on stress and human health. Springer, New York

Lindesay J, Briggs K, Lawes M, Macdonald A, Herzberg J 1991 The domus philosophy: a comparative evaluation of a new approach to residential care of the demented elderly. International Journal of Geriatric Psychiatry 6: 727–736

Macpherson R, Eastley R J, Richards H, Mian I H 1994 Psychological distress among workers caring for the elderly. International Journal of Geriatric Psychiatry 9: 381–386

Maslach C 1982 Burnout – the cost of caring. Prentice Hall, New York

Maslach C, Jackson S 1981 The measurement of experienced burnout. Journal of Occupational Behaviour 2: 99–113

Menzies I 1960 A case study of the functioning of social systems as a defence against anxiety. Human Relations 13(2): 95–121

Morris R G, Morris L W, Britton P G 1988 Factors affecting the emotional wellbeing of the caregivers of dementia sufferers: a review. British Journal of Psychiatry 153: 147–156

Nolan M, Grant G 1993 Rust out and therapeutic reciprosity: concepts to advance the nursing care of older people. Journal of Advanced Nursing 18: 1305–1314

Norfolk B, Stirton J 1987 An investigation into stress at work: a survey of 10 psycho-geriatric wards at High Royds hospital, 2nd edn. National Union of Public Employees, London

Norman A 1987 Severe dementia: the provision of long-stay care. Centre for Policy on Ageing, London

Norton D, McClaren R, Exton-Smith A N 1962 (reprinted 1979) An investigation of geriatric nursing problems in hospital. Research Report NCCOP. Churchill Livingstone, Edinburgh

Oaklander H, Fleishman E 1964 Patterns of leadership related to organizational stress in hospital settings. Administrative Science Quarterly 16 March: 520–532

Office of Population Census and Surveys 1978 Occupational mortality: the Registrar General's decennial supplement of England and Wales 1970–1972. HMSO, London

Oswin M 1978 Children living in long-stay hospitals. Heinemann, London

Parkes K 1994 Personality and coping as moderators of work stress processes: models, methods and measures. Work and Stress 8(2): 110–129

Pearlin L, Schooler L 1978 The structure of coping. Journal of Health and Social Behaviour 19: 2–21

Pennington R E, Pierce W L 1985 Observations of empathy of nursing home staff: a predictive study. International Journal of Aging and Human Development 21(4): 281–290

Pines A, Aronson E, Kafry D 1981 Burnout: from tedium to personal growth. The Free Press, New York

Poulin J E, Walter C A 1993 Burnout in gerontological social work. Social Work 38(3): 305–310

Revicki D, May H 1989 Organisational characteristics, occupational stress and mental health in nurses. Behavioural Medicine 15(1): 30–36

Ritter S A, Tolchard B, Stewart R 1995 Coping with stress in mental health nursing. In: Carson J, Fagin L, Ritter S (eds) Stress and coping in mental health nursing. Chapman and Hall, London

Royal College of Nursing, British Geriatric Society and Royal College of Psychiatrists 1987 Improving care of elderly people in hospital. RCN, London

Shouksmith G, Wallis D 1988 Stress amongst hospital nurses. In: Wallis D, de Wolff C J (eds) Stress and organisational problems in hospitals. Croom Helm, London

Sullivan P J 1993 Occupational stress in psychiatric nursing. Journal of Advanced Nursing 18: 591–601

Tomlin S 1989 Abuse of elderly people: an unneccessary and preventable problem. A Public Information Report from the British Geriatrics Society, London

Trygstad L N 1986 Stress and coping in psychiatric nursing. Journal of Psychosocial Nursing 24(10): 23–27

Wagner G 1988 A positive choice: report of the independent review of residential care. HMSO, London

Walker E 1986 Stress and nursing. Unpublished MSc Thesis, UWIST, University of Wales, Cardiff

Wallis D 1986 Satisfaction, stress and performance: issues for occupational psychology in the 'caring professions'. Keynote address to the BPS Occupational Psychology Conference, University of Nottingham, January 1986

Wells T 1980 Problems in geriatric nursing care: a study of nurses' problems in care of old people in hospital. Churchill Livingstone, Edinburgh

Wright R, Williams B, Dill J 1992 Interactive effects of difficulty and instrumentality of avoidant behaviour on cardiovascular reactivity. Pyschophysiology 29(6): 677–686

Wynne R, Clarkin N, McNieve A 1993 The experience of stress amongst Irish nurses – a survey of Irish Nurses Organisation members. Irish Nurses Organisation and National Council of Nurses of Ireland, Dublin

Youll P J, McCourt-Perring C 1993 Raising voices: ensuring quality in residential care. An evaluation of the Caring in Homes Initiative, Brunel University and HMSO, London

RECOMMENDED READING

Payne R, Firth-Cozens J (eds) 1987 Stress in health professionals. Wiley & Sons, Chichester. *This edited volume, published almost a decade ago, remains a standard text on stress in the health professions. The introductory chapter provides a general framework for looking at occupational stress and subsequent chapters discuss the main elements in the stress model in relation to different health care occupations. The authors address how much strain there is in an occupation, the major sources of stress and what might be done to remove these stressors. Paid carers of elderly people are not singled out, but several chapters refer to the strains involved.*

Work and Stress 1993 7(1) Special Issue: Coping with stress at work. Taylor & Francis, London. *Work and Stress is an international, multidisciplinary quarterly journal of stress, health and performance at work. This whole issue is devoted to coping with stress at work. The editorial laments the lack of empirical research on the construct of coping with stress at work. Two issues, the editorial tells us, have impeded this research: the difficulties of measuring coping strategies, and the emphasis of previous research into negative features at work that cause stress rather than positive features to help workers cope with stress. This special issue of the journal provides a comprehensive review of occupational stress research and a coherent picture of current understanding of the stress process and coping strategies.*

Work and Stress 8(2) Special Issue: A healthier work environment. Taylor & Francis, London. *This special issue*

of Work and Stress is devoted to promoting healthier work environments. The issue contains a collection of scientific papers delivered at a meeting in Stockholm in 1991 that explored the concepts and methods of measurement involved in the promotion of a healthier work environment. The editorial argues that further research in the field of occupational safety and health, together with its application in the workplace, will promote healthy work environments, healthy workers and healthy organisations.

27

Supporting residents in long-stay settings

Sally J Redfern

When residential or nursing home care becomes the best option for clients and their carers it is important that institutions provide the most beneficial environment possible: 'Living in a residential establishment should be a positive experience ensuring a better quality of life than the resident would enjoy in any other setting' (Wagner 1988, p. 114). We need an understanding of the effects of institutional environments on the wellbeing of confused residents. The problem is, how can you tell what these effects are?

This chapter focuses on support of residents in long-stay settings. We look first at the values that underpin a supportive approach to quality of life and quality of care, specifically values relating to residents' rights and the opportunity to live ordinary lives even when disabled. We consider what it is like to live in residential and nursing homes and whether elderly mentally infirm people are better off in segregated or integrated accommodation. This is followed by a brief appraisal of the long-stay hospital closure programme and some of the settings that replaced hospital care. A review of different models of care in residential settings conveys an idea of the range of facilities available and we describe the kind of support that an old person should expect from the physical and social environment and the caring regime. The final section of the chapter discusses how support in residential settings can be measured, either as a continuing audit activity or as part of a research-based evaluation.

First, a few facts and figures. The Department of Health compiles statistics on local authority supported residents in homes for people with mental illness in England based on the returns submitted by local authorities. Its report based on information at March 1993 (Department of Health 1994) reveals that, since 1983, there has been a decrease of 24% in local authority supported residents in homes and hostels making a total in 1993 of just 3700. Half (52%) of these residents lived in local authority homes, 26% in voluntary homes, 15% in private homes and the rest in other accommodation. As the number of supported residents decreased in local authority homes over the decade 1983 to 1993, the number in voluntary homes also decreased and the number in private homes increased by 61%. Most (89%) of the local authority supported residents with mental illness are aged under 65, and there has been little variation in this level between 1983 and 1993. Of those aged over 65 supported by local authorities, 48% lived in local authority homes, 26% in voluntary homes, 20% in private homes and 7% in other accommodation.

These figures say nothing, of course, about the number of elderly mentally ill people living in private or voluntary homes at their own, or their family's, expense or those in health authority funded hospital wards. Nor do they indicate the proportion – the majority – who live at home with family carers. Chapter 24 discusses service provision more widely and Chapter 25 looks at support of old people living at home and their carers.

VALUES UNDERPINNING A SUPPORTIVE APPROACH TO QUALITY OF LIFE AND QUALITY OF CARE

Residents' rights

There are two basic questions that need to be asked with respect to long-stay care in residential settings (Smith 1989, p.1): ' ... how do we know what a high quality service looks like for residents; and secondly, how can we bring about positive changes in working practices?'

Smith puts forward five principles for long-stay psychiatric care:

Principle 1. 'People in long-stay wards have the same human values as others and have a right to respect and privacy' (p. 2).

Residents, like all of us, want a homely place to live in, their own personal space, their own possessions. They want access to other people, to be asked about their quality of life and the services received, not to be fearful of reprisals from the staff, to have choice and make their own decisions, and to be acknowledged and appreciated. Caring staff assume these values are held by residents who cannot express them themselves and will alter their assumptions only when given firm evidence to the contrary.

Principle 2. Residents have the right to an individual care plan with planned interventions and treatment, a long-term agenda, clear goals for maximum independence, involvement of the family in care planning, regular review of the plan and appropriate amendment as a result.

Principle 3. Service provision should ensure that residents can participate fully in the community.

They want to go out as they wish, to be taken out from time to time, to have their own money to spend, to be treated as worthy individuals, not as members of a group and, above all, not to stand out as abnormal. This means that staff do not wear uniforms or badges, especially when taking residents out, they accept flexible working hours – including weekends and evening trips – they help residents use local facilities – shops, banks, hairdresser, dentist, church, clubs – they treat residents as they would like to be treated themselves, and they avoid compulsory 'mass recruitment'.

Principle 4. 'A person has a right to sufficient and individualised support so as to respond to their unique and constantly changing needs, and their potential for change' (p. 7).

Residents want the opportunity to learn and interact with others of their own choosing, protection from exploitation yet reasonable risk-taking, not to be blamed if things go wrong and help to do the things they want to do. They do not want to be told that there are insufficient resources. They want to know about changes planned that will affect them, and to be involved in planning the changes.

Just as residents need support so do staff. Staff need support and training to be able to achieve what residents want. A means of information exchange and consultation is necessary so that views can be expressed and decisions acted upon (see Ch. 26).

Principle 5. Residents have a right to expect a positive image of them to be projected within and outside the institution.

They want to be self-determining human beings, able to make their own decisions and mistakes, to be treated as adults and not to be labelled in derogatory terms or as helpless, and to live in an environment that, as far as possible, reflects home.

These principles could be said to go without saying; they are what we all would want in these circumstances. But can they be achieved for residents living in long-stay psychiatric institutions and, if so, why are they so uncommon there? Residential living in the community has put insufficient emphasis on what people in general would call normal and ordinary. Living arrangements need to be outward looking, closely linked and integrated into the community and not so big that large-scale institutionalisation is inevitable. There is the view that the Registered Homes Act operates against ordinary living arrangements. The Act applies to all homes that provide personal care and catering and its regulations are bound, it is said, to damage the quality of life of residents who seek ordinary living: 'The application of these rules to ordinary life situations strips away the ordinary home atmosphere and imposes an institutional model on people seeking to escape it' (Collins 1993, p. 15).

Normalisation

What is ordinary life and how does it differ from institutional living? (The characteristics of institutional living are listed in Box 27.1.)

Box 27.1 Characteristics of institutional living

- denial of humanity and individuality
- no personal space
- no privacy
- little choice
- little comfort
- little personal safety
- few possessions
- no dignity
- pauperised
- dependent
- no control, no participation, no decision making
- cannot function as ordinary human beings.

(Source: Collins 1993)

By contrast to institutional living (Box 27.1), the 'ordinary life principle':

- provides opportunities we all take for granted
- provides the opportunity to live alone or in small groups in ordinary houses where residents can interact with neighbours
- enables residents to participate fully in managing their own lives
- allows residents to be accepted as part of the community because they are seen as ordinary people (Collins 1993).

People who live in large groups – a religious community, new age commune, old people's home – are not accepted as valued members of society in this country because the norm is not to live in large groups. Their mode of living sets them apart, people are uneasy in the presence of large numbers, even more so if members have visible disabilities. But once ordinary people see people with disabilities being treated as

respected citizens with ordinary living responsibilities, they will treat them likewise. Therefore everyone's sense of personal worth and development will rise.

Ramon's book, *Beyond Community Care* (1991), provides the conceptual underpinnings to the notion of ordinary living. She focuses on three related principles: 'normalisation', 'social role valorisation' and 'integrated living' for improving the quality of life of people with disabilities (that is to say, people with developmental, or learning, disabilities, physical disabilities or mental distress or illness). Ramon's view is that, if we all – the public, carers, professionals, policy makers – acknowledge these principles, then people with disabilities will be able to lead a normal life in ordinary settings.

The notion of normalisation originated in Scandinavia in the 1950s and moved to North America in the late 1960s, then Australia in the 1970s and to Europe, including Britain, in the 1980s (Ramon 1991). The development of the concept has been attributed to Wolfensberger (1972) and Ramon describes it as: ' … the principle by which people with a disability have the right to lead a valued ordinary life, based on the belief in their equality as human beings and citizens' (Ramon 1991, p. 6).

As Ramon, and others (e.g. Baxter et al 1990) demonstrate, normalisation includes what few of us stop to think about; we take these things for granted (see Box 27.2).

These expectations are compatible with the notion of an ordinary life outlined earlier and with the principles of good relationships, choice, participation, personal development and greater mixing highlighted by Brandon and Jack in Chapter 14. This is the stuff of

---

Box 27.2 Components of normalisation

- patterns and conditions of everyday life that everyone else has
- access to ordinary services that other people use – ordinary houses, schools, leisure facilities, employment
- normal rhythm of days, weeks, years
- normal sized living units
- adequate privacy
- normal growing-up experiences
- normal access to social, emotional and sexual relationships
- the possibility of doing paid work
- choice and participation in decisions affecting one's future.

(after Ramon 1991)

---

ordinary living; the opportunity for control over one's life, to have choices, social encounters and the possibility of avoiding poverty. Even though ordinary living may not be glorious, most of us regard it as qualitatively better than the lifestyle currently available to people with disabilities.

Having choice, though, can backfire. Baxter et al (1990) talk about the 'conservative corollary' to normalisation, in that people who are devalued are more likely than others to attract adverse comment if they dress unconventionally, for example. Therefore, it is best, they say, to veer on the side of conservatism in order to be regarded as normal. This advice can be a particular problem, for example, for black and other ethnic minority people if they are encouraged to be 'conservative' in their dress when that dress is abnormal and pretty radical for them.

Ramon (1991) describes four concepts that together define normalisation – deinstitutionalisation, social role valorisation, opportunities for ordinary living and the meaning of disability. We draw from her work in considering them here.

Deinstitutionalisation

Supporters of the normalisation principle are unanimous in arguing against people with disabilities living in institutions. As indicated in Box 27.1, they see institutions as anathema to ordinary living because institutional living includes:

- segregation from the rest of the population
- total dependence on the institution
- no choice
- social control and isolation
- the stigma of being different.

Deinstitutionalisation was described by Wing in the early 1960s to counter what he saw as the passive, regimented lifestyle of people in long-stay hospitals leading to the secondary impediments of deficiency in social and self-care skills. Other observers of the time concurred with this view by describing the life apart of people living in psychiatric hospitals, geriatric hospitals, old people's homes and prisons (Goffman 1961, Kleemeier 1961, Pincus 1968, King et al 1971). Ramon's (1991) view is that it is the structural nature of these places rather than 'badness' of staff or administrators which leads to oppression of residents, and also of staff. It is also the case that just physically moving people out of an institution is not enough to prevent institutionalisation. Ramon is scathing about the rhetoric behind 'community care', believing that

its usefulness has been outlived because its proponents have failed to define it in terms of precise and specific criteria.

Social role valorisation (SRV)

Social role valorisation is the highest goal of normalisation in that it creates, supports and defends valued social roles for people at risk of social devaluation. Wolfensberger & Thomas (1994, p. 53) define SRV thus:

Briefly, Social Role Valorisation (SRV) is a broad theory of social relationships, deviancy reversal and human service ... that is based on, but supersedes, the principle of normalization. ... SRV posits: (a) that people are highly apt to be accorded the good things of life if they are seen in positive, valued roles in society; (b) that devalued people tend to be cast, even forced into, and kept, in very devalued roles; and that therefore (c) people who are societally devalued, or at risk of such devaluation, need to be helped to obtain and maintain valued social roles.

Ramon highlights the 'double act of devaluation' that occurs for people with disabilities. That is to say, people with disabilities are:

- perceived as different in a negative sense – are devalued
- segregated from ordinary people and living patterns
- prevented from performing socially valued roles and behaviour, and
- further devalued as a result.

Devaluation includes: 'rejection, distantiation, segregation, congregation, discontinuity, loss of autonomy, deindividualisation, disenfranchisement, dependency on artificial, paid relationships, involuntary systemised poverty, being suspected of multiple problems, being negatively imaged, brutalisation and awareness of oneself as devalued and as a burden to others' (Ramon 1991, p. 9).

SRV takes the opposing stance. It promotes people's self-perception and social standing so that they feel socially valued. For a person with disabilities, SRV is meaningful only if it is reciprocated by people without disabilities; the relationship must be an equal one. SRV covers the same ground as normalisation except that SRV conforms less to the 'statistical and largely mythical majority' which underlies normalisation (Ramon 1991). Many proponents agree with Wolfensberger that SRV supersedes normalisation.

SRV is derived from the symbolic interactionist school within sociology and social psychology and is strongly influenced by the labelling approach to deviance (Ramon 1991). Deviants are degraded; deemed as bad or mad and incapable of making socially valued decisions. They are stripped of their rights and prescribed treatment or sanctions which they must accept if they are to be 'cured' or their deviancy prevented. All this leads to labelling and stigma, plus probable segregation in an institution where everyone is so devalued by others that they come to devalue themselves.

Labelling theorists regard this process as largely irreversible because the 'deviant' has internalised the devalued image and cannot lose it even when having moved out of the institution; the so-called self-fulfilling prophecy. Thus a vicious cycle is set up – the 'double act of devaluation' referred to earlier. The SRV approach takes a less pessimistic view. It regards the process of labelling and being devalued as reversible; it is possible for a person to be valued again and to lose the internalised devalued image. Much of the current practical work involved in the normalisation and SRV process is attempting to reverse this process (Ramon 1991).

Opportunities for ordinary living

Living an ordinary, non-institutional life is crucial for being socially valued. Opportunities for ordinary living should cover all areas of everyday life – income, housing, work, education, health services, recreation and social interaction. Support services that promote ordinary living should therefore be located within the range of communal services available to everyone rather than ghettoised. This questions the wisdom of segregating elderly patients with multiple problems in geriatric rather than general hospital wards and elderly mentally ill people in units separated from the physically frail. We look at the case for and against segregation later.

The meaning of disability

A disability is something that limits a person in some way and requires effort to sort it out so that the person can live ordinarily. Sorting out may be to accept the limitation as a given; after all, we mostly accept that we cannot do anything about it if we lack a specific skill or talent. As Ramon puts it, disability is 'part of everyone's socially acceptable imperfection' (Ramon 1991, p. 12). A minority view is that disabled people are special because the struggle to live with the disability makes them better people. Another view is that disability is meaningless because what matters is

dignity within one's life, not whether you are disabled or not.

Values underlying normalisation and social role valorisation

Bearing in mind these four concepts – deinstitutionalisation, SRV, opportunities for ordinary living and the meaning of disability – the values underlying normalisation and SRV have been defined by Ramon (Box 27.3).

Box 27.3 Values underlying normalisation and social role valorisation

- people first
- respect for persons
- right to self-determination
- right to be dependent
- empowerment.

(after Ramon 1991)

Lumping people with disabilities into categories – 'the chronically mentally ill', 'the mentally handicapped' – negates the simple value that people with disabilities are people as much as anyone else. Proponents of normalisation and SRV credit people with dignity and rights even if their level of performance falls short of that reached by people without the disability. Respect for persons involves belief in their personhood; respect is one of the sanctions attached to socially valued people in the SRV approach.

People who have the right to self-determination make decisions for themselves. This right accepts that they have more knowledge about themselves than anyone else does, so that it is not the case that the professional knows best. Many professionals have difficulty accepting that people with disabilities have the right to make mistakes too; difficulty because of their investment in success at all costs and expectation by society that professionals do not make mistakes.

Social work is the helping profession most likely to be concerned with these values and to apply them to their work; they see it as unrealistic and patronising to protect people with disabilities from making mistakes (Ramon 1991). Nurses could adopt these values more than they do. They could integrate these values into their work without losing their important role, along with medicine, in cure and damage limitation. A certain amount of risk-taking by service providers, and allowing people the right to fail, is necessary if service users are to be able to be reasonably autonomous and take responsibility for their lives.

Do we have the right to be dependent? Our society sees independence as the ideal; dependence conveys weakness and failure. But many of us are encouraged to be financially and socially dependent – wives, mothers, young people, old people – even if they have no disability. People with disabilities are encouraged all the more; they are encouraged to be dependent on informal carers and service providers much more so than before they had a disability. 'Good' patients are passive, dependent, acquiescent, uncritical, happy, accepting of routine and loss of control over their lives.

On the surface, SRV calls for autonomy and discards dependency. But its emphasis on the right to *mutual* and professional support implies the right to be dependent at times. As Ramon makes clear, if autonomy is a value within SRV, then accepting interdependence as a positive state of being is implicit. Dependence might also be a way of achieving some degree of independence and control. We all know of instances when old people in residential homes and hospitals have refused to do things for themselves even when they would agree that they are capable of the task. Refusing to do what they know they can do may be the only way they can keep any independence.

For people with disabilities to be really empowered, the power must be transferred to them from those with the power – professionals, informal carers, friends, central and local government, voluntary activists. Empowerment is about presence, choice, autonomy, competence, status, participation (O'Brien 1988). Ramon (1991) sees empowerment as synonymous with self-determination if it is to be taken seriously.

SRV challenges cherished traditional values held by professionals about people with disabilities; values to do with professional expertise, professional power, professional conduct, segregation and integration. SRV threatens the divide between professionals and users. It takes issue with the traditional way of relating to clients as vulnerable and disadvantaged; instead, it focuses on their strengths, abilities and advantages. It reduces the gap between client-expressed need and professionally defined need. Proponents of SRV strive to guide professionals through an attitude change so that they accept their clients as valid partners in the helping process and recognise their right to an ordinary life. It has to be said, though, that organisational change is also necessary if SRV is to work; professionals cannot succeed alone.

Summarising thus far, we have considered the values that guide residential care practices. We move on to discuss the reality of residential life for elderly people and how these values can be translated into practice.

Living in residential settings

Geographical, professional and social isolation of large hospitals leads to a framework of behaviours and an ethos peculiar to the hospital (Collins 1993). The large isolated hospital is so different to the rest of the community that societal norms no longer apply. Instead, standards that emphasise the distance between the institution and society make each a separate world. Residents and staff develop ways of coping with the unique pressures of the institutional environment and behave in ways that would not be accepted outside, yet their attitudes and actions are seen as an integral part of institutional life. Collins writes about mental handicap hospitals, now scheduled for, or having completed, closure programmes. The institutional frame is as relevant to geriatric and psychogeriatric hospitals, and also to many much smaller residential and nursing homes which have absorbed, or have continued, the institutional ethos.

Moving into 'the community' does not automatically instil a way of life that is ordinary and non-institutional. Staff who move with residents without any preparation will still treat the institution and the outside world as separate entities when they cross the boundary. They find the standards and criteria in one quite irrelevant in the other and trying to reduce the dissonance between them is too difficult to cope with without help. Staff who can cope with these different worlds keep them separate and independent; if they try to merge them, they find they cannot continue to work in that setting (Collins 1993).

Consistent underfunding over the years has reinforced this separateness so that standards of comfort, amenities, care and staffing have been lower than what society would expect. Collins describes the consequences of this underfunding. First, people with disabilities (Collins refers to people with learning disabilities but the argument applies equally to elderly people with mental health problems) are perceived as having few needs or rights. Secondly, the lack of a stimulating and educative environment accentuates a person's disabilities even more. We can see a vicious cycle here: underfunding prevents users from benefiting from the service, overworked staff are discouraged from attempting to improve the service, deprived residents become unable to take advantage of what help there is, so that injecting more funds into the institution is seen as lacking any benefit and a low priority.

Many residents of large hospitals remain in the same place (ward, lounge) virtually all day long doing nothing (Godlove et al 1982, Collins 1993). Their interactions with others are confined to meal times, bath time and toileting, with the emphasis on getting the task done. Lack of stimulation leads to stunted personal growth and loss of the skills they had before admission, such as speech.

Residents' hospital records are often inadequate because of their medical orientation. There is usually very little information on how they have spent their lives over the years. Collins observes that, even in progressive long-stay hospital environments, medicine dominates still and much more so than in community homes that take an ordinary life approach. Labelling occurs more readily in hospitals; people are defined by virtue of the label – dementia, paralysis, blindness, epilepsy – rather than as a person. And behaviour labelled as 'challenging' can be equally harmful.

Individualised care

Planning the care of vulnerable residents will be most supportive if it is individualised. Supportive carers recognise each resident as unique with a unique set of needs and wants regardless of disability. Individualised care is fundamental to 'primary nursing' (Ersser & Tutton 1991), and to the 'individual programme approach' (IPP) designed for vulnerable people with learning disabilities (Baxter et al 1990). IPP provides a systematic approach to support and care designed to help people with disabilities achieve goals appropriate to their needs, wishes and circumstances. A variation on IPP is 'shared action planning' which emphasises mutuality in care planning, is more egalitarian than IPP and less likely to lose sight of the priorities of the user (Brechin & Swain 1987).

Individualised patient care in nursing sees the patient as unique, deserving of respect, with the right to be treated with dignity, to have a say in the assessment of need and the plan of care, and to receive continuity of care. Factors that facilitate individualised patient care include: personal qualities of nurses, shared understanding by the nursing team of the goals of nursing care and what constitutes good practice, adequate staffing levels and skill mix, and supportive leadership and management of nursing work (Redfern 1996).

There is a growing emphasis, in the care of people with disabilities who need continuing care, on individualised, culture-relevant, life-relevant, holistic approaches to assessment and care, so placing the user centre stage. Fundamental to shared action planning and to primary nursing is that users, their families and providers are involved equally in planning care, although this can be difficult to achieve given unequal user-professional status. Individualised care can be reduced to tokenism if users and their families are not included in discussions and are expected to accept whatever is offered with gratitude. An added problem is the impotence providers feel, in today's climate of cuts to community care funds, when they cannot deliver what they, the users and their families have agreed to be the best course of action.

Segregation or integration?

Should demented residents be segregated in specialist homes or units, or integrated with other residents within ordinary residential homes? Those favouring segregation argue that it provides a safe and planned environment and avoids distress often found amongst alert residents. Proponents of integration argue that moderately demented residents, who do not have difficult behavioural problems, do well in integrated settings and do not upset other residents (Netten 1993). The Wagner review (1988) recommends an increase in specialist provision to improve the quality of life of lucid and demented residents. The question remains, however, whether there should be specialist homes or specialist provision within integrated homes.

The literature reveals that confused residents in 'integrated' homes tend to be a separate population and be 'loners', although it is not known whether that is their choice (Netten 1993). Netten found from her study of seven integrated homes that five were designed for communal living and only one had a lounge used primarily by confused residents. In only two did confused residents eat separately from the alert, but alert residents were reported by the managers as 'accepting' of confused residents in none of the homes; in two they were tolerated but in five they were rejecting or openly antagonistic. No association was found between the attitudes of alert to confused residents and the proportion of confused residents in the home, which ranged from 5–41% in the seven integrated homes.

So, whether to develop special services for people with disabilities or to expand generic services remains a thorny issue. Proponents of normalisation advocate the latter but the users' movement sees the former as the way forward as is the case with services for some ethnic minorities (Ramon 1991). It remains the case, though, that there is a long way to go before the values specified earlier are translated into practice in all residential settings, segregated or integrated. First the barriers of social stigma, labelling, medical dominance and insufficient resources must be overcome.

FROM HOSPITAL TO COMMUNITY CARE

In this section we consider the process of closure and resettlement that occurred in the move from hospital to community living. In particular, was the transition done in a way that supported residents and helped them to benefit from the profound changes to their way of living? Or did they merely move from one institutional life to another?

The background

The move to run down the large mental and mental handicap hospitals has its roots in the 1950s with voluntary admissions, more discharges, an open door policy and the growing belief that patients need to retain links with the outside world (Knapp et al 1992). Post war publications were strongly critical of hospitals (Goffman 1961, Wing & Brown 1970) and there was an associated rise in therapeutic communities, half-way houses, hospital-hostel wards, community mental health programmes and supportive intensive care programmes. Public attitudes were becoming more tolerant of people with learning disability and mental illness and it was shortsighted to inject funds into decaying Victorian hospitals that psychiatrists were convinced could no longer be effective in the treatment of these people (Knapp et al 1992). Enoch Powell, Minister of Health, announced in 1961 the intention to work towards removing the long-stay in-patient population but proper community care provision, that is over and above formal residential and day care, did not begin before the late 1980s. 30 years later the hospital closure policy has not been completed even though government documents have continued to advocate it and to increase provision of services in the community (see Ch. 24 for further discussion).

Experimental nursing homes for elderly mentally frail people

Before the hospital closure programme started in any significant way, the Department of Health set up three experimental NHS nursing homes for elderly mentally ill people. Their aims were to provide individualised care in homely, domestic living environments in contrast to the long-stay hospital wards that were currently available for this client group. The homes were well staffed compared to typical ward establishments and funds were made available for improving the quality of care. The scheme was evaluated by the Institute of Human Ageing at Liverpool University (Copeland et al 1990).

The findings showed that the additional funds were put into routine physical care activities (hygiene, dressing, feeding) rather than the 'life enhancing' care (social interaction and activities) that was intended. The reason for this failure was seen as more to do with difficulty in motivating the residents than anything else although use of activity organisers and occupational therapy aides encouraged social interaction. Responsibility for client care was devolved to care assistants who acted as key workers and there was no evidence that the residents were disadvantaged by this. The pattern of daily life was unstructured, flexible and individualised. It is significant that management support was high, with careful staff recruitment, inservice training and quality assurance procedures.

Although encouraged by their key workers, residents rarely exercised choice or took the initiative to be autonomous in any activity. Dependency learned in hospital would have been difficult to destroy. Most (60%) of the residents spent their time doing nothing or dozing, wandering or engaged in disturbed behaviour, but a substantial minority (40%) took part in purposeful activity. The new way of living clearly benefited some residents in that their level of cooperation increased and agitation and aggression decreased. The residents' level of dependence gradually increased over time, as would be expected, although a few improved in cognitive functioning and activities of daily living before eventually deteriorating.

Community links – with families and the wider society – remained low, although the relatives who did visit were most positive about the move, maintaining that standards of care were higher and the staff more caring than in hospital. Most important to relatives was the homeliness of the settings, a decrease in guilt when the resident was admitted, the relief from constant worry and continuous caring when the resident had been living at home, and knowing she is well cared for.

Death rates in all three homes were low. One of the homes catered for day attenders, whose mortality rate was much higher (59%) than the residents' (24%) over the 2-year study period. A lower death rate in the residents, who are usually frailer than day attenders, suggests that specialist, protective residential settings promote longevity; not necessarily an indication of a higher quality of life though.

The success of the hospital closure programme

Ramon (1991) observed the deinstitutionalisation policies and processes that have occurred in the USA and Europe. The main impetus for most governments, with the notable exception of Italy, was to cut costs by transferring residents from large expensive hospitals to community facilities; the assumption was that community care is cheaper. The aim was to complete the transfer with the minimum of fuss and cost. Only Italy, Denmark and Sweden, Ramon tells us, explicitly incorporated principles of normalisation and SRV into their community care policies. Most countries paid little attention to the wishes of residents in the transfer process although there were exceptions, most notably for people with learning disabilities, in which assessment schemes took account of normalisation/ SRV principles. Similarly for staff; little account was taken of their skills and wishes when institutions closed. Preparing residents and staff for a new style of living and working that resembles ordinary living was an add-on extra to the main process of closure.

Italy took a different approach to hospital closure. Long before the closure date, day-to-day planning, implementation and re-planning took place during communal meetings between staff and residents, both of whom were committed to changing and dismantling the institution. New skills and satisfaction emerged in areas of work considered stagnant and doctors and nurses shed their power. The hospital sites were not sold but were used for community purposes – a school, a nursery, a riding school staffed by ex-patients. The Italian approach used SRV to focus on ordinary life principles that respected the dignity and rights of service users. Ramon's view is that there has been little commitment to deinstitutionalisation in the UK and the USA. Instead, a transfer has occurred from one total institutional style of living to another. There are exceptions, for children and people with learning disabilities, but not, generally speaking, for people in mental distress.

Most people who leave institutions require supported accommodation in hostels, adult placement schemes with landladies, group homes or small nursing homes. Increasingly the commercial sector is taking over this group, encouraged by central government in its drive to reduce public expenditure. Planners have not shown much interest in the lifestyle of relocated residents; their privacy, separation of living, working, education and recreation spaces, and control over finances and shopping are not what would be found in an ordinary home. Instead, staff

control, lack of individuality and a regimented way of life continue (Ramon 1991).

Ramon specifies the factors that should be taken into account when closing an institution:

- coordinate and consult with all agencies involved
- adequate financial support from central government for the transition period
- invest in motivating and backing workers so that they see the change as positive
- avoid a mechanical, administrative approach that is doomed to fail; leaders need flexibility to innovate creatively
- recognise and identify the barriers to change; learn how to disarm any opposing power brokers and how to enthuse people into changing their perception of themselves as losers to enthusiastic converts and gainers
- give users more than lip service during the change; users, informal carers and the local community must be properly involved in the whole process.

The new funding arrangements for community care from April 1993 had a major impact on the resettlement programme and quality of care because the residential care home allowance, which had been an automatic entitlement under Department of Social Security regulations, became a discretionary payment under local authority social service departments (Collins 1993). Since 1993, people moving out of hospitals have had to compete for the allowance – with elderly people, people with learning disabilities, people with special needs – and local authorities do not have sufficient funds for all. The result has been a reduction in service provision and slow down of the hospital closure programme now that it is realised that the costs of maintaining people who need a high level of services in the community is not a cheap option.

Collins investigated the extent and reasons for the slow progress being made in the closure of mental handicap hospitals and whether ordinary life principles were used when resettling residents. The findings showed that Ramon's factors listed above were often not taken into account. For example, the hospital staff and the community resettlement officers often had different agendas. The recommendations made by hospital staff about residents' suitability for community resettlement were tempered by their scepticism towards the community as a suitable place for residents to live compared to hospital and their own vulnerability about the move. This led to an unwillingness by some hospital staff to cooperate in the resettlement process and community staff distrusting or ignoring hospital assessments and views.

The result was often conflict between resettlement officers who wanted the best value for money and purchasers who wanted the cheapest option.

The 'peas in pods' single model approach to resettlement, based on the assumption that what works for some will work for all, is doomed to fail. It does not work for everybody else so why should it work for hospital residents? Some provider trusts offer a range of types of provision which residents are expected to fit into, but the services may not change and adapt to the changing needs of individual users. Collins describes an example where a trust was faced with an elderly resident who was developing dementia and whose needs were outstripping available services. There was no suitable nursing home in the area and the trust saw no option but to re-admit the resident to hospital.

Just as much retraining is needed for resettling staff as it is for residents. Although some hospital nurses are enthusiastic and can adopt new policies and approaches to care, others cannot cope with flexibility, weak inter-professional boundaries and user choice and power. The safety they found in a dominant medical and nursing hierarchy with its organisation-led rules and regulations is lost. Some staff prefer to take redundancy than to face the stress of change but hospital managers may not offer redundancy payments because of the expense and expect unsuitable staff to move and adapt. Intensive training before relocation followed by continued retraining after the move can mitigate the negative consequences of redeploying unsuitable staff, but swamping the community with unskilled, unprepared staff will reduce the quality of life of the people community care is supposed to serve (Collins 1993).

The Department of Health and Social Security commissioned the Personal Social Services Research Unit at the University of Kent to 'promote, monitor and evaluate' the *Care in the Community* demonstration programme which consisted of 28 projects designed to help long-stay hospital residents move to community residential settings (Knapp et al 1992, 1994). Three of these projects catered for elderly physically frail people and four for elderly mentally ill people, mostly with dementia. Three of the four for the mentally frail provided residential home care with some day care. The fourth had a home care support service designed to delay or prevent admission to residential homes by supporting elderly people in sheltered housing.

Given that very few elderly residents in long-stay hospital care move into community settings, these four projects were unusual, particularly in that most of the residents suffered from dementia. All moved into a residential home or sheltered housing complex and so the danger of transferring to institutional 'congregate community care' existed, but the researchers saw no evidence of this. There were no significant differences in the residents' skills and behaviour after the move compared to before, which could be regarded as a success given that deterioration would be expected in this group. By contrast, the elderly physically frail group showed significantly greater social disturbance and more apathy when living in the community than in hospital. The staff in all the projects had difficulty in persuading elderly residents to take part in activities but there was a marginally increased level of participation after moving to the community, especially for the elderly mentally frail group compared to the elderly physically frail group. Contact with family and friends remained high and morale and life satisfaction increased and depression decreased after the move compared to before for both groups.

This project by Knapp and his colleagues was different from many community care projects in that elderly physically and mentally frail people were helped to move permanently to residential homes or sheltered housing, rather than take short respite stays in residential homes. Each of the community projects had case-managed services designed to meet clients' needs and preferences. The authors concluded that community care run on these lines is cost effective.

MODELS OF CARE IN RESIDENTIAL SETTINGS

According to Netten (1993), Denmark has stopped all new building of nursing homes and favours independent homes in small housing complexes. This is a significant change in policy given the impressiveness of Denmark's design of old people's homes in the past (Millard 1983). Sweden uses group living units in blocks of flats which are staffed 24 hours a day by specially trained staff (see the section on group living below). In the UK there are advocates for high, medium and low health care input homes, each of which would emphasise small group living, a positive philosophy of care and multi-professional working. Nursing homes would give a high input of care, social services homes would cover medium care needs and modified housing with extra care would suit low care needs (Lodge 1990).

Group living

The idea of living in small groups, of about eight residents, within residential settings has become increasingly popular over the last 10 years or so. It is seen to overcome the lack of activity, dependency and depression common in anonymous large group environments (Rothwell et al 1983, Hodgkinson 1988). The principle underlying group living is to increase social interaction of residents through sharing activities, avoiding side-by-side seating common in anonymous lounges and promoting self-support. The residents decide on the composition of the groups, as far as possible, and carry out everyday activities themselves (serving meals, washing up, tidying the living areas). A large space is retained for gatherings of all the residents but, for everyday activities, they keep to their small groups.

Advantages of group living are that friendships develop, the more able-bodied look after the more infirm, and the setting is more homely and closer to ordinary living than large residential environments (Hodgkinson 1988). Rothwell et al (1983) investigated social activity, life satisfaction and orientation of residents before and after a home for the elderly in Newcastle, England changed to group living. Most of the residents were ambulant and many were mildly or moderately demented, although none severely so. The residents were free to organise their own groups as long as there was a mix of dependency level across the groups. The results showed that engagement in social activity and life satisfaction were significantly higher after the changeover compared to before, but level of orientation was much the same. It was at mealtimes, particularly, when social activity increased; conversation between residents increased and able-bodied residents helped the less able.

Group living has been shown to be beneficial for demented residents and staff in Sweden (Wimo et al 1991, Annerstedt 1993, Annerstedt et al 1993a, 1993b, Alfredson & Annerstedt 1994). The Swedish model differs from group living found in the UK in that the residents are housed in flats in ordinary residential blocks rather than in residential homes. The approach used is to optimise holistic care in homely settings which adopt normalisation principles. Each resident owns a private area with his or her own furniture and belongings, and there are common areas for social activities. Wimo's team found that quality of life was higher for half the residents after they had been living in the group compared to the baseline (measured when they were living at home, alone or not, or in a nursing home or psychiatric hospital). These residents were more cheerful, more confident, calmer, more active, they slept better and they took more initiatives. Moreover, group living was cheaper than hospital care.

The research by Annerstedt's group found that the residents in group living accommodation were more able and less behaviourally disturbed than comparable residents in traditional institutional care; baseline measures had shown no differences between the two groups. The research had incorporated an educational programme for the staff and improvement in the residents was explained by the increase in staff expertise and the strategies of care used in the group living environment which helped residents to cope well given their disabilities. The staff, who provided 24-hour care, were more satisfied, more motivated to work with demented residents and the quality of their care was higher than the traditional institutional care staff. The findings of this and previous research has led the Swedish government to recommend group living for demented elderly people who need continuing care (Alfredson & Annerstedt 1994).

The hotel model

Some old people prefer a more solitary existence than that provided by group living models, arguing that hotel living is more like living at home (Hodgkinson 1988). Residents' lives centre on their own rooms where care is provided discreetly. Meals are taken at individual tables in the dining room. For this model to be successful, the rooms should be large enough to be bed-sitting rooms. Hodgkinson describes the advantages of hotel living as freedom to move at will between public and private space, freedom to be alone or with someone of your own choice, residents with unpleasant habits can be avoided and personal care is given on an individualised basis when needed. Disadvantages include little likelihood of helping or receiving help from other residents, participating in activities or making friends, and relationships with staff are likely to be formal. Loneliness is common, although the forced intimacy that can occur in group living and residential home environments is unlikely to occur.

Mixed group and hotel living

An argument has been made for both approaches operating in the same setting, so that residents can choose from both (Norman 1984). The hotel model would provide access to small sitting rooms and kitchenettes, self help would be encouraged in the dining room and there would be opportunities for residents to participate together in social and educational activities. The group living model would allow residents to eat alone in a public dining room or have meals served in their own rooms if they wish.

Both models would have lockable bedrooms and cupboards for valuables, residents would bring in their own furniture if they wished and would buy their own luxuries (TV, telephone).

Hodgkinson (1988) reminds us that the entrance halls of residential homes are often a wasted space when they could be a popular gathering point. It is often easier to talk to others in passing than in a formal lounge. So, the entrance area should be warm and light with attractive seating placed so that sitters can view the outside world and passers-by. A notice-board is a good idea, in a place where people can congregate to discuss activities. The lounge should contain mixed seating arrangements so that residents have a choice of being alone or with others.

Mixed models present challenges for staff and residents who are used to more institutional environments. The greater flexibility requires them to learn new ways of working. Meals are not taken at set times and keeping residents' rooms tidy is not the prime responsibility of staff. Residents learn not to hand themselves over body and soul to the staff; instead they participate in their own care and in the daily work and life of the place as long as they can. Staff learn to take risks, be flexible in their working hours, develop good communication skills, take responsibility and accountability for their care and be open to change and continual learning. There has to be good communication between staff, day and night, and regular meetings are necessary to keep everyone informed and to discuss care, progress and activities.

Domus residential units

These are small-scale NHS-managed residential units developed in London for mentally frail elderly people who were living in psychogeriatric wards (Lindesay et al 1991). The domus philosophy was set up to improve the quality of care by focusing on the anxieties and attitudes of staff that promote 'institutional maintenance' practices. That is to say, policies, procedures and routines that fulfil the institution's needs rather than the residents'. Many studies have demonstrated preoccupation of the staff with safety, hygiene and administration and have neglected the personalised individualised care of the 'horticultural' model in favour of the impersonal routines of 'warehousing' (Wells 1980, Evers 1981, Godlove et al 1982, Baker 1983, Miller 1985, Willcocks et al 1987).

The domus philosophy has four assumptions (Lindesay et al 1991, p. 274):

1. 'That the domus is the residents' home for life

2. That the needs of the staff are as important as those of the residents
3. That the domus should aim to correct the avoidable consequences of dementia, and accommodate those that are unavoidable
4. That the residents' individual psychological and emotional needs may take precedence over the physical aspects of their care.'

Priority is given to staff training and adequate staffing levels and the emphasis is on homeliness and ordinary living, rather than clinical hospital standards, and residents are encouraged to retain their independence and take part in the activities of the domus. Residents have their own bedrooms and they share washing facilities, living rooms, kitchen and garden. Meals are taken in the dining room. The staff consists of nurses and care assistants, an occupational therapy aide to help with activities and a visiting general practitioner. Access to the multi-professional community psychogeriatric team is available when necessary.

In their comparison of the domus with two long-stay psychogeriatric hospital wards, all of which catered for severely disturbed elderly demented people, Lindesay et al (1991) found significantly higher levels of staff-resident interaction and resident activity in the domus. The domus staff expected residents to function as independently as possible, to have choice and control and to take part in social and recreational activities if they wished. The domus residents, who were comparable to the ward residents in severity of cognitive impairment and depression, were significantly more independent in dressing, washing, feeding and toileting. They were also more adept in orientation, recognition of visitors and communication. The level of job satisfaction of the staff was higher in the domus, although not significantly so.

A later study by the same research group compared two domus settings – one for demented elderly people and the other for elderly people with chronic schizophrenia – with baseline psychogeriatric and psychiatric wards where the residents had lived before moving to the domus (Dean et al 1993). 1 year after the move, the domuses were providing significantly more choice over policy, control by residents, privacy and opportunities for social and recreational activity than occurred in the baseline wards. What was exceptional was that the residents' cognitive function improved after the move, significantly so in the domus for demented residents. One resident spoke within a week of moving to the domus when she had been completely mute for 5 years. They also improved in some activities of daily living and in communication skills over time and were more active and interpersonally engaged than they had been in the wards. As the authors observed: 'The rapid and significant improvement of these demented individuals demonstrates that traditional institutional care can seriously exacerbate their already severe cognitive impairment and that it is possible to reverse this by improving their social environment' (Dean et al 1993, p. 815).

Staff morale was higher in the domus for demented residents, probably because there were more of them, which gave them more time to be with the residents. The staff particularly valued autonomy in decision-making, the greater sense of self-esteem and fulfilment after the move to the domus compared to before.

The costs of domus care were examined by Beecham et al (1993). As they observed, if this group of highly dependent elderly people is to be cared for in the community, as dictated by national policy, then it is easy to predict that their service needs will far outstrip currently available resources. Their cost evaluation of the two domuses studied by Dean et al was comprehensive in that it included all components of individual care packages, it looked at differences in costs between residents, it attempted to compare like with like and it combined costs with information on outcomes. Beecham's group estimated the average (median) cost per resident week in the domus for the elderly folk with dementia to be £951 (range £951–£1017) and, for the elderly people with chronic schizophrenia, to be £909 (range £908–£1038) (adjusted to 1992–1993 prices). Lower costs are reported by Copeland et al (1990) in an earlier study and so allowances would have to be made for inflation. There the average cost per week of care in three experimental nursing homes for elderly mentally ill people was £308, for a specialist hospital that included acute care £313, for a hospital for the elderly mentally infirm £288, for NHS rotating and day care, £180–£223, and for care in a private home, £75–£230. The significant differences in the Copeland study were in staffing levels. Similarly, in the domus study, nearly three-quarters of the total went on staff costs which were much higher than in the hospital wards from which the residents came, which were 56% of the total costs. There is no doubt that the domuses cost more than hospital wards (median, £833 per week for the demented residents and £781 for the chronic schizophrenic group in the domus study) but the quality of care in the domuses and the cognitive and self-care abilities of the residents were higher. The authors conclude:

The results suggest that reducing long-stay hospital provision by replacing it with a *range* of community-based alternatives would bring about overall cost savings, mostly accruing to health authorities, and promote a more cost-effective service. The cost implications of providing domus-style care, however, are not inconsequential, but these clients are among the most dependent in hospital and many patients moving from hospital will require a lower level of community support.
>   (Beecham et al 1993, p. 831, their emphasis)

Thus, even though costs are high, the domus model does enable very dependent mentally frail elderly people to be supported in the community with a high quality of care and a high quality of life, and so 'points a way forward for service developments' (Beecham et al, p. 831).

Night and weekend homes

Current policy favours keeping patients in their own homes with intermittent care provision – day hospitals, day centres, respite care, night sitters, etc. (see Ch. 25).

Also, night hospitals: we know of one night hospital in south London for elderly people with dementia, known as CREST, which was developed to give carers respite and a good night's sleep (Watkins 1994). The old people are collected from home in the evening, given all care needed and helped to bed, are helped to bath and dress in the morning and returned home. If they wish to be up and doing things during the night, that can be accommodated. The great advantage of CREST over a day hospital is that the carer is not left to get the old person up in the morning and to bed at night. Watkin's (1994) evaluation showed that CREST was extremely popular with most of the carers and the behaviour of most of the old people did not change significantly over a 6-month to 2-year period. This she interpreted as a positive outcome in that people with dementia would be expected to deteriorate over time. CREST is now attached to a day hospital so that a combination of day and night care for part of the week can be offered.

There is every likelihood that, for people with dementia, admission to permanent care will occur sooner or later, most often when the informal carer has reached breaking point (unless the old person dies first). One means of looking after the needs of caring relatives, is to provide residential facilities in which the informal carer looks after the old person during the day but hands over the care to paid staff during the nights and weekends. The facility would run along the lines of a domus home and be situated close to the relative's home (Netten 1993). The informal carer would continue to be the key worker and would retain prime responsibility in the facility for the resident during the day. Thus, the person who has been looking after the elderly resident for years and would like to continue to do so, can. These informal carers would 'work' a 5-day week, would use their tremendous skills and knowledge of the resident's needs and wishes, yet have time off at nights and weekends. Professionals would be available for support and advice and they and care assistants would take over the care as and when the informal carer could no longer, or no longer wanted to, cope. This model would be ideal in bridging the difficult transition period for old person and carer, between provision of care at home with insufficient support for informal carers and permanent residential care where staff take over completely.

SUPPORT FROM THE PHYSICAL ENVIRONMENT

Everyone would agree that the physical design of homes should be comfortable, offer privacy and choice and yet be economically viable. Recommendations on the optimum size and design have varied over the years but the personal and public space provided should be conducive to group living (Netten 1993). Group living homes accommodate about 40 people divided into groups of about eight residents. Flatlets, rather than bedrooms, maximise personal privacy, dignity and independence (Peace et al 1982, Willcocks et al 1987), although some residents prefer open public places to their bedsitting rooms or flats (Norman 1984).

Netten refers to the report by the Scottish Action on Dementia (1986) which recommends that environments should meet the principles of normalisation, compensation, individualisation, and integration into the community. But, as we have seen, these principles could be contradictory. It is not 'normal' to have clear signs labelling different rooms but signs do 'compensate' for cognitive deficits; and 'redundant cueing' – making a message available through more than one space – can overcome these conflicting objectives and meet the needs of the cognitively impaired.

There is very little by way of policy recommendations for design of environments for people with dementia, although there is a growing consensus that buildings for people with orientation difficulties should 'make sense' domestically, be small and local with different rooms for different purposes, should create clarity, provide many cues, reduce disorienting features and provide plenty of space for residents and staff (Marshall 1992, Netten 1993).

Norman (1984) identified four types of residential home design – purpose-built single unit, group living unit, ward-like unit and the converted private home.

About a third of the homes in the PSSRU survey of residential accommodation for older people (Darton 1986) were classified as group or semi-group living units in that separate areas existed for daily living, eating and sleeping but were clustered together for small groups of residents. Communal homes or single units, on the other hand, have a single dining area for all residents and several sitting areas and communal areas some distance away from bedrooms.

A clear and easily understood design of home is essential for confused residents to find their way about, and it is the converted home that tends to be the most complex and confusing in layout. Communal homes are often the least confusing although group homes score high on clarity if residents do not stray from their group (Netten 1993).

In her study of residential homes, Netten investigated ambience, personal territory and complexity of the environment.

Ambience

A quiet atmosphere and bright surroundings make it much easier for elderly people with reduced sensory and cognitive abilities to find their way around. Residents who can will find a quiet place or will turn on the light. But reduced competence or environmental restriction will lead to social disturbance, withdrawal or disorientation. Netten found that purpose-built homes are lighter, especially in their communal areas. All the homes in her sample were quiet although in some sitting rooms TV noise dominated. In no home was there quiet music or a hum of conversation; talk was confined to isolated remarks or questions.

Personal territory

Even demented elderly people can be active participants in their physical environment and be affected by it. Officers in charge of homes have been known to place chairs in communal sitting areas in groups only to find them mysteriously moved to positions with their backs to the walls, done, they find, by residents who are there to 'keep an eye on things', not to interact socially (Netten 1993).

Netten distinguishes between physical privacy and territory. Privacy consists of visual, acoustic and olfactory dimensions. Territory is a person's own space, such as where she or he always sits; it need not be private.

Most (around 60%) residential homes have single bedrooms these days (Darton 1986, Netten 1993) which means that residents have access to private as well as public space, although daytime use of bedrooms can be restricted. Demented residents are more likely to find themselves sharing a bedroom and are more likely to be pushed out of their favourite chairs than lucid residents. These residents are likely to be the ones who are allotted less than the minimum of 10 square metres recommended by local authority guidelines. Some authorities advocate residential flatlets rather than single bedrooms because residents spend most of their time in their own rooms (Willcocks et al 1987).

Residents who are surrounded by personal possessions are perceived less negatively by staff than those without (Millard & Smith 1981) and confused residents, in particular, need help in personalising their own space. Observation windows into bedrooms and a change of room will undermine a resident's sense of territory. Reasons given by staff for a change of room are deterioration in a resident's, or co-occupant's, behaviour or a move to a more attractive room (Netten 1993). Any change will reduce the sense of continuity and so can be detrimental to confused residents. In eight out of 13 homes in Netten's study, nearly all the residents had their 'own' chair in the sitting room but only half of the confused residents always sat in the same chair.

Complexity of the environment

Ability to orientate spatially is essential if confused residents are to have any control over their environment (e.g. finding their bedroom or the toilet). In most homes bedroom doors look no different from other doors. Netten (1993) found three aspects influenced residents' ability to find their way around the home:

- personal factors – e.g. degree of intellectual impairment
- social factors – e.g. type of regime in the home
- physical factors – e.g. the layout of the home.

She used regression analysis to analyse the association between the physical environment and the residents' ability to find their way around the home. The factors that were the most significant predictors were the residents' level of orientation, mental ability, physical ability, number of zones to be negotiated, number of complex route-finding decisions to be made, number of exits from the route and level of lighting.

Although her findings were not totally clear-cut, they do support the current preference for group rather than communal living designs. There were two reasons for this. First, residents living in group designs had

more control over their routes in that there were fewer exits where route-finding decisions had to be made than was the case in communal living homes. Second, when physical and mental disability were held constant, more group living homes predicted a higher 'find' score for residents than communal living homes did. That is to say, resident success in finding their way was higher in the group living homes. Netten emphasises that her 'find' measure needs validation but it looks a promising tool for assessing the impact of the physical environment on demented elderly people.

The two homes that had been converted from private housing were the least confusing of all Netten's homes, perhaps because they were the most 'normal'; most like living at home where the bedrooms are upstairs and the living rooms downstairs. One of the most significant factors in Netten's analysis is the number of landmarks, or meaningful decision points, in a route. If each decision point has a landmark that is meaningful to residents then they are likely to make a 'correct' decision. Meaningful landmarks might be an ornament or a picture on the wall or an architectural feature of some kind that attracts attention. Long neutral corridors with identical doors are not meaningful, even for the most lucid of residents.

SUPPORT FROM THE SOCIAL ENVIRONMENT: THE CARING REGIME

Early research showed that the social environment of homes has a major effect on residents' quality of life; promoting, for example, institutional neurosis (Barton 1966) and the negative outcomes of the 'total institution' (Goffman 1961, Kleemeier 1961, Pincus 1968, King et al 1971). Studies such as these suffer from methodological difficulties such as selective intakes, interactive effects between residents and their environment, the multiple variable problem and difficulties in measuring outcome (Netten 1993).

Confused residents are treated differently than lucid residents by staff and other residents and often occupy the least favourable parts of the home. For her research into the quality of life of elderly confused residents of old peoples' homes, Netten (1993) drew from Booth (1985) and Moos and Lemke (1985) to measure the following dimensions using the Sheltered Care Environment Scale (Moos et al 1979), observation and interview:

- relationships: integration into the life of the home, privacy and cohesion and conflict between staff and residents

- personal growth: stimulation (keeping active and participative), freedom and independence (to use the facilities and come and go from the home at will) and continuity (knowledge by the staff of the residents' life histories)
- system maintenance and change: planned care (thought through care plans and policies), regimentation (tasks are staff rather than resident oriented), control by residents over their lives and physical comfort.

Relationships

Friendship

Close friendship is regarded as one of the most important factors in promoting residents' wellbeing, but whether this applies to confused residents too is uncertain. Netten (1993) asked staff for information about friendships they had observed and found that 36% of the residents in seven homes associated regularly with another resident. However, the staff were doubtful that the relationship was true friendship. They argued that true friendship would have a noticeable impact when one of the pair died, but they had noticed no signs of grieving by the survivor. Perhaps it is common for very old people to resist close friendships to protect themselves from the grief of another loss when the friend dies. Close relationships occurred in Netten's study between residents and staff in 27% of cases; but usually residents who had friendships with staff got on well with everybody.

Sometimes confused people are rejected by other residents and become isolated. It is difficult to know how far this rejection occurs in segregated homes and how far friendships are made there. An example of being rejected occurred to my mother who lives in an integrated residential home. She could not understand why another resident, with whom she had shared the same table at mealtimes, had now moved to another table. She blamed the staff, saying that it was unfair and they were punishing her for no good reason. The staff felt unable to tell her that the other resident had asked to be moved because he could not stand my mother's incessant and, to him, meaningless chatter. For her, though, this was yet another loss in her life, the loss of a friend, to add to the loss of her husband, my father, who she claims had 'abandoned' her for another woman and now ignores her when they pass in the street (in fact my father died at this time but my mother has always denied his death).

Privacy

It is likely to be the case that staff will respect the privacy of confused residents less than lucid residents because of the need, they say, to keep a close eye on the confused for their own safety. Netten (1993) reported that most residents (61%) had their own rooms and 9% shared with more than one other. In nearly all the homes in her study residents were able to receive visitors in private.

Only about 25% of residential homes have lockable bedrooms although a similar proportion have access to a lockable drawer (Booth 1985). Netten's study confirms this; the one home she reported to have lockable bedrooms was a specialist home for confused residents. One wonders whether the concern by staff to protect confused residents' safety is always necessary or an unacceptable invasion of their privacy.

Personal growth

Personal growth is not often considered to be relevant to old people, particularly demented old people, even though reality orientation, validation therapy and reminiscence can improve functioning (see Chs 20, 21 and 22). Netten (1993) looked at participation in communal activities, individual activities and freedom allowed to residents as measures of personal growth. She found that organised communal activities have a positive and stimulating effect on residents who are keen to participate but a negative, confusing effect on those who prefer not to take part. Most frequent were group therapy sessions, clubs and live entertainment by staff although the variation between homes was high; some organised 48 activities per month, others only one and specialist homes for confused residents had more activities. Netten found a high correlation between the number of organised activities and the proportion of residents in the home who were confused but, generally speaking, the level of organised activity was not high.

Staff in homes face conflict in getting the balance right between allowing residents freedom to roam in and outside the home at will and restricting their freedom through concern for their safety. How much can homes afford to take risks and let confused residents roam freely? Box 27.4 shows the dilemma the staff of the residential home face in getting the balance right with my mother.

Netten found that residents in most of the homes she studied are given free access to communal spaces in the home and to bedrooms, although some homes restrict daytime bedroom use. In practice, unaccom-

Box 27.4 Striking a balance between safety and risk-taking

My mother could be described as a 'purposeful wanderer' in that she objects strongly if prevented from going out at any time of day or night. For a long time the staff did not restrict her. She always had an objective they knew – shopping, church, to look after the children – which she could not articulate, and she would find her way back – usually. But sometimes she did not; she would get lost and be brought back to anxious staff by the police. It was only when she began wanting to go out in the middle of the night and became aggressive and angry if prevented, that a psychogeriatrician was called, and that led to chemical restraint in the form of a psychotropic drug. Now she is more acquiescent, less agitated and less likely to wander. The staff say she is more peaceful and much easier to handle; their relief is obvious. The family sees a changed, deteriorating but calmer person. We are also relieved except when there is evidence of drug overdose and she cannot control her bladder and bowel. Who is the beneficiary of the drug – my mother or the home and family?

panied use of the grounds occurred in only 27% of her sample even though 94% said residents could roam freely in the grounds. Only four out of 13 homes had an enclosed and secure outside area and, for many staff, running the risk of residents wandering off and getting lost was inexcusable.

Another aspect of personal growth is what Netten refers to as continuity, or knowledge by the staff of the resident's background. The more the staff know about residents – their life histories, their families, their personalities – the better able they are to handle stress and negative behaviour (see Ch. 21 on validation therapy for more on this). Netten identified retention of their own GP, having their own possessions in their rooms and visitors as indicators of continuity. Most of the residents in her sample had not kept their GP but used the one assigned to the home, and only in half the homes could personal items of furniture be accommodated. Most residents (70%) received visitors at least monthly but only 64% of the demented residents did. Only 11% of the demented residents went out with visitors and weekends or holidays away were rare.

System maintenance and change

The balance between flexibility and regimentation is an important part of the caring regime. For demented

people, a high level of organised routine may not be a negative feature; organisational clarity (e.g. regular care planning and review) is positive as long as it is compatible with residents' needs. A rigid approach, however, indicates low tolerance of residents' 'challenging' behaviour (Netten 1993) and the more dependent residents are, the more likely will they be regimented (Booth 1985).

Netten measured regimentation by recording whether care tasks were done at the resident's or the staff's convenience. For example, she found 'block toileting' – done for the convenience of staff irrespective of the resident's expressed wish – to be carried out in eight out of 13 homes, but 85% of incontinent residents were toileted regularly. 10 of the homes said they had set getting up and bathing times; in practice no resident had choice although the homes did try to allocate key workers on a regular basis. Bedtime was a more relaxed affair with only those who needed help being put to bed at times that suited the staff.

Being in a position to retain control over our lives enhances quality of life. Netten measured residents' control by the existence of a resident's committee, choice of food at mealtimes, existence of a payphone or telephone extensions in bedrooms and choice of clothing. She found that only one home had a residents' committee, although two others had tried but failed, choice of menu occurred in only two out of the 13 homes, a payphone was available in 11 but no-one had a telephone extension in their bedroom and, although all the homes encouraged residents to choose their own clothes, 29% of the confused residents had new clothes chosen for them.

Some writers are pessimistic about the degree of control staff have over quality of care in residential homes (e.g. Booth 1986). Netten (1993, p. 108), however, challenges this pessimism, saying: 'Many of the influences found to be of importance for outcomes of elderly demented people are well within the control of staff, given sufficient motivation and resources. The conflicting needs of elderly people with confusional difficulties mean that providing good quality care will always be a balancing act, but one that is clearly possible to accomplish'.

All types of long-stay care for elderly people – hospital and residential – aim to promote residents' quality of life, choice, privacy, dignity, fulfilment and homeliness of the environment but not all achieve these aims. Challiner et al (1994) compared quality of care in 116 long-stay settings using a postal questionnaire that they had developed and validated. They found quality of care to be significantly lower in

NHS hospital continuing care wards compared to local authority residential homes and private residential and nursing homes. The wards catered for residents with the highest dependency levels which confirmed the hypothesis that resident dependency is negatively related to quality of care. The authors' explanation for the findings was that residents living in old 'workhouse back wards' with poor amenities have high dependency, more residential homes are modern, purpose-built and attractive, and staff in high dependency settings have to spend more time on physical needs so that the sociorecreational aspects of care suffer. There is, though, no good reason why dependent residents should not enjoy the same quality of care as the more able.

Macdonald et al (1990) investigated physical dependence and confusion levels of residents in hospital long-stay wards together with the physical state of the wards and the residents' perception of their physical and social surroundings. The study sample covered 808 elderly residents in 61 wards in 32 hospitals in what was then the South West Thames Regional Health Authority in England. 51% of the residents were aged over 85 and 60% had occupied a hospital bed for over 1 year. As found by Challiner et al (1994), the residents were very dependent on staff for help with bathing, dressing, toileting, transferring from bed to chair and maintaining continence, but they were able to feed themselves. Over half had a 'low level of awareness'. 36% only (291 of the 808) were fit enough to be interviewed and, although there were wide variations between districts, most of the residents were positive about the social environment, saying that the atmosphere was cheerful and homely, they could get a good night's sleep, they had visitors, they could go out as they liked and they were not lonely. Less positive was that there was not enough to do and time passes too slowly.

The residents were generally satisfied with the physical amenities – clothing was kept in good repair, meals were large enough, they could bathe and use the toilet in private, the ward appearance was acceptable and they were able to control the ambient temperature. More negatively, there was nowhere to meet visitors in private and no place to be alone.

The degree of personal autonomy was high, residents saying that they could do as they please, go to bed when they liked, wear their own clothes, have their own possessions, choose who to sit with and have a say in ward affairs. Most (90%), though, said that visiting time was insufficient; unrestricted visiting is not universal, it seems. Perceptions of the staff were positive and negative. Generally speaking, nurses were kind and would respond to complaints, they could see the doctor when they wished, and the staff were polite and respectful. But a substantial minority of residents were critical of doctors for losing interest in them or for not being available when wanted and some residents were afraid of the staff because they made fun of them. These findings might be overly positive because of the reluctance of patients and residents to criticise through fear of reprisal. The findings do show that residents who live in hospital are treated as, and take the role of, patients.

A good atmosphere is essential in influencing positive staff-resident relationships. Without it residents and staff do not communicate; they look bored, unhappy and apathetic. Environments with a good atmosphere are different; there is more activity, more communication and interest, and more team working (Smith 1989). Flexible leadership, a degree of risk-taking and supportive managers contribute to this atmosphere.

Is there any difference in care regime in homes with a high proportion of nurses compared to those with few? Netten (1993) found that the proportion of staff with nursing qualifications was associated with an increase in residents' apathy but their level of orientation improved. It may be that nurses are more likely to regard quiet residents as 'good' and 'no trouble', and their knowledge of dementia enables them to work more effectively than other staff in promoting orientation.

One of the homes in Netten's study that emerged with poor resident outcome scores was run in a way that was oriented more to staff than residents. There was no choice over clothes and bedtimes, and staff took residents to the toilet in a wheelchair for convenience rather than encouraging them to walk. The home was noisy, and more of the staff were nurses than was the case in other homes. This home had low staff turnover and sickness and a low level of psychotropic drug prescribing, but there was a tendency to underestimate residents' abilities. Over-control and over-protectiveness seems to be characteristic of this kind of home.

The association between number of care staff and quality of care is not clear. Willcocks et al (1987) found that positive resident-oriented care practices occurred with higher staff ratios and more part-time staff, but Lemke and Moos (1986) found no association between staffing and quality of care. It is probably the case that staffing above a certain level has little effect on quality but below that level, care suffers (Bond et al 1989).

We can sum up the principles of care required in residential care settings for elderly people with mental disorders settings by quoting from the statement published by the Social Services Inspectorate and Department of Health (1993). This document specifies 19 minimum standards of residential care for elderly people (Box 27.5). It draws on the views of users and providers of residential care and follows the earlier documents, *Home Life* (Avebury 1984) and *A Positive Choice* (Wagner 1988).

Other guidance for promoting quality of life for residents in old people's homes can be found in Youll & McCourt-Perring (1993) who evaluated the Caring

---

Box 27.5 Principles of residential care for elderly people

Residential care for mentally frail older people should:
1. Offer residents the opportunity to enhance their quality of life.
2. Involve residents in all decisions unless there are good reasons against this.
3. Assume residents are capable of making choices about their own lifestyle unless it is clear that they cannot.
4. Provide each resident with a written contract agreeing terms of residence and the services provided.
5. Require a trial period before a decision about long-term residence is made.
6. Offer residents the opportunity to review their situation regularly.
7. Inform residents in writing of the complaints procedure which includes consultation with officials outside the home.
8. Ensure residents retain their citizens' rights and help them to exercise these.
9. Ensure residents have unrestricted access to all community support services.
10. Ensure residents have continuity in personal care and in maintaining their former links.
11. Provide private accommodation, preferably single lockable rooms.
12. Ensure residents' needs and wishes are respected, particularly with regard to ethnic, religious and cultural factors.
13. Ensure residents can retain and be treated with dignity.
14. Ensure that staff regard the needs of residents as paramount.
15. Avoid institutional practices that restrict residents' rights and choices.
16. Specify the home's functions, objectives and services clearly.
17. Monitor and evaluate performance against its aims and objectives.
18. Ensure day care and other activities do not interfere with the lifestyle of residents.
19. Involve residents in the use of the home for activities (e.g. fund raising).

(from SSI/DH 1993, pp. 48–50)

---

in Homes Initiative set up by the Department of Health to follow up recommendations of the Wagner review (Wagner 1988).

MEASUREMENT

Knowing what the best model of care for elderly mentally frail people in residential settings is poses enormous challenges for care providers, particularly when residents cannot express their views. How can the quality of life of elderly residents with dementia be measured and what affects their quality of life? These are questions that Netten (1993) sought to answer. She developed a 'model of environmental effect' to show the association between demented residents and their care environment.

Her approach emphasises the demands of the environment on the resident, described as 'environmental press' and the 'environmental docility hypothesis' (Lawton 1982). A positive affect and adaptive behaviour by residents depends on their competence and aspects of the environment working interdependently. The environmental docility hypothesis states that the lower the resident's competence, the more likely will his or her behaviour be influenced by environmental forces. This suggests that getting the environmental forces right is of crucial importance to the quality of life of elderly residents with dementia, in particular.

Netten developed Moos and Lemke's (1985) model ' ... in which the personal and environmental influences are linked to adaptive behaviour by means of cognitive appraisal and coping response' (Netten 1993, p. 17). She made use of Lawton's (1982) four dimensions of the environment – the supra-personal, personal, social and physical – and attempted to link these causally to residents' individual experience, coping, stability and change.

Using Moos et al's (1979) Sheltered Care Environment Scale, Netten (1993) compared the homes for lucid and confused elderly people in her sample to US norms in nursing and residential homes. Netten's homes scored significantly higher, on average, on conflict between residents and their influence over the home's rules and regulations, and significantly lower on cohesion between staff and residents, resident independence and organisational order. There was no significant difference on any of the dimensions for the confused compared to lucid residents.

Social climates of homes have been classified into categories according to the openness of their regimes. For example, Netten refers to Timko and Moos's (1991) classification of homes into six categories:

- supportive, self-directed
- supportive, well organised
- open conflict
- suppressed conflict
- emergent positive
- unresponsive.

Booth's (1985) classification is simpler:

- positive homes – high freedom, high choice
- mixed homes – high in some areas, low in others
- restrictive homes – low freedom, low choice.

Netten (1993) did a cluster analysis on her 13 homes based on their Sheltered Care Environment Scale scores and found that four were positive in regime, six were mixed and three were restrictive. The positive homes had significantly higher resident influence, independence, cohesion and conflict scores. So, where residents had influence in the running of the home, for example, the level of conflict in the home was relatively high. Netten put the profile of her positive homes on a par with Timko and Moos's emergent-positive type. Her restrictive and mixed homes were closest to their open conflict type.

Netten argues persuasively for her method's potential as a measure of home regime using the Sheltered Care Environment Scale. A home scoring over 30 on independence and over 80 on resident influence, for example, would, she says, be positive in its regime. A home scoring less than 12 on independence would be restrictive.

Audit and quality assurance

Smith (1989) provides advice on assessing the quality of life and quality of care of people in long-stay psychiatric hospitals by drawing from guidance on quality assessment for people with learning disabilities. She identifies six stages:

- Stage 1: identify the stake-holders – residents, relatives, care staff, managers, representatives of voluntary organisations, etc. – and formulate a group of workable size; large enough to represent all interests but small enough to work effectively (about 8–10 people).
- Stage 2: agree the principles of care that are important about the residents' lives rather than service principles.
- Stage 3: define what it means for residents and staff to put the principles into practice. This can stimulate creative ways of working and identify what changes are needed.

- Stage 4: take a small number of issues at a time and record current working practices.
- Stage 5: specify action goals that accord to the principle.
- Stage 6: monitor the goals regularly to ensure that the changes are implemented.

This guidance applies equally to any long-stay group. It follows the audit cycle of identifying the problem, setting standards, assessing or measuring the care, identifying change needed, implementing the change and monitoring its effects.

When assessing quality of services for people with severe disabilities, including elderly people with dementia, two questions asked by Smith (1989) are: how do you know what to change and how do you change it? In deciding what to change, Smith's advice is to ask and observe the residents. Never underestimate people's ability, even demented people, to communicate; learn to 'listen' through gesture, expression and other behaviour as well as through speech; get to understand how people experience a service by 'shadowing' them over long periods and joining in 'getting to know you' exercises; use role play with staff so that they understand what it is like to be dependent and controlled; and set up an independent advocacy service for people who cannot speak for themselves. In deciding how to change things, the underlying principle is about empowering residents and staff. If they are involved in collecting the evidence, suggesting changes and evaluating their effects, they are likely to take ownership and work to implement change. Smith sums the outcome of this kind of approach thus:

It would seem to us that if nurses are skilful, discreet, communicative, genuine, warm, a team, respectful, respected, informative, consultative, ordinary people, understanding, teachers, listeners, share decision-making, risk-takers, not possessive, approachable, democratic [and] confident [then] residents feel safe, have dignity, feel trusted, feel trust, feel warmth, feel secure, feel respected, feel respectful, feel informed, feel powerful, are ordinary people, feel understood, can learn, feel like talking, have control, have freedom, have self-esteem, less isolated, can have autonomy. (Smith 1989, p. 19)

Collins (1993) gives similar advice in assessing the quality of life of people who cannot communicate or understand and argues that assessments be made by whoever knows the resident best. Rules and regulations required to achieve environmental health standards result in loss of homeliness and ordinariness; not allowing the cat into the kitchen, heavy fire doors and fire extinguishers, for example. The regulations requiring these standards make it impossible for group living homes to be like home.

Since the NHS and Community Care Act (1990), the importance of service evaluation has been emphasised strongly (Ramon 1991). Professionals have, Ramon tells us, traditionally evaluated a service by focusing on user outcomes and programme outcomes and not the process that led to the outcome. In normalisation and SRV the process is as important as the outcome because the way in which a service is delivered is so significant in social evaluation. SRV proponents look at the extent to which the principles of normalisation and its values, incuding its administration and cost effectiveness, are implemented. For example, they consider:

- examples of physical and social integration
- appropriateness of structures and interpretations for residents of different ages
- quality of the setting – physical comfort, environmental beauty, individualisation and interaction (Ramon 1991).

Staff, users and community representatives are included in this quality assurance process. Wolfensberger & Glenn (1978) developed the Program Analysis of Service Systems (PASS) as a quantitative method for evaluating human services that takes these aspects into account.

Wagner (1988) recommended that a system of self-regulation and performance review should be a condition of registration for all residential and nursing homes, which would require all homes to have a good understanding of what constitutes good quality and

how it can be assessed. The focus of the Department of Health/Social Services Inspectorate (1989, cited in Netten 1993) is increasingly on residents' quality of life, quality of care and quality of management in the home. Basic values they look for include privacy, dignity, independence, choice, rights and fulfilment but, as Wagner (1988) recognises, it is difficult to measure whether these values are put into practice when their indicators are difficult to define and when there is no direct evidence of what is important to elderly mentally ill people. Netten (1993) points out that what is appropriate for confused elderly people might reveal apparent contradictions in these values. For example, is it better to allow a resident the choice to dress in a bizarre fashion or to promote her dignity by persuading her to wear the clothes she wore quite appropriately before she developed dementia? This contradiction aside, Netten recommends the Sheltered Care Environmental Scale (Moos et al 1979) as a useful tool for inspectors of homes to use.

The Social Services Inspectorate/Department of Health (1993) report offers guidance to people who purchase, register, inspect or manage residential service provision on what to look for and how to decide whether acceptable standards are practised. The report specifies standards, their criteria and evidence that would show whether the criteria have been met. The standards refer to values (of privacy, dignity, independence, choice and rights), decision-making, risk-taking, restraint, the environment, health care, relatives and friends and equal opportunities. As an example, Table 27.1 includes some of the criteria and evidence to look for specified under the health care standard.

Table 27.1 Extract from the health care standard recommended by the Social Services Inspectorate and Department of Health (1993)

Standard: elderly people with mental disorders have the same rights of access to necessary health care facilities as any other citizen

Criteria	Evidence to look for
Full health care information and health care history is gathered at the time of admission	Pre-admission information on file
Specialist doctors and GPs contribute to assessment in appropriate cases	Assessment and individual programme plan records
Relationships with health care professionals are well developed	Evidence in assessment records and individual programme plans Views of users, relatives and friends Appropriate staff are seen to be involved during inspection
The hearing of users is maintained to the highest possible level and remaining hearing is optimised	Regular hearing tests Hearing aids fit and are worn Hearing aids are kept clean Batteries are regularly checked and replaced when necessary Staff notice, and take action, when users appear to be hearing less well

Methods of measurement for use with elderly mentally frail people

Quality of life in residential settings requires knowledge of the resident's value system and involves measurement of living arrangements, resident-environment fit, residents' perceptions of their care and the degree of restrictiveness of practices in the home (Bowling 1995). Assessment scales completed by residents are continually being developed and the reader is referred to Bowling (1995) for a recent review of symptom scales, quality of life instruments and role functioning measures for use with people with psychiatric conditions and psychological morbidity. Many elderly mentally infirm people can complete scales with help (Macdonald et al 1988) but the only feasible way to assess the quality of life of severely demented people is to use observation.

Observation schedules can record quantitative information (such as promptness of staff response to residents' requests, refreshments available, activities performed) and more qualitative information (such as content of conversations, non-verbal behaviour and facial expressions). Another approach is to collect vignettes of the everyday life of the old person from observations of the sufferer and interviews with family members. Kitwood (1990, 1993, Kitwood & Bredin 1992) took this approach in his development of a dialectic theory of the dementing process.

Balogh et al (1993) analysed six systems used in assessing the quality of psychiatric nursing in mental health settings:

- the Central Nottinghamshire Psychiatric Nursing Audit (CNPNA) (Howard & Hurst 1987)
- Standards of Care and Practice Audit (SCAPA) (Worcester District Health Authority 1987)
- Quality Review Teams (QUARTZ) (Hill & Lieper 1992)
- Achievable Standards of Care (City & Hackney Health Authority 1987)
- Psychiatric Monitor (Goldstone & Doggett 1989)
- Quality Evaluation of Standards (QUEST) (Jardine et al 1987).

Balogh's team do not recommend a best buy. Instead, they take the view that each system has advantages and disadvantages and will be more or less useful in different settings. Their analysis addressed six dimensions:

- status of the system – publication details, manual or computer application, verification of reliability and validity, etc.
- sphere of application – client group, professionals, settings
- constitution – identity of auditor, staff involvement, etc.
- advice and guidance – training required, guidance on auditing and data collection, etc.
- data collection – data sources, collection format, sample size, topics covered, etc.
- results – analysis method, presentation, ownership, dissemination, etc.

Copeland et al (1990) evaluated care provision of three experimental homes for elderly mentally infirm people. They could not employ an experimental method with random allocation of residents to facilities and a control group but they could make comparisons between the experimental homes and other units on staff resources, the social and physical environment, resident dependence and the social regime. They used a comprehensive range of measures:

- the Clifton Assessment Procedures for the Elderly (CAPE) (Pattie & Gilleard 1979) for asessing patient dependency
- the Crichton Royal Behavioural Rating Scale (CRBRS) (Charlesworth & Wilkin 1982) for physical and mental functioning, ADL task ability, behavioural problems
- interview and self-completion questionnaires for staff opinions and attitudes (included interviews with psychogeriatricians and nursing officers)
- interview for relatives' views
- diaries for staff activity analysis in which their interactions with residents were described as 'demanding' (crisis intervention), 'routine' (day-to-day supportive care) or 'positive' (care designed to enhance quality of life)
- observation – of two day shifts in each home divided into half-hour periods. The observer recorded the activity of everyone seen – residents, staff, visitors – together with the location of the individual, what she was doing, interaction with others, nature of any speech, details of direct care by staff and whether it was 'demanding', 'routine', or 'positive', observable signs of residents' state of mind (sadness, irritation, anxiety). The observation was used to validate the diaries and record patterns of living and social interaction
- Booth's (1985) Institutional Regimes Questionnaire to measure the social environment (personal choice, privacy, segregation, participation)
- Robinson et al's (1984) architectural checklist to distinguish homely from institutional characteristics of the building and layout

- documentation – case notes, reports, minutes of meetings, local area statistics and financial information
- costs of each home compared to a psychogeriatric ward.

Knapp et al (1992, 1994) used the following methods in their evaluation of the 28 projects in the Care in the Community demonstration programme, four of which were for elderly mentally frail people:

- the CAPE Behaviour Rating Scale (Pattie & Gilleard 1979) which contains four subscales for staff to assess residents' skills and behaviour: physical disability, apathy, communication difficulties and social disturbance
- Cantril's (1965) Ladder and the PGC Morale Scale (Lawton 1975, adapted for England by Challis & Knapp 1980) to assess resident morale and life satisfaction
- Snaith et al's (1971) Depression Inventory
- an author developed Personal Presentation Checklist to cover residents' clothes, general appearance and unusual traits
- Henderson's Interview Schedule for Social Interaction (Henderson et al 1981)
- items from Raynes et al (1979) and Wykes (1982) to assess residents' lifestyle and living environment
- interviews with residents for their participation in daily activities.

Challiner et al (1994) developed and validated a method for evaluating the quality of long-stay hospital and residential care by brief postal survey which they adapted from the schedule for quality measurement in local authority homes developed by Willcocks and her colleagues (1987). The questionnaire contains 18 items, selected by residents and staff as the most important indicators of quality of care, which were answered by care staff. The items include resident freedom (to use their rooms when they choose, to come and go outside the home, to have privacy, go to bed when they wish); resident growth (taught new skills, encouraged to maintain their self-care skills and to help themselves, staff are encouraged to sit and talk with residents); and environmental facilities (separate toilets for men and women, lockable cupboards in bedrooms, opportunity to make telephone calls in private, accessible bedside lights, a lounge with no TV, an accessible garden, a place to meet visitors in private).

Intra-rater and inter-rater reliability of the measures were high and validity, assessed by correlating scores with those from an interview with the home/ward manager and the quality of care delivered by care workers, was also high. The scale was considered sensitive in that it discriminated significantly between settings with different levels of resident dependence (using the Barthel Index, Mahoney & Barthel 1965). Although the authors argue that more research on quality of care of demented residents is needed, they regard this brief measure as a cost-effective way of monitoring quality in a large number of settings. It could, they say, be used as a screening tool by the local authority inspectorate or by home managers as a regular audit tool. High and low scoring homes could then be studied in greater depth so that the successes can be understood and the deficiencies rectified.

Disturbed behaviour in dementia sufferers can be assessed using Patel and Hope's (1992) Rating Scale for Aggressive Behaviour in the Elderly (RAGE), a 23-item scale completed on the basis of observations over 3 days. 19 of the items refer to the behaviour of residents and four items focus on methods used to control them. Using this scale in Victoria, Australia, Martin et al (1994) found the highest level of disturbed behaviour in nursing homes catering for elderly mentally infirm people but there was no correlation between RAGE score and degree of cognitive impairment.

Measuring activities, quality of care and quality of life of elderly mentally frail people is clearly extremely difficult, particularly if they cannot communicate. When asking the resident directly is impossible, direct observation and interviews with staff and family members are the most appropriate proxy measures. As we have seen from the study of the three experimental nursing homes for the mentally frail (Copeland et al 1990) and the Care in the Community demonstration programme (Knapp et al 1992, 1994), a comprehensive evaluation demands multiple methods.

CONCLUSION

This chapter has looked at support of old people living in residential settings. The principles of high quality continuing care for elderly mentally ill people emphasise that they have the same human values and rights as anyone else, they have the right to be treated as ordinary people and to participate in their communities, and they have the right to an individual plan of care that meets their needs and is regularly reviewed with them and their families and amended as necessary. We have considered what ordinary living is all about and how it differs from institutional living.

Should demented residents be segregated in special homes or integrated with other old people in ordinary residential homes? Proponents of normalisation reject segregation and argue most persuasively that integration is a necessary, if not sufficient, requirement for achieving the principles of ordinary living. Others, including user pressure groups, favour an increase in specialist provision to improve the quality of life and quality of care of mentally frail old people. The debate is not clear cut. Mildly or moderately demented old people are probably happier living in integrated settings. Severly demented people are probably better off in special accommodation, like domus units, where their needs are given priority.

The hospital closure programme and development of alternative accommodation have paid little attention to the wishes of residents. Policies and procedures for transferring elderly mentally ill people could do well to study the approach taken by Italy and the successful transfer process developed for some people with learning disabilities. Models of care that seem to be most beneficial for demented residents favour group living, in ordinary residential flats as in Sweden or in domus units as introduced in one London borough.

The approach in domus units, that puts as much emphasis on the needs and development of staff as it does on the residents, has shown that a good quality of life and high quality of care can be achieved for this vulnerable group.

Assessing the quality of care provision for elderly people in residential settings is extremely difficult, especially for those whose communication skills have failed them. Multiple methods of measurement, including observation, are complex and expensive but necessary. Self-regulation and performance monitoring should be a condition of registration for all residential and nursing homes and made explicit within their contracts with residents. The guidance now offered by the Social Services Inspectorate and Department of Health (1993) makes it likely that more homes will demonstrate that acceptable standards are met and that fewer unscrupulous homes can get away without detection. Legal and ethical issues surrounding elderly people living in residential care, and the mental health care of elderly patients, are the subject of the next chapter.

REFERENCES

Alfredson B, Annerstedt L 1994 Staff attitudes and job satisfaction in the care of demented elderly people: group living compared with long-term care institutions. Journal of Advanced Nursing 20: 964–974

Annerstedt L 1993 Development and consequences of group living in Sweden: a new mode of care for demented elderly. Social Science and Medicine 37: 1529–1538

Annerstedt L, Fournier K, Gustafson L et al 1993a Group living for people with dementia. Dementia Services Development Centre, Department of Applied Social Science, School of Human Sciences, University of Stirling

Annerstedt L, Gustafson L, Nilsson K 1993b Medical outcome of psychosocial intervention in demented patients. International Journal of Geriatric Psychiatry 8: 833–841

Avebury K 1984 Home life. Report of a working party chaired by Kina, Lady Avebury, Centre for Policy on Ageing, London

Baker D E 1983 'Care' in the geriatric ward: an account of two styles of nursing. In: Wilson-Barnett J (ed) Nursing research: ten studies in patient care. Wiley and Sons, Chichester

Balogh R, Bond S, Simpson A, Quinn H 1993 An analysis of instruments and tools used in psychiatric nursing audit. Centre for Health Services Research, University of Newcastle, Newcastle

Barton R 1966 Institutional neurosis, 2nd edn. Wright, Bristol

Baxter C, Poonia K, Ward L, Nadirshaw Z 1990 Double discrimination: issues and services for people with learning difficulties from black and ethnic minority communities. King's Fund Centre Commission for Racial Equality, London

Beecham J, Cambridge P, Hallam A, Knapp M 1993 The costs of domus care. International Journal of Geriatric Psychiatry 8: 827–831

Bond J, Bond S, Donaldson C, Gregson B, Atkinson A 1989 Evaluation of an innovation in the continuing care of very frail elderly people. Ageing and Society 9(4): 347–382

Booth T 1985 Home truths: old people's homes and the outcome of care. Gower, Aldershot

Booth T 1986 Institutional regimes and induced dependency in homes for the aged. The Gerontologist 26(4): 418–423

Bowling A 1995 Measuring disease. Open University Press, Buckingham

Brechin A, Swain J 1987 Changing relationships: shared action planning with people with a mental handicap. Harper and Row, London

Cantril H 1965 The pattern of human concerns. New Brunswick, Rutgers University Press, New Jersey

Challiner Y, Watson R, Julious S, Philp I 1994 A postal survey of the quality of long-term institutional care. International Journal of Geriatric Psychiatry 9: 619–625

Challis D J, Knapp M R J 1980 An examination of the PGC Morale Scale in an English context. In: Goldberg E M, Connelly N (eds) 1982 The effectiveness of social care for the elderly, Heinemann Educational Books, London

Charlesworth A, Wilkin D 1982 Dependency among old people in geriatric wards and residential homes. Research Report No. 6. Psychogeriatric Unit, University of Manchester, Manchester

City and Hackney Health Authority 1987 Achievable standards of care for the elderly patient cared for in acute assessment wards, continuing care wards, nursing homes and day hospitals within the City and Hackney Health Authority. King's Fund Centre, London

Collins J 1993 The resettlement game: policy and procrastination in the closure of mental handicap hospitals. Values into Action report. Joseph Rowntree Foundation, London

Copeland J R M, Crosby C, Sixsmith A J, Stilwell J 1990 Three experimental homes for the elderly mentally ill. Final Report. Institute of Human Ageing, University of Liverpool, Liverpool

Darton R 1986 Methodological report of the PSSRU survey of residential accommodation for the elderly, 1981. PSSRU Discussion Paper 422. Personal Social Services Unit, University of Kent, Canterbury

Dean R, Briggs K, Lindesay J 1993 The domus philosophy: a prospective evaluation of two residential units for the elderly mentally ill. International Journal of Geriatric Psychiatry 8: 807–817

Department of Health 1994 Residential accommodation for people with mental illness and learning disabilities: local authority supported residents at March 1993, England. Government Statistical Service, Department of Health, London

Department of Health/Social Services Inspectorate 1989 Homes are for living in. HMSO, London

Ersser S, Tutton E 1991 Primary nursing – a second look. In: Ersser S, Tutton E (eds) Primary nursing in perspective. Scutari Press, Harrow, Middlesex

Evers H 1981 The creation of patient careers in geriatric wards: aspects of policy and practice. Social Science and Medicine 15A: 581–588

Godlove C, Richard L, Rodwell G 1982 Time for action: an observation study of elderly people in four different care environments. Joint Unit for Social Services Research, University of Sheffield, Sheffield

Goffman E 1961 Asylums. Doubleday Anchor Books, New York

Goldstone L A, Doggett D P 1989 Psychiatric Nursing Monitor: an audit of the quality of nursing care in psychiatric wards. Poly Enterprises (Leeds) Ltd, Leeds

Henderson S, Byrne D G, Duncan-Jones P 1981 Neurosis and the social environment. Academic Press, Sydney

Hill R G, Lieper R 1992 Evaluating QUARTZ: a research evaluation of a quality assurance programme. RDP Publications, London

Hodgkinson J 1988 Residential living: lifestyle or life sentence? Booklet No. 2, Homework: meeting the needs of elderly people in residential homes. Centre for Policy on Ageing, London

Howard D, Hurst K 1987 The central Nottinghamshire psychiatric nursing audit, Central Nottinghamshire Health Authority

Jardine C D, Forrest J, Wells J 1987 QUEST: quality evaluation of standards. Grampian Health Board Mental Health Services, Scotland

King R D, Raynes N V, Tizard J 1971 Patterns of residential care. Routledge & Kegan Paul, London

Kitwood T 1990 The dialectics of dementia – with particular reference to Alzheimer's disease. Ageing and Society 10(2): 177–196

Kitwood T 1993 Towards a theory of dementia care: the interpersonal process. Ageing and Society 13(1): 51–67

Kitwood T, Bredin K 1992 Towards a theory of dementia care: personhood and well-being. Ageing and Society 12(3): 269–287

Kleemeier R 1961 The use and meaning of time in special settings. In: Kleemeier R (ed) Ageing and leisure. Oxford University Press, New York

Knapp M, Cambridge P, Thomason C, Beecham J, Allen C, Darton R 1992 Care in the community: challenge and demonstration. Ashgate, Aldershot

Knapp M, Cambridge P, Thomason C, Beecham J, Allen C, Darton R 1994 Residential care as an altermative to long-stay hospital: a cost-effectiveness evaluation of two pilot projects. International Journal of Geriatric Psychiatry 9: 297–304

Lawton M P 1975 The Philadelphia Geriatric Center Morale Scale: a revision. Journal of Gerontology 30: 85–89

Lawton M P 1982 Competence, environmental press and the adaptation of older people. In: Lawton M, Windley P, Byerts T (eds) Aging and the environment: theoretical approaches. Springer, New York

Lemke S, Moos R 1986 Quality of residential settings for elderly adults. Journal of Gerontology 41: 268–276

Lindesay J, Briggs K, Lawes M, Macdonald A, Herzberg J 1991 The domus philosophy: a comparative evaluation of a new approach to residential care for the demented elderly. International Journal of Geriatric Psychiatry 6: 727–736

Lodge B 1990 Alternative homes for people with dementia: new directions in service principles and design. British Association for Service to the Elderly, Newcastle

Macdonald L, Sibbald B, Hoare C 1988 Measuring patient satisfaction with life in a long-stay psychiatric hospital. The International Journal of Social Psychiatry 34(4): 292–304

Macdonald L D, Higgs P F D, Ward M D, Millard P H 1990 Long stay wards for the elderly: the patients and their views. Report to SW Thames Regional Health Authority, St George's Hospital Medical School, London

Mahoney F I, Barthel D W 1965 Functional evaluation: the Barthel Index. Maryland State Medical Journal 14: 61–65

Martin C, McKensie S, Ames D 1994 Disturbed behaviour in dementia sufferers: a comparison of three nursing home settings. International Journal of Geriatric Psychiatry 9: 393–398

Marshall M 1992 Designing for disorientation: guidelines from the Dementia Services Development Centre. In: Coles R, Duncan I, Kelly M, Marshall M, Wightman A (eds) Signposts not barriers. Dementia Services Development Centre, University of Stirling

Millard P H 1983 Long-term care in Europe: a review. In: Denham M J (ed) Care of the long-stay elderly patient. Croom Helm, London

Millard P, Smith C 1981 Personal belongings – a positive effect? The Gerontologist 21(1): 85–90

Miller A F 1985 A study of the dependency of elderly patients in wards using different methods of nursing care. Age and Ageing 14: 132–138

Moos R, Lemke S 1985 Specialised living environments for older people. In: Birren J, Schaie K (eds) Handbook of the psychology of aging. Van Nostrand Reinhold, New York

Moos R, Gauvain M, Lemke S, Max W, Mehren B 1979 Assessing the social environments of sheltered care settings. The Gerontologist 19: 74–82

NHS and Community Care Act 1990. HMSO, London

Netten A 1993 A positive environment? physical and social influences on people with senile dementia in residential care. Ashgate, Aldershot, Hants

Norman A 1984 Bricks and mortals: design and lifestyle in old people's homes. Centre for Policy on Ageing, London

O'Brien J 1988 Framework for accomplishment. Responsive Systems Associates, Decatur, Georgia

Patel V, Hope R 1992 A rating scale for aggressive behavior in the elderly – the RAGE. Psychological Medicine 22: 211–221

Pattie A, Gilleard C 1979 Manual of the Clifton assessment procedures for the elderly (CAPE). Hodder and Stoughton, London

Peace S M, Kellaher L A, Willcocks D M 1982 A balanced life: a consumer study of residential life in 100 local authority old people's homes. Research Report No. 14. Survey Research Unit, Polytechnic of North London

Pincus A 1968 The definition and measurement of the institutional environment in institutions for the aged and its impact on residents. International Journal of Ageing and Human Development 1: 117–126

Ramon S (ed) 1991 Beyond community care. Macmillan in association with MIND, Basingstoke and London

Raynes N V, Pratt M, Roses S 1979 Organisational structure and care of the mentally retarded. Croom Helm, London

Redfern S J 1996 Individualised patient care: its meaning and practice in a general setting. NT research 1(1): 23–33

Robinson J W, Thompson T, Emmons P, Graff M, Franklin E 1984 Towards an architectural definition of normalization: design principles for housing severely and profoundly retarded adults. Center for Urban and Regional Affairs, University of Minnesota, Minneapolis

Rothwell N A, Britton P G, Woods R T 1983 The effects of group living in a residential home for the elderly. British Journal of Social Work 13: 639–643

Scottish Action on Dementia 1986 Principles relating to the design of residential environments for dementia sufferers. Discussion Paper. Scottish Action on Dementia, Edinburgh

Smith H (ed) 1989 Commitment to quality: safeguarding quality of care in long stay psychiatric hospitals. Community Living Development Team Discussion Paper, KFC No 89/44. King's Fund Centre, London

Snaith R P, Ahmed S N, Mehta S, Hamilton M 1971 Assessment of the severity of primary depressive illness. Psychological Medicine 1: 143–149

Social Services Inspectorate, Department of Health 1993 Inspecting for quality: standards for the residential care of elderly people with mental disorders. HMSO, London

Timko C, Moos R 1991 A typology of social climates in group residential facilities for older people. Journal of Gerontology 46(3): 160–169

Wagner G 1988 Residential care: a positive choice. National Institute of Social Work, HMSO, London

Watkins M 1994 An evaluation of CREST, a night hospital for elderly people suffering from dementia. Unpublished PhD thesis, Department of Nursing Studies, King's College London

Wells T 1980 Problems in geriatric care. Churchill Livingstone, Edinburgh

Willcocks D, Peace S, Kellaher L 1987 Private lives in public places: a research-based critique of residential life in local authority old people's homes. Tavistock, London

Wimo A, Wallin J O, Lundgren K, Rönnbäck E, Asplund K, Mattsson B, Krakau I 1991 Group living, an alternative for dementia patients: a cost analysis. International Journal of Geriatric Psychiatry 6: 21–29

Wing J K, Brown G W 1970 Institutionalism and schizophrenia. Cambridge University Press, Cambridge

Wolfensberger W 1972 The principle of normalisation in human services. National Institute on Mental Retardation, Toronto

Wolfensberger W, Glenn L 1978 PASS 3, Program Analysis of Service Systems: a method for the quantitative evaluation of human services. Field Manual. National Institute on Mental Retardation, York University, Toronto

Wolfensberger W, Thomas S 1994 Obstacles in the professional human service culture to implementation of social role valorisation and community integration of clients. Care in Place 1(1): 53–56

Worcester and District Health Authority 1987 Standards of Care and Practice Audit (SCAPA) Psychiatry. Department of Quality Assurance, Worcester and District Health Authority

Wykes T 1982 A hostel for 'new' long-stay patients: an evaluative study of a 'ward in a house'. In: Wing J K (ed) Long-term community care: experience in a London borough. Psychological Medicine, Monograph Supplement 2: 57–97

Youll P J, McCourt-Perring 1993 Raising voices: ensuring quality in residential care. HMSO, London

RECOMMENDED READING

Booth T 1985 Home truths: old people's homes and the outcome of care. Gower, Aldershot. *This is an account of an empirical study of the environment and care regime in residential homes for elderly people and their effects on outcomes of care. It looks at resident dependency and caring practices and assesses whether the caring regime has a measurable effect on the wellbeing of residents. Although over 10 years old now, it continues to be useful reading both for its methodology and the policy implications that emerged.*

Bowling A 1995 Measuring disease. Open University Press, Buckingham. *This is a companion volume to Ann Bowling's earlier book,* Measuring Health: a review of quality of life measurement scales. Open University Press, Milton Keynes, 1991. *Together they contain a huge number of scales designed to measure symptoms of ill health, wellbeing and quality of life, role functioning, stress and coping, and so on. Also included are reviews of the strengths and weaknesses of each scale together with its reliability and validity, if evidence is available. So, a very useful source book for readers who are searching for outcome measures for their evaluation of care.*

Knapp M, Cambridge P, Thomason C, Beecham J, Allen C, Darton R 1992 Care in the Community: challenge and demonstration. PSSRU, University of Kent, Ashgate, Aldershot. *This team, from the Personal Social Services Research Unit, University of Kent, was commissioned by the Department of Health and Social Security to monitor and evaluate the Care in the Community demonstration programme consisting of 28 pilot projects which moved 900 people with long-term care needs from hospital to community settings. The book describes the pilot projects and the processes of care in each. It evaluates the projects in terms of outcomes and costs for each client group (people with mental health problems, elderly people, people with physical disabilities and people with learning disabilities). The book is recommended for its guidance on carrying out meticulous research on a complex, multidimensional topic.*

Netten A 1993 A positive environment? physical and social influences on people with senile dementia in residential care. Ashgate, Aldershot. *This is a study of local authority residential care for elderly people with dementia. Netten explored how quality of life of demented elderly people can be measured and what affects quality of life of this group. She developed a model of the relationship between the resident and the care environment – the 'model of environmental effect'. This book is recommended for its methodological approach and its policy implications. Netten developed a route-finding measure to*

analyse the relationship between the physical environment and demented residents' ability to find their way around the home.

Ramon S (ed) 1991 Beyond Community Care: normalisation and integration work. Macmillan in association with MIND, Basingstoke and London. *This collection provides a comprehensive account of the principles and theory of normalisation, and experience of normalisation and social role valorisation from the service user's and service provider's perspective. It debates controversial issues and offers solutions to many obstacles that users and their professional and lay carers face.*

Raynes N V, Wright K, Shiell A, Pettipher C 1994 The cost and quality of community residential care: an evaluation of the services for adults with learning disabilities. David Fulton Publishers, London. *This book looks at ways of measuring cost and quality in residential homes. It focuses on homes for people with learning disabilities but its ideas for encouraging cost effective care apply to all residential settings.*

Youll P J, McCourt-Perring 1993 Raising voices: ensuring quality in residential care. HMSO, London. *This is an evaluation and commentary on the national programme of research on residential care – the Caring in Homes Initiative – that was commissioned by the Department of Health following the Wagner Review. The account of the experiences of residents and staff led to a critique of many approaches to care and ideas for improving services to meet residents' needs and wishes.*

28

Legal and ethical issues in mental health care of elderly patients

Phil Fennell

INTRODUCTION

This chapter discusses some of the practical issues which arise in caring for elderly mentally disordered patients in the UK. Elderly patients make up a significant percentage of the psychiatric in-patient population of NHS hospitals and private mental nursing homes. Estimates published by the Department of Health (1993a) for the financial year 1990–1991 show that of 200 300 psychiatric admissions to NHS hospitals, 23 300 (11.6%) were of patients aged between 65 and 74, and 40 200 (20%) were aged 75 and over. The characteristic mental health problems of old age tend to be dementia and depressive disorders. Although many of the ethical and legal questions relating to the care of elderly patients apply equally to others, there are some problems which have a particular impact on this group.

The basic legal and ethical framework for the mental health system is provided by the Mental Health Act 1983, common law rules and principles developed through case-law, the Mental Health Act *Code of Practice* issued by the Department of Health and the Welsh Office, and guidance on various aspects of care issued by the Mental Health Act Commission (MHAC) or professional bodies such as the BMA or the UKCC. Codes are a form of 'soft law', in the sense that they are not legally binding, but in the event of legal proceedings arising out of failure to follow relevant guidance, professionals would be expected to produce a reason for their conduct. As the *Code of Practice* on the 1983 Act points out, the legislation does not impose a duty to comply with the Code, but failure to follow it may be referred to in evidence in legal proceedings (Department of Health 1993b, para. 1.1).

The chapter begins by looking at the considerations to be taken into account in deciding whether to use the powers of detention in the 1983 Act or to admit a patient informally. This is followed by a discussion of the legal and ethical importance of seeking consent to treatment as a reflection of the right of self-determination, and the legal duty of doctors and others to obtain consent to treatment from adults who are capable of making their own treatment decisions. The mere fact that someone is diagnosed as suffering from mental disorder or is detained under the Mental Health Act does not necessarily mean that person is incapable of making a legally valid decision about their own medical treatment.

The third section of the chapter deals with the provisions of Part IV of the Mental Health Act 1983 on consent to treatment. After outlining the basic scheme of Part IV, this section describes the operation of section 57 of the 1983 Act, which provides that certain more serious treatments such as psychosurgery may only be given with valid consent from the patient and a favourable second opinion from an independent doctor. The discussion then turns to the provisions of Part IV governing the circumstances in which treatment may justifiably be given without consent to detained patients. Once the possibility exists of treating people who cannot speak for themselves without first explaining what is proposed and seeking their consent, an additional ethical burden arises of ensuring that the proposed intervention is necessary, is genuinely in the person's interests, and above all is not harmful. Section 58 of the 1983 Act institutes a system of second opinions to provide a safeguard where treatment is given without consent, and the roles of different health care professionals and the second opinion doctor in this process are outlined. This is followed by a discussion of the common law provisions relating to the treatment of mentally incapacitated patients without consent. The chapter concludes with an analysis of the possibilities for elderly patients to make advance treatment directives and the vexed question of 'do not resuscitate' (DNR) orders.

THE DECISION TO USE COMPULSORY POWERS UNDER THE MENTAL HEALTH ACT 1983

At the heart of the 1983 Act is the distinction between informal and detained patient status. Section 131 provides that nothing in the Act shall prevent a patient requiring treatment for mental disorder from 'being admitted to any hospital ... in pursuance of arrangements made in that behalf without any application, order or direction rendering him liable to be detained'. Over 90% of psychiatric patients are admitted informally. In the year ending 31 March 1993

there were 263 400 admissions, of which 21 356 were compulsory (Department of Health, *Statistical Bulletin* 1995). Whilst admissions, including compulsory admissions, have risen steadily since 1983, psychiatric beds have reduced from 85 000 in 1981 to 47 000 in 1992 (Jewesbury 1994, para. 5.1). Informal admission does not necessarily mean that they have admitted themselves voluntarily. It is frequently used in cases where patients lack the capacity to consent to going into hospital, and this is often the case with confused elderly patients, with detention being reserved for those who actively object to admission.

The 1983 Act provides safeguards for detained patients. They have to be informed as soon as practicable after admission of the fact that they are detained and made aware of their rights (s 132). They are entitled to apply for review of their detention by a Mental Health Review Tribunal, and if they do not apply within specified periods, their case is automatically reviewed (ss 66 and 68). If they are to be given certain treatments without consent, they are entitled to an independent second opinion (s 58). They are visited by the Mental Health Act Commission (MHAC) which has power to ensure that their complaints are properly investigated (s 120).

As they are not subject to any formal compulsion to remain in hospital or to accept treatment, informal patients do not have access to these safeguards, even though in practice many of them are not consenting to hospital treatment. There are significant numbers of elderly patients whose status is informal but who have no practical means of exercising their theoretical right to leave the hospital because they lack the mental capacity to survive outside. The decision to detain often presents difficult ethical dilemmas, requiring professionals to ensure that they understand the criteria set down in the legislation and the *Code of Practice* and can steer the difficult course between over-zealous use of their powers and undue hesitancy which may put a patient at risk.

There are three basic civil admission procedures under the 1983 Act: admission for assessment with or without treatment for up to 28 days, which is not renewable (Mental Health Act 1983, s 2); emergency admission for assessment for up to 72 hours (s 4); and admission for treatment for up to 6 months, renewable for a further 6 months, and thereafter for periods of up to 12 months at a time (s 3).

Compulsory admission under the 1983 Act may take place where the patient is suffering from mental disorder and detention is necessary in the interests of his or her own health *or* safety *or* for the protection of other people (Department of Health 1993b, para. 2.6).

Only one of these grounds needs to be met, and a person need not be behaving dangerously to be compulsorily admitted. The *Code of Practice* states that detention may be justified in the interests of the patient's own health, 'even if there is no risk to his own or other people's safety' (Department of Health 1993b, para. 2.9). A patient may be admitted under section 3 for treatment only if the necessary treatment cannot be provided without detention in hospital.

Patients are usually detained under the Act only if they are unwilling to be admitted informally. The *Code of Practice* states that:

Where admission to hospital is considered necessary and the patient is willing to be admitted informally, this should in general be arranged. Compulsory admission should, however, be considered where the patient's current medical state, together with reliable evidence of past experience, indicates a strong likelihood that he will change his mind about informal admission prior to his actual admission ... with a resulting risk to his health or safety or to the safety of others.　　　(Department of Health 1993b, para. 2.7)

Elderly patients more usually enter hospital informally, unless they express clear objections to admission. Mental illnesses associated with old age such as advanced dementia or Alzheimer's disease ultimately have the effect of removing people's capacity to take elementary care of themselves, which means that constant supervision may be necessary to avoid patients coming to harm. This poses legal and ethical problems where patients are informal, are mentally incapacitated, and may need to be restrained from leaving the ward or hospital and putting themselves at risk.

The Reports of the Health Service Commissioner frequently contain accounts of complaints that confused elderly patients have not been adequately supervised, have wandered off and have later been found dead from hypothermia or some other accident (Health Service Commissioner 1989, pp. 303–321). Yet the care of informal patients in wards which are routinely locked raises the issue described by the MHAC (1985, para. 8.10) as 'de facto detention', where patients are physically unable to leave the hospital or ward, but have none of the opportunities for review which would be available if they were detained under the Act. Adequate staffing of elderly care wards is the key to avoiding a custodial style of care, and the *Code of Practice* (Department of Health 1993b, para. 18.23) emphasises that authorities and managers are 'responsible for trying to ensure that staffing is adequate to prevent the need for the practice of locking patients in wards, individual rooms or any other area'. However, the Code goes on to say (para. 18.24) that it

is the nurse in charge of the shift who is responsible for the care and protection of patients and staff, and the maintenance of a safe environment.

The best ways to maintain such an environment are by adequate staffing levels and a vigilant caring staff rather than by reliance on technology which, unless used properly as an adjunct to personal care rather than the basis of the safety policy, can lead to a reduction in the interactions between patients and staff which are such an essential part of mental health care. There is a widespread practice of fitting elderly care wards with double handled doors or combination locks to prevent patients from wandering out. The *Code of Practice* (para. 18.27) says that these should be used as little as possible and only in units where there is a regular and significant risk of patients wandering off accidentally and, as a result, being at risk of harm. Attaching a tag to an elderly person which sets off an alarm seems ethically questionable, as it demeans the person concerned, and is a poor substitute for adequate staffing levels to ensure that those who may be at risk do not wander. Experience shows that buzzer systems to alert staff every time the door of a ward is opened are likely to prove ineffective because their sound eventually becomes so commonplace as to be ignored as background noise or so irritating that staff are tempted to disable the device. The Code states that units should have clear policies on the use of locks and other devices, and a mechanism for reviewing decisions.

In some cases what is described as 'wandering' may be a reaction to the restrictive horizons of a care regime which is unduly ward bound, and there will be less incentive for patients to do it if they are regularly escorted on walks in the hospital grounds and beyond. Where security devices are used, the Code distinguishes between those who are not deliberately trying to leave a ward, who may be legitimately deterred by combination locks or double handles, and those who persistently and purposefully try to leave, regardless of whether they understand the risk involved. In the latter case, the Code says that consideration must be given to assessing whether they might more appropriately be formally detained rather than remain as informal patients, hence entitling them to review of the decision to make them stay in hospital (para. 18.27).

The 1983 Act provides holding powers for doctors and nurses where it is considered that an informal patient should be detained. It introduced the possibility that a nurse could detain a *psychiatric* in-patient for up to 6 hours in limited circumstances. The doctor in charge of an informal patient's treatment has the power to hold that person for up to 72 hours if it is considered that an application for compulsory admission should be made, and that power can be delegated to another doctor nominated for the purpose (Mental Health Act 1983, ss 5(1), (2)). If neither the doctor in charge nor his or her nominee is available, the hospital managers have the power to detain an in-patient who is receiving treatment for mental disorder if a nurse of the prescribed class furnishes a written report (Mental Health Act 1983, s 5(4)). The report must state that it appears to the nurse that: (a) the patient is suffering from mental disorder to such a degree that it is necessary for his health or safety or for the protection of others that he be immediately restrained from leaving the hospital; *and* (b) that it is not practicable to secure the immediate attendance of a doctor who can exercise the holding power under s 5(2). It is the personal decision of the nurse, who cannot be instructed to exercise the power by anyone else. The nurse must be of the prescribed class, which is a nurse registered in Part 3, 5, 13 or 14 of the register, or a nurse qualified following a course of preparation in mental health or mental handicap nursing (Mental Health Act 1983, s 5(7); Mental Health (Nurses) Order 1983 as amended by the Mental Health (Nurses) Amendment Order 1993).

The completion of the form recording the exercise of the nurses holding power (Mental Health (Hospital, Guardianship and Consent to Treatment) Regulations 1983, reg 4(1)(h), Form 13) renders the patient immediately liable to be detained for a period of 6 hours or until the earlier arrival of a doctor with the power to hold the patient under section 5(2), whichever is the sooner. The *Code of Practice* states that the nurse must enter the reasons for invoking the power in the patient's nursing and medical notes and must send an incident report form to the managers (Department of Health 1993b, para. 9.4). A nurse invoking the holding power is entitled to use the minimum force necessary to prevent the patient from leaving hospital (Department of Health 1993b, para. 9.6). It is important to remember that the purpose of the holding powers is to enable a full assessment to be made of the need for detention by an approved social worker, who must interview the patient in a suitable manner and determine whether detention is necessary, and by two doctors who must provide reports on the patient's mental condition. The period of detention authorised under the holding powers are maxima, and the relevant professionals should be summoned to carry out their assessment as soon as the holding power is instituted, as the full assessment may conclude that detention is not warranted after all.

THE LEGAL AND ETHICAL IMPORTANCE OF CONSENT-SEEKING

The common law recognises the right of competent adult patients to decide what medical treatment they will have. The right is based on ideas of self-determination and the sanctity of the person. An early statement of these principles came from Cardozo J in the 1905 case of *Schloendorff* v *Society of New York Hospitals* ((1905) 21 NY 125 at 128) where he said: 'Every human being of adult years and sound mind has the right to determine what shall be done with his own body; and a surgeon who performs an operation without his patient's consent commits an assault'.

The principle has since been endorsed in a number of English cases, most notably *Re T (adult: refusal of medical treatment)* ([1992] 4 All ER 649) where Lord Donaldson MR said:

An adult patient who ... suffers from no mental incapacity has an absolute right whether to consent to medical treatment, to refuse it or to choose one rather than another of the treatments being offered ... This right of choice is not limited to decisions which others might regard as sensible. It exists notwithstanding that the reasons for making the choice are rational, irrational, unknown or even non-existent.

The *Code of Practice* defines consent as (Department of Health 1993b, para. 15.12) 'the voluntary and continuing permission of the patient to receive a particular treatment, based on adequate knowledge of the purpose, nature and likely effects of that treatment including the likelihood of success and any alternatives to it. Permission given under any unfair or undue pressure is not "consent"'.

Patients' rights to self-determination and to give or withhold consent are protected by the law of battery and the law of negligence. A battery occurs when there is an invasion of a person's bodily integrity without their consent. Because the tort of battery exists to protect the right of bodily autonomy, the plaintiff need not prove that he or she has suffered harm as a result of the treatment, and a doctor may still be guilty of battery even though acting in what he or she believed to be the patient's interests. Undoubtedly a finding that a doctor has been guilty of battery represents a severe stigma, and there has been what Kennedy & Grubb (1994, p. 171) describe as a 'determined effort' by the courts in England and elsewhere to limit the scope of the tort of battery in modern medical law, leaving it with a 'virtually vestigial role'. Nevertheless, they also make the important point that, 'As a mechanism for compensating injured patients ... it remains a powerful symbolic and actual deterrent against doctors ignoring the right of autonomy of their patients'.

Adult patients who have the necessary mental capacity have the right to make their own treatment decisions. To give such patients treatment which involves touching them without obtaining their consent is a battery. If the doctor has obtained consent following an explanation in broad terms of the nature, purpose and likely effects of the treatment, there can be no liability in battery (*Chatterton* v *Gerson* 1980, *Sidaway* v *Bethlem Royal Hospital Governors* 1985). However, there may be liability in negligence if insufficient information about the treatment has been given. In *Sidaway* (1985) two of the Law Lords (Keith and Brandon) said that the disclosure of a serious adverse risk might be so obviously necessary for the patient to make a true choice that no reasonably prudent doctor would fail to disclose it. However, in the same case the House of Lords held that, as a general rule, the amount of information to be given is a matter for the discretion of the doctor, who will not be found negligent if he or she has acted in accordance with a responsible body of medical opinion, skilled in the specialty, the test in *Bolam* v *Friern Barnet Hospital Management Committee* (1957).

When considering the amount of information to be given to a mentally disordered person, we must also consider the doctrine of therapeutic privilege, a concept of uncertain scope, whereby a doctor may decide not to give information about a treatment to a patient because to do so might put that person's health at risk. In such a case it would be for the doctor to make out the grounds for non-disclosure and to show that his or her decision accorded with a responsible body of medical opinion. If a patient asks general questions the amount of information to be given in response is a matter for the clinical judgment of the doctor concerned, who must act in accordance with a responsible body of medical opinion. In 1985, in *Blyth* v *Bloomsbury*, Leonard J held that the defendants had been negligent in not advising the plaintiff of the risks of treatment with Depo Provera, in the light of her manifest and reasonable request to be advised. However, the decision was overturned in 1987 by the Court of Appeal, where Kerr LJ said that the question of what a plaintiff should be told in answer to a general inquiry could not be divorced from the *Bolam* test, any more than when no such inquiry is made. Neill LJ too held that the amount of information to be given in response to questions must depend on the circumstances, and as a general proposition was governed by the *Bolam* test.

Consent-seeking is an important ethical and legal requirement. It enables patients to weigh for themselves the benefits and risks of treatment and make their own decisions about what is in their interests. When treating mentally disordered patients it is important to remember that the fact that they are mentally disordered does not necessary mean that they are incapable of giving a valid consent to treatment. There is a presumption that a patient is capable until the contrary is shown.

The *Code of Practice* sets down a number of criteria to be used in deciding whether a patient is capable of making a treatment decision. They require understanding, not only of the likely effects of the treatment, but also of the likely consequences of not having it. An individual must have the ability to (Department of Health 1993b, para. 15.10):

- understand what medical treatment is and that somebody has said that he needs it and why the treatment is being proposed
- understand in broad terms the nature of the proposed treatment
- understand its principal benefits and risks
- understand what will be the consequences of not receiving the proposed treatment
- possess the capacity to make a choice.

Every attempt should therefore be made to explain what is proposed in suitable language and to secure patients' agreement to their treatment. It is particularly important for clinical staff to ensure that they distinguish between difficulties of communication which may be overcome and lack of mental capacity to consider whether to have treatment.

The *Code of Practice* (Department of Health 1993b, para. 15.4) notes that for the purposes of the 1983 Act, medical treatment includes 'nursing, and also includes care, habilitation and rehabilitation under medical supervision'. This includes physical treatment such as ECT and the administration of drugs and psychotherapy.

The *Code of Practice* (Department of Health 1993b, paras. 15.5–7) stipulates that it is essential for both informal and detained patients to have a treatment plan which should be formulated by the multi-disciplinary team under the coordination of the patient's consultant and recorded in the clinical notes. The treatment plan should include a description of the immediate and long-term goals for the patient, and indicate clearly the treatment and methods of treatment proposed. Wherever possible the plan should be discussed with patients, with a view to eliciting their contribution, and giving them an opportunity to say whether they agree with it. The Code also emphasises the importance of discussing the treatment plan with appropriate relatives concerned about the patient, but stresses that, where the patient is capable of providing consent, his or her consent should always be sought to such discussions. The common law principle requiring consent applies to 'adult patients of full capacity'. Exceptions are made to permit treatment without consent for those who lack capacity to decide for themselves, or whose resistance to treatment may be irrational because of their mental disorder. Part IV of the Mental Health Act 1983 provides for detained patients to be given treatment for mental disorder without their consent. The common law empowers doctors to give treatment to mentally incapacitated patients without their consent if that treatment is necessary to alleviate or prevent serious deterioration in their physical or mental health. The following two sections discuss those statutory and common law provisions.

CONSENT AND PART IV OF THE 1983 ACT

The Scheme of Part IV

Part IV of the 1983 Act has two basic purposes. First, to make it clear that treatment may be given to detained patients without their consent, and second, to subject certain treatments to regulation by a system of second opinions. The second opinions are binding, not advisory.

Two groups of treatments require a second opinion: 'section 57 treatments', psychosurgery or the surgical implantation of hormones, which require *both* valid consent *and* approval by a second opinion doctor; and section 58 treatments, ECT or psychotropic medicines, which require *either* consent *or* a second opinion. Section 57 applies to all patients detained and informal, section 58 only to those who are 'liable to be detained'. A patient's consent or a second opinion may authorise a plan of treatment under which one or more of the forms of treatment mentioned in the relevant section may be given (Mental Health Act 1983, s 59). A patient may withdraw consent at any time before the completion of the treatment (Mental Health Act 1983, s 60). If this happens, subject to the emergency provisions of section 62, a second opinion will be required before the treatment can be resumed. Progress reports must be furnished by the doctor in charge of the treatment of each patient who has received treatment following a second opinion under section 57 or 58 (Mental Health Act 1983, s 61). If treatment is immediately necessary to meet one of a number of defined emergency situations it may be given without prior compliance with the second opinion procedures (Mental Health Act 1983, s 62).

Finally, the consent of a patient is not required for treatments other than those covered by the section 57 and 58 procedures if those treatments are given by or under the direction of the Responsible Medical Officer (RMO) (Mental Health Act 1983, s 63). RMO is the legal term for the psychiatrist in charge of the treatment of a detained patient. Section 63 applies to patients who are liable to be detained with the exception of those listed in section 56, principally those detained for 72 hours or less, who may not be treated without consent under Part IV, although they might be under common law (Mental Health Act 1983, s 56).

Psychosurgery and surgical implants of hormones

Section 57 treatments require *both* the patient's consent *and* approval of a second opinion doctor. The procedure applies to both informal and detained patients. The treatment may only be given if the patient can understand its nature, purpose, and likely effects, and has consented. The decision as to capacity and the validity of consent is made by a team of three people, a psychiatrist and two others appointed by the Mental Health Act Commission. Even if the patient has given valid consent, the treatment may not proceed unless the medical member of the team certifies that it ought to be given, having regard to the likelihood that it will alleviate or prevent deterioration in the patient's condition (Mental Health Act 1983, s 57 and the Mental Health (Hospital, Guardianship and Consent to Treatment) Regulations 1983 SI 1983 No 893, reg 16(1)). Although the non-medical members of the appointed panel have no involvement in the second part of the decision, there is some concession to multidisciplinariness in that, before making it, the second opinion doctor must consult two other people who have been professionally concerned with the patient's medical treatment, one of whom must be a nurse, and the other neither a nurse nor a doctor (Mental Health Act 1983, s 57(3)).

As Table 28.1 shows, since the 1983 Act there have been between 50 and 65 applications under section 57 per 2 year period from 1983–1991, although this declined to 46 between 1991 and 1993 because of difficulties during 1991 experienced by the main psychosurgery centre, the Geoffrey Knight Unit at the Brook Hospital, in obtaining yttrium rods with which to carry out the operations. Of the 274 referrals since 1983, psychosurgery was authorised in 218 cases (79.6%), authority was refused in 10 cases (3.7%), 42 (15.3%) were withdrawn, and 4 (1.4%) were pending at the end of 1993.

Although psychosurgery was extremely popular in

Table 28.1   Requests for psychosurgery second opinions

Period	Referrals	Authorised	Refused	Withdrawn*
1983–1985	57	34	4	17
1985–1987	54	32	4	18
1987–1989	52	44	1	7
1989–1991	65	56	1	8
1991–1993	46	42	0	4

* Includes cases pending at end of 2 year period of report.
Source: Mental Health Act Commission, *First–Fifth Biennial Reports* (1985),
(1987), (1989), (1991), (1993).

the 1940s and early 1950s, at least 12 000 operations being carried out in England and Wales between 1942 and 1954 (Ministry of Health 1961), nowadays it is a treatment of last resort which is rarely given. The MHAC does not publish information about the age of patients put forward for psychosurgery, so it is not possible to say what proportion is elderly. Section 57 requires the patient's consent. Section 58 allows medicines and ECT to be given without consent, subject to a second opinion.

Medicines and ECT

Whilst the section 57 procedures apply to both detained and informal patients, section 58 applies only to the treatment of detained patients with medicines and ECT. Patients detained under provisions which authorise detention for 72 hours or less (Mental Health Act 1983, ss 4, 5(2) or 5(4), 135 and 136) cannot be given treatment without consent for mental disorder under the Mental Health Act (Mental Health Act 1983, s 56). The same is true of offender patients who have been remanded for psychiatric reports to hospital (Mental Health Act 1983, s 35), who are being detained in a place of safety pending admission under a hospital order (Mental Health Act 1983, s 37(4)), or who are subject to a restriction order or direction and have been conditionally discharged from hospital (Mental Health Act 1983, ss 42(2), 73 or 74). In the absence of consent these people can only be treated under common law (discussed below).

Section 58 treatments include ECT at any time, or medicines for mental disorder after 3 months from the time medicine was first given during that detention. These require *either* the patient's consent *or* a second opinion. Section 58 applies only to patients who are *liable to be detained*, who may be treated without consent, subject to the approval of a second opinion approved doctor (SOAD) if they are incapable of

consenting (i.e. of understanding the treatment's nature, purpose and likely effects) or are refusing it. The SOAD must consider the likelihood of the treatment alleviating or preventing deterioration in the patient's condition. In recognition of 'the multidisciplinary principle', that the decision as to whether the treatment should be given is not purely medical, before deciding that a treatment ought to be given, SOADs must consult a nurse and another person who has been professionally concerned in the patient's treatment.

The role of the patient's responsible medical officer (RMO)

The Mental Health Act *Code of Practice* emphasises that although Part IV can be used to authorise treatment without consent, nevertheless the RMO must always seek the patient's valid consent before giving treatment (Department of Health 1993b, 16.9, 16.11, 16.13). If the patient is capable of consenting and has consented to ECT or medicine, the RMO certifies this on Statutory Form 38 (Mental Health (Hospital, Guardianship and Consent to Treatment) Regulations 1983 SI 1983 No 893, reg 16(2)(b) and Schedule 1). Unlike the consent forms used in general medicine, the statutory consent form does not require the patient's signature, only that of the RMO. The RMO must certify that two criteria are met: that the patient is capable, and that he or she consents to the treatment. The RMO is the gatekeeper of the system since, where patients agree to treatment, there will only be a second opinion if their RMOs consider them to lack capacity to consent. Where the patient refuses, a second opinion will only be needed if the RMO decides to persist with the treatment.

In assessing capacity, the patient's RMO must have regard to the requirements of the Code discussed earlier. Both the *Code of Practice* and the Law

Commission's recent proposals in their *Mental Incapacity* report (Law Commission 1995, para. 3.18) import into the test of capacity an implied right to be told about the principal benefits and risks of the treatment, and in that regard represent an attempt to move away from the common law doctor-centred approach to disclosure of risks.

In addition to certifying that the patient is capable and has consented, the RMO must give a brief description of the treatment consented to. The *Code of Practice* requires the RMO to indicate on the Form 38 certificate of consent the drugs prescribed by the classes described in the British National Formulary (BNF), the method of their administration, and the dose range, indicating the dosages if they are above the BNF limit. The BNF is not the only prescribing guide available to doctors but, under DDL(84)4 and the *Code of Practice*, it plays an important part in the second opinion process. Not only do RMOs describe the drugs consented to in terms of BNF categories, so too do the SOADs when they authorise treatment without consent.

The BNF is published jointly by the British Medical Association and the Royal Pharmaceutical Society and updated biannually. It describes the effects and side-effects of each drug, specifying recommended maximum dosage levels, determined on the advice of medical advisers working mainly from the manufacturer's data sheet, and produced after the available information has been considered by the Committee for the Safety of Medicines in the process of deciding to give the drug a product licence. Some of the less sedative antipsychotics have no BNF recommended maximum. The BNF is intended for the guidance of doctors, pharmacists and others who have the necessary training to interpret the information it provides. Each category (for example 4.2.1 anti-psychotic drugs, or 4.2.2 depot antipsychotics) includes a large number of different drugs, so this method of describing treatment consented to confers considerable scope for the RMO to change medication within categories, or to give more than one drug within the same category at the same time. If the patient is incapable of refusing treatment, it is the personal responsibility of the RMO to ensure that a second opinion visit is requested (Department of Health 1993b, paras. 16.23 and 16.26).

The role of the nurse

In February 1994 the Mental Health Act Commission issued Practice Note 2 entitled *Nurses, the Administration of Medicine for Mental Disorder, and the*

Mental Health Act, urging health authorities and trusts to include information about consent procedures under the 1983 Act in their policies and guidelines about the administration of medicines. The Note emphasises that the 3 month stabilising period begins to run from the first time when medicine was given during any continuous period of detention, so that if a patient is initially admitted for 28 days under section 2 and then the detention is continued using section 3, the 3 months starts to run from the first time when any medicine is given during the currency of the section 2. Medicine can only be given after the 3 months if there is a statutory Form 38 stating that the patient is capable and has consented, or if a second opinion doctor has authorised the medication on Statutory Form 39. The Practice Note stresses that (Mental Health Act Commission 1994):

The nurse administering the prescribed medication to patients ... subject to the provisions of section 58 ... must ensure that he or she is legally entitled to administer that medication by ensuring that all necessary legal requirements have been met. Following the 3 month period the legal authority is embodied in Forms 38 and 39. The nurse should fully understand the legal significance of these documents. A copy should be kept with the medicine card and reference made to it at the time of the administration of any medication used for the treatment of mental disorder. The nurse should:
(i) check the medicine card for date of entry of prescription and dosage;
(ii) ensure, if within the 3 month rule that the 3 month period has not been exceeded by checking the date of first administration;
(iii) ensure that where a patient has consented to medication beyond the 3 month rule that there is a Form 38 in place;
(iv) ensure that when a second opinion has been obtained that Form 39 is in place and has been correctly completed; and
(v) ensure that the administration of medicine is consistent with the guidance contained in the documents 'Scope of Professional Practice' (UKCC 1992) and 'Standards for the Administration of Medicines' (UKCC 1993).

The two UKCC documents mentioned impose important professional obligations on nurses. Both documents quote the passage from the UKCC Code of Professional Conduct stating that registered nurses are professionally accountable for their practice, and requiring them, in the exercise of their professional accountability, inter alia, to:

1. Act always in such a manner as to promote and safeguard the interests and wellbeing of patients and clients.
2. Ensure that no action on their part, or within their sphere of responsibility, is detrimental to the interests, condition or safety of patients or clients.

Standards for the Administration of Medicines specifies in detail what nurses may expect of doctors and pharmacists, as well as their own obligations when giving drugs. The booklet contains important provisions regarding the administration of medicines on the oral authority of a doctor, and the prescribing of medicines PRN (pro re nata – as the circumstances dictate) to be administered on the authority of the nursing staff on the spot. These state that nurses can reasonably expect the following (UKCC 1993, paras. 6.10–6.12):

6.10 that the registered medical practitioner understands that the administration of medicines on verbal instructions, whether he or she is present or absent, other than in exceptional circumstances, is not acceptable unless covered by the protocol mentioned in Para 6.11;
6.11 that it is understood that, unless provided for in a specific protocol, instruction by telephone to a practitioner to administer a previously unprescribed substance is not acceptable, the use of fax being the preferred method in exceptional circumstances or isolated locations; and
6.12 that, where it is the wish of the professional staff concerned that practitioners in a particular setting be authorised to administer, on their own authority, certain medicines, a local protocol has been agreed between medical practitioners, nurses ... and the pharmacist.

There must therefore be local protocols on telephone prescription and the administration of PRN medication if these practices are to take place.

Nurses also have an important role in the second opinion procedure, because the SOAD must consult a nurse and one 'other person' who has been professionally concerned with the patient's treatment before treatment can be authorised. In the light of their professional responsibilities it is vitally important for nurses to have a basic understanding of Part IV of the 1983 Act and its operation.

The role of the second opinion approved doctor (SOAD)

SOADs are appointed by the Mental Health Act Commission (MHAC), whose secretariat nominates, from a panel of approximately 150 consultant psychiatrists, a doctor who is independent of the hospital where the patient is receiving treatment to undertake the second opinion visit. The relationship between the MHAC and the second opinion doctors is 'at arm's length'. Although the MHAC arranges regular training seminars for SOADs, it has no control over their decisions, and there is no appeal to the MHAC against a decision to refuse or grant authority to treat.

The SOAD must visit the patient and interview him or her in private, but others may be present if the patient and SOAD agree or if the doctor would be at significant risk of physical harm from the patient (Department of Health 1993b, para. 16.28b). The Mental Health Act *Code of Practice* describes the SOAD's role as (Department of Health 1993b, para. 16.38):

to provide an additional safeguard to protect the patient's rights. He must at the time of the interview determine whether the patient is capable of consenting and giving valid consent, or, if the patient does not give his consent or is not capable of giving his consent, whether the treatment proposed by the patient's RMO is likely to alleviate or prevent deterioration of the patient's condition and should be given.

If at the time of the visit the patient is capable of consenting and consents, the SOAD will complete a Form 38 to this effect. If there is no valid consent, the Code stresses that SOADs act as individuals and must reach their own judgment as to whether the proposed treatment is reasonable in the light of the general consensus of appropriate treatment for such a condition, taking account not only of the therapeutic efficacy of the proposed treatment but also (where a capable patient is withholding his consent) the reasons for such withholding, which should be given their due weight (Department of Health 1993b, para. 16.39). DHSS circular letter DDL (Dear Doctor Letter) 84(4), issued in 1984 to all RMOs, described the purpose of the second opinion as 'to protect the patient's rights by ensuring that a treatment given without his consent is justified and in his interests' (Mental Health Act Commission 1984, para. 16).

In many jurisdictions in the United States proxy decision-makers are required to operate on the basis of substituted judgment when making decisions about the treatment of an incapacitated person. This means that they must take account of the patient's known views, religious and other beliefs, and general outlook on life in an attempt to make the decision that the person him or herself would have made. This test centres on an attempt to give effect to the patient's known or projected wishes. If such information is lacking, then the best interests test, the favoured approach of English common law on treatment decisions, is applied. Best interests tests depend on the views of professionals, usually doctors, as to what is best for the patient. However, at least they require that the likely benefits be weighed against the risks, and may incorporate some concept of the least invasive alternative.

The Law Commission (1993, p. 57) has proposed a useful definition of best interests which requires the treatment provider to take into account the known wishes of the patient, whether there is a less intrusive alternative to the treatment, and the other factors which the incapacitated person might be expected to consider if able to do so, such as the treatment's likely effect on life expectancy, health, happiness, freedom and dignity. The statutory test of likelihood that the treatment will alleviate or prevent deterioration is much looser even than the best interests test, and it has been further diluted in guidance. In deciding whether treatment ought to be given, the SOAD must have regard to (Mental Health Act 1983, s 58(3)(b)) 'the likelihood that it will alleviate or prevent deterioration in the patient's condition'. DDL(84)4 made it clear that SOADs' role is not to substitute their own decision as to what the treatment should be for that of the RMO making the treatment proposal. Where there is no consent, the question for the SOAD is 'whether or not the treatment plan is one which should be followed even if it is not necessarily the one which the appointed doctor would make himself'.

The Guidance goes on to say that (Mental Health Act Commission 1984, para. 17) 'doctors vary in their therapeutic approach and appointed doctors should feel able to support a consultant proposing a programme which others would regard as one which should be followed'. In other words, the approach is based on similar principles to those by which a doctor would be adjudged not to have been negligent under English law – the doctor-friendly *Bolam* test (*Bolam* v *Friern Barnet Hospital Managers* [1957] 1 WLR 582) whereby a doctor is not negligent who behaves in accordance with practice accepted at the time by a responsible body of medical opinion (however small) skilled in the specialty concerned. Here too the question is in effect, 'Would the treatment be supported by a responsible body of opinion skilled in the specialty?' Given the test to be applied by the SOADs in deciding whether to authorise treatment, it will come as no surprise that the concordance rate between SOADs and RMOs is high. Every MHAC Biennial Report has mentioned the high level of agreement, putting it between 94% and 96% (Mental Health Act Commission 1985, para. 11.4; 1987: 22, 1989: 5; 1991: 31, 1993: 37). The importance of the Bolam-based approach was evident in the MHAC's explanation in their *Second Biennial Report* (Mental Health Act Commission 1987, p. 22): 'No doubt a substantial part of the concordance can be explained by the facts that second opinions prove generally to be requested in respect of well-established and widely agreed treatment procedures, and that the role of the appointed doctor is not to impose his own views as to

which treatment can properly be supported as an acceptable form of treatment'.

The SOAD must consult a nurse and one 'other person' who has been professionally concerned with the patient's medical treatment, broadly defined in section 145(1) of the 1983 Act to include nursing, and care, habilitation and rehabilitation under medical supervision. This reflects Parliamentary concerns that the decision should have a multidisciplinary element. The consultees 'may expect a private discussion with the SOAD (again only in exceptional cases on the telephone) and to be listened to with consideration' (Department of Health 1993b, para. 16.36). The Code lists a number of issues which consultees should consider commenting upon (Department of Health 1993b, para. 16.37):

— the proposed treatment and the patient's ability to consent to it;
— other treatment options;
— the way in which the decision to treat was arrived at;
— the facts of the case, progress, attitude of relatives etc;
— the implications of imposing treatment on a non-consenting subject and the reasons for the patient's refusal of treatment;
— any other matter relating to the patient's care on which the consultee wishes to comment.

The nurse consultee must be qualified. Nursing assistants, auxiliaries and aides are excluded.

The duty to consult the 'other person' professionally concerned with the patient's treatment has been much discussed. The RMO is responsible for ensuring that someone is available who must be professionally concerned with the patient's 'medical treatment'. The Act, DDL(84)4 and the *Code of Practice* all make it clear that the certificate (Form 39) cannot be issued unless the two people designated have been consulted. The hospital managers, in consultation with the RMO, are responsible for ensuring that the patient is available to meet the SOAD, and that the RMO and the two consultees are available (although it is recognised that in exceptional circumstances this may not be possible). They must also ensure that primary copies of the section papers and the patient's case notes are available (Department of Health 1993b, para. 16.25).

Difficulties in finding someone to consult have frequently led to SOADs accepting people whose knowledge of the patient is scanty or non-existent, who could by no stretch of the imagination be said to have been 'professionally involved' in the patient's treatment, or who had known the patient for a very short time. Where the patient had just been admitted, this may be difficult to avoid, but not all cases fall into this category. In some cases the nurse and the other person have first met the patient no more than a couple of hours before the SOAD's visit, having been brought in specially 'to get to know the patient in order to fulfil the requirements of the Act' (Fennell 1995a, Ch. 12).

The MHAC *Fifth Biennial Report* (Mental Health Act Commission 1993, p. 38) states that 'to require the statutory other consultee to be invariably professionally qualified and included in a professional register would be unnecessarily restrictive'. However, they also express grave doubts about the validity of some certificates which refer to consultation of ward clerks, 'gymnasium technicians' or 'occupational therapy aides'. They propose that SOADs should endeavour to meet with somebody whose qualifications, experience and knowledge of the patient enable them to make an effective contribution to the work of the multidisciplinary team. However, they then suggest a watering down of the statutory requirement by saying that this could include those who are not professionally qualified but who are working under the direction of someone who is, who would take responsibility for their actions and whose name would appear on the statutory form, which would appear to allow the occupational therapist to sign on behalf of the occupational therapy aide.

The second opinion doctor gives a broad description of the treatment which he or she is prepared to authorise on Statutory Form 39. Where the treatment is ECT a maximum number of administrations is specified. Where it is medicine the authorised treatment is expressed in terms of the classes described in the British National Formulary (BNF), the method of their administration, and the dose range, indicating the dosages if they are above the BNF recommended limit. The SOAD must expressly indicate if more than one drug at a time from any BNF category may be given.

Reviews

The House of Commons Special Standing Committee expressed the view that when a second opinion had been given to authorise a course of treatment without consent, the authorisation should not, in Kenneth Clarke's words, be 'a timeless authorisation for the treatment to continue, but should be subject to a periodic review', the suggestion for this coming from representatives of the psychiatric profession themselves (Hansard H.C. Debs ser 6 vol. 29, cols 57–60, 18 October 1982). Section 61 of the 1983 Act requires the RMO to furnish a progress report on Form MHAC 1 to the MHAC each time the detention of a patient who has had a second opinion is renewed. The reports are then monitored by the MHAC National Standing

Committee on consent, which decides whether to send another SOAD to visit the patient.

Emergency treatment

Once a patient is detained under section 2 or 3, emergency treatment may be given under section 62 pending the arrival of a second opinion doctor. Section 62 of the 1983 Act authorises treatment to be given in certain defined types of emergency, without prior compliance with the second opinion procedures. It provides that the procedures in section 57 and 58 do not apply to any treatment which is:

(a) immediately necessary to save the patient's life; or
(b) which (not being irreversible) is immediately necessary to prevent a serious deterioration in his condition; or
(c) which (not being irreversible or hazardous) is immediately necessary to alleviate serious suffering by the patient; or
(d) which (not being irreversible or hazardous) is immediately necessary and represents the minimum interference necessary to prevent the patient behaving violently or being a danger to himself or others.

A treatment is deemed irreversible if it has unfavourable irreversible physical or psychological consequences and hazardous if it entails significant physical hazard.

The purpose of the section is to allow treatment to be given if a second opinion cannot be arranged sufficiently speedily to meet the demands of an emergency, whilst at the same time protecting patients against hazardous or irreversible treatments unless their lives are in serious danger or their health is about to suffer serious deterioration. Hence the MHAC has consistently maintained the view that where it is invoked, a request should simultaneously be made for a second opinion, so that repeated use does not arise (Mental Health Act Commission 1987, p. 23).

Section 62 does not apply to patients who are detained under powers authorising detention for 72 hours or less, such as the doctor's holding power, or the emergency admission for assessment under section 4. Treatment without consent under Part IV may only be given to a patient admitted under section 4 if the admission has been converted to a section 2 by the furnishing of a second medical report (Mental Health Act 1983, s 56). The MHAC have expressed concerns about treatment purportedly being given under section 62 when the patient is either not detained or is held under the short-term holding powers to which the section does not apply (Mental Health Act Commission 1993, p. 37). In these circumstances, if treatment is to be given it must be under common law. In such cases, the *Code of Practice* (Department of Health 1993b, para. 15.24) suggests that authority for emergency treatment may be found in common law, described in the following terms: 'on rare occasions involving emergencies where it is not possible immediately to apply the provisions of the ... Act the common law authorises such treatment as represents the minimum necessary to avert behaviour by the patient that is an immediate danger to self or to other people'.

The *Code of Practice* urges hospital managers to ensure that a form is devised to monitor the use of section 62, to be completed by the patient's RMO every time urgent treatment is given, recording details of the proposed treatment; why it is of urgent necessity to give it; and the length of time for which it is given (Department of Health 1993b, para. 16.19). The *Fifth Biennial Report* noted that although hospitals have been asked to do this for at least 5 years, 'many ... have still not instituted an effective recording system', particularly when the treatment involved is medicine (Mental Health Act Commission 1993, p. 37).

Other treatments

An important concern behind Part IV was the need to clarify the powers of staff to treat without consent. Section 63 provides that any medical treatment for mental disorder not specifically identified as requiring a second opinion may be given to a detained patient without consent by or under the direction of the patient's RMO. 'Medical treatment for mental disorder' is defined broadly to include 'nursing, and care, habilitation and rehabilitation under medical supervision', extending beyond those treatments which require a second opinion. Section 63 was included, in the words of Lord Elton, Government spokesman in the Lords, 'to put the legal position beyond doubt ... for the sake of the psychiatrists, nurses and other staff who care for these very troubled patients' (Lord Elton 1982, cols 1064–5). When faced with the criticism that this provision might authorise a disturbingly wide range of interventions, Lord Elton (1982, col 1071) emphasised that this provision was not intended to apply to 'borderline' or 'experimental' treatments but 'things which a person in hospital for treatment ought to undergo for his own good and for the good of the running of the hospital and for the good of other patients ... perfectly routine, sensible treatment'.

In fact subsequent case law (*F v Riverside Health Trust* 1993; *Re KB (adult) (mental patient: medical treatment)* 1994) has established that anorexia nervosa is a form of mental disorder and that forcible feeding

of anorexic patients is treatment for mental disorder within the meaning of section 145(1) of the 1983 Act, which may be given without the patient's consent under section 63. In *B v Croydon Health Authority* (1995), the patient suffered from a borderline personality disorder rather than anorexia, but the Court of Appeal held that section 63 applied to treatment directed at the symptoms or sequelae of mental disorder just as much as to treatment directed to remedying B's underlying personality disorder which caused her compulsion not to eat. Section 63 was not intended to apply to controversial treatments like force feeding. The question which must now be addressed by the Department of Health is whether the section 58 procedure should be extended by regulation to include force feeding, or whether they are content to leave the position as it is (Fennell 1995b).

The operation of the section 58 second opinions

The MHAC publishes statistics of second opinions biennially. The figures from the five Biennial Reports published since the 1983 Act are shown in Table 28.2, which shows a clear increase since the 1983 Act came into force.

The MHAC's figures show the following gender breakdown of second opinions (Table 28.3).

There have been consistently more second opinions for women since Part IV came into force. Table 28.4 shows the type of treatment for which second opinions have been given.

In the period 1991–1993, for the first time since the 1983 Act came into force, second opinions for medicines outnumbered those for ECT. Well over 90% of all patients having second opinions under section 58 are suffering from mental illness. Since 1989 the MHAC has produced statistics of second opinions for patients with a diagnosis of mental illness by gender and type of treatment, showing that women far outnumber men as second opinions for ECT, and the

Table 28.2 Total second opinions under section 58

Year	Second Opinions
1983–1985	4032
1985–1987	5845
1987–1989	7592
1989–1991	7169
1991–1993	8839

Source: *First, Second, Third, Fourth, and Fifth Biennial Reports* of the Mental Health Act Commission (1985), (1987), (1989), (1991), (1993).

Table 28.3   Second opinions by gender of patient

Year	1983–85	1985–87	1987–89	1989–91	1991–93
Males	1781	2472	3152	3048	4010
Females	2251	3373	4440	4121	4829
Total	4032	5845	7592	7169	8839

Source: Mental Health Act Commission, *First–Fifth Biennial Reports.*

Table 28.4   Second opinions under section 58 by type of treatment

Year	1983–85	1985–87	1987–89	1989–91	1991–93
Medicine	1886	2483	3138	3023	4627
ECT	2146	2455	4203	3978	4067
Both		907	251	166	145
Total	4032	5845	7592	7169[1]	8839

Source: Mental Health Act Commission, *First–Fifth Biennial Reports.*

Footnote

[1] These are the figures from the *Fourth Biennial Report*, p. 34. The total is correct, but they do not add up correctly.

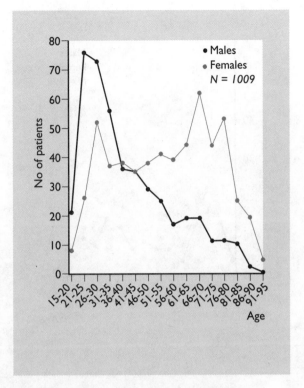

Figure 28.1   Second opinions: age and gender.

reverse is the case for medicines. Between 1989 and 1991, 71.4% (2827) of the mental illness second opinions for ECT were for women and 61.6% (1671) of those for medicines were for men. Between 1991 and 1993 women were 67.4% (2614) of the second opinions for ECT, whilst men were 59.6% (2546) of those for medicines.

Elderly patients and the second opinion process

A significant number of the consultations for ECT are for elderly patients, mainly women, with severe depressive illness. A study carried out in 1992 by the author of 1009 second opinions under section 58 contained 566 female patients and 443 men (Fennell 1995a, Ch. 12). Figure 28.1 shows the gender breakdown of the sample.

Whilst 60% of the men were 40 or under, and 80% of them were 55 or under, women tended to be more concentrated in the older age groups, with 70% over 40, and more than 50% over 55. As for treatment, 490 were for ECT, 497 were for medicines, and 22 were for both. The gender split for ECT was 73% (357) women and 27% (133) men, whilst for medicines it was

reversed (although not exactly) with 61% (301) men and 39% (196) women. Nine men and 13 women were having second opinions for both ECT and medicines.

Figure 28.2 shows the gender and age of patients having second opinions for ECT. For women there is a steep increase after 40, with high concentrations in the 61–80 age group. Once we reach the over 80 age group, the vast majority of second opinions for both sexes are for ECT. 42 of the 48 women over 80 and 7 of the 12 men in that age group were having second opinions for ECT. No less than 17 women in the ECT group were in the 86–90 age bracket, and 2 were over 91.

The equivalent figures for medicines are given in Figure 28.3, which shows a decline in second opinions after 45, with the fall being more pronounced for men.

These figures show that elderly patients given treatment under section 58 are much more likely to be receiving ECT than medicines. They also lend support to the MHAC statement in their *Third Biennial Report* (Mental Health Act Commission 1989, p. 24) that a large proportion of the ECT work of second opinion doctors 'takes place on old persons with severe depression who have been detained because they

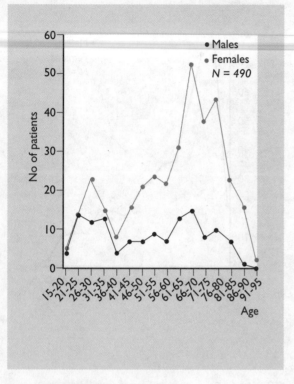

Figure 28.2 Second opinions: ECT.

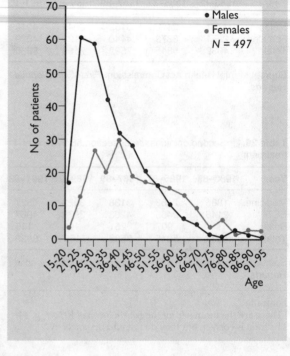

Figure 28.3 Second opinions: medicines.

cannot consent to ECT, even though they are already unprotestingly in hospital and the treatment is required because they are refusing food and fluids'. For these patients the reason for detention is to authorise treatment without consent, not to prevent them from leaving hospital. The second opinion doctors considered that detention was 'an unnecessary stigma' that could be avoided if treatment without the patient's consent could be arranged in another way, and expressed the fear that harmful delay in treating the patient could occur whilst the formalities of detention were being completed and before a second opinion visit can be arranged.

The section 62 emergency treatment power is used to a considerable extent in relation to elderly patients having ECT. Of the 1009 cases surveyed, no less than 11.5% (116 patients) had received treatment under section 62 (85 women and 31 men), and in all but four cases the emergency treatment was ECT. In all the emergency ECT cases, the reason for the administration of emergency ECT was either the immediate need to save life, or to prevent serious deterioration in the patient's condition. Patients having

emergency ECT were frequently described in terms such as 'refusing food and fluids, inaccessible and beyond reassurance', and the treatment as 'necessary to save the life of the patient'. In one case the patient had been tube fed from admission, had lost 15 pounds in the past week, and her physical state had become critical.

By the time the second opinion doctors were brought in in the emergency cases there was little alternative to ECT. The seemingly large number of very elderly patients being detained for ECT treatment raises a number of questions. Patients often appeared to be seriously deteriorated by the time they were admitted compulsorily for depressive illnesses. Where they are admitted direct from the community, this raises questions about the effectiveness of community care and illustrates the need for effective preventive programmes. In some cases they are already in hospital informally and deteriorate to the extent that their doctors consider them to need ECT. In the context of elderly care there are many difficult ethical dilemmas to face, most notably the momentous decision to override a person's refusal of ECT. There is also a difficult calculation to be made between the risks associated with severe depressive illness and those attaching to anaesthetics which are essential to the safe administration of ECT. These increase dramatically with age.

Sections 58, 62 and 63 authorise the treatment of patients detained under sections 2 and 3 without consent. Informal patients are presumed to be entitled to refuse these treatments, although if they refuse treatment for mental disorder deemed necessary in their own interests or for the protection of others, their RMO has the legal power to detain them. We have already seen how there is a reluctance to use powers of detention with elderly mentally incapacitated patients to enable them to be treated lawfully without consent. Part IV enables detained patients to be treated for mental disorder without consent. Since Part IV was enacted, there have been developments in the judge-made common law enabling mentally incapacitated patients to be treated for physical or mental disorder without their consent where it is necessary in their best interests.

TREATMENT WITHOUT CONSENT AND THE COMMON LAW

Undoubtedly the emergent case law on consent in the 1970s and early 1980s, and the introduction of the second opinion procedures in the 1983 Act led to increased awareness of consent issues among those treating mentally disordered people. There was also growing awareness that the provisions of Part IV apply only to treatment for mental disorder, and they do not authorise the treatment of informal patients without consent. This gave rise to considerable disquiet about the legal position when treatment was given to an informal, incapacitated patient without consent. Whilst the 1983 Act allows for treatment of the detained without consent, it does not provide authority to treat for mental or physical disorder the multitude of informal patients who are incapable of making a decision. In 1989 in *Re F (Mental Patient: Sterilisation)* the House of Lords declared that no-one else has the power to consent to treatment on behalf of an incapacitated patient, but that at common law doctors have a power, and in certain circumstances a duty to give treatment to incapacitated adults which is necessary in their best interests. Treatment is necessary in a patient's best interests if it is carried out in order to save life or to ensure improvement or prevent deterioration in his or her physical or mental health.

In deciding whether a treatment is necessary in a patient's best interests, the doctor must act in accordance with a responsible and competent body of medical opinion skilled in the specialty, the so-called *Bolam* standard. If the doctor decides that treatment is in the patient's best interests, there is not only a power, but in certain circumstances there may also be a duty to give it, and there can be no liability in battery. The corollary is that if the doctor, again according with the *Bolam* standard, believes the treatment not to be in the incapacitated patient's best interests, to give it is a battery.

The principle in *Re F* allows diagnostic procedures to be carried out and treatment to be given to an incapacitated patient without coming to court if they are necessary in the patient's best interests (*Re H (Mental patient)* 1992). It is possible at common law for a person who is clearly refusing treatment to be deemed to lack capacity (*Re C (Mental patient: Medical Treatment)* (1994)). C, a 68-year-old patient detained in Broadmoor and suffering from paranoid schizophrenia, sought court recognition of his current capacity to refuse amputation of a gangrenous leg and prospective validation of his advance directive. He refused to consent to amputation in any circumstances, even if it meant death. The immediate danger to his health was averted by surgery to remove the area of infected tissue without amputation. The hospital authorities refused the undertaking sought by his solicitor that they would recognise C's repeated refusals and would not amputate in any future circumstances, so he sought a declaration that he was capable of refusing amputation and an injunction restraining Heatherwood Hospital from amputating his right leg without his express written consent. Thorpe J granted the orders sought, and in so doing laid down a test for determining capacity to make treatment decisions at common law. The question to be decided here was whether C's capacity was so reduced by his chronic mental illness that he did not sufficiently understand the nature, purpose and effects of the proffered amputation. Thorpe J held that the presumption that C was capable had not been displaced even though he was detained and his general capacity was impaired by schizophrenia. He had delusions of a successful international career in medicine. He felt that he would not die if his leg was not amputated, because God would protect him. Dr Nigel Eastman, a consultant forensic psychiatrist who appeared as an expert witness for the plaintiff, expressed the view that three elements had to be considered:

1. whether the patient could comprehend and retain the treatment information

2. whether he was capable of believing it
3. whether he could weigh it in the balance to arrive at a choice.

Thorpe J adopted this test, and found that it had not been established that C did not understand the nature, purpose and likely effects of the amputation he was refusing. He understood and retained the relevant treatment information and in his own way he believed it, even though he did not accept the doctors' assessment that the vascular disease of his foot would lead to a return of his gangrene and threaten his life. In fact, he is still alive 2 years after the court action. He had arrived at a clear choice. So although it was questionable whether C 'believed' the relevant treatment information, in the sense that he did not accept the doctors' assessment of the likely consequences of not having his leg amputated, he was nevertheless found to not be incapable because 'in his own way he believed it'.

Re C is an important reminder that it is for those alleging incapacity to displace the presumption of capacity, and that the mere fact that someone is suffering from mental disorder does not necessarily mean they are incapable of making a treatment decision. It has also enshrined the 'Eastman' test of incapacity as part of the common law. This may be difficult to implement in practice because of the second criterion, that the patient must believe the relevant treatment information. It does not mean that, in order to be capable, the patient must accept the medical evaluation of the likely outcome of having the treatment or not having it and of the trade-off between risks and benefits. As Thorpe J would later put it in *B v Croydon District Health Authority* (1994, p. 21), 'there is a difference between outright disbelief (due to mental disorder) which meant being impervious to reason, divorced from reality, or incapable of adjustment after reflection', and 'the tendency which most people have when undergoing medical treatment to self-assess and then to puzzle over the divergence between medical and self-assessment' (*B v Croydon Health Authority* 1994, p. 20). If a person is to be given treatment without consent under common law, this must be preceded by an assessment that they lack capacity in accordance with the above common law tests. The Law Commission (1995) has proposed placing the common law authority to treat incapacitated adults on a statutory footing.

In the case of certain treatments, such as non-therapeutic sterilisations (i.e. those with a purely contraceptive purpose, *Re GF (Medical treatment)* 1992) and the withdrawal of artificial hydration and nutrition from permanently insensate patients (*Airedale NHS Trust v Bland* 1993), the Law Lords have advised that a High Court declaration should be sought and guidance on the procedure to be adopted in each type of case has been provided by the Official Solicitor (1993, 1994).

Advance statements

Dramatic developments in upholding patient autonomy have occurred in the recognition of advance statements about medical treatment. Advance statements, also known as living wills, enable people who currently have the capacity to consent to or refuse treatment to make provision for their medical treatment in the event of their future incapacity by stating in advance the type of treatment which they would want or not want in certain circumstances. The term advance directive, which was widely used for a time, is now felt to be inappropriate because a patient cannot order a doctor to give treatment which is contrary to that doctor's clinical judgment of the patient's best interests or which is contrary to law, such as an injection intended to shorten life. Model forms on which such directives can be made are distributed by a number of organisations such as the Terence Higgins Trust and the Voluntary Euthanasia Society.

In 1992 the BMA issued a statement supporting the principle of advance directives, but resisting the idea of legislation to make them binding. However, judicial dicta in *Re T (adult) (medical treatment)* and *Airedale NHS Trust v Bland* had already indicated that advance refusals of specific treatment could in certain circumstances be binding. In *Re C (Mental patient: Medical Treatment)* Thorpe J put their validity beyond doubt by stating that C's advance refusal of amputation was valid because he was capable at the time he made it, it was clear in its terms and sufficient in scope to bind a doctor in future circumstances. This was the first occasion where an English court had been invited to rule directly on the validity of an advance refusal. The House of Lords Select Committee on Medical Ethics which reported in January 1994, after the decision in *Re C*, also commended advance statements but did not see any need for legislation, recommending instead that the colleges and faculties of the health care professions should jointly develop a code of practice (1994, p. 54). A major benefit in their Lordships' view was that their preparation should stimulate discussion about patients' preferences between doctors and patients. The Committee suggested (House of Lords 1994, p. 54) that the 'informing premise' of any new code should be that advance statements would be:

[R]espected as an authoritative statement of the patient's wishes in respect of treatment ... [and] ... those wishes should be overruled only where there are reasonable grounds to believe that the clinical circumstances which actually prevail are significantly different from those which the patient had anticipated, or that the patient has changed his or her views since the directive was prepared. A directive may also be overruled if it requests treatment which the doctor judges is not clinically indicated or if it requests any illegal action.

The Select Committee (House of Lords 1994, p. 55) also recommend that the code should encourage professionals to disseminate information about advance directives, and procedures should be established to lodge directives with patients' GPs, who would be required to produce them for other health care professionals who assume the care of the patient, such as when the patient is admitted to hospital. The existence of a statement should be indicated by a card which the patient would carry. Finally, they recommend that the proposed code should encourage but not require regular review and re-endorsement by patients of their directives, which might help to eliminate the danger of a statement becoming out of line with medical practice or the patient's current wishes, whilst at the same time reinforcing the patient's continuing commitment to it.

Following *Bland* and *Re C*, the BMA issued a new statement in January 1994 supporting 'limited legislation to translate the common law into statute and clarify the non-liability of doctors who act in accordance with an advance directive' (British Medical Association 1994, para. 1). In April 1995 the BMA published *Advance Statements about Medical Treatment* (1995), a response to the House of Lords invitation to develop a code of practice on advance statements for health professionals, defining different types of advance statement and explaining their legal and ethical status. The Commission propose legislation for the recognition and enforceability of advance refusals of treatment. Their draft Bill would recognise advance refusals by anyone over 18. These would be presumed to be valid if made in writing and signed by the person and at least one other person as a witness to his signature, and could be revoked or altered by the person at any time while he has the capacity to do so. The BMA's request for a statutory defence would be met by the Law Commission's Bill which would provide that (Law Commission 1995, Draft Mental Incapacity Bill, cl 9(4)):

No person should incur liability for (1) the consequences of withholding any treatment or procedure if he or she has reasonable grounds for believing that an advance refusal of treatment applies; or (2) for carrying out any treatment or procedure to which an advance refusal applies unless he or she knows or has reasonable grounds for believing that an advance directive exists.

An advance statement clearly now has legal force provided the person has the necessary capacity which, in cases where doubts may be raised later, entails an assessment of capacity at the time it is drawn up. The statement should be drawn up in close consultation with the patient's own doctor who can advise of the likely forms of treatment which may arise after the onset of incapacity, and to whom it will probably fall to implement it. Finally, at the time of implementing the statement, especial care will be needed to ensure that the refusal of consent is still applicable in the circumstances which have subsequently occurred.

Although advance statements are potentially an important means of upholding patient autonomy, their use does raise difficult practical issues (House of Lords 1994, pp. 38–44). There need to be effective safeguards to ensure that patients, particularly vulnerable elderly people, are not pressured into making advance statements, and solicitors and health care professionals involved in their preparation must be vigilant to ensure that this does not happen. If a patient made an advance refusal of psychiatric treatment and was subsequently detained under the Mental Health Act 1983, the detention would override the directive and treatment for mental disorder could be given without consent subject to compliance with Part IV of the Act.

Do not resuscitate or 'Not for the 222s' orders

Although in some cases cardiopulmonary resuscitation may prolong a life which retains worthwhile quality, in others it may be, in the words of the House of Lords Select Committee (1994, p. 46), 'a traumatic and undignified interruption of the natural process of dying'. In some cases patients themselves ask not to be subjected to the trauma of resuscitation because they feel that the quality of life which they subsequently have is not worth the ordeal. However, these decisions are not always the patients', and there is long-standing practice of marking certain patients' clinical notes with a statement that cardiopulmonary resuscitation should not be attempted. This gives rise to many difficult ethical questions, and is a cause of considerable anxiety both for patients and their relatives. The orders take a number of forms from the comprehensible 'Do Not Resuscitate' (although this often appears in the notes as 'DNR', which is much less obvious to the layperson) to the coded 'Not for the 222s' or whatever internal telephone number the hospital uses to summon the crash team. There have been complaints to the Health Service Commissioner (1991, p. 50) by relatives of patients who have been incapable of deciding for themselves and whose notes were marked 'Not for the 222s', where the decision appears to have been taken by a junior doctor. The relatives also complained that they had not been consulted. There were also fears that the decision may be taken on the basis of illegitimate criteria being smuggled into the concept of quality of life, such as the patient's age or mental health status.

The BMA and the RCN have developed guidelines in conjunction with the United Kingdom Resuscitation Council on the subject of these orders, which state that the responsibility for making them rests with the consultant in charge of the patient's treatment. They suggest (discussed in House of Lords 1994, p. 47) that a Do Not Resuscitate Order could be considered where the patient's condition indicates that resuscitation is unlikely to be successful, where it is not in accord with the clearly established wishes of the patient expressed at a time when he or she was legally competent, or where successful resuscitation is likely to be followed by a length and quality of life which is unlikely to be acceptable to the patient. Any decision should be made in consultation with the whole health care team, and the patient where appropriate, and the reason for the decision should be thoroughly recorded. This is an example where an advance directive could be of significant assistance, where the type of treatment being refused could be clearly specified. Where the patient has not indicated any wishes, the matter is one of clinical judgement which should be based on the likely outcome for the patient, not his age or mental health status. The views of relatives, whilst relevant and a possible source of important indications of what

the patient might have wanted, should not be taken as determinative, since relatives' and patients' interests may not always coincide.

CONCLUSION

As John Harris (1988, p. 39) has put it, 'The problem for all who care about others is how to reconcile respect for the free choices of others with real concern for their welfare when their choices appear to be self-destructive or self-harming', and we may include in that group those who are unable to make any choice due to mental incapacity. Over the past two decades there have been remarkable developments in the law and ethics regarding the treatment of elderly people with mental disorder, including the provisions of the Mental Health Act and its codes of practice, a growing body of judge-made common law, and increasing numbers of professional codes of guidance governing ethically difficult aspects of care. These various provisions have as their aim the achievement of a system of mental health care where the autonomously expressed wishes of patients are given adequate weight, and where patients are not denied necessary treatment because they are not capable of expressing their wishes or are irrationally objecting due to their mental disorder. Most important, they aim to remind us that when someone becomes a psychiatric patient they do not thereby forfeit all rights and claims to respect for their individuality. As the House of Lords Select Committee put it (House of Lords 1994, p. 57): 'Long term care of those whose disability or dementia makes them dependent should have special regard to need to maintain the dignity of the individual to the highest possible degree'.

REFERENCES

Airedale NHS Trust v *Bland* [1993] 2 W.L.R. 316; (1992) 12 BMLR 64

B v *Croydon Health Authority* Fam D (1994) 22 BMLR 13

B v *Croydon Health Authority* CA [1995] 1 All ER 683

Blyth v *Bloomsbury* 1985 The Times 24 May 1985 (QBD)

Blyth v *Bloomsbury* 1987 [1993] 4 Med LR 151 (CA). The Times 11 February 1987 (CA)

Bolam v *Friern Barnet Hospital Management Committee* [1957] 1 WLR 582; (1957) 1 BMLR 1

British Medical Association 1992 Statement on advance directives. BMA, London

British Medical Association 1994 Statement on advance directives. BMA, London

British Medical Association 1995 Advance statements about medical treatment. BMJ Publications, London

Chatterton v *Gerson* [1981] 1 QB 432; (1980) 1 BMLR 80

Department of Health 1993a Health and personal social services statistics for England. HMSO, London

Department of Health 1993b The Mental Health Act code of practice. HMSO, London

Department of Health 1995 Statistical bulletin: in-patients formally detained in hospitals under the Mental Health Act 1983 and other legislation, England: 1987–8 to 1992–3.

Lord Elton 1982 Hansard H.L. Debs, Ser. 5, Vol. 426, cols. 1064–71, 1 Feb 1982

F v *Riverside Health Trust* (1993) 20 BMLR 1

Fennell P W H 1995a Treatment without consent: law psychiatry and the treatment of mentally disordered people since 1845. Routledge, London

Fennell P W H 1995b Force feeding and the Mental Health Act 1983 (1995) NLJ 145: 319–320

Harris J 1988 Professional responsibility and consent to treatment. In: Hirsch S R, Harris J (eds) Consent and the incompetent patient: ethics, law and medicine. Gaskell/Royal College of Psychiatrists, London

Health Service Commissioner 1989 Selected investigations completed November 1988–March 1989 HC 393. HMSO, London

Health Service Commissioner 1991 Selected investigations completed October 1990–March 1991. HMSO, London

House of Lords 1994 Report of the select committee on medical ethics, vol. 1. HMSO, London

Jewesbury I 1994 Supervision registers and supervised discharge. IBC conference paper 11th November 1994

Kennedy I, Grubb A 1994 Medical law: text with materials, 2nd edn. Butterworths, London

Law Commission 1993 Mentally incapacitated adults and decision-making: medical treatment and research, consultation paper no 129. HMSO, London

The Law Commission 1995 Mental incapacity law, com no 231. HMSO, London

Mental Health Act 1983. HMSO, London

Mental Health Act Commission 1984 Guidance for responsible medical officers: consent to treatment. DDL(84)4

Mental Health Act Commission 1985 First biennial report 1983–1985. HMSO, London

Mental Health Act Commission 1987 Second biennial report 1985–1987. HMSO, London

Mental Health Act Commission 1989 Third biennial report 1987–1989. HMSO, London

Mental Health Act Commission 1991 Fourth biennial report 1989–1991. HMSO, London

Mental Health Act Commission 1993 Fifth biennial report 1991–1993. HMSO, London

Mental Health Act Commission 1994 Nurses, the administration of medicine for mental disorder, and the Mental Health Act practice note 2. Mental Health Act Commission, Nottingham

Mental Health (Hospital, guardianship and consent to treatment) regulations 1983 SI 1983 No 893

Mental Health (Nurses) Order 1983 S.I. 1983 No 891 as amended by the Mental Health (Nurses) Amendment Order 1993, S.I. 1993 No 2155

Ministry of Health 1961 Leucotomy in England and Wales. Reports on Public Health and Medical Subjects No. 104. HMSO, London

Official Solicitor 1993 Practice note: (sterilisations: minors and mental health patients) [1993] 3 All ER 222

Official Solicitor 1994 Practice note persistent vegetative state: withdrawal of treatment [1994] 2 All ER 413

Re C (Mental patient: medical treatment) [1994] 1 WLR 290

Re F (Mental patient: sterilisation) [1990] 2 A.C. 1; Sub nomine *F v West Berkshire Health Authority* (1989) 4 BMLR 1; [1989] 2 All ER 545

Re GF (Medical treatment) [1992] 1 F.L.R. 293

Re H (Mental patient) (1992) 9 BMLR 71

Re KB (adult) (mental patient: medical treatment) (1994) 19 BMLR 144

Re T (Adult: refusal of treatment) [1992] WLR 782

Schloendorff v Society of New York Hospitals (1905) 21 NY 125

Sidaway v Bethlem Royal Hospital Governors [1985] AC 1; [1985] 2 WLR 480; (1985) 1 BMLR 132

United Kingdom Central Council for Nursing and Midwifery 1992 The scope of professional practice. UKCC, London

United Kingdom Central Council for Nursing and Midwifery 1993 Standards for the administration of medicines. UKCC, London

RECOMMENDED READING

Gordon Ashton 1994 The elderly client handbook: the Law Society's guide to acting for older people. The Law Society, London. *Written primarily for solicitors. A useful outline of the legal issues which affect elderly people, including community care, care and treatment in hospital and management of property and affairs.*

British Medical Association 1995 Advance statements about medical treatment. BMJ Publications, London. *Guidance for health professionals on drafting advance statements (living wills) about medical treatment. Essential reading for all doctors and those advising the elderly on their future medical treatment should they become incapacitated.*

The Law Commission 1995 Mental incapacity law com no 231. HMSO, London. *Proposals for legislation to provide a comprehensive legal framework for decision-making of all kinds – financial, living, treatment – on behalf of mentally incapacitated adults.*

Richard Gordon 1993 Community care assessments: a practical legal framework. Longman, London. *Summarises in accessible language the provisions of the National Health Service and Community Care Act 1990 on community care,* *discussing the criteria for assessment and service provision, the requirements of the law regarding fairness, legal remedies, and the financial implications of assessment.*

House of Lords 1994 Report of the Select Committee on medical ethics, vol 1. London, HMSO. *Report of the House of Lords Select Committee appointed to consider the legal, clinical, and ethical implications of a person's right to withhold consent to life-prolonging treatment, and the position of patients who are no longer able to give or withhold consent. An important summary of the views of different interested groups, together with recommendations on how medical decisions which have the effect of shortening life should be taken. Conclusions include: strong endorsement of competent patients to refuse consent to any medical treatment; recommendation of no change in the law to permit euthanasia; rejection of creation of new offence of 'mercy killing'; recommendation of abolition of mandatory life sentence for murder; treatment limiting decisions should not be determined by considerations of resource availability; commend development of advance directives; suggest that no legislation necessary to recognise advance directives, but recommend that code of practice should be developed.*

R M Jones 1994 Mental Health Act manual, 4th edn. Sweet and Maxwell, London. *The full text of the* Mental Health Act 1983, *relevant regulations, the* Mental Health Act Code of Practice, *and* Mental Health Act Commission Practice Notes, *with helpful explanatory annotations.*

Kennedy I, Grubb A 1994 Medical law: text with materials, 2nd edn. Butterworths, London. *An excellent discussion of the central issues of medical law and ethics, with a very detailed section on consent to treatment.*

Law Commission 1993 Mentally incapacitated adults and decision-making: medical treatment and research, consultation paper no 129. HMSO, London. *An important discussion paper outlining provisional proposals for a system of powers to enable treatment decisions to be taken on behalf of incapacitated patients. This would include a statutory authority for treatment providers to give treatment which is in the patient's best interests, advance directives, and treatment proxies, where the patient could nominate in advance someone to be involved in treatment decisions. Disputes and controversial treatments would be referred to a 'judicial authority'.*

Letts P 1990 Managing other people's money. Age Concern, London. *An extremely useful guide, written in lay person's language, to the administration of the finances of people with problems of mental ill health.*

29

Reflections

Ian J Norman
Sally J Redfern

In this final chapter we draw upon the previous chapters in an attempt to summarise some of what strikes us as the main issues and challenges facing mental health care workers concerned with elderly people. Our aim is to highlight what is good about current practice and what changes are needed to improve health care for sufferers, informal carers and paid workers.

WHO ARE 'THE ELDERLY'?

Kendrick and Warnes' (Ch. 1) analysis of demographic changes throws light on old people's experiences of their social conditions and mental health. The widespread perception of a relentless and limitless growth in the number of old people in the UK population is misleading. As a proportion of the total population there is likely to be an increase, particularly the oldest old, but in absolute terms the number of elderly people is expected to fluctuate. Although the major increases in life expectancy achieved in previous centuries are unlikely to be repeated, there is scope for significant improvement in mortality rates. There are striking differences in mortality rates internationally and across geographical regions in the UK; North America and some European countries have better rates than the UK, and southern England enjoys lower rates than Scotland and Northern Ireland. Also for social class. Substantial improvements in mortality rates would be achieved if the whole population enjoyed the lifestyle of the more privileged. It is interesting that although frailty, disablement and chronic sickness are concentrated in older members of the elderly population, the ages at which a given proportion of the population is severely impaired rises in line with mean life expectancy.

As for composition of the elderly population, women are over-represented and the oldest people are mostly widows living alone on low incomes. Over the next decade and beyond, the elderly population will be joined by increasing numbers of people who were born in other cultures and came to the UK in early life. These old people often suffer from what Norman (1985), over a decade ago, referred to as the 'triple jeopardy' of old age – racial or cultural discrimination, and lack of access to suitable services. Research suggests that these people are particularly at risk of mental disorder in old age and are less likely than people in the indigenous population to have such disorders recognised and treated (Norman 1988).

THE EXPERIENCE OF OLD AGE

What emerges from the chapters in Part 1 is that the personal and social experience of ageing depends on people's own experiences and capacities on the one hand and societal attitudes and policies on the other. Individual variation increases in late life and emerges as a major theme in all three chapters. There are great differences in the experience of ageing between individuals, depending on their health and vitality, savings and income, the quality of their housing and its location, their social networks and responsiveness of social services. However, according to Kendrick and Warnes (Ch. 1), some generalisations have been confirmed:

- real average living standards have improved
- on transition from work to retirement, the income of most people declines
- wealth differentials established during working lives tend to increase in retirement years.

As well as individual variability, there are great differences in the experience of ageing across historical cohorts. The impact of higher living standards is difficult to predict but it is likely that old people of future generations will be healthier than their parents and grandparents. Even more likely is that new generations of elderly people will have higher expectations of their life and functioning and they will make more demands on health and social care services.

It is clear that the pessimistic, stereotyped view of physical and mental decline as unavoidable consequences of ageing is overstated. Herbert and Thomson (Ch. 3) point to the misleading results of cross-sectional studies which compare people of different generations at one point in time and therefore do not account for cohort effects (e.g. diet, educational background, trends in smoking, different lifestyles).

More recent longitudinal studies now paint a more complex and sophisticated picture of human ageing. For most of us, as we get older, there is some deterioration in physical and mental functioning but there is greater heterogeneity between individuals in older than younger ages. Lifestyle differences play an important role in how people age and individual variability is marked; no two individuals show the same degree of physiological or pathological change, and chronological age is a poor predictor of loss of physiological function or performance.

What emerges from Herbert and Thomson's chapter is that the biological process of ageing cannot be considered in isolation from economic, environmental and psychosocial factors when seeking to understand the experience of old age. Rentoul (Ch. 2) explains that developmental psychologists conceive old age as a stage of development in the life cycle with its own tasks and challenges. In the psychoanalytic tradition the work of Erikson is particularly notable. His model of characteristics of an ideal old age has stood the test of time and continues to underpin the work of theorists and researchers, although it has also been criticised for failing to acknowledge all the forces that oppose human development, with the result that integrity – the positive pole of the integrity–despair dimension – is rarely fully achieved. Rentoul, though, argues that Erikson's theory of the last stage of life is more complex and sophisticated than the notion of integrity versus despair implies. What is important is the way in which the earlier tasks were experienced and handled and their impact on future development. Thus, a recurrent theme in this book, which has implications for health care professionals, is that to understand older people it is important to see them in the context of their whole life history; in particular to consider the ways in which important issues were either resolved or were not.

Rentoul (Ch. 2) tells us that recent work on personality and ageing has confirmed that people's behaviour remains stable over spans of 10 years or more; people tend to enjoy the same interests and activities as before and to hold the same ideas and values. Recognising that personality traits are likely to be preserved into later life is important if carers are to avoid confounding awkward or unpleasant behaviour with early signs of mental disorder. As Johnson puts it: 'nice younger people tend to become nice older people. Those who were cantankerous, intolerant, spiteful, mean, narrow minded, selfish or indolent will continue to be' (Johnson 1988, p. 143).

Intellectual functioning and cognitive performance are often assumed to decline with age and to become worse in old age. However, this view is closely associated with negative stereotypes of elderly people and relies on experiments conducted under artificial laboratory conditions rather than in real life situations. The evidence on cognitive change across the life cycle is equivocal. Some factors other than age which affect cognitive performance are more likely to apply to older than younger people; for example, lack of familiarity with tests used, lack of confidence in one's own intellectual abilities, feeling overwhelmed by the tester or the test situation, and poor health. Slowing of response is the most marked cognitive change with ageing. There is some evidence to suggest that this may worsen when information irrelevant to the task in hand is presented. It may be that older people find it more difficult than younger people to ignore irrelevant material. This has obvious implications for carers when giving information to elderly people.

The cognitive abilities of some old people are adversely affected by deteriorating physical and mental health. Others show no evidence of cognitive decline until at least the age of 75, and draw upon their experience and wisdom into very late life to the benefit of their community and society. The performance of some old people on psychological tests can be outstanding. Rentoul (Ch. 2) reports Rabbitt's finding that 10–15% of people in their eighties perform on fluid intelligence tests at the same level as the best of those 20 years younger. The underlying factors which maintain this level of functioning in old age have yet to be fully articulated.

A clear finding of the research studies described in Chapter 2 is that elderly people who are socioeconomically more privileged cope better with widowhood and other life stresses than those worse off. The well off enjoy better health, more extensive social networks and more coping resources. In widowhood gender differences feature in the capacity of older people to adapt, with men at higher risk than women of mortality, especially from suicide. Widowhood is an expected transition for women but not for men and so its impact is likely to be greater for men. Men may enjoy fewer extensive social networks than women and are less able to use those available. Also men feel under pressure not to express their feelings and are thus less able than women to do active grief work and thereby avoid some of widowhood's deleterious effects. Whether this will be true of future generations of men remains to be seen.

Retirement is now regarded as not directly linked to physical or mental decline, although not everyone perceives it positively and for some it is associated with financial problems and health decline. Relocation to an institutional setting, though, is recognised as a stressful event, and is associated with increased morbidity and mortality. However, the evidence again suggests large individual differences in response to relocation linked to individual and, more importantly, institutional (environmental) factors which can predict positive adjustment; Rentoul (Ch. 2) refers to research that shows the quality of nursing care to be the most important predictor. There are clear implications from this research for nurses and others concerned with creating therapeutic and supportive environments for elderly people in residential settings.

Problems of physical and mental health are significant sources of stress for elderly people, and can leave them depressed and failing in health. A consistent finding, Rentoul reveals, is that people are more likely to become depressed in response to chronic stress (e.g. chronic illness or long-term financial problems) than in response to sudden stressful life events. As with younger people, social support acts as a buffer for elderly people in moderating the impact of stress, and there is some evidence to show that the expectation of certain experiences in old age (increases in ill health and widowhood, for example) may weaken the beneficial impact of social support.

The relationships between life events, social support and wellbeing are complex. Some generalisations can be made, but there are many unanswered questions about the mechanisms involved. As Kendrick and Warnes (Ch. 1) point out, we know that people's reactions to the losses of ageing and their adjustments to changed capacities are, to some extent, conditioned by their expectations of old age, which in turn will be influenced by social norms and comparisons made with their parents and peers. But the complexities of these relationships are little understood. What emerges, particularly from Chapter 3, is that there may be a difference between the factors perceived by health care professionals as important in affecting health and wellbeing and what elderly people themselves consider important. The large Swedish study by Lindgren and colleagues, discussed by Herbert and Thomson, which considered the prevalence of a range of problems and their effects on wellbeing, found that the most important factors related to perceived health were activity, contentment and mobility problems. Contentment was affected by the activity score and loneliness, and loneliness was affected by the age and type of housing. The important message from these findings is that interventions to improve old people's satisfaction are probably more important than those that seek marginal improvements in their medical condition. This has implications for mental health promotion with elderly people, as discussed by Armstrong and Sparkes in Chapter 15.

In summary, the strong messages that come across, particularly from Part 1, are:

- the importance of individual variability
- the need to consider current circumstances of elderly people
- the powerful influence of personal history.

Decline in most aspects of functioning is not an inevitable part of ageing; and rewarding social relationships and independence and autonomy can go a long way towards reducing emotional disturbance and health deterioration. The inverse association between socioeconomic status and the ability to cope with life stresses and mental disorder, in particular depression, is well established. The mechanisms involved are complex, but a general improvement in living standards and financial provision is most likely to reduce depression in old age. The correlates of positive adjustment to living healthy lives in institutional environments, together with a range of coping strategies, are increasingly recognised as important to the wellbeing of elderly people.

Overall, successful ageing seems to be characterised by continuity between late life and earlier periods. Emotional wellbeing is most likely to persist if we can sustain into late life our own idiosyncratic patterns of social relationships, self-image, values, activities and living arrangements which we have built up over a lifetime (Johnson 1988). To understand the experience of ageing for any of us, it is important to consider old age in the context of our personal histories as individuals and as members of a specific cohort.

DEPRESSION – A MAJOR PUBLIC HEALTH PROBLEM

Of the functional mental disorders discussed in this volume, depression emerges as a major public health problem. Kendrick and Warnes (Ch. 1) report an incidence of depression in elderly people of 15–30 cases per thousand per year, high prevalence rates and also a relatively high proportion of people with symptoms of depression not reaching case level. For example, Copeland et al found that 10.7% of their sample had depressive symptoms in addition to the 11.3% who were 'cases'. Most at risk are women, with approximately double the prevalence of men, and people living in deprived inner cities areas. Other associations between social factors, life events and depression are more contentious; Kendrick and Warnes quote studies showing conflicting results. However, Hughes (Ch. 8)

points to the especially high prevalence rates found in studies of, for example, people receiving home care services, medical in-patients, GP attenders, people in residential homes and Alzheimer's disease sufferers. The implication is that people working with these groups should be extra vigilant for signs of depression. This is particularly important, given the evidence that many depressed elderly people receive no treatment or support and that depression is frequently overlooked or dismissed as an understandable and untreatable response to the vicissitudes of late life.

According to Kendrick and Warnes (Ch. 1) and Hughes (Ch. 8), the prognosis for depression in late life is poor. Both chapters report the study by Copeland et al in Liverpool which found that two-thirds of over-65-year-olds with depression were still ill or had died after 3 years of follow-up. In discussing principles of care and treatment Hughes highlights the importance of a problem-solving approach involving family members and employing a combination of physical, psychological and social interventions to promote recovery and, importantly, to prevent relapse. A multidisciplinary approach is usually needed, with attention given to the timing and sequencing of interventions and to physical problems which should be treated.

Psychological interventions

Several chapters in Part 3 describe psychological interventions for depressed elderly people. In Chapter 16 Scrutton identifies counselling as an underused intervention which can help people resolve their grief following loss and bereavement and can promote feelings of life satisfaction and fulfilment. Thus counselling can help depressed elderly people move towards a clearer understanding of their situation and their options, raise their expectations and reduce their fears. For Scrutton, many of the counselling agendas of old age derive from dominant social attitudes about ageing and old people that are now recognised as contributing to the negative stereotype of old people which undermines their social status and self-esteem. Some old people accept this stereotype and resign themselves to unrewarding social roles. Others reject it but in so doing may adopt strategies that are self-defeating; rejecting offers of help from relatives and friends and striking out at professional carers. These old people become socially isolated and increasingly unhappy.

One task of the counsellor is to help the demoralised person to distinguish between factors which are part of the reality of old age and those which are part of the social construction of ageing, that is the personal acceptance of social attitudes which limit the potential of elderly people to lead fulfilling lives. The counselling agenda may also focus on late life tasks such as those identified by Bergmann (1978) as:

- accepting the proximity of death
- coping and coming to terms with physical disability and ill health
- accepting that some degree of dependence on support systems is inevitable, in all stages of life
- sustaining mutually rewarding relationships with family and friends at a time of life in which interpersonal conflict and dissatisfaction are common themes in the experience of unhappy elderly people.

Scrutton identifies reminiscence as an ally to counselling unhappy elderly people, being both a means of conversation and a way of cementing the counselling relationship. However, research on reminiscence with elderly depressed people has produced mixed results. It may be counter-productive if what is recalled is always negative events (Hanley and Baiklie 1984). Reminiscence is reviewed in detail by Bornat in Chapter 22. She criticises the early policy of discouraging older people from talking about the past. As she observes, 'it now seems cruel to expect events evoking pain and guilt to be silently endured in isolation'. Her views are supported by Fry (1983) who used reminiscence to focus on unhappy memories and found that the expression of unresolved fears and feelings and strong emotions was associated with less self-reported depression and increased self-confidence.

In Chapter 19 Wells and Wells discuss cognitive therapy, perhaps the most firmly established psychological intervention for depression. The principle underlying cognitive therapy is that depression arises from errors of cognition, judgement, reasoning and remembering. The result is that depressed people make incorrect assumptions about themselves and others and feel worthless. The therapist works at forming a collaborative relationship with depressed people to ground their distress in specific problems so that they can become capable of resolution. By learning to review their irrational and maladaptive beliefs, critically depressed people come to discover the incorrectness of their interpretations for themselves.

According to Wells and Wells the evidence in support of cognitive therapy as an effective intervention for depression in old age is promising but as yet inconclusive. There are many difficulties involved in conducting double-blind, placebo-controlled trials involving psychotherapies, particu-

larly with elderly people who may have a number of medical problems that may affect outcome. Even so, cognitive therapy is an attractive treatment option. Its short-term nature and problem-solving focus make it suitable for older people, particularly for those who are sensitive to medications or who suffer from medical conditions that contraindicate the prescription of psychoactive drugs. Further, cognitive therapy is grounded in collaboration and partnership; principles which underpin the best therapeutic relationships. And it combats therapeutic nihilism by providing a rationale for depressed elderly people to take control of their lives once again, rather than wait passively for the drugs to work or for something to come along to raise their mood.

Prevention and treatment strategies

In sum, depression emerges as a major health problem for elderly people, and one which demands much more attention to prevention and treatment strategies than it currently gets. Kendrick and Warnes (Ch. 1) refer to the World Health Organization's conclusion that the primary medical care team is the cornerstone of community psychiatry. They point to well organised and efficient primary health care teams as offering the best hope for combating depression in old age. True multidisciplinarity, in which all members besides the general practice (GP) are fully involved and work to their full potential, is crucial if mental health care for elderly people is to have maximum benefit. Our experience suggests that community psychiatric nurses attached to primary health care teams are effective in providing short-term cognitive therapy and advising GPs and other non-specialists in the management of resistant cases. Other community nurses also have an important role to play. They regularly visit old people who are physically ill and at risk of depression and so are well placed to identify depression in their patients if trained properly to do so. However, the evidence from the study in south London by Gilleard suggests that most nurses do not have these skills. They tend to over-diagnose depression in housebound elderly patients and therefore cannot identify accurately which patients need extra support and treatment.

Another underused resource is practice nurses, who are at present little involved in psychiatric care apart from administering depot injections to people with chronic schizophrenia. They are increasingly involved in screening over-75-year-olds, as part of GPs' contracts, and, as with their community nursing colleagues, they need training to identify depression as well as dementia. According to Kendrick and Warnes (Ch. 1) there is some evidence from the study by Wilkinson that practice nurses are a valuable resource for GPs in promoting compliance with treatment and advising on the side-effects of antidepressants; however, the efficacy of this collaborative work is yet to be established.

THE NEW CULTURE OF DEMENTIA CARE

We turn now to consider treatment approaches to dementia – a disorder that is much less prevalent in old age than commonly thought, but which has devastating effects on the lives of sufferers and carers. What comes across strongly from chapters in this volume is that psychological interventions for those suffering from dementia are therapeutic and that a new culture of dementia care is emerging. Morton (Ch. 21) refers to this new culture as person-centred, which has three key features, all of which resonate with values currently held by the caring professions:

- A shift in the traditional power relations away from the therapist and towards the client. The therapist ceases to give direction or advice or offer insight, but takes on a facilitating role designed to help clients get in touch with and use their own inner resources.
- Increasing interest in the dementing person's perception of reality.
- Emphasis on the act of successful communication as crucial to high quality care.

Thus the onus is on the caregiver to encourage the dementing person's attempts to communicate and ensure successful completion. Through this, the dementing person experiences increased self-esteem and enhanced quality of life.

Validation therapy

Validation therapy (discussed by Morton, Ch. 21) was developed by Feil in the 1960s but has attracted attention in the UK only relatively recently. In addition to Rogerian person-centredness, validation is described by Morton as having three further key ingredients:

- a psychoanalytic orientation
- a four-stage model of disorientation
- the addition of a final life stage and task to Erikson's eight-stage developmental model.

Morton's critique of validation therapy highlights weaknesses in its theoretical base. Thus Feil's assumption that all behaviour of the dementing person, no matter how bizarre, has a rational basis is questioned. So is her four-stage theory of dementia, her final life stage and her view that disorientation in dementia is a process by which the ego loses contact with objective reality and retreats into a subjective reality inhabited by psychologically significant material and people. Morton's critique demonstrates that the theoretical underpinning of validation therapy becomes increasingly vulnerable as it departs from its person-centred assumptions and seeks to combine them with psychodynamic ideas.

The communication techniques advocated by Feil make sense to many of us who have worked with dementing people, particularly those with severe dementia, but the benefit of validation therapy for dementing people remains uncertain. Feil makes a range of claims for validation therapy. She reports (Feil 1992, 1992a, 1992b) that after 6 months of once-weekly sessions, patients demonstrated improved gait, less need for physical and chemical restraints, less crying, pounding, blaming, swearing and acting out of sexual behaviours, and that eye contact improved. However, there have been few attempts to test these claims empirically. The research that has been done (for example, Robb et al 1986, Scanland & Emershaw 1993), failed to establish significant changes in patients following validation therapy. The standardised outcome measures used may have been insufficiently sensitive to the small changes that might occur with severely disabled people with a progressive illness. Moreover, they adopted an experimental design which, with small samples, suffers from the masking effect of group analysis; that is, positive responses in some individuals may be cancelled by negative responses in others.

An alternative to the experimental design is to use single-case study designs which allow analysis within and across cases to draw attention to the characteristics of individuals who respond positively to psychological interventions and those who do not. Morton and his colleague Christine Bleathman, in a small-scale study at the Maudsley Hospital (Morton & Bleathman 1991) used a single-case study cross-over design to compare the benefits of reminiscence therapy and group validation therapy. A number of observation instruments and behaviour rating scales were used but the results were inconclusive. Only three out of five patients completed the study. Two showed a marked increase in interaction in the post-validation therapy period. In one of the patients this was due to an increased length of and number of patient-initiated interactions. In the other it was due to an increase in duration of interaction. In both there was a decrease in interaction in the reminiscence therapy phase. The third subject showed a rise in frequency and duration of interactions following reminiscence therapy, but not following validation therapy.

A more recent small-scale study, in which one of us (IJN) was involved, adopted a similar research design to compare the effects of validation therapy with involvement in another group activity (Harris 1995). Harris's observations of the activities of dementing people in the validation therapy groups support Morton's findings (discussed in Ch. 21) that we tend to underestimate hugely the latent social abilities of dementing elderly people. Harris's results also support Morton & Bleathman (1991), in that they showed an increase in interaction in some patients following validation therapy. Harris also found that patients who had the greatest problems expressing themselves responded more positively to validation therapy than those who had fewer problems. However, these findings are tentative. The single-case study design, as drawn on by Morton and Bleathman, and by Harris, has the potential to reveal changes in individuals, but the small sample size in both studies was not capable of illuminating any clear pattern of responses relevant to patient characteristics.

Reality orientation

Morton (Ch. 21) points out that validation therapy developed as a reaction to the dominant psychological therapy of the time, reality orientation, which Feil saw as inappropriate for all dementing people except for those with mild confusion. For Feil reality orientation is not only a waste of time and effort with dementing people, in that it has few positive benefits in bringing about increased orientation, but it has a negative impact; sudden insight into reality bringing pain (momentary realisation of their desperate situation), withdrawal and increased dependency. Reality orientation also represents for Feil a missed opportunity to discover the true reasons behind disordered speech and behaviour. In Chapter 20 Holden rejects these criticisms. She argues that critics misunderstand what reality orientation is all about or, more precisely, has become in the late 1990s. If catastrophic reactions do occur it is because common sense and sensitivity have not been used by the therapist; these reactions arise from poor technique, rather from the reality orientation therapy itself.

The picture of reality orientation painted by Holden shows just how far it has changed since its development by Folsom in the late 1950s. Its goal in those early years was to address the unmet emotional needs of psychiatric patients in long-stay residential care (Hanley 1984, Holden & Woods 1988). The emphasis was on building relationships and spending time in one-to-one contact with patients. It was not long, however, before other aspects of the therapy took primacy over this inter-personal aspect. The guidelines of the American Hospitals Association (1976, cited in Hanley 1984), demonstrate clearly a shift in emphasis: staff were urged to 'correct residents when they ramble confusedly in speech and actions' ... and to ... 'show residents that you expect them to comply'. This was done showing 'kindness and politeness, while being matter-of-fact' (AHA 1976, cited in Hanley 1984, p. 187). This suggests that by the mid 1970s reality orientation had lost touch with its person-centred origins and bore the hallmarks of a rigid form of behaviour therapy. When introduced into the UK in the 1970s reality orientation was greeted with enthusiasm because it offered hope to care staff on behalf of dementing people, where previously there had been none. Much research into the benefits of reality orientation followed (reviewed in Holden & Woods 1988), largely as a formal classroom therapy; much of it was inconclusive. But by the early 1980s the popularity of reality orientation had begun to wane. Woods (1994) suggests that this resulted from the corrective and prescriptive nature of the therapy, which was often practised in a rigid and patronising manner without respect for the adult individual. It seems likely that Feil's disillusion with reality orientation was with a therapy that no longer sought to meet the emotional needs of dementing people.

Holden's contribution to this volume (Ch. 20) suggests that reality orientation has come full circle, returning to its origins as a person-centred therapy. As described, reality orientation now emphasises:

- An individual focus incorporating realistic and relevant assessments and a planned individualised programme with clear goals and regular monitoring of individual achievement.
- Maximising use of retained skills, abilities and experience and maintaining individual routines. No longer is the emphasis simply on promoting orientation.
- Environmental modifications which extend beyond the physical environment to incorporate aspects of the psychological environment of care settings; and organisational factors, such as morale and motivation of staff, which exert great influence on the way that reality orientation is carried out.

- Education of therapists to ensure they hold the right attitudes, values and principles, for example:
  - respect for the dementing person and for the principle of normalisation
  - a commitment to improve the physical and psychological aspects of care environments.

  Also, knowledge of the effects of ageing and medical conditions affecting older people to enable realistic goals to be set for individuals and achievements to be realistically evaluated.
- Eclecticism: incorporating a variety of modes and methods including activities, reminiscence, exercise and skills and memory training. Also recognition that reality orientation is not antagonistic to other psychological interventions, such as reminiscence therapy, but provides a valuable backdrop to them.

We conclude that reality orientation as practised in the 1990s is now part and parcel of the new culture of dementia care, having once represented the antithesis to person-centred approaches.

Reminiscence

Evidence of the new culture of dementia care, in which one focus is on the experience of dementia for the sufferer, is also found in Bornat's (Ch. 22) review of reminiscence with dementing elderly people. She describes the work of Gibson, whose reminiscence work seeks to encourage conversation and increase sociability of dementing people and build a picture of their lives which can lead to more sensitive and appropriate care. Reminiscence work can result in small improvements in the behaviour of dementing people. It can also challenge staff preconceptions, enhance the quality of relationships between dementing people and their carers and increase carers' job satisfaction. From Bornat's chapter, reminiscence offers one way of helping us to understand what dementing people are feeling and saying, and may postpone the parting of the ways between dementing people and their carers which almost inevitably occurs as the illness progresses.

Disorientation in dementia

Theories of disorientation in dementia are discussed in several chapters. Herbert and Thomson (Ch. 3) describe Grimley Evans' model of Alzheimer's disease, which postulates interaction between genetic susceptibility and environmental agents and seeks to explain why the outcome of the same disease process can and does vary from one individual to the next.

Thus Grimley Evans postulates that some people who develop Alzheimer's disease have a genetic endowment which gives them 70 years or more before they accumulate a toxic dose of environmental factors. Others (a minority) have a genetic endowment that affects their brains in later life. The functional impairment which results is influenced by both genetic and environmental factors. 'Better brains' (from genetic endowment or improved by education) may be better at compensating for the damage from the disease process, and environmental factors, such as the quality of input from social and health services, will also influence social functioning. Models such as this are valuable since they seek to reconcile the fact of a disease process with environmental factors, which either promote or inhibit wellbeing and social competence, in a way that Feil's account of dementia fails to do. They are worth testing and developing to draw out implications for care and treatment.

Of the models of disorientation in dementia the work of Kitwood and the Bradford Dementia Research Group receives particular attention, being raised by Adams (Ch. 11) and considered in detail by Morton (Ch. 21). Kitwood and his team hypothesise a dialectical interplay between physical (neurological) factors and the social psychology which surrounds dementing people and increasingly robs them of self-confidence and social status. Kitwood's other important contribution to our understanding of dementia, also discussed by Morton (Ch. 21), is his account of communication in dementia, which clearly draws upon social psychology and interactionist sociology in emphasising the importance of seeking to understand people's intentions and interpretations of the actions of others.

Kitwood is critical of some psychological therapies, including validation therapy and reality orientation, since both define the 'problem' of dementia as residing with the sufferer and do not recognise that 'we' – the therapist or carer – come to the situation as part of the problem. Morton argues, though, that Kitwood's work is squarely in the person-centred tradition and its practical implications are not qualitatively different or more advanced than other attempts to bring person-centred principles and values to the work of dementia care. Recommendations of the Bradford group reflect commonly held notions of good practice, communication skills, empathy and social sensitivity.

A future agenda for dementia care

Morton (Ch. 21) points out that we all need personal

relationships to sustain our sense of being part of the human world and, if we develop dementia, we need them even more. He concludes with two key questions which we emphasise here as setting the future agenda for dementia care. First, the practical problem of how to spread the new person-centred agenda for dementia care beyond conference-attending, journal-reading professionals to those who deliver hands-on care to dementing people. As discussed by Norman (Ch. 26), these people are often poorly paid, inadequately trained and supervised, and undervalued. In addition, they experience stress from quantitative overload (too much to do) and qualitative underload (understimulating) care settings. It is not surprising that, for many, 'getting through the day' is more important than the quality of their care.

The second problem which prevents person-centred ideals having an impact on quality of life for significant numbers of dementing people is that of identifying and developing communication methods that have a positive and demonstrable impact. As Morton points out, Feil's attempt to describe communication strategies associated with her four stages of dementia may not have been totally successful but she did at least address the real issue of what works with whom. As we have seen, single-case study designs as used by Morton & Bleathman (1991) and Harris (1995) have shown promising results, but the sample sizes were too small to demonstrate significant effects. Larger scale single-case studies, conducted over a longer time-scale and employing methods sensitive to the small changes that may arise from psychological interventions with elderly dementing people whose capabilities are in decline, are a priority for researchers.

DEVELOPMENTS IN SERVICE PROVISION

We turn finally to reflect upon directions for services for elderly mentally ill people. Most chapters discuss the UK context, but, in so doing, illustrate the impact of forces which are affecting health and social care professionals in other parts of Europe, and elsewhere. Tinker (Ch. 24) identifies four policy changes which have guided service developments for elderly people:

- preventing people from going into institutions
- returning people from institutions to the community
- improving conditions in institutions
- building up community care.

We address each of these in turn.

Preventing people from going into institutions

Tinker points out that it is easy to prevent people from entering institutions if the number of beds is declining. The real questions are whether elderly mentally ill people are living successfully in the community, and how their carers are coping. Brandon and Jack (Ch. 14) and Askham (Ch. 25) shed light on these questions.

Brandon and Jack's chapter on struggling with services sums up at least one family's experience of trying to care for, and care about, a dementing relative. Brandon concludes his personal account of caring for his father-in-law thus: 'I had met a man with whom I ordinarily wouldn't have spent 5 minutes in conversation and gained some sort of mysterious commitment to him through marriage – a commitment I never properly understood and failed to honour. For me, it was and continues to feel a massive personal failure. It is hard to imagine a way to let down another human being more comprehensively.'

Jack's analysis of Brandon's experience demonstrates that the failure was not Brandon's alone. The major failure was in the services offered to disabled people and their family carers. Jack draws attention to two preoccupations of studies and descriptions of informal care which have negative consequences for carers and cared for. First, just listing the effects of disabilities and needs of the cared for on the carer leads to an over-simplified carer/dependant model which cannot reflect the interdependent reality which most families experience. Thus, informal caring is seen as an unrewarding and unreciprocated non-relationship which is almost inevitably damaging for the carer. Second, comparing the relative impact of different levels of service provision on carer wellbeing neglects the relationship between informal and formal carers. Thus, the professional relationship may be part of the so-called burden of caregiving rather than its solution.

There are many lessons in Chapter 14 for all of us who are part of the formal caring apparatus. One major source of distress for Brandon arose from the failure of professional carers to attend to the relationship between informal carers and those they care for, assuming that it was a non-relationship which offered no possibility of mutual reward. Instead the professionals colonised this relationship; severed it in the rush to provide services, resulting in later abandonment and guilt which Brandon and his wife endured alone. Jack attributes this, at least in part, to the dominance of the individually-oriented pathology model of professional social work which, he argues, is positively damaging to the practice of social care. The result is an emphasis on:

- assessment of disorder and dysfunction without recognising the importance of promoting health and coping strategies
- needs assessment rather than the advocacy of rights
- the search for 'insight' rather than providing education, information and practical help
- the imposition of treatment rather than practising a partnership.

Brandon and Jack reject the individual pathology model and advocate models of social work more suited to the practice of social care. These models are not new but so far have had limited influence on social work practice; Brandon and Jack's chapter indicates the need for a re-evaluation.

Askham (Ch. 25) points to the issues and problems of supporting elderly people at home. Her analysis of the state of current provision resonates with some of the aspects of service provision discussed by Brandon and Jack. Askham concludes that support services of any kind are valued by informal carers, particularly practical services that give them most relief or relieve the burden of daily tasks. If asked, most people say they are happy with the level of provision they receive, but this may reflect the limited resources that are made available and the possibility that it suits professionals to turn a blind eye. Under-provision is evident in the most common types of support service: community nursing, home care, day care and institutional respite care, and also for the support of older people and their carers when the diagnosis is functional mental disorder rather than dementia. Overall, the sort of services provided seem to be the right ones. The gaps in service provision most often identified are to do with the inadequacy of existing services rather than their scope. The most pressing research questions are, however, concerned not with user satisfaction or scale of provision, but with the efficacy of support services: whether they are beneficial to the mental health of elderly people and their informal carers; and whether they can help people, who might otherwise be in institutions, to live longer at home. The whole question of what different types of support provide what benefits to which people in what circumstances needs further investigation.

Returning people from institutions to the community

Tinker's (Ch. 24) second theme of policy change which

has guided service developments for elderly people is concerned with returning people from institutions to the community. This theme is discussed by Tinker and also by Redfern (Ch. 27) and by Morley and Sellwood (Ch. 13) specifically in relation to people with a diagnosis of schizophrenia who may also suffer from institutionalisation.

Morley and Sellwood distinguish between elderly people with schizophrenia who find themselves resident in institutions as the result of two different events. The first group entered large hospitals suffering from schizophrenia when younger and, following repeated episodes, stayed on to become long-stay patients. The second group are older people with schizophrenia who live in institutional care in the community. Thus, although Tinker focuses in Chapter 24 on resettlement (that is, moving from a large hospital to a community setting), Morley and Sellwood remind us that small-scale residential services may have as institutionalising an effect on residents as the large hospitals they were designed to replace. Elderly people in nursing homes, hostels, hostel wards and staffed group homes may be especially at risk. The characteristic problems created by institutional care are well known: the routinisation of daily life, separation of staff and inmates and segregation from the outside world. These characteristics make the caring task more manageable for staff: they can maintain emotional distance from patients, ensure their compliance, cope with a large number of tasks and avoid difficult or embarrassing encounters between inmates and the world outside.

Family carers may face similar problems and stresses to those faced by paid staff in institutions. For example, problems in getting dependent family members to do what they want them to, problems in relating to them, in coping with the volume of tasks presented by caring for someone who is dementing, and handling potentially embarrassing encounters between the person and others coming to the home. In an effort to manage their stress, family carers may develop institutional-type care by, for example, developing a routinised day, maintaining a distance between themselves and the sufferer, or segregating the sufferer from others in the household. We cannot assume that, because research suggests that most people want to remain at home even if they become frail or disabled (Salvage et al 1989), care at home – even when such care really exists – is always a positive experience. However, we know almost nothing about these matters. The social organisation of care for elderly mentally disordered people living in their own homes has yet to be understood. We are not even certain that institutional-type care at home is undesirable. It is conceivable that, for some dementing elderly people, some institutional-type care is a good thing because it lends stability to their lives and enhances their sense of security. However, any such argument is itself a research question and cannot be answered before we understand more fully the nature of home care for dependent elderly people.

Tinker points to the available evidence which shows that people now left in the large hospitals are the oldest and the most physically and mentally disabled; those who will need the most support to live as normal a life as possible in the community. If they are moved from the old institution, 24-hour community provision has to be available. To this end, in the UK, the National Health Service and Community Care Act 1990 requires each person who needs care to have an individual discharge plan. Under the provisions of the Care Programme Approach (CPA), which was launched by the UK government in 1991, health authorities are required to appoint a key worker and formulate a plan in collaboration with other agencies. Tinker points out that monitoring of CPA is, at time of writing, virtually non-existent.

The provision of adequate primary health care services is crucial to the success of resettlement schemes, and it is envisaged by the Audit Commission (1994) that only those with the most serious mental health problems should be treated in hospital. Tinker's chapter underlines our earlier remarks about the central place of the primary health care team in community psychiatry and the need for the skills of team members to be strengthened.

Adequate supportive housing is also essential to the success of a resettlement scheme and there has been an increase in both hostels and small houses in the community in which a number of ex-residents can live together. As mentioned above, it is easy for small residential settings to become isolated from the community even when located on an urban street. Morley and Sellwood (Ch. 13) also refer to Perkins et al's criticism of residential and nursing accommodation for older people as offering little choice and flexibility. For example, many elderly people with schizophrenia end up relocated into residential homes in which there are a large proportion of confused residents. Moreover, many homes are very large. Morley and Sellwood (Ch. 13) cite a survey by Willcocks et al, in 1986, of 100 residential homes which showed that 65% had more than 40 residents and 50% had more than 50. Since homes like these are noted for low levels of social interaction and activity, leading to the development of passivity and dependence, one must question their suitability for elderly people with chronic schizophrenia resettled from the old hospitals. According to Morley and Sellwood, small scale homely accommodation which offers residents greater control over their lifestyle and privacy is preferred for resettlement of these people. Also, intensive preparation of both staff and patients before any move has been shown to result in improved patients' functioning.

Redfern (Ch. 27) raises the thorny problem of integration or segregation; whether dementing people should be segregated in special homes or integrated with other old people in ordinary residential homes. She points to strong arguments on both sides. Proponents of normalisation argue that integration is a necessary, if not sufficient, condition for achieving the principle of ordinary living. Others, including users' pressure groups, claim that segregation provides the best opportunity for well planned care regimes to meet the special needs of dementing patients, and avoids distress to alert elderly residents. The literature suggests that there is no clear-cut answer. The degree of confusion experienced by the resident is an important factor to be considered in making placement decisions in individual cases, as is the proportion of confused to alert residents in the home and the mental health problems experienced by other residents. Redfern concludes that mildly or moderately demented residents are probably happier living in integrated settings and, as long as they do not have behaviour problems, are not likely to upset other residents. Severely demented people, on the other hand, are probably better off in segregated settings in which their particular needs are given priority.

Drawing on work by Ramon, Redfern (Ch. 27) points to the very different ways in which hospital closure and resettlement has been managed in the USA and most countries of Europe, compared to Italy, Denmark and Sweden. In the former large group the main impetus for hospital closure was financial, the aim being to 'transfer' residents from large expensive hospitals to community facilities without fuss and at minimum cost. The result was that little attention was paid to the views and wishes of residents or staff, and preparing both groups for new ways of living and working which would enhance opportunities for ordinary living was an add-on extra to the main programme of closure. In contrast, Italy's hospital closure programme was underpinned by ordinary life principles that respected residents' rights and dignity and was well planned, involving considerable consultation with staff and residents to harness their motivation for dismantling institutional ways of working and living. Predictably, the consequences for residents of UK hospital closure programmes, particularly the earlier programmes, were disastrous. Often transfer occurred from one total institutional style of living to another, and often at the cost of relationships and social networks built up over many years of hospital life. Only relatively recently has it been recognised that maintaining people who need high levels of support in the community is not a cheap option. This realisation, along with new funding arrangements for community care from April 1995, are amongst pressures which have resulted in reduced services for mentally ill people in the community and a slowing down of the hospital closure programme.

Despite the hard lessons learned from hospital closures, the research studies discussed by Tinker (Ch. 24) and Redfern (Ch. 27) which have evaluated resettlement schemes for elderly people are reasonably encouraging. Both of these chapters draw attention to research by the Personal Social Services Research Unit at the University of Kent which evaluated the *Care in the Community* demonstration programme consisting of 28 projects designed to help long-stay hospital residents to move into community residential settings. Four of these projects catered for elderly people, mostly with dementia, providing residential home care with some day care or, in one project, a support service to delay or prevent admission to residential homes through provision of supportive sheltered housing. The evaluation showed that community living is most often preferred by the residents themselves, coordinated individual care planning can work well and the costs of community care need not be prohibitively expensive. Tinker concludes that essential elements of a successful resettlement programme are individual care plans and adequate support services, including medical, social and housing provision. In addition, half-way provision (a smaller hospital or hostel) and/or special financial help to the individual or to other service providers may be required. Drawing on Ramon, Redfern (Ch. 27) adds: good coordination and consultation between agencies involved; flexibility and creativity by service planners; recognition of barriers to change and a strategy to disarm opposing powers and change the self-perception of those involved from losers to enthusiastic converts and gainers; and users' involvement in the whole process.

Improving conditions in institutions

Brandon's experience of struggling with services (Ch. 14) is, for the most part, a sad reflection on the state of nursing care for long-stay patients. His account of his father-in-law's 'care' in hospital is instructive:

We visited dutifully each weekend. Some staff were welcoming and others openly hostile. Carefully, I had made some comment about the radio being very loud so we couldn't converse with the confused old man. The charge nurse responded with a grim smile, all teeth: 'You can always take him home – can't you?' Now we were abject beggars asking for favours ... We were never asked about any of his likes or dislikes, anything of his personal character or history. They knew absolutely nothing about him and didn't feel any lack of knowledge ... He lost his rights of citizenship in becoming a long-stay patient.

This account resonates with the findings from studies of hospital care for elderly people referred to by Norman (Ch. 26), most of which describe undesirable environments, activities and patterns of (nursing) care and highlights, in particular, poor psychosocial care including: lack of concern with individual needs of elderly people; lack of attention to principles of choice, privacy and dignity; and low levels of patient activity and nurse-patient interaction, particularly for confused elderly people. Norman argues (Ch. 26) that these poor care practices are associated with depressed and demoralised staff whose behaviours towards long-stay and continuing care patients reflect the syndrome of burnout and the lesser known syndrome of rustout. Burnout and rustout have similar features – isolation and emotional detachment – but have different causes. Burnout arises from quantitative and qualitative overload (stressful work with patients under tight time constraints), whereas rustout results from qualitative underload (unstimulating and routine work with patients). Both overload and underload are stressful features of direct care work with elderly mentally ill people and have negative consequences for workers, particularly for the many care assistants who have little control over their work. Strategies for increasing coping and thereby improving the quality of care include psychological strategies such as problem solving and positive reappraisal, and organisational supports such as clinical supervision and staff support groups and training programmes, particularly those that involve residents themselves. In short, high quality care environments are those in which care workers are valued and supported as much as the residents.

In Chapter 27 Redfern asks two basic questions with respect to long-stay care:

- what does a high quality service look like for residents?
- how can working practices be improved?

The first of these questions requires attention to principles and values underpinning residential care, specifically values relating to residents' rights and opportunities to lead ordinary lives, even when disabled. Normalisation, social role valorisation and integrated living are seen by Ramon (cited by Redfern, Ch. 27) as the bedrock of good care practice. If these principles are acknowledged by all in society then elderly disabled people will be enabled to lead normal lives in ordinary settings.

The extent to which these three principles are reflected in the reality of life for most elderly mentally ill people in long-stay care varies. But the evidence suggests that some models of residential care offer a better chance of these principles taking root and being reflected in practice than others. Redfern discusses the relative merits of several models. The first of these, which was developed in the UK before the large hospital closure programme got into full swing, was three experimental Department of Health-funded NHS nursing homes for elderly mentally ill people which aimed to provide individualised care in a homely living environment. The evaluation of these nursing homes by Copeland and his team at Liverpool University showed mixed results for the residents themselves but, importantly, highlighted some key issues relevant to high quality residential care including:

- the importance of management support for care workers, such as careful staff recruitment, in-service training and audit procedures
- the untapped potential of care assistants as key workers
- setting realistic goals which recognise the limited potential of residents whose illnesses sap their motivation for social interaction and activities.

Redfern (Ch. 27) points out that the nursing home, as a setting for long-stay residential care, has now been superseded, in some European countries at least, by other sorts of provision which are built on a smaller scale. Drawing on work by Netten, she observes that Denmark, once noted for its impressive design of old people's homes, now favours independent homes in small housing complexes. In the UK the trend is also towards smaller units offering a positive care philosophy and multiprofessional working and different levels of health care input. Thus nursing homes give a high input of care, social services homes a lower input and modified housing with extra care suits people with low care needs. Models of care most suited to dementing residents involve small group living; in flats in ordinary residential blocks as in Sweden, or in domus units as introduced in one London borough.

Evaluations of the domus model are encouraging.

Redfern (Ch. 27) refers to research by Lindesay and his team who compared the domus with two long-stay psychogeriatric wards catering for residents with similar levels of cognitive impairment and depression. They found:

- significantly higher staff–resident interaction and resident activity in the domus
- significantly greater independence of domus residents in some daily living activities
- more positive attitudes of domus staff who expected residents to function as independently as possible and to choose whether or not to take part in social and recreational activities.

The financial cost of the domus model is higher than long-stay hospital provision, but it does seem to offer the possibility of high quality life and high quality care to a vulnerable group of elderly people.

The success of the domus approach is in part the outcome of its care philosophy, set out in Chapter 27, which emphasises that the needs of the staff are as important as those of the residents and gives high priority to staff training and support. The important issue of staff training as a prerequisite of high quality residential care is taken up by Norman (Ch. 26), who highlights work training as a way of helping carers to cope with stress and as a cost-effective way of increasing carers' knowledge about residents, so creating more favourable attitudes towards them, increasing competence and motivation and improving job satisfaction and quality of work. Norman (Ch. 26) reports an evaluation of the Institute of Social Work's Training for Care Staff Programme (TCSP) by Youll & McCourt-Perring which drew important conclusions for guiding the development of training for residential care staff. As they said, successful staff training is integral to service provision and cannot be 'bolted-on' to a care establishment without taking account of its values, practices and purposes. The receptiveness of staff to training depends on the climate of the home and attitudes of staff. Training will not have beneficial effects in care settings in which staff feel undervalued and unappreciated. Training cannot solve what are essentially management's problems and, since successful training leads to an empowered and critical workforce, management must be prepared to change too and become more open and responsive to staff development.

Whatever model of provision is preferred, high quality care in residential homes depends on a supportive physical environment and a caring regime. Redfern (Ch. 27) discusses these aspects in detail. The physical design of homes should be comfortable, offer privacy and choice and be economically viable. Homes should also be conducive to group living, provide each resident with personal territory (such as a personal space, private or otherwise, for sitting) and be personalised with possessions. For dementing people, homes need to 'make sense' domestically; they should be small and local, but with plenty of space for staff and residents, have rooms for different purposes and provide discreet cues (e.g. meaningful landmarks, such as ornaments), a quiet atmosphere and bright surroundings which promote orientation.

In discussing the caring social environment Redfern (Ch. 27) points to the importance of providing opportunities for friendship between residents and between residents and staff. Also offering opportunities for personal growth, which inevitably means striking the balance between the rights of residents to come and go as they please and the risks of injury. Striking the right balance between flexibility and regimentation is crucial. Routine is important to most of us, and particularly to elderly dementing residents since it increases the predictability of events and thereby allows them more control over their lives. But if the routine becomes rigid dementing people are most vulnerable because they are unable to express their needs and preferences and the routine may ride roughshod over them. Our experience suggests that it is best to let residents establish their own daily routine and then support it with a structured and dependable programme to which changes are introduced only gradually.

Overall, the literature reviewed by Redfern suggests that direct care staff do have more control than is often supposed over the quality of care in residential homes, given motivation and sufficient resources, and leadership which creates a positive environment and attitudes for care. The literature also suggests that overall quality of care in hospital wards is worse than in local authority and private residential homes and nursing homes. This may, in part, be because residents in long-stay wards are treated as, and take the role of, 'patients'. Nurses may be more likely than workers with a different occupational background to treat patients in this way, but the evidence is mixed. Redfern refers to Netten's finding that the proportion of staff with nursing qualifications in residential homes for dementing people was associated with an increase in residents' apathy, but improved levels of orientation. Nurses may ignore residents who are quiet and sitting comfortably, but their training enables them to work more effectively than other staff in promoting orientation.

In sum, there seems to be a consensus about aspects of residential care environments which are important to high quality care. The evidence suggests that this care can be provided for elderly people with different levels of dependency, in segregated or integrated settings, if adequate resources are provided and steps taken to overcome barriers of social stigma, pejorative labelling and care regimes which lead elderly people to be treated as patients first, rather than as people.

Building up community care

Tinker's (Ch. 24) fourth theme guiding service developments is building up community care. Community care is provided mostly by families, with support from statutory and voluntary services which have long been acknowledged as inadequate. Tinker charts the growing critique of UK community care provision in official reports culminating in the National Health Service and Community Care Act 1990, which set the organisational framework for present day services. One of the main changes introduced by the Act was the creation of an internal market for health care, which involved distinguishing between purchasers (district health authorities, general practitioners) and providers of services, i.e. hospitals and community health units, either directly managed by the district health authorities, or transferred into NHS trusts, or the independent sector. An internal market also operates in social services and Tinker (Ch. 24) notes the need for joint commissioning between health and social services of mental health services, for example of residential and nursing home facilities.

One main effect of the internal market is an expanding role for the independent sector, that is private (for profit) and voluntary (not for profit) organisations. The expansion of services provided by the private sector has been mainly in acute medical care. Old people, particularly those who are mentally ill, have not been perceived as 'profitable' and the expansion of private services for them has been predominantly restricted to private residential and nursing home care rather than in the provision of domiciliary services. In contrast, the voluntary sector, which has a long history of providing services for elderly mentally ill people, is likely to take on an increasing service provider role as services are contracted out, and to combine this with their traditional pressure group activities. We can expect increasing independent provision of day care and also advice and support for old people and their carers at home.

The functioning of this internal market is complex and continually evolving. Concerns about it are not independent of political viewpoints. Tinker (Ch. 24) points out that the market does provide scope for innovations to take place and the variety of providers guards against a monopoly. However, she raises the following concerns: the contracts between service providers and purchasers might be too tight to allow innovation; the profit element may force down service quality to an unacceptable level; and it is not clear who will monitor and enforce service standards.

SUMMARY AND CONCLUSION

In this chapter we have drawn from other chapters to reflect on some of the major developments in mental health care for elderly people and the challenges that lie ahead. The considerable expansion in knowledge of the experience of old age is crucial to understanding the distinction between normal experiences of, and reactions to, the final stage of life on the one hand, and the impact of pathology on the other. We have drawn attention to the prevalence of depression in old age and the challenge it presents to health and social care workers. Nurses working in GP practice and general community nurses, given adequate training, could do much more in identifying old people who are at risk and in monitoring their progress. Community psychiatric nurses are too scarce a resource to be able to identify more than the tip of the iceberg. The modern therapeutic interventions available offer an encouraging new culture for dementia care which will benefit sufferers and their families. It is imperative that the culture of enthusiasm reaches all care workers, especially the care assistants who do the bulk of the day-to-day work. They need and deserve as much support as dementing people and their families but, without this support, burnout and rustout will continue.

We have described developments in service provision for elderly mentally frail people under the four categories identified by Tinker (Ch. 24): preventing people going into institutions, returning people from institutions to the community, improving conditions in institutions and building up community care. There are many lessons to be learned before policy makers and purchasers and providers of health care get it right as regards service provision in the whole community, including care in institutions, for elderly people and their carers.

Mental health care for elderly people is an increasingly complex enterprise which demands con-tributions from a range of academic and professional disciplines. The range includes members of the health and social care professions, social policy analysts, gerontologists, epidemiologists, natural scientists and social scientists who contribute to the theoretical development of the speciality. And also from elderly people and their carers at home who are experts and, given the chance, could advise on the mix of services and modes of care and treatment which are most helpful.

The benefits of multiprofessional teamwork are well-established although all too often it is given only lip-service in practice. There is a huge difference between the rhetoric of multiprofessional teams and true interprofessional working that puts elderly mentally disturbed people and their families where they should be, at the centre of service provision. Placing service users centre stage enhances the possibility of effective therapies – reminiscence, reality orientation, validation therapy, resolution therapy, cognitive therapy, dementia care mapping and so on – reaching them.

Mental health care for elderly people is becoming a defined discipline with professionals from many occupational groups claiming membership. As a discipline it has great potential to assist the professional in being able to avoid the professional 'protectionism' and 'reductionism' sought by existing disciplines (Nolan 1994). The drive by each discipline to underline its power and status by claiming certain territory as its own does not serve the best interests of service users. Elderly people and their families can be utterly confused by the range of carers they meet – district nurses, community psychiatric nurses, occupational therapists, social workers, psychogeria-tricians, general practitioners, care assistants, home helps – that is, if they see anyone at all. How much better it would be for them if one professional worker looked after all their needs. The 'gerocomist' or trans-disciplinary professional would be one solution (Hollingberry 1993). This generic worker would have qualified from a broad-based educational programme that combined nursing, social work, medicine, physiotherapy, occupational therapy with gerontology and the biological and social sciences. The outcome would be a generic worker with a broad education in gerontology and care of elderly people who could assess, diagnose, plan, meet and manage all the health and social care needs that most old people and their families require. More specialist needs would be referred to gerocomists who had taken further training.

Established and fledgling disciplines are likely to greet this suggestion of a generic worker as heretical;

established disciplines because of the challenge to their hallowed ground, and fledgling disciplines because they are only just beginning to carve out their own territory. In the meantime, let us encourage opportunities for shared learning amongst students of different professions. As these students qualify and

some choose to practise in the elderly mental health care field, maybe the idea of a gerocomist will not feel so far-fetched. Open-minded multiprofessional team working is the answer for the mental health care of older people. We hope this book has made a contribution to that ambition.

REFERENCES

Audit Commission 1994 Finding a place: a review of mental health services for adults. HMSO, London

Bergmann K 1978 Neurosis and personality disorder in old age. In: Isaacs A D, Post F (eds) Studies in geriatric psychiatry. Wiley, New York

Feil N 1992 V/F Validation: the Feil method. Feil Productions, Cleveland

Feil N 1992a Validation therapy. Geriatric Nursing May/ June: 129–133

Feil N 1992b Honesty, the best policy. Nursing the Elderly 4(5): 10–12

Fry P S 1983 Structured and unstructured reminiscence training and depression among the elderly. Clinical Gerontologist 1: 15–37

Hanley I 1984 Theoretical and practical considerations in reality orientation therapy with the elderly. In: Hanley I, Hodge J (eds) Psychological approaches to the care of the elderly. Croom Helm, Beckenham

Hanley I, Baikie E 1984 Understanding and treating depression in the elderly. In: Hanley I, Hodge J (eds) Psychological approaches to the care of the elderly. Croom Helm, Beckenham

Harris R 1995 Group validation therapy with elderly demented people: a small scale experimental study of its effects. Unpublished BSc Nursing Dissertation, King's College London

Holden U, Woods R 1988 Reality orientation: psychological approaches to the confused elderly, 2nd edn. Churchill Livingstone, Edinburgh

Hollingberry R 1993 Gerocomist: a new trans-disciplinary profession. Paper presented at the British Society of Gerontology Conference, Norwich, September

Johnson M 1988 Biographical influences on mental health in old age. In: Gearing B, Johnson M, Heller T (eds) Mental health problems in old age: a reader. Wiley/Open University, Chichester

Morton I, Bleathman C 1991 The effectiveness of validation therapy in dementia: a pilot study. International Journal of Geriatric Psychiatry 6: 327–330

Nolan M 1994 Geriatric nursing: an idea whose idea has gone? A polemic. Journal of Advanced Nursing 20: 989–996

Norman A 1985 Triple jeopardy: growing older in a second homeland. Centre for Policy on Ageing, London

Norman A 1988 Mental disorder and elderly members of ethnic minority groups. In: Gearing B, Johnson M, Heller T (eds) Mental health problems in old age: a reader. Wiley/Open University, Chichester

Robb S, Stegman C, Opal Wolanin M 1986 No research versus research with compromised results: a study of validation therapy. Nursing Research 35(2): 113–118

Salvage A, Jones D, Vetter N 1989 Opinions of people aged over 75 years on private and local authority residential care. Age and Ageing 18(6): 360–386

Scanlon S, Emershaw L 1993 Reality orientation and validation therapy. Journal of Gerontological Nursing 19(6): 7–11

Woods R 1994 Reading around ... reality orientation. Journal of Dementia Care, March–April: 24–25

Index